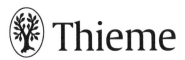

Pharmacology Test Prep

1500 USMLE-Style Questions & Answers

Mario Babbini, MD, PhD
Professor
Department of Pharmacology
Ross Medical School

Mary Thomas, PhD
Professor Emeritus
Department of Pharmacology
University of Texas Medical Branch at Galveston

Thieme
New York • Stuttgart • Delhi • Rio

Vice President and Editorial Director, Educational Products: Anne Vinnicombe
Developmental Editor: Julie O'Meara
Editorial Assistant: Huvie Weinreich
Senior Vice President, Editorial and Electronic Product Development: Cornelia Schulze
Production Editor: Barbara A. Chernow
International Production Director: Andreas Schabert
International Marketing Director: Fiona Henderson
Director of Sales, North America: Mike Roseman
International Sales Director: Louisa Turrell
Vice President, Finance and Accounts: Sarah Vanderbilt
President: Brian D. Scanlan
Compositor: Carol Pierson, Chernow Editorial Services, Inc.

Library of Congress Cataloging-in-Publication Data

Babbini, Mario, author.
  Pharmacology test prep : 1500 USMLE-style questions & answers / Mario Babbini, Mary Thomas.
    p. ; cm.
    ISBN 978-1-62623-041-5 (alk. paper) — ISBN 978-1-62623-042-2 (eISBN)
    I. Thomas, Mary (Professor of pharmacology), author. II. Title.
    [DNLM: 1. Pharmacological Phenomena—Examination Questions. QV 18.2]
    RS97
    615.1076—dc23   2014027117

© 2015 Thieme Medical Publishers, Inc.
Thieme Publishers New York
333 Seventh Avenue, New York, NY 10001 USA
+1 800 782 3488, customerservice@thieme.com

Thieme Publishers Stuttgart
Rüdigerstrasse 14, 70469 Stuttgart, Germany
+49 [0]711 8931 421, customerservice@thieme.de

Thieme Publishers Delhi
A-12, Second Floor, Sector-2, Noida-201301
Uttar Pradesh, India
+91 120 45 566 00, customerservice@thieme.in

Thieme Publishers Rio, Thieme Publicações Ltda.
Argentina Building 16th floor, Ala A, 228 Praia do Botafogo
Rio de Janeiro 22250-040 Brazil
+55 21 3736-3631

Cover design: Thieme Publishing Group

Printed in the United States of America by Sheridan Books   5 4 3 2 1

ISBN 978-1-62623-041-5

Also available as an e-book:
eISBN 978-1-62623-042-2

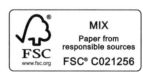

Contents

Section IV: Cardiovascular and Renal Systems

Section V: Endocrine System

Section VI: Respiratory, Gastrointestinal, and Hematopoietic Systems

Section VII: Inflammation and Immunomodulation

Section VIII: Chemotherapeutic Drugs

Preface

This book is a collection of multiple choice questions (MCQs) to promote the learning of pharmacology in the framework of preclinical and clinical disciplines. The main features of the book are the following:

- The MCQs are all of the type that is used for the step 1 medical board exams in the United States and are written according to United States Medical Licensing Examination (USMLE) guidelines (i.e., patient-centered vignettes). All questions are "one best answer"; in most cases, there are five answer choices, but in some cases six or seven answer choices are given.
- Because the MCQs are about pharmacology, each question mentions a drug or a drug class either in the stem or as the answer choices.
- Each MCQ is provided with a level of difficulty, a learning objective, the correct answer, and an explanation.
- There are three levels of difficulty: easy, medium, and hard.
- The learning objective is a brief behavioral statement written using an action verb. If a student can perform that action, then he or she should be able to answer the question correctly. The explanation includes both the reasons why a given answer is correct and why the distractors are wrong.
- Many questions are related to the highest levels of Bloom's taxonomy (e.g., interpretation of data and solution of problems) rather than being simple recall questions.
- For each drug or drug class, the concepts asked by the MCQs are related to mode of action, pharmacokinetics, pharmacodynamics, adverse effects, interactions, or clinical uses.
- Most MCQs are integrated questions, and a good knowledge of the relevant human physiology, biochemistry, pathology, microbiology, and/or elementary clinical medicine is a necessary prerequisite to determine the right answer to the question. Therefore, the question with its answer explanation can also be used as a powerful tool for reviewing and integrating the medical science disciplines.
- The MCQs are grouped in chapters covering most topics presented in standard pharmacology textbooks. There are 20 to 50 MCQs in each chapter, totaling over 1500 questions.

MCQs are the learning tool most frequently used by medical students. This book is intended as an integrated tool for both course study and board exam preparation. Because the book is organized along clinical rather than strictly pharmacological lines, it should be useful for both step 1 and step 2 exam preparation.

Pharmacology is a fast-evolving discipline. The authors have checked sources believed to be reliable, in order to provide information that is in accordance with the currently accepted standards. However, the authors are aware that in several instances the pharmacotherapy of disease is still controversial. They have tried, as much as possible, to avoid questions addressing controversial issues.

This book is not intended to be a substitute for pharmacology textbooks. Students are strongly advised to consult their textbooks of pharmacology for more in-depth coverage of the subject matter.

Mario Babbini, MD, PhD
Mary Thomas, PhD

1 General Principles of Pharmacology

Questions: 1-1 Pharmacokinetics

1. A 22-year-old woman suffering from asthma was prescribed albuterol by inhalation. Albuterol is a bronchodilating drug with a molecular weight of 239 daltons. Which of the following permeation processes most likely accounted for the transfer of the drug through the bronchial mucosa?

   A. Aqueous diffusion
   B. Lipid diffusion
   C. Facilitated diffusion
   D. Endocytosis
   E. Active transport

Difficulty level: Easy

2. A 34-year-old man on vacation in Mexico was admitted to the hospital because of vomiting, double vision, and muscular paralysis. The man reported that he had eaten some canned food from a local vendor the previous day. After a physical examination, a presumptive diagnosis of botulism was made. It is known that botulinum toxin causes paralysis by getting inside the axon terminals of motor nerves, where it inhibits the release of acetylcholine. Botulinum toxin is a protein with a molecular weight greater than 100,000 daltons. Which of the following permeation processes most likely accounts for the transfer of the toxin through the nerve cell membrane?

   A. Aqueous diffusion
   B. Lipid diffusion
   C. Facilitated diffusion
   D. Endocytosis
   E. Filtration

Difficulty level: Easy

3. A 51-year-old woman suffering from hyperthyroidism was administered an oral solution of radioactive iodine to destroy her thyroid gland. Which of the following permeation processes most likely accounted for the transfer of the drug across the thyroid cell membrane?

   A. Active transport
   B. Lipid diffusion
   C. Facilitated diffusion
   D. Endocytosis
   E. Aqueous diffusion

Difficulty level: Easy

4. A 12-year-old boy recently diagnosed with type 1 diabetes started a therapy with two daily subcutaneous administrations of insulin. Which of the following permeation processes best explains the absorption of insulin from the site of injection?

   A. Bulk flow transport
   B. Lipid diffusion
   C. Facilitated diffusion
   D. Endocytosis
   E. Active transport

Difficulty level: Hard

5. An 85-year-old man was recently admitted to a nursing facility. Diseases listed in his medical record on admission were depression with anxiety symptoms, atrial fibrillation, chronic obstructive pulmonary disease, and osteoarthritis. Medications taken orally by the patient included the following:

   Sertraline (base, $pK_a = 9.5$)

   Diazepam (base, $pK_a = 3.0$)

   Amiodarone (base, $pK_a = 7.4$)

   Theophylline (acid, $pK_a = 8.8$)

   Ibuprofen (acid, pK_a 4.8)

   Shortly after administration, which of the following drugs was most likely concentrated inside the patient's gastric cells?

   A. Sertraline
   B. Diazepam
   C. Amiodarone
   D. Theophylline
   E. Ibuprofen

Difficulty level: Medium

6. A 17-year-old boy took a tablet of naproxen for a headache. Naproxen is a weak acid with a pK_a of 5.2. What percentage of the drug was most likely water soluble in the patient's plasma?

   A. 1%
   B. 24%
   C. 50%
   D. 76%
   E. 99%
   F. > 99%

Difficulty level: Medium

7. A 69-year-old woman was brought to a local hospital emergency department by her son, who reported that his mother was found lethargic, disoriented, and combative a few hours earlier. Additional history revealed that she had ingested a large number of aspirin tablets in a suicide attempt. An appropriate therapy was instituted, which included the administration of sodium bicarbonate to increase the elimination of salicylate. Which of the following best explains the mechanism of this increased elimination?

    A. Decreased tubular active transport of salicylate
    B. Decreased renal biotransformation of salicylate
    C. Decreased bioavailability of salicylate
    D. Urinary ion trapping of salicylate
    E. Increased glomerular filtration of salicylate

Difficulty level: Medium

8. A 63-year old man recently diagnosed with hypertension started a therapy with hydrochlorothiazide, one tablet daily. Hydrochlorothiazide is an acidic drug with a pK_a of about 9. Which of the following parts of the digestive tract most likely represents the main site of absorption of that drug?

    A. Oral mucosa
    B. Stomach
    C. Small intestine
    D. Colon
    E. Rectum

Difficulty level: Easy

9. The pharmacokinetic properties of five new drugs (P, Q, R, S, and T) were studied in healthy volunteers. The same dose of each drug was administered intravenously (IV) and orally to the same subject on two separate occasions. The results were the following:

Drug	AUC$_{Oral}$ (mg h/L)	AUC$_{IV}$ (mg h/L)
P	50	600
Q	200	2000
R	30	400
S	100	120
T	45	90

Abbreviations: AUC, area under the curve; IV, intravenous.

Which of the following drugs most likely has the highest oral bioavailability?

    A. Drug P
    B. Drug Q
    C. Drug R
    D. Drug S
    E. Drug T

Difficulty level: Easy

10. During a phase 1 clinical trial, four different oral dosage forms of the same dose of a drug were administered to a healthy volunteer on four separate occasions. The plasma concentration–time curves are plotted below.

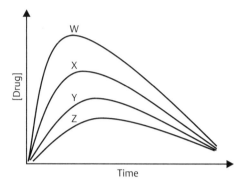

Which of the following features best explains why formulation W produces the largest plasma concentration–time curve of the drug?

    A. Highest absorption through gut wall
    B. Lowest first-pass effect
    C. Lowest hepatic clearance
    D. Highest volume of distribution
    E. Lowest drug elimination

Difficulty level: Easy

11. A 26-year-old man became inebriated after drinking several glasses of alcoholic beverages at a party. Ethanol is a polar, nonionizable drug with an approximate molecular weight of 46 daltons. Which of the following permeation processes mediated the man's intestinal absorption of ethanol?

    A. Aqueous diffusion
    B. Bulk flow transport
    C. Facilitated diffusion
    D. Active transport
    E. Endocytosis

Difficulty level: Hard

12. A 44-year-old man took a large dose of acetaminophen in aqueous solution to treat an excruciating headache. Two hours later, the pain was not diminished. Because acetaminophen should be effective in about 30 minutes after its oral administration, which of the following conditions most likely delayed the oral absorption of the drug in this patient?

    A. A moderate increase in intestinal peristalsis
    B. The presence of strong pain
    C. The administration of the drug in aqueous solution
    D. A large volume of distribution of the drug
    E. A very low clearance of the drug

Difficulty level: Medium

13. A 22-year-old woman was admitted to the emergency department after a car accident. The woman had extensive brain trauma and multiple fractures. She complained of severe pain, and the attending physician planned to administer morphine. The physician knew that the dose should be carefully titrated because the entry of morphine into the patient's central nervous system (CNS) was most likely higher than normal. Which of the following factors is most likely to have increased morphine entry into the CNS of this patient?

   A. The high first-pass effect of the drug
   B. The brain trauma of the patient
   C. The young age of the patient
   D. The low clearance of the drug
   E. The high ionization of the drug

Difficulty level: Easy

14. A 67-year-old woman recently diagnosed with atrial fibrillation started treatment with atenolol, 100 mg/d. With this dose, the percentage of atenolol bound to plasma proteins is about 5%. Which of the following would have been the bound percentage of atenolol if a dose of 50 mg/d had been administered to the same patient?

   A. 2.5%
   B. 5%
   C. 10%
   D. 1.25%
   E. 2%

Difficulty level: Hard

15. A 34-year-old man recently diagnosed with grand mal epilepsy started treatment with valproic acid, an antiseizure drug with a pK_a of 5. What percentage of the drug was most likely lipid soluble in the patient's duodenal lumen (assuming pH = 7 in the lumen)?

   A. 1%
   B. 24%
   C. 50%
   D. 76%
   E. 99%

Difficulty level: Easy

16. A 4-year-old boy suffering from acute lymphoblastic leukemia was about to receive an intrathecal injection of methotrexate, a drug that cannot cross the blood–brain barrier.

Which of the following statements best explains why several drugs, including methotrexate, cannot easily enter the brain?

   A. Cerebrospinal fluid pressure is lower than cerebral perfusion pressure.
   B. The pH of cerebrospinal fluid is lower than plasma pH.
   C. Many drugs are bound to protein and cannot cross brain capillaries.
   D. Endothelial cells of brain capillaries and choroid plexus have tight junctions.
   E. Most drugs are completely ionized in blood.

Difficulty level: Medium

17. The ability of five different drugs (P, Q, R, S, and T) to cross the placenta was studied in laboratory animals. The following data were obtained.

Drug	Molecular Weight (daltons)	Protein Bound in Maternal Plasma (%)	Ionized in Maternal Plasma (%)
P	20	0	100
Q	250	99	50
R	4500	25	10
S	500	10	90
T	2000	15	30

Which of the following drugs most likely crossed the placenta at the fastest rate?

   A. Drug P
   B. Drug Q
   C. Drug R
   D. Drug S
   E. Drug T

Difficulty level: Medium

18. A 52-year-old woman suffering from rheumatoid arthritis started a treatment that included infliximab, a monoclonal antibody against tumor necrosis factor-α (TNF-α). The drug has a volume of distribution of about 3 L. Which of the following is most likely the main site of distribution of this drug?

   A. Fat tissue
   B. Plasma
   C. Extracellular fluids
   D. Cell cytosol
   E. Total body water

19. A 36-year-old woman recently diagnosed with trichomoniasis started a treatment with metronidazole. The drug has a hepatic clearance of 4.86 L/h and a renal clearance of 0.54 L/h. On the assumption that only the liver and kidney are involved in the elimination of this drug, what percentage of the administered drug will be eliminated by the liver?

    A. 20%
    B. 40%
    C. 50%
    D. 60%
    E. 70%
    F. 90%

20. The pharmacokinetic properties of five new drugs (P, Q, R, S, and T) were studied in laboratory animals. The drugs were given orally, and the results are shown below.

Drug	Percentage of Drug Reaching the Portal Vein	Hepatic Clearance (mL/min)
P	90	20
Q	86	1000
R	50	450
S	2	100
T	10	30

Which of the following drugs most likely has the highest oral bioavailability?

    A. Drug P
    B. Drug Q
    C. Drug R
    D. Drug S
    E. Drug T

21. When studied in healthy volunteers, the oral bioavailability of a new drug turned out to be 20%. Knowing that in this case the entire administered drug reached the portal circulation, which of the following will be the hepatic clearance (in mL/min) of the drug?

    A. 500
    B. 800
    C. 1200
    D. 1500
    E. 2000

22. A new drug was studied in a healthy volunteer during a phase 1 clinical trial. Urine and plasma samples were collected 1 hour after the intravenous administration of a test dose. Drug concentration was 40 mg/mL in urine and 1 mg/mL in plasma. The urine output of this subject was 1.44 L/d. Which of the following was most likely the renal clearance of the drug, in mL/min?

    A. 40
    B. 30
    C. 20
    D. 50
    E. 60
    F. 10

23. A 10-mg dose of a new drug that follows first-order, one-compartment model kinetics was given intravenously to healthy subjects in a phase 1 clinical trial. The volume of distribution (V_d) of the drug turned out to be 80 L. Which of the following would have been the volume of distribution of the drug (in liters) if the administered dose were 20 mg?

    A. 40
    B. 80
    C. 240
    D. 160
    E. 120

24. A 45-year-old man suffering from epilepsy had been receiving carbamazepine, one tablet daily. The drug has a total clearance of 63 L/h and a hepatic clearance of 62 L/h. The man was recently diagnosed with a skin infection due to *Mycobacterium marinum,* and treatment with rifampin and ethambutol was started. Knowing that rifampin is a potent inducer of microsomal enzymes, which of the following changes most likely occurred to the pharmacokinetics of carbamazepine?

    A. The hepatic clearance of the drugs decreased.
    B. The first-pass loss of the drug decreased.
    C. The renal clearance of the drug decreased.
    D. The volume of distribution of the drug increased.
    E. The half-life of the drug decreased.

25. A 59-year-old Japanese man with atrial fibrillation presented to his physician complaining of red urine. The man had been receiving a standard dose of warfarin, which is an anticoagulant drug biotransformed by CYP2C9 isozyme. Which of the following was the most likely cause of the patient's disorder?

A. Increased protein binding of warfarin
B. Decreased renal excretion of warfarin
C. Genetic polymorphism of CYP2C9
D. Decreased metabolism of CYP2C9
E. Increased CYP2C9 synthesis in a person of Asian origin

Difficulty level: Easy

26. The pharmacokinetics of a new drug was studied in laboratory animals. The drug was given orally, and the following results were obtained:

    Percent reaching the portal circulation: 40%

    Liver clearance: negligible

    Liver blood flow in the animal was 1000 mL/min. Which of the following would be the oral bioavailability of the drug?

    A. 1.0
    B. 0.4
    C. 0.1
    D. 2.2
    E. 0.6
    F. 0.8

Difficulty level: Medium

27. A 35-year-old Caucasian man complained to his physician of tingling sensation in his limbs and noted that his arms sometimes felt heavy. The man, recently diagnosed with pulmonary tuberculosis, had been receiving isoniazid and rifampin for 2 months. He was diagnosed with peripheral neuropathy, a known adverse effect of isoniazid. Which of the following events most likely caused the patient's symptoms and signs?

    A. Rifampin-induced inhibition of isoniazid metabolism
    B. Worsening of the disease, despite the therapy
    C. Allergic reaction to rifampin
    D. Inherited deficiency of N-acetyltransferase
    E. Allergic reaction to isoniazid

Difficulty level: Medium

28. A 49-year-old obese man recently diagnosed with vasospastic angina started a treatment with nifedipine. The drug has a volume of distribution (V_d) of about 55 L in a 70-kg person, but in this obese patient, the V_d turned out to be 110 L. The standard loading dose of nifedipine for a patient weighing 70 kg is 30 mg. Which of the following should be the therapeutic loading dose administered to this patient (in mg) in order to achieve the same target concentration?

    A. 20
    B. 40
    C. 60
    D. 90
    E. 120
    F. 150

Difficulty level: Easy

29. A 22-year-old man suffering from adult autism and violent behavior started a treatment that included buspirone, a drug with a large first-pass effect. Which of the following pharmacokinetic properties of the drug was most likely affected by this large first-pass effect?

    A. Volume of distribution
    B. Oral bioavailability
    C. Renal clearance
    D. Sublingual bioavailability
    E. Intramuscular bioavailability

Difficulty level: Easy

30. A 47-year-old man recently diagnosed with systolic heart failure started a treatment that included furosemide. The drug has a total clearance of about 136 mL/min, and about 66% of the drug is excreted as such in the urine. On the assumption that, in this case, only the liver and kidneys are involved in drug elimination, which of the following was most likely the renal clearance of furosemide (in mL/min)?

    A. 90
    B. 70
    C. 110
    D. 25
    E. 81
    F. 16

Difficulty level: Hard

31. The pharmacokinetics of a new drug that followed first-order, one-compartment model kinetics was studied in a healthy volunteer. A 20-mg dose was given intravenously. The plasma concentration of the drug turned out to be 2 mg/L initially and 1 mg/L 2 hours later. Which of the following was most likely the total clearance of the drug (in L/h)?

    A. 2.5
    B. 8.4
    C. 5.5
    D. 6.7
    E. 3.5
    F. 4.9

Difficulty level: Easy

32. The pharmacokinetic properties of five new drugs (P, Q, R, S, and T) were studied in laboratory animals. A 100-mg dose of each drug was administered intravenously to the same animal on five separate occasions. The plasma concentration–time curves for each drug are depicted in the figure below:

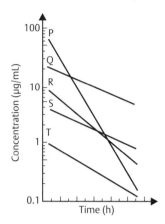

Which of the following drugs has the largest volume of distribution?

A. Drug P
B. Drug Q
C. Drug R
D. Drug S
E. Drug T

Difficulty level: Easy

33. The pharmacokinetics of a new drug was studied in healthy volunteers. It was found that the drug followed first-order, one-compartment model kinetics and had a volume of distribution of 100 L. After the oral administration of 200 mg, the theoretical plasma concentration at time 0 turned out to be 1 mg/L. Which of the following was most likely the oral bioavailability of the drug?

A. 0.1
B. 0.5
C. 0.8
D. 1.0
E. 2.3
F. 1.6

Difficulty level: Hard

34. A 32-year-old male cocaine addict was brought unconscious to the emergency department. A friend stated that the man had intravenously self-injected an unknown dose of cocaine 2 hours earlier. An immediate lab analysis indicated that the plasma level of cocaine was 0.75 mg/L. Cocaine has a volume of distribution of about 130 L and a half-life of about 1 hour. Which of the following was most likely the injected dose of cocaine (in mg)?

A. 250
B. 390
C. 420
D. 315
E. 180
F. 115

Difficulty level: Hard

35. A 23-year-old healthy male volunteer received an intravenous dose of 2 mg of a new drug during a clinical trial. The drug followed a first-order, one-compartment model kinetics and had a volume of distribution of 10 L. After 6 hours the plasma concentration of the drug was 50 µg/L. Which of the following was most likely the half-life of the drug (in hours)?

A. 1
B. 2
C. 3
D. 4
E. 5
F. 6

Difficulty level: Medium

36. The figure below depicts the plasma concentration–time curves for four drugs (W, X, Y, and Z) given by IV infusion to the same laboratory animal on four separate occasions.

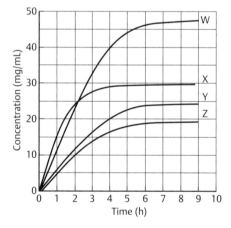

Which of the following drugs has the shortest half-life?

A. Drug W
B. Drug X
C. Drug Y
D. Drug Z

Difficulty level: Hard

37. The pharmacokinetics of a new drug was studied in a healthy volunteer. The drug was given by intravenous infusion at a rate of 30 mg/h. The plasma concentration–time curve of the drug is depicted below.

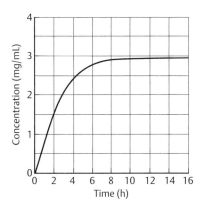

Which of the following is most likely the total clearance of the drug (in L/h)?

A. 4
B. 6
C. 2
D. 10
E. 14
F. 16

Difficulty level: Easy

38. The pharmacokinetics of a new drug following zero-order kinetics was studied in a healthy volunteer. Three hours after the intravenous administration of a test dose, the plasma concentration of the drug was 8 mg/L, and 1 hour later it was 7 mg/L. Which of the following was most likely the plasma concentration of the drug (in mg/L) immediately after drug administration?

A. 9
B. 32
C. 11
D. 16
E. 64
F. 5

Difficulty level: Medium

39. The figure below depicts the concentration–time curve of a new drug after a single intravenous dose of 20 mg was administered to a laboratory animal.

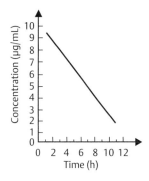

Which of the following drugs does the new agent most resemble?

A. Atropine
B. Propranolol
C. Ethanol
D. Phenylephrine
E. Clonidine
F. Dobutamine

Difficulty level: Hard

40. The pharmacokinetics of a new drug was studied in a healthy volunteer. The drug followed first-order, one-compartment model kinetics and had a half-life of 3 hours. An intravenous infusion of the drug was started at 8:00 a.m. A blood sample taken at 2:00 p.m. of the same day showed a plasma drug concentration of 60 µg/mL. Which of the following was most likely the plasma concentration of that drug (in µg/mL) at the steady state?

A. 100
B. 60
C. 80
D. 30
E. 40
F. 120

Questions: I-2 Pharmacodynamics

Difficulty level: Medium

1. A 68-year-old man recently diagnosed with atrial fibrillation started therapy with atenolol, a β-receptor blocker. Which of the following changes most likely occurred in cardiac myocytes during the first 2 weeks of therapy?

A. Spare β receptors became activated.
B. The G-protein number decreased.
C. The β-receptor number increased.
D. Most β receptors became phosphorylated.
E. The ability to respond to intracellular cyclic adenosine monophosphate (cAMP) declined.

2. A new drug was tested in an in vitro system. It was found that only one enantiomer of the racemic pair bound substantially to a specific receptor, whereas the other enantiomer showed negligible binding. Which of the following terms best defines this property?

   A. Intrinsic activity
   B. Affinity
   C. Stereoselectivity
   D. Potency
   E. Variability
   F. Maximal efficacy

3. A 14-year-old girl suffering from seasonal rhinitis started a therapy with loratadine, a drug that binds to H_1 histamine receptors. Which of the following terms describes a characteristic of loratadine binding to the H_1 receptor?

   A. Intrinsic activity
   B. Potency
   C. Maximal efficacy
   D. Affinity
   E. Receptor activation

4. Two new drugs were tested in laboratory animals. Which of the following drug parameters was most likely recorded to estimate the relative potency of both drugs?

   A. The therapeutic index of both drugs
   B. The maximal responses produced by each drug
   C. The graded log dose–response curve of both drugs
   D. The volume of distribution of both drugs
   E. The clearance of both drugs

5. A 65-year-old man suffering from osteoarthritis has been taking naproxen, 500 mg daily for 1 month. The drug was effective, but the patient suffered from nausea and heartburn. The physician decided to try another nonsteroidal antiinflammatory drug (NSAID) and prescribed celecoxib, a drug ~5 times more potent than naproxen, with negligible gastrointestinal side effects. Which of the following would be the most appropriate daily dose of celecoxib (in mg) to prescribe to the patient?

   A. 50
   B. 1000
   C. 10
   D. 25
   E. 100
   F. 75

6. A 2-year-old boy was admitted to the emergency department after a generalized tonic-colonic seizure. His mother reported that the boy apparently ingested several tablets of propranolol, a β-blocker, which he had found in his father's dresser drawer. Vital signs on admission were blood pressure 85/50 mm Hg, heart rate 40 beats per minute (bpm), respiratory rate 20/min. The boy received an intramuscular injection of glucagon, a hormone that activates glucagon receptors in the heart, causing a significant increase in heart contractility. Which of the following terms best defines the antagonism between glucagon and β-blockers?

   A. Chemical
   B. Functional
   C. Competitive
   D. Pharmacokinetic
   E. Pharmacological

7. The effect of a new autonomic drug was tested on a healthy volunteer during a clinical trial. The subject was treated with saline or with the drug, and cardiac rate was recorded at rest or after exercise. The results are reported below.

Treatment	Heart Rate (bpm)	
	At Rest	After Exercise
Saline	70	150
Drug	85	100

Abbreviation: bpm, beats per minute.

Which of the following terms best defines the tested drug?

   A. Noncompetitive antagonist
   B. Competitive antagonist
   C. Partial agonist
   D. Physiologic antagonist
   E. Full agonist
   F. Chemical antagonist

8. A 65-year-old woman suffering from atrial fibrillation had been taking a drug to treat this condition for 6 months. The drug had no intrinsic activity and bound reversibly to $β_1$ receptors. Which of the following terms best defines this drug?

   A. Partial agonist
   B. Functional antagonist
   C. Inverse agonist
   D. Noncompetitive antagonist
   E. Competitive antagonist
   F. Full agonist

Difficulty level: Medium

9. A new β-blocker was tested in healthy volunteers. The cumulative frequency distribution of subjects showing a decrease of 10 bpm in the heart rate was plotted against the log dose. Which of the following drug parameters can be determined from this cumulative frequency distribution?

A. Receptor affinity
B. Median effective dose
C. Therapeutic index
D. Therapeutic window
E. Maximal efficacy

Difficulty level: Easy

10. In the figure below, curve X depicts the in vitro log dose-response curve for a full α_1 agonist on contraction of vascular smooth muscle. Which of the curves best depicts the log dose-response curve of that agonist when a fixed dose of a competitive α_1 antagonist is given concomitantly?

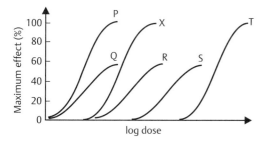

A. Curve P
B. Curve Q
C. Curve R
D. Curve S
E. Curve T

Difficulty level: Medium

11. The figure below depicts the in vitro log dose-response curves of five different drugs (P, Q, R, S, and T). Which of the following pairs of drugs can fully activate the same receptors?

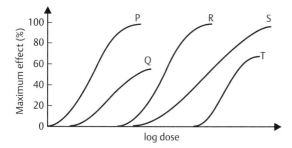

A. Drugs P and Q
B. Drugs P and R
C. Drugs P and S
D. Drugs Q and T
E. Drugs Q and S
F. Drugs R and S

Difficulty level: Easy

12. The figure below depicts the in vitro log dose-response curves of five different drugs (P, Q, R, S, and T) acting on the same receptor.

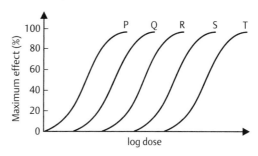

Which of the following drugs has the highest ED_{50}?

A. Drug P
B. Drug Q
C. Drug R
D. Drug S
E. Drug T

Difficulty level: Easy

13. A 65-year-old woman who had been admitted to the hospital with a myocardial infarction developed ventricular tachycardia and received an intravenous injection of lidocaine. Her cardiologist knew that the dose given must be within the range of doses that have a high probability of therapeutic success. Which of the following terms best defines this range?

A. Intrinsic activity
B. Efficacy
C. Potency
D. Therapeutic index
E. Therapeutic window
F. Response variability

Difficulty level: Medium

14. A 67-year-old man suffering from terminal cancer started analgesic treatment with an opioid drug. Knowing that tolerance to opioids is pronounced, which of the following drug parameters was most likely increased after a few days of treatment?

A. Maximal efficacy
B. Median effective dose
C. Therapeutic index
D. Potency
E. Half-life

Difficulty level: Medium

15. A 17-year-old girl started smoking 1 month ago, and now she is smoking 5 to 10 cigarettes daily. She has noticed that the first cigarette of the day often causes mild tachycardia, which does not usually occur with the following cigarettes. Which of the following terms best defines this tolerance pattern?

A. Cross-tolerance
B. Tachyphylaxis
C. Pharmacokinetic tolerance
D. Innate tolerance
E. Sensitization

Difficulty level: Medium

16. A 64-year-old man with terminal cancer had been suffering from continuous pain and started treatment with morphine. After a few days of treatment, the initial dose was no longer effective, and the physician gradually increased the dose, knowing that pharmacodynamic tolerance most likely had occurred. Which of the following best explains the mechanism of tolerance in this patient?

A. Accelerated morphine metabolism
B. Increased affinity of receptors to morphine
C. Decreased binding of morphine to plasma proteins
D. Decreased morphine receptor density
E. Decreased concentration of morphine in the brain

Difficulty level: Medium

17. A 17-year-old boy drank increasing amounts of alcohol when attending parties. He noticed that lately he was able to better tolerate alcohol effects and asked his physician the reason for this. The physician said that pharmacodynamic tolerance had probably occurred. Which of the following actions most likely mediated this tolerance?

A. Decreased concentration of the drug at the site of action
B. Homeostatic adaptive changes that counteract the drug effect
C. Decreased bioavailability of the drug
D. Increased biotransformation of the drug
E. Increased number of drug receptors

Difficulty level: Easy

18. A 46-year-old woman complained to her physician that the sedative effect of the drug she was taking had increased substantially. The woman, who was suffering from generalized anxiety disorder, had been taking diazepam, one tablet daily. A few days earlier, she had started taking cimetidine to treat her heartburn. Cimetidine is an inhibitor of the cytochrome P-450 system in the liver. Which of the following terms best defines this cimetidine–diazepam interaction?

A. Additive effect
B. Potentiation
C. Synergism
D. Sensitization
E. Reverse tolerance

Difficulty level: Easy

19. A 45-year-old woman recently diagnosed with a urinary tract infection started therapy with a trimethoprim–sulfamethoxazole combination. Both trimethoprim and sulfamethoxazole are bacteriostatic drugs when given alone. However, a bactericidal effect is obtained when the two drugs are given in combination. Which of the following terms best defines this drug interaction?

A. Additive effect
B. Potentiation
C. Synergism
D. Reverse tolerance
E. Sensitization

Difficulty level: Easy

20. A 2-year-old girl was rushed to the emergency department after ingesting several tablets of a medication containing iron. An emergency treatment was started that included the intravenous administration of deferoxamine. This drug is able to combine with iron in plasma to form an inactive complex and therefore to antagonize iron effects. Which of the following terms best defines this antagonism?

A. Competitive
B. Noncompetitive
C. Functional
D. Chemical
E. Pharmacokinetic

Difficulty level: Easy

21. A new drug was tested in an in vitro system. The relationship between the concentration of the drug and the association and dissociation of the drug–receptor complex was evaluated. Which of the following factors regulates this relationship?

A. The pharmacological response
B. The volume of distribution of the drug
C. The total clearance of the drug
D. The law of mass action
E. The rate of signal transduction

Difficulty level: Easy

22. An 83-year-old woman suffering from overflow urinary incontinence started a therapy with a cholinergic drug that was able to relieve leaking. Which of the following best defines the molecular event initiated by drug–receptor binding and ending with the therapeutic effect in this patient?

A. Receptor upregulation
B. Drug efficacy
C. Signal transduction pathway
D. Drug–receptor interaction
E. Drug potency

Difficulty level: Easy

23. A 9-year-old boy suffering from mild asthma used a β_2 agonist "as needed" by inhalation. Which of the following was most likely the immediate consequence of the activation of β_2 receptors?

A. Opening of ligand-gated K^+ channels
B. Increased synthesis of cAMP
C. Decreased synthesis of cAMP
D. Conformational change of a G protein
E. Phosphorylation of a G protein

Difficulty level: Easy

24. A 57-year-old man who was in the hospital after a surgical procedure complained of a severe abdominal pain. The physician decided to start analgesic treatment with an opioid. The drugs he was considering were morphine (10 mg IM) and buprenorphine (0.3 mg IM). Morphine is a full agonist at mu (μ) opioid receptors, whereas buprenorphine is a partial agonist at the same receptors. The above-mentioned doses of the two drugs are equieffective. Which of the following pairs of statements correctly defines the potency and efficacy of morphine and buprenorphine?

A. Morphine is more potent. Buprenorphine is more effective.
B. Morphine is more potent. Buprenorphine is less effective.
C. Morphine is less potent. Buprenorphine is more effective.
D. Morphine is less potent. Buprenorphine is less effective.

Difficulty level: Easy

25. A series of new β agonists was tested in laboratory animals. Heart rate was measured after treatment with different doses of each drug. The results are given below:

Drug	ED_{50} (mg)	Maximal Increase in Heart Rate (bpm)
A	2	+15
B	10	+22
C	15	+30
D	5	+40
E	20	+55

Abbreviations: bpm, beats per minute; ED_{50}, effective dose that produces a response in 50% of subjects.

Which of the following drugs was the most potent?

A. Drug A
B. Drug B
C. Drug C
D. Drug D
E. Drug E

Difficulty level: Easy

26. Two new diuretics were tested in healthy volunteers. They were given singly or together on separate occasions. The results are given below:

Drug	Dose (mg)	Daily Urine Output (L)
A	20	5
B	5	3
A + B	20 (A) + 5 (B)	8

Which of the following terms best defines the type of drug–drug interaction that has occurred?

A. Synergism
B. Potentiation
C. Additive
D. Functional antagonism
E. Pharmacokinetic antagonism

Difficulty level: Medium

27. A 45-year-old woman recently diagnosed with lupus erythematosus started a treatment with a synthetic steroid. Which of the following is the most likely time lapse expected between receptor activation and therapeutic response?

A. Few milliseconds
B. Few seconds
C. Few minutes
D. One or 2 hours
E. Several hours or days

Difficulty level: Medium

28. The figure below depicts the in vitro log dose–response curves of different drugs acting on the same receptor.

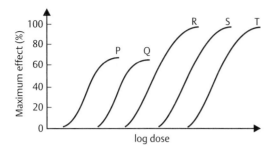

Which of the drugs has the highest affinity for the receptor?

A. Drug P
B. Drug Q
C. Drug R
D. Drug S
E. Drug T

Difficulty level: Easy

29. Some new drugs acting on the same receptor were studied in laboratory animals. It was found that

- Drug X was able to decrease the constitutive level of activity of the receptor.
- Drug Y was able to increase the constitutive level of activity of the receptor.

- Drug Z was able to antagonize the effects of both drug X and drug Y.

Which of the following terms best defines drug X?

A. Competitive antagonist
B. Partial agonist
C. Inverse agonist
D. Irreversible antagonist
E. Full agonist

Difficulty level: Medium

30. A clinical trial was conducted by orally administering a new analgesic drug to a group of patients suffering from arthritic pain. One hour after administration, the patients were questioned about pain relief, and a sample of blood was collected from each patient to measure plasma drug levels. Pain relief generally correlated well with plasma levels, but three patients whose plasma levels were equal to zero reported good pain relief. Which of the following is the most likely explanation of the analgesic effect of the drug in those three patients?

A. High bioavailability of the drug
B. Small volume of distribution of the drug
C. Very low clearance of the drug
D. Poor patient compliance
E. Placebo effect

Questions: 1-3 Adverse Effects of Drugs

Difficulty level: Easy

1. A 23-year-old woman complained to her physician that the diphenhydramine she used to prevent motion sickness when traveling by boat was effective in preventing vomiting but caused drowsiness and dry mouth. Which of the following terms best explains the underlying cause of these drug-related adverse effects?

A. Genetic predisposition
B. Nonspecific cytotoxicity
C. Drug–receptor interaction
D. Immunologic response
E. Preexisting pathology

Difficulty level: Medium

2. Five new anticonvulsant drugs (P, Q, R, S, and T) were tested in laboratory animals. It was found that all of the drugs had approximately the same lethal dose that produces death in 50% of subjects (LD_{50}). The median effective dose of each drug is reported below:

Drug	Median Effective Dose (mg)
P	3
Q	10
R	24
S	35
T	50

Which of the drugs most likely has the highest risk of overdose toxicity?

A. Drug P
B. Drug Q
C. Drug R
D. Drug S
E. Drug T

Difficulty level: Easy

3. A 51-year-old man reported to his physician that in the morning he noticed his urine was cloudy and red. The man had been taking an oral anticoagulant for 3 weeks to treat a deep venous thrombosis. If the patient's symptoms were caused by the anticoagulant, which of the following adverse drug reactions was most likely involved?

   A. Overdose toxicity
   B. Autoimmune reaction
   C. Idiosyncratic reaction
   D. Pseudoallergic reaction
   E. Immediate allergic reaction

Difficulty level: Hard

4. A 23-year-old woman scheduled for surgical dilation and curettage was anesthetized with thiopental. Shortly after recovery from the anesthesia, the woman had generalized seizures followed by a deep coma. Further information given by her husband indicated that the patient's mother had suffered from acute intermittent porphyria. If the coma was caused by thiopental, which of the following drug reactions was most likely involved?

   A. Type II allergic reaction
   B. Delayed allergic reaction
   C. Idiosyncratic reaction
   D. Pseudoallergic reaction
   E. Overdose toxicity

Difficulty level: Medium

5. A 28-year-old woman who had had a mitral valve replacement for rheumatic heart disease 2 years ago had her suspected pregnancy confirmed by a positive pregnancy test. Her current medications include the anticoagulant warfarin (U.S. Food and Drug Administration [FDA] category for teratogenic risk D) and amoxicillin (FDA category B). Which of the following would be the best course of action to be implemented by her family physician?

   A. Stop all medications throughout pregnancy
   B. Suspend warfarin for the first trimester of pregnancy
   C. Replace warfarin with heparin and continue amoxicillin
   D. Continue warfarin and replace amoxicillin with penicillin G
   E. Reduce the dose of warfarin and continue amoxicillin

Difficulty level: Medium

6. Five new antihypertensive drugs were tested in healthy volunteers. All of the drugs were found to be equally effective in controlling hypertension. The minimum effective plasma concentrations and the minimum toxic plasma concentrations were determined for each drug. The results are reported below:

Drug	Plasma Concentration (mg/L)	
	Minimum effective	Minimum toxic
P	5	20
Q	1	10
R	30	60
S	0.6	3
T	20	80

Which of the drugs has the highest probability of therapeutic success?

   A. Drug P
   B. Drug Q
   C. Drug R
   D. Drug S
   E. Drug T

Difficulty level: Medium

7. A 32-year-old African American man who worked as a Peace Corps volunteer in Ghana presented with weakness, fatigue, yellowing of his skin and sclera, and slight fever. He recently was given chloroquine as a prophylaxis for malaria. Laboratory findings confirmed the diagnosis of hemolytic anemia likely due to chloroquine treatment. This patient's disease was most likely mediated by genetic polymorphism of which of the following enzymes?

   A. N-acetyltransferase
   B. Glucose-6-phosphate dehydrogenase
   C. Reduced form of nicotinamide adenine dinucleotide (NADH)–methemoglobin reductase
   D. Pseudocholinesterase
   E. Glucuronosyltransferase

Difficulty level: Medium

8. A 61-year-old woman complained to her physician of a burning sensation when she urinated. Past history of the patient was significant for serious hypersensitivity to sulfa drugs. Urinalysis revealed abundant gram-negative bacteria, and a sensitivity test showed that they were sensitive to amikacin, piperacillin, trimethoprim-sulfametoxazole, ciprofloxacin, and ceftriaxone. A diagnosis of urinary tract infection was made, and an antibiotic therapy was prescribed. Which of the following antibiotics should be avoided in this patient?

   A. Trimethoprim-sulfamethoxazole
   B. Piperacillin
   C. Amikacin
   D. Ciprofloxacin
   E. Ceftriaxone

Difficulty level: Easy

9. A new hypnotic drug was tested in laboratory animals. It was found that the ED_{50} for inducing sleep was 2 mg/kg. Which of the following best explains the meaning of that dose?

   A. The mean dose able to elicit sleep induction
   B. The dose with a 50% probability of causing sleep
   C. The dose that elicits sleep in 50% of animals
   D. The mean dose with a good probability of sleep induction
   E. The dose that elicits a median therapeutic sleep response in most animals

Difficulty level: Medium

10. A newborn boy whose mother had epilepsy presented with microcephaly, a broad nasal bridge, short nose, cleft palate, and hypoplasia of the distal phalanges. Drugs used by the mother during pregnancy included phenytoin for seizures, methyldopa for pregnancy-induced hypertension, and erythromycin for an upper respiratory infection during the first trimester. During the delivery, the woman was treated with diazepam and had epidural anesthesia with lidocaine. Which of the drugs taken by the mother most likely caused the baby's presenting syndrome?

    A. Methyldopa
    B. Phenytoin
    C. Erythromycin
    D. Lidocaine
    E. Diazepam

Difficulty level: Medium

11. A 75-year-old woman complained to her physician of increased need to urinate during the night. The woman had been receiving gentamicin for 2 months to treat a urinary tract infection. Lab tests revealed a serum creatinine level of 5 mg/dL (normal 0.5–1.2 mg/dL). Serum gentamicin concentration obtained just before the last dose was 9 mg/dL (normal < 2 mg/dL). The patient was most likely suffering from which of the following adverse drug reactions?

    A. Type II allergic reaction
    B. Type III allergic reaction
    C. Idiosyncratic reaction
    D. Pseudoallergic reaction
    E. Overdose toxicity

Difficulty level: Medium

12. A 34-year-old man was admitted to the hospital because of sudden onset of fever (102.2°F, 39.0°C), oliguria, and a skin rash. The man had been receiving ampicillin for primary syphilis. Laboratory findings showed eosinophiluria, proteinuria, and increased serum levels of urea nitrogen and creatinine. A diagnosis of drug-induced tubulointerstitial nephritis

was made. Which of the following adverse drug reactions best explains the disease of this patient?

    A. Overdose toxicity
    B. Tachyphylactic reaction
    C. Idiosyncratic reaction
    D. Allergic reaction
    E. Pseudoallergic reaction

Difficulty level: Medium

13. A 15-year-old boy was admitted to the hospital with fever (103.1°F, 39.5°C), a morbilliform skin eruption, lymphadenopathy, angioedema, and arthralgia. The boy had been receiving ampicillin for a pulmonary infection for 2 weeks. Lab data revealed elevated circulating immune complexes. Which of the following adverse drug reactions best explains the patient's disorder?

    A. Overdose toxicity
    B. Anaphylactoid reaction
    C. Idiosyncratic reaction
    D. Autoimmune reaction
    E. Serum sickness

Difficulty level: Hard

14. A 69-year-old man presented to the hospital with a skin eruption over his neck, arms, and legs. The patient reported that he was diagnosed with senile pruritus 3 week earlier, and he had been applying a topical doxepin cream to relieve itching. Physical examination revealed red, swollen skin covered with blisters, and a patch test confirmed that the skin eruption was due to doxepin. Which of the following adverse drug reactions best explains the patient's disorder?

    A. Type I allergic reaction
    B. Type II allergic reaction
    C. Idiosyncratic reaction
    D. Pseudoallergic reaction
    E. Type IV allergic reaction

Difficulty level: Hard

15. A 38-year-old woman went to her physician because of a bluish discoloration of her lips. Medical history was significant for an inherited deficiency of the reduced form of nicotinamide adenine dinucleotide (NADH)–methemoglobin reductase. One week earlier, she had started therapy with trimethoprim-sulfamethoxazole to treat a urinary tract infection. Physical examination showed cyanosis of the oral mucosa, and a blood test revealed a high level of methemoglobinemia. The physician suspected that sulfamethoxazole was the cause of the patient's cyanosis. Which of the following adverse drug reactions best explains the patient's disorder?

A. Type I allergic reaction
B. Type IV allergic reaction
C. Idiosyncratic reaction
D. Pseudoallergic reaction
E. Overdose toxicity

Difficulty level: Easy

16. A 32-year-old woman complained to her physician of urticaria. Three days earlier, the woman had started therapy with amoxicillin for infectious tonsillitis. The physician suspected an allergic reaction to the drug. Which of the following was most likely the main determinant of that drug reaction?

A. Dose of the drug
B. Chemical structure of the drug
C. Oral bioavailability of the drug
D. Genetic pedigree of the patient
E. Liver and kidney functions of the patient

Difficulty level: Easy

17. An 85-year-old woman was admitted to the hospital with an infected decubitus ulcer. Cultures revealed *Staphylococcus aureus* that was sensitive to some β-lactam antibiotics, namely, oxacillin, cephalexin, and imipenem. Which of the following would be the first procedure to undertake in order to minimize the risk of an allergic reaction to these antibiotics?

A. Start the therapy with a very small dose
B. Perform a skin sensitivity test
C. Pretreat the patient with an antiallergic drug
D. Use another β-lactam antibiotic active against *S. aureus*
E. Get a detailed drug history

Difficulty level: Medium

18. A 32-year-old pregnant woman was found to have a red blood cell count of $3.2 \times 10^6/mm^3$ (normal $3.5–5.5 \times 10^6$) and a positive direct Coombs test during a regular clinic visit. The woman had started a treatment with methyldopa 4 months earlier because of stage 1 hypertension. Which of the following mechanisms most likely mediated the drug-induced reaction of this patient?

A. Deficiency of the reduced form of nicotinamide adenine dinucleotide (NADH)–methemoglobin reductase
B. Production of autoantibodies against red blood cells
C. Drug-induced deficiency of folic acid
D. Drug-induced bone marrow suppression
E. Deficiency of glucose-6-phosphate dehydrogenase

Difficulty level: Easy

19. A 64-year-old man was hospitalized for treatment of *Staphylococcus aureus* bacteremia and was given an intravenous infusion of vancomycin. A few minutes later he developed symptoms of an anaphylactic-like reaction. The patient was not aware of previous exposure to vancomycin, and a search for antibodies to the suspected drug was negative. Which of the following types of drug reaction was most likely experienced by the patient?

A. Type I allergic reaction
B. Autoimmune reaction
C. Genetically mediated reaction
D. Pseudoallergic reaction
E. Overdose toxicity

Difficulty level: Medium

20. A 43-year-old man had to undergo surgery to remove a biliary calculus. The anesthesiologist chose to supplement the anesthesia with succinylcholine, a paralyzing agent that has a rapid onset and a short duration of action. In this patient, however, the drug-induced paralysis lasted several hours, necessitating the anesthesiologist to continue the anesthesia and continue artificial respiration. Which of the following adverse drug reactions best explains the patient's disorder?

A. Type II allergic reaction
B. Immediate allergic reaction
C. Idiosyncratic reaction
D. Pseudoallergic reaction
E. Overdose toxicity

Answers and Explanations: I-1 Pharmacokinetics

Learning objective: Describe the main features of lipid diffusion of drugs across cell membranes.

1. **B** Lipid diffusion is by far the most common transport system of drugs across cell membranes. Because albuterol has a low molecular weight, lipid diffusion most likely accounts for the transfer of albuterol through the bronchial mucosa.

A, C–E See correct answer explanation.

Learning objective: Identify the mechanism of permeation of botulinum toxin through nerve cell membranes.

2. **D** Very large molecules cannot permeate cell membranes by diffusion or filtration. The only way they can cross cell membranes is by endocytosis, a process by which a substance is bound to the cell surface, engulfed by the cell membrane, and carried into the cytosol, where the substance can be released by breakdown of the vesicle membrane.

   A–C, E See correct answer explanation.

Learning objective: Describe the main features of active transport of drugs across cell membranes.

3. **A** About one fifth of the iodides ingested with foods are selectively removed from the circulating blood by the Na^+-dependent secondary active transport system that concentrates iodide in thyroid cells 30 to 100 times its concentration in the blood. Because radioactive iodine is essentially the same as iodide taken with foods, it is transported into the thyroid cells by the same secondary active transport system.

   B–E See correct answer explanation.

Learning objective: Describe the main features of bulk flow transport of drugs across cell barriers.

4. **A** A drug administered subcutaneously will initially be located primarily in the extracellular fluid. In order to be absorbed, the drug must enter the general circulation; that is, it must cross the capillary wall. Capillaries have very wide fenestrae that permit the passage of molecules with a molecular weight as high as 30,000 daltons (D). Therefore, most drugs given by the subcutaneous or intramuscular routes will enter the general circulation by bulk flow transport (or filtration; also known as solvent drag) through capillary fenestrae. Moreover, insulin is a protein with a molecular weight of about 6000 D, so it cannot cross the capillary wall by lipid or aqueous diffusion through aquaporins (water channels) of cell membranes. Bulk flow transport is a passive process and is directly proportional to the pressure gradient across the capillary wall. It does not depend on the structure of the drug but only on its molecular size (both lipid- and water-soluble drugs can be filtered provided the molecule is not too large).

   B See correct answer explanation.

   C–E Facilitated diffusion, endocytosis, and active transport do not seem to be involved in the absorption of insulin from the site of injection.

Learning objective: Explain the main mechanistic features of ion trapping.

5. **E** The Henderson-Hasselbalch equation predicts that a weak acid will be more nonionized, and therefore more lipid soluble, when pK_a is greater than pH. Because the pH of the stomach lumen is less than 2, ibuprofen, an acid drug with a pK_a of 4.8, will be mainly nonionized in the gastric lumen and will readily penetrate the gastric mucosal cell membranes. Inside the mucosal cells, however, the pH is about 7, and the drug will become mainly ionized because now the pK_a is less than the pH. Consequently, the concentration gradient of the nonionized, lipid-soluble form will remain high, and the drug will continue crossing cell membranes. At equilibrium, the concentration of the nonionized moiety of the drug will be the same on both sides, but the concentration of the ionized moiety inside the cell can be 15 to 20 times higher than that in the gastric lumen, as the ionized moiety is "trapped" inside the cell (ion-trapping mechanism). Therefore, the total drug concentration inside the cell will be high.

   A–C Basic drugs are mainly ionized when the pK_a is higher than the pH; therefore, most of the drug will stay in the stomach lumen.

   D Theophylline, an acidic drug with a pK_a of 8.8, is mainly nonionized in the stomach lumen and therefore can readily penetrate the gastric cell membranes. Inside the gastric cells, however, the drug remains mainly non-nonionized (i.e., lipid soluble) because the pK_a is greater than the pH. Therefore, the drug will be able to diffuse through the basolateral membrane of the cell, thus reaching the extracellular fluids. No ion trapping occurs, and the drug will not concentrate inside the cells.

Learning objective: Explain why the lipid and water solubilities of a drug are related to their pK_a and to the pH of the solvent.

6. **F** An acidic drug is mainly water soluble when its pK_a is lower than the pH of the medium. The amount of water solubility is proportional to the difference between pH and pK_a, according to the following table

Difference between pH and pK_a	> 2.0	2.0	1.0	0.5	0.0
Percentage	> 99	99	90	76	50

Because the pH of plasma is about 7.4, the drug will be greater than 99% water soluble in the patient's plasma.

   A–E See correct answer explanation.

Learning objective: Describe the ion-trapping mechanism of drugs.

7. **D** Aspirin is an acidic drug. As a rule, the excretion of an acidic drug can be accelerated by alkalinizing the urine, because an acidic drug dissociates to its charged, polar form in alkaline solution. This form, being water soluble, is "trapped" in the tubular lumen and cannot be transported back into the blood across the renal tubular cells. Conversely, the urinary excretion of a weak base may be accelerated by acidifying the urine.

   A Salicylates do not undergo active transport.

   B Salicylate biotransformation by the kidney is negligible.

C Aspirin was already absorbed, so bioavailability is not relevant.

E Glomerular filtration of a drug is strictly related to the renal glomerular filtration rate (GFR). It is very rare for drugs to significantly increase GFR.

Learning objective: Identify the main site of absorption of drugs administered by the oral route.

8. **C** All drugs given by the oral route are primarily absorbed by the small intestine. This is because of the very large surface area of the small intestine, which is about 250 m² and represents about 80% of the total area of the gastrointestinal tract. Hydrochlorothiazide is an acidic drug with a pK_a of about 9, so it will be more lipid soluble in the stomach (where the pH is less than 2) than in the small intestine (where the pH is around 7). Nevertheless, absorption will take place mainly in the small intestine because of its enormous absorptive surface area.

    A Because a drug given orally is swallowed, the oral mucosa does not contribute to absorption.

    B, D, E See correct answer explanation.

Learning objective: Calculate the oral bioavailability of a drug, given sufficient data.

9. **D** Oral bioavailability is measured by the ratio AUC_{Oral}/AUC_{IV}. Drug S gives an oral bioavailability of 0.83, the highest of all the listed drugs.

    A–C, E See correct answer explanation.

Learning objective: Explain why the dosage form of a drug formulation can affect the oral bioavailability of that drug.

10. **A** The amount of drug reaching the portal circulation after oral administration can be strongly influenced by the dosage formulation. Because only single molecules of the drug can pass through the gut wall, the drug must be in solution in order to enter the intestinal epithelial cells. For example, a tablet must be disintegrated and dissolved before reaching the portal circulation. The efficiency of this process depends on several factors, including the way the tablet is manufactured and the excipients used. Once in the portal circulation, the drug can be metabolized by the liver, but the hepatic clearance will be the same, regardless of the different dosage forms. Because in this case the same dose of the drug was administered, the concentration of the drug in the portal vein will be directly proportional to the oral bioavailability of the different formulations, which is indicated by the different AUCs depicted in the figure.

    B–D See correct answer explanation.

Learning objective: Describe the main characteristics of drug permeation across cell membranes.

11. **A** Being a polar drug, ethanol is readily water soluble. Because its molecular weight is small, it can cross cell membranes by aqueous diffusion through aquaporins.

    B–E See correct answer explanation.

Learning objective: List the main factors affecting the absorption of drugs administered by the oral route.

12. **B** Strong pain can substantially decrease gastric emptying, likely because of the activation of the sympathetic nervous system. Because the absorption of drugs by the stomach is very small, gastric emptying is a major factor influencing the rate of intestinal drug absorption, and its decrease can significantly delay this absorption.

    A, C These factors usually speed up, not delay, the intestinal absorption of drugs.

    D, E The distribution and elimination (clearance) of drugs have nothing to do with absorption.

Learning objective: Describe the main factors that can increase the entry of drugs into the central nervous system.

13. **B** The permeability of the blood–brain barrier can be increased by several factors. Damage to the brain by any cause (trauma, infections, tumors, metabolic disorders, cerebrovascular disorders) is one of the most common causes of increased blood–brain barrier permeability.

    A, D The first-pass effect is related to the bioavailability of a drug. Clearance is related to the elimination of a drug. Passage into the brain is related to the distribution of the drug. Bioavailability, distribution, and elimination are independent processes.

    C The permeability of the blood–brain barrier is physiologically increased only in the fetus and the newborn.

    E The high ionization of the drug decreases, not increases, the drug entry into the brain.

Learning objective: Describe the main features of drug–protein binding.

14. **B** Drugs bind primarily to albumin (if acidic) or to α_1 acid glycoprotein (if basic).The extent to which drugs are bound to protein is highly variable (e.g., 0% for lithium, 99% for warfarin). Drugs ordinarily bind to protein in a reversible fashion and in dynamic equilibrium, according to the law of mass action, as shown by the equation

$$[Free\ drug] + [Protein] \rightleftarrows [Drug-protein\ complex]$$

Mass action kinetics predicts that a constant percentage of the drug is bound; therefore, binding is independent of the dose (i.e., the kinetics of binding is first order).

    A, C–E See correct answer explanation.

Learning objective: Calculate the degree of ionization of a drug in cell fluids using the Henderson-Hasselbalch equation.

15. **A** The answer can be found using the Henderson-Hasselbalch equation:

$$\text{Weak acid:}\quad \log \frac{\text{Nonionized}}{\text{Ionized}} = pK_a - pH$$

In the present case, the equation becomes

$$\text{Log} \frac{\text{Nonionized}}{\text{Ionized}} = -2$$

Taking the antilog on both sides, the equation becomes

$$\frac{\text{Nonionized}}{\text{Ionized}} = \frac{1}{100}$$

and remembering that the total drug (i.e., 100% = 1) is the sum of the ionized and nonionized form:

$$\frac{1 - \text{Ionized}}{\text{Ionized}} = \frac{1}{100}$$

that is:

$$\text{Ionized} = \frac{100}{101} = 0.99$$

Therefore, the ionized form will be 99%, and the nonionized, lipid-soluble form will be 1%.

B–E See correct answer explanation.

Learning objective: Describe the main factors that can hinder the entry of drugs into the central nervous system.

16. **D** Drugs may enter the central nervous system (CNS) by crossing the cerebral capillaries (i.e., from plasma to the extracellular fluid [ECF]) or by crossing the choroid plexus (i.e., from plasma to the cerebrospinal fluid [CSF]). The composition of CSF is essentially the same as that of brain ECF, and there appears to be free communication between the brain ECF and CSF. In both of these cases, the drug must cross the blood–brain barrier (BBB). The main reasons that this barrier limits the transfer of drugs into the CNS are (1) endothelial cells of brain capillaries are connected to each other by occluding zonulae and do not have fenestrae, and (2) epithelial cells of the choroid plexus are connected by occluding zonulae.

A, B These statements are correct, but they do not explain the low drug permeability of the blood–brain barrier.

C Drugs are variably bound to plasma proteins; because the bound and free drugs are in equilibrium, even very extensively bound drugs can appreciably enter the brain.

E Very few drugs are completely ionized in the blood.

Learning objective: Outline the main drug factors that can affect the placental transport of a drug.

17. **A** The membranes separating fetal blood from maternal blood in the intervillous space resemble cell membranes elsewhere in their general permeability behavior. Therefore, drug factors affecting placental transport include the molecular size of the drug (drugs with molecular weight greater than 1500 D cross the placenta poorly), its physicochemical properties (lipophilic drugs diffuse readily; highly ionized drugs with molecular weight greater than 200 D cross the placenta slowly), and its degree of protein binding (drugs highly protein bound cross the placenta slowly).

Drug P has a very small molecular weight and is not protein bound. Because it is 100% ionized, it will be completely water soluble and will easily cross the placenta by aqueous diffusion through aquaporins.

B Drug Q will cross the placenta slowly because it is highly protein bound.

C, E Drugs R and T will cross the placenta with difficulty because of their high molecular weight.

D Drug S will cross the placenta with difficulty because it is primarily ionized (i.e., water soluble) and is too big to permeate the membranes by aqueous diffusion.

Learning objective: Explain why the volume of distribution (V_d) can predict, to a certain extent, the pattern of distribution of a drug in the body.

18. **B** Because the volume of plasma in a person weighing 70 kg is about 3 L, it can be deduced that drugs with a volume of distribution of about 3 L distribute in plasma. In fact, infliximab is a large molecule that cannot leave the vascular compartment. It binds to and neutralizes TNF-α in the blood, thus preventing the actions of this cytokine.

A, D In these cases, the volume of distribution would be greater than 42 L.

C In this case, the volume of distribution would be about 13 L.

E In this case, the volume of distribution would be about 42 L.

Learning objective: Calculate the percentage of a drug eliminated by the liver, given sufficient data.

19. **F** Because the total clearance is 5.4 L/h, and the hepatic clearance is 4.86 L/h, the hepatic clearance will be 90% of the total clearance (4.86/5.40 = 0.9, or 90%). Therefore, 90% of the drug will be eliminated by the liver.

A, C–F See correct answer explanation.

Learning objective: Describe the factors affecting the oral bioavailability of a drug.

20. **A** A large fraction of drug P reaches the portal vein and is poorly metabolized by the liver (as seen by the low hepatic clearance). This means that a large fraction of the drug can reach the systemic circulation; that is, the oral bioavailability of the drug is high.

B About the same fraction of both drug P and drug Q reaches the portal vein. However, the hepatic clearance of drug Q is much higher than that of drug P. Therefore, the oral bioavailability of drug Q will be lower than that of drug P.

C–E A lower fraction of these drugs reaches the portal vein. Therefore, their oral bioavailability must be lower than that of drug P.

Learning objective: Calculate the hepatic clearance of a drug, given sufficient data.

21. **C** By definition, clearance is the volume of blood from which all the drug is removed per unit of time. If all of the drug were removed by the liver, the liver clearance would equal the liver blood flow (volume per unit of time), that is, 1500 mL/min. Because 20% of the drug can reach the general circulation, it follows that 80% of the drug is removed by the liver, that is, the drug contained in 80% of the blood flow. Therefore, the liver clearance will be 80% of the liver blood flow (0.8 × 1500 mL/min = 1200 mL/min).

A, B, D, E See correct answer explanation.

Learning objective: Calculate the renal clearance of a drug, given sufficient data.

22. **A** If the daily urine output is 1.44 L/d (24 h), the urine flow in that subject will be

$$\text{Urine flow } 1440 \text{ mL}/1440 \text{ min} = 1 \text{ mL/min}$$

Remembering that the renal clearance (CL_r) of a substance is given by

$$CL_r = (\text{Urine flow} \times \text{Urine concentration})/\text{Plasma concentration}$$

the renal clearance of that drug will be

$$CL_r = (1 \text{ mL/min} \times 40 \text{ mg/mL})/1 \text{ mg/mL} = 40 \text{ mL/min}$$

B–F See correct answer explanation.

Learning objective: Calculate the volume of distribution (V_d) of a drug, given sufficient data.

23. **B** The volume of distribution (V_d) of a drug is independent of the dose. In fact,

$$V_d = D \times F/\text{Cp}_0,$$

where D = dose, F = fraction absorbed, and Cp_0 = plasma concentration at time 0.

If the dose is increased by a certain proportion, the plasma concentration will also be increased by the same proportion, and the V_d will remain the same.

A, C–E See correct answer explanation.

Learning objective: Explain the consequences of drug induction or inhibition of microsomal enzymes.

24. **E** When microsomal enzymes are induced, the hepatic clearance of a drug increases. Because the hepatic clearance of carbamazepine is close to the total clearance, the total clearance of the drug will also increase substantially. Remembering that

$$t_{1/2} = 0.7 \, V_d/CL,$$

where $t_{1/2}$ = half-life, V_d = volume of distribution, and CL = clearance, the half-life of the drug will decrease.

A–C These parameters are increased, not decreased, when microsomal enzymes are induced.

D The volume of distribution of a drug does not change when the amount of drug reaching the general circulation changes.

Learning objective: Describe how the genetic polymorphism of P450 isozymes can influence the effects of drugs.

25. **C** P450 isozymes show genetic polymorphism, and different subgroups have been characterized as poor, intermediate, extensive, and ultra-rapid metabolizers. In the case of CYP2C9 isozyme, more than 20% of Asians are poor metabolizers. Therefore, the hematuria of the patient was most likely related to the fact that he was a poor metabolizer of warfarin, so the anticoagulant effect of the drug was too pronounced.

A, D, E All these reasons would cause a decrease, not an increase, in the warfarin effect.

B Theoretically, decreased renal excretion of warfarin would cause an increase in the warfarin effect. However, more than 95% of warfarin is metabolized, so adverse effects of warfarin due to variation in renal excretion are unlikely.

Learning objective: Calculate the oral bioavailability of a drug, given sufficient data.

26. **B** The liver clearance was negligible, so all of the drug reaching the portal circulation will reach the systemic circulation. Because only 40% of the drug reaches the portal circulation, the oral bioavailability of the drug is 0.4. (*Note* that the liver blood flow rate is not needed to solve the problem.)

A, C–F See correct answer explanation.

Learning objective: Explain the reason for increased toxicity of drugs biotransformed by acetylation.

27. **D** Isoniazid is biotransformed mainly by hepatic acetylation, which is under genetic control. About one half of people of Caucasian origin are slow acetylators because they have an inherited deficiency of N-acetyltransferase. Slow acetylators have a higher risk of adverse effects with isoniazid.

A Rifampin can increase, not reduce, the biotransformation of many drugs by increasing the synthesis of microsomal enzymes.

B, C, E These pathologic conditions do not cause peripheral neuropathy.

Learning objective: Calculate the therapeutic loading dose of a drug, given sufficient data.

28. **C** The dose of a drug can be calculated using the equation

$$\text{Dose} = V_d \times Cp_0/F$$

where V_d = volume of distribution, Cp_0 = plasma concentration at time 0, and F = fraction absorbed. Because the V_d of the obese patient is twice the V_d of a normal-weight person, the dose must be doubled to 60 mg to achieve the same plasma concentration.

A, B, D–F See correct answer explanation.

Learning objective: Explain the relationship between first-pass effect and oral bioavailability.

29. **B** If an orally administered drug is extensively biotransformed during its first pass through the gut wall and/or the liver, less drug will reach the general circulation. That is, its oral bioavailability will be reduced. In fact, buspirone has an oral bioavailability of about 5%.

A Absorption (measured by bioavailability) and distribution (measured by volume of distribution) are independent processes; therefore, volume of distribution is not affected by the absorption of the drug.

C Renal elimination (measured by renal clearance) and bioavailability are independent processes; therefore, renal clearance is not affected by the absorption of the drug.

D, E Sublingual and intramuscular administrations avoid the first-pass effect.

Learning objective: Calculate the renal clearance of a drug, given sufficient data.

30. **A** If 66% of the drug is excreted as such in the urine, its renal clearance will be 66% of the total clearance (0.66 × 136), or about 90 mL/min.

B–F See correct answer explanation.

Learning objective: Calculate the total clearance of a drug, given sufficient data.

31. **E** The plasma concentration (Cp) of the drug is 2 mg/L initially and 1 mg/L after 2 hours; therefore, the half-life ($t_{1/2}$) of the drug is 2 hours.

The volume of distribution of the drug (V_d) is given by

$$V_d = 20 \text{ mg}/2 \text{ mg/L} = 10 \text{ L}$$

Thus, the total clearance (CL) will be

$$CL = 0.7 \times V_d/t_{1/2},$$
$$CL = 0.7 \times 10 \text{ L}/2 \text{ h} = 3.5 \text{ L/h}$$

A–D, F See correct answer explanation.

Learning objective: Estimate the magnitude of a volume of distribution of a drug using information from a graph.

32. **E** The volume of distribution (V_d) of a drug is given by

$$V_d = D/Cp_0,$$

where D = dose and Cp_0 = theoretical plasma concentration at time 0. Because the dose is the same for all drugs, the drug with the lowest Cp_0 (drug T, as seen in the graph) will have the largest V_d.

A–D See correct answer explanation.

Learning objective: Calculate the oral bioavailability of a drug, given sufficient data.

33. **B** The bioavailability can be calculated as

$$V_d = D \times F/Cp_0,$$

where V_d = volume of distribution, D = dose, F = oral bioavailability, and Cp_0 = theoretical plasma concentration at time 0. Therefore, rearranging:

$$F = (V_d \times Cp_0)/D = (100 \text{ L} \times 1 \text{ mg/L})/200 = 0.5$$

A, C, D See correct answer explanation.

E, F These options are irrational. Bioavailability cannot be higher than 1 (or 100%).

Learning objective: Calculate the administered dose of a drug, given sufficient data.

34. **B** Because the half-life of cocaine is 1 hour, the plasma concentration of the drug should have been 1.5 mg/L 1 hour after the injection and 3 mg/L immediately after the injection. To determine the dose,

$$D = Cp \times V_d = 3 \text{ mg/L} \times 130 \text{ L} = 390 \text{ mg},$$

where D = dose, Cp = plasma concentration, and V_d = volume of distribution.

The lethal dose of cocaine is about 500 mg in a nonaddicted person. Hence the dose taken by the patient was most likely high enough to induce coma.

A, C–F See correct answer explanation.

Learning objective: Calculate the half-life of a drug, given sufficient data.

35. **C** The initial plasma concentration (Cp) of the drug would be

$$Cp = D/V_d = 2000 \text{ µg}/10 \text{ L} = 200 \text{ mg/L},$$

where D = dose and V_d = volume of distribution. Therefore, the Cp will be 100 µg/L after one half-life and 50 µg/L after two half-lives. Because this is the concentration after 6 hours, the half-life of the drug will be 3 hours.

A, B, D–F See correct answer explanation.

Learning objective: Identify the half-life of a drug from a graph.

36. **B** When a drug is given by intravenous infusion, it will reach 50% of steady state after 1 half-life. The steady-state plasma concentration for drug X is about 30 mg/mL. From the graph it can be seen that 15 mg/mL is reached in 1 hour.

    A The steady state for drug W is about 47 mg/mL. Half of this value (about 23 mg/mL) is reached in 2 hours.

    C The steady state for drug Y is about 25 mg/mL. Half of this value (about 12 mg/mL) is reached in 2 hours.

    D The steady state for drug Z is about 20 mg/mL. Half of this value (about 10 mg/mL) is reached in 2 hours.

Learning objective: Calculate the total clearance of a drug, given sufficient data.

37. **D** The steady-state plasma concentration (C_{ss}) is reached when the rate of infusion is equal to the rate of elimination, that is,

$$D/T = Css \times CL,$$

where D = dose, T = time, and CL = clearance. From the graph, we have C_{ss} = 3 mg/L.
    Therefore,

$$CL = (D/T)/C_{ss}, 30 \text{ mg/h/3 mg/L} = 10 \text{ L/h}$$

    A–C, E, F See correct answer explanation.

Learning objective: Calculate the plasma concentration of a drug, given sufficient data.

38. **C** The kinetics of drug absorption, distribution, and elimination is defined as zero order (or saturation kinetics) when a constant amount of the drug is absorbed, distributed, or eliminated per unit of time. If the plasma concentration of the drug was 8 mg/L 3 hours after the administration and 7 mg/L 1 hour later, this means that 1 mg/L of the drug is lost every hour. Therefore, the drug was 9 mg/L 2 hours after

the administration, 10 mg/L 1 hour after the administration, and 11 mg/L immediately after the administration.

    A, B, D–F See correct answer explanation.

Learning objective: Estimate the order kinetics of a drug from a graph.

39. **C** The concentration–time curve is a straight line, which indicates that a constant amount of a drug is eliminated per unit of time. Therefore, the drug follows zero-order kinetics. The three main drugs that follow zero-order, rather than first-order, kinetics are ethanol, salicylic acid, and phenytoin.

    A, B, D–F All these drugs, like most drugs used clinically, follow first-order kinetics.

Learning objective: Calculate the plasma concentration of a drug at the steady state, given sufficient data.

40. **C** Because the half-life of the drug is 3 hours, 75% of the plasma concentration of the drug at the steady state will be reached in two half-lives, that is, at 2:00 p.m. The plasma concentration of the drug at 2:00 p.m. is 60 µg/mL. This represents 75% of the plasma concentration of the drug at the steady state. Therefore, at the steady state the plasma concentration will be 80 µg/mL (60 ÷ 0.75).

    A, B, D–F See correct answer explanation.

PHARMACOKINETICS Answer key							
1.	B	6.	F	11.	A	16.	D
2.	D	7.	D	12.	B	17.	A
3.	A	8.	C	13.	B	18.	B
4.	A	9.	D	14.	B	19.	F
5.	E	10.	A	15.	A	20.	A
21.	C	26.	B	31.	E	36.	B
22.	A	27.	D	32.	E	37.	D
23.	B	28.	C	33.	B	38.	C
24.	E	29.	B	34.	B	39.	C
25.	C	30.	A	35.	C	40.	C

Answers and Explanations: I-2 Pharmacodynamics

Learning objective: Explain the most likely consequence of chronic blockade of drug receptors

1. **C** When receptors are chronically blocked, the number of those receptors may increase over time, a process called receptor upregulation. The effector response will be greater than usual if the blockade is abruptly removed.

    A By definition, spare receptors are not involved in receptor activation or blockade.

    B G-protein synthesis is not under β-receptor control. Blockade of β receptors prevents the activation, not the synthesis, of G proteins.

    D Phosphorylation desensitizes the receptor. This can occur after repeated activation of the receptor, not after repeated blockade.

    E Beta-receptor blockade can affect the synthesis of cAMP but not the ability of the cell to respond to cAMP that has already been synthesized.

Learning objective: Define the term *stereoselectivity*.

2. **C** A peculiar property of receptors is stereoselectivity, meaning that they often bind only one enantiomer of a racemic pair.

    A Intrinsic activity refers to the ability of a drug (once bound to a receptor) to initiate changes that lead to a biologic response.

    B Affinity refers to the strength of drug binding to a receptor.

    D Potency refers to the dose of a drug required to produce a given effect.

    E Variability refers to the fact that the number of receptors can vary with time.

    F Maximal efficacy refers to the maximal effect that can be produced by a drug.

Learning objective: Define the term *affinity* (of a drug).

3. **D** Affinity is the tendency of a drug to bind to a receptor. According to the occupation theory, binding to a receptor is driven by the law of mass action; that is, the number of bound receptors increases when the number of available drug molecules increases. Suppose that 100 receptors are exposed to 1000 molecules of drug A or to 1000 molecules of drug B. Also suppose that, in this instance, 40 molecules of drug A are found to be bound to the receptors, but only 10 molecules of drug B are bound to the receptors. It can be concluded that receptor affinity of drug A is greater than that of drug B.

    A Intrinsic activity (often intrinsic efficacy is used as a synonym) refers to the ability of a drug (once bound to a receptor) to initiate changes that lead to a biologic response.

    B Potency refers to the dose of a drug required to produce a given effect. The lower the dose required to produce the effect, the higher the potency.

    C Maximal efficacy refers to the maximum effect produced by the drug.

    E Receptor activation is related to the drug's intrinsic activity (the higher the intrinsic activity of a drug, the higher the amount of receptor activation brought about by that drug).

Learning objective: Explain how the graded log dose–response curve can be used to determine the relative potency of two drugs.

4. **C** By definition, potency refers to the dose needed to produce a given effect. In a graded log dose–response curve, potency can be readily estimated by reading the dose on the abscissa (x-axis) corresponding to a given effect read on the ordinate (y-axis). Potency is inversely proportional to the dose needed to produce a given effect; the lower the dose, the greater the potency.

    A Unless the toxic doses of the two drugs are the same, therapeutic index can tell nothing about the relative potency of the two drugs.

    B The maximal response of each drug is termed its maximal efficacy. Potency and efficacy are independent variables.

    D, E Volume of distribution and clearance are pharmacokinetic variables. Potency is a pharmacodynamic variable.

Learning objective: Calculate the equieffective dose of a new drug given to a patient when the old drug must be suspended because of adverse effects.

5. **E** Because naproxen was therapeutically effective, it is rational to start the therapy with an equieffective dose of the new drug. Celecoxib is ~5 times more potent than naproxen, so a dose 5 times lower, or 100 mg, should be equieffective.

    A–C, D, F See correct answer explanation.

Learning objective: Define the term *functional antagonism*.

6. **B** Glucagon is sometimes used to treat β-blocker overdose. By blocking β_1 receptors in the heart, β-blockers lead to a dose-dependent decrease in heart contractility. Glucagon-induced activation of glucagon receptors leads to an increase in heart contractility. When a drug response mediated by the activation of a receptor is antagonized by an opposite response produced by another drug acting on a different set of receptors, the antagonism is defined as functional (also called physiologic).

    A, C–E See correct answer explanation.

Learning objective: Define the term *partial agonist*.

7. **C** Because, by definition, a partial agonist can activate each receptor only partially, it will produce less than the full effect even when it has occupied 100% of receptors. Moreover, in the presence of a full agonist, a partial agonist will behave as an agonist when the concentration of the full agonist is low, but it will behave as an antagonist when the concentration of the full agonist is high.

    The tested drug was most likely a partial agonist at β_1 receptors. At rest, when the norepinephrine levels are low, the drug causes a little increase in heart rate by partially activating β_1 receptors. After exercise, when the levels of norepinephrine are high, the drug behaves as an antagonist, thus decreasing the heart rate.

    A, B, D–F See correct answer explanation.

Learning objective: Define the term *competitive antagonist.*

8. **E** By definition, a drug without intrinsic activity is one that is able to bind receptors but is not able to activate them. Therefore, it is defined as an antagonist. When the binding is reversible, the antagonism is referred to as competitive, and the drug is a competitive antagonist.

    A–D, F See correct answer explanation.

Learning objective: Describe the drug parameters that can be determined from a plot of a cumulative frequency distribution of responders versus log dose.

9. **B** The cumulative frequency distribution of subjects showing a desired effect when treated with increasing doses of a drug is called a quantal log dose–response curve. From this curve, the dose that can produce that effect in 50% of individuals (called the median effective dose) can be read on the abscissa (x-axis).

    A Affinity is the tendency of a drug to bind to a receptor. It can be measured by plotting the fraction of receptors bound by a drug against the log of the drug concentration. It cannot be measured from a quantal log dose–response curve.

    C, D The therapeutic index is a ratio between the toxic (TD_{50}) and the effective (ED_{50}) dose of a drug. The therapeutic window is the interval between the minimum effective dose (ED_1) and the minimum toxic dose (TD_1). In order to measure these variables, two quantal log dose–effect curves are needed.

    E Maximal efficacy is the maximal effect a drug can produce. It can be measured with a grade log dose–response curve, but not with a quantal log dose–response curve.

Learning objective: Identify the log dose–response curve of an agonist when a fixed dose of a competitive antagonist is given concomitantly.

10. **E** When a dose of a competitive antagonist is given in the presence of a dose of a full agonist, the apparent affinity of the agonist for its receptor is decreased, as some receptors will be occupied by the antagonist. Therefore, the dose-response curve of an agonist in the presence of a fixed dose of a competitive antagonist will be shifted to the right, but the maximal response will not be affected because the competitive antagonism is surmountable. In other words, all the receptors can be occupied by the agonist even in the presence of a competitive antagonist, provided that the amount of the agonist is high enough to displace all of the antagonist that is present (remember that the interaction between drugs and receptors is driven by the law of mass action).

    A–D See correct answer explanation.

Learning objective: Identify the log dose–response curves of two drugs that can fully activate the same receptors.

11. **B** Drugs P, R, and S can all produce the same maximal effect. However, curves P and R are parallel, whereas curve S is not. This suggests that drugs P and R act on the same receptors, whereas drug S most likely acts through different receptors.

    A, C–F See correct answer explanation.

Learning objective: Identify the highest ED_{50} of a drug from a graph of multiple log dose–response curves.

12. **E** The depicted curves are graded log dose–effect curves. In this type of curve, the ED_{50} of a drug is defined as the dose producing 50% of the maximum effect. It can be estimated from the dose on the abscissa (x-axis) that corresponds to the 50% of maximum effect on the ordinate (y-axis). From the graph it can be seen that drug T has the highest ED_{50}.

    A–D See correct answer explanation.

Learning objective: Define the therapeutic window of a drug.

13. **E** The therapeutic window is the interval between the minimum therapeutic dose (or plasma concentration) and the minimum toxic dose (or plasma concentration) of a drug. Because doses below the minimum therapeutic dose are by definition ineffective, and doses above the minimum toxic dose are, by definition, toxic, this window defines the range of doses that have a high probability of therapeutic success.

    A Intrinsic activity refers to the ability of a drug (once bound to a receptor) to initiate changes that lead to a biologic response.

    B Efficacy refers to the maximal effect that a drug can produce.

    C Potency refers to the dose of a drug required to produce a given effect.

    D The therapeutic index is a ratio between a toxic dose and an effective dose of a drug. Like the therapeutic window, it is an index of the safety of a drug, but it is a single value and therefore cannot predict the range of doses that are both safe and effective.

    F Response variability refers to the range of responses, not to the doses eliciting the responses.

Learning objective: Identify the drug parameter that is increased when a drug effect undergoes tolerance.

14. **B** By definition, tolerance is a decreased responsiveness to the action of a drug. Therefore, a higher dose of that drug will be necessary to obtain the given effect in 50% of the population (the median effective dose [ED_{50}]) when tolerance has occurred.

A The maximal efficacy refers to the maximum effect achievable if the dose is taken to very high levels. In tolerant subjects, maximal efficacy may still be achieved, even if higher doses are needed to obtain it.

C The therapeutic index is the ratio between a toxic dose and an effective dose. Because the effective dose is increased as a result of tolerance, the therapeutic index is expected to decrease or to remain the same (if the toxic dose is also increased).

D Potency, which refers to the dose of the drug needed to produce a given effect, is decreased when tolerance has occurred.

E Tolerance can be due to increased metabolism of the drug. In this case, however, the half-life would be decreased, not increased.

Learning objective: Explain the meaning of the term *tachyphylaxis.*

15. **B** Tachyphylaxis refers to a drug tolerance that appears rapidly (in a matter of hours) and also disappears rapidly when the drug is withdrawn. So, the first cigarette caused tachycardia because tolerance to nicotine effects disappeared overnight, but tolerance to those effects was rapidly resumed when smoking was reinstated.

A Cross-tolerance refers to tolerance to a drug that is shared by other drugs with similar chemical structure and/or similar pharmacological effects.

C Tolerance is called pharmacokinetic when it is due to a decrease in the effective concentration of the drug at the site of action.

D Innate tolerance refers to a genetically determined lack of sensitivity to a drug that is observed the first time the drug is administered.

E Sensitization refers to a drug response that increases with the repetition of the same dose of that drug.

Learning objective: Explain the mechanisms of pharmacodynamic tolerance.

16. **D** Opiates exhibit pharmacodynamic tolerance, which can be defined as the decreased responsiveness to the action of a drug whose concentration at the site of action remains the same. The most common mechanism underlying pharmacodynamic tolerance is receptor downregulation; a decrease in receptor density.

Other listed mechanisms refer to homeostatic adaptive changes of the organism that counteract the drug effect.

A, E Tolerance due to increased metabolism of the drug and to decreased concentration of the drug at the site of action is called pharmacokinetic, not pharmacodynamic, tolerance.

B, C These events would have increased, not decreased, the effects of morphine.

Learning objective: Explain the mechanisms of pharmacodynamic tolerance.

17. **B** Tolerance can be defined as a state of decreased responsiveness to the action of a drug that results from prior exposure to that drug or to a related drug. Drug tolerance can involve a decreased concentration of the drug at the site of action, due mainly to an increased biotransformation of the drug (pharmacokinetic tolerance), or it can occur even when the concentration of the drug at the site of action is not modified (pharmacodynamic tolerance). In the latter case, the underlying mechanism can be either a decreased number of receptors (the most common), a change in the postreceptor mechanisms, or homeostatic adaptive changes that counteract the drug effect. Homeostatic adaptive changes seem especially important in tolerance to ethanol. In fact, central nervous system (CNS) effects are more pronounced when ethanol concentrations reaches a certain level than when the same concentration is present during recovery from drunkenness. This indicates that homeostatic adaptive changes occurred in the CNS during the intoxication period.

A, C, D These mechanisms explain pharmacokinetic, not pharmacodynamic, tolerance.

E A decreased, not increased, number of receptors can explain pharmacodynamic tolerance.

Learning objective: Define the term *drug potentiation.*

18. **B** Although benzodiazepines are no longer first-line agents for generalized anxiety disorder, they are still used when other drugs are poorly tolerated or ineffective, as most likely occurred in this case. Potentiation occurs when a drug enhances the effect of another drug but is devoid of that effect when given alone. Cimetidine is devoid of sedative effects but can increase the sedative effect of diazepam by inhibiting hepatic metabolism of diazepam metabolism.

A Additive effect occurs when the response elicited by combined drugs is equal to the combined responses of the individual drugs.

C Synergism occurs when the response elicited by combined drugs is greater than the combined responses of the individual drugs.

D, E These terms refer to drug effects that increase over time when the drug is given chronically.

Learning objective: Define the term *drug synergism.*

19. **C** A drug interaction is defined as synergistic when the response elicited by combined drugs is greater than the combined responses of the individual drugs. In other words, the response elicited by the drug combination is more than simply additive. In the present case, the effects of the individual drugs are bacteriostatic, whereas the effect of the combined drugs is more than an additive bacteriostatic effect (by definition, a bactericidal effect is greater than a bacteriostatic effect). The interaction is therefore defined as synergism.

    A Additive effects occur when the response elicited by combined drugs is equal to the combined responses of the individual drugs.

    B Potentiation occurs when a drug enhances the effect of another drug but is devoid of that effect when given alone.

    D, E These terms refer to drug effects that increase over time, when the drug is chronically given.

Learning objective: Define the term *chemical antagonism.*

20. **D** Chemical antagonism is said to occur when a drug combines chemically with the drug to be antagonized, making that drug pharmacologically inactive, as in the present example. A chemical antagonist does not act on receptors or on the pharmacokinetics of the drug to be antagonized.

    A–C, E See correct answer explanation.

Learning objective: Identify the law that regulates the relationship between drug concentration and the association and dissociation of the drug–receptor complex.

21. **D** According to the law of mass action, the number of receptors occupied by a drug depends on the drug concentration and the affinity of the drug–receptor complex. In other words, the higher the concentration (i.e., mass) of the drug, the higher the number of receptors occupied by the drug.

    A, E These factors depend on receptor activation and on the association and dissociation of the drug–receptor complex, but they do not regulate them.

    B, C These are pharmacokinetic parameters. Pharmacokinetic changes do not regulate pharmacodynamic properties.

Learning objective: Define the process initiated by drug–receptor binding and ending with the therapeutic effect.

22. **C** The detailed molecular pathway that starts from the drug binding to its receptor and leads to a measurable pharmacological effect is called the signal transduction pathway. It can include several steps that occur following the activation of the receptor and are termed *postreceptor mechanisms.* An example of a postreceptor mechanism is the opening of ion channels, or the activation of G proteins, which in turn causes the increased or decreased synthesis of second messengers. These messengers ultimately produce a pharmacological effect, often through the activation of different protein kinases.

    A, B, D, E See correct answer explanation.

Learning objective: Describe the immediate consequence of the activation of metabotropic receptors.

23. **D** When a metabotropic receptor, e.g., the β_2 receptor, is activated, it binds to a G protein, which undergoes a conformational change leading to a free guanosine triphosphate (GTP)-α subunit that can regulate a membrane enzyme or an ion channel.

    A–C These are consequences of G-protein activation, not the immediate event following the activation of metabotropic receptors.

    E Activation of a G protein can ultimately cause phosphorylation of many proteins, thus controlling their function, but the G protein does not undergo phosphorylation.

Learning objective: Identify which drug is more potent and which drug is more effective, given sufficient data.

24. **D** Potency of a drug refers to the dose of that drug needed to obtain a given effect. Because 10 mg of morphine is needed to get an analgesic effect equal to that given by 0.3 mg of buprenorphine, morphine is less potent than buprenorphine.

    Efficacy refers to the maximal effect produced by a drug. By definition, partial agonists have a maximal efficacy lower than that of full agonists. Because morphine is a full agonist and buprenorphine a partial agonist at the same receptor, buprenorphine is less effective than morphine.

    A–C See correct answer explanation.

Learning objective: Identify the most potent among different drugs, given sufficient data.

25. **A** Potency refers to the dose needed to achieve a given effect. Therefore, the lower the dose, the higher the potency. Because the ED_{50} is the dose needed to obtain a given effect in 50% of individuals receiving the drug, drug A is the most potent. Potency has nothing to do with efficacy, which refers to the maximum attainable effect, irrespective of the dose given. In fact, in the present case, drug A is the most potent and the least effective.

    B–E See correct answer explanation.

Learning objective: Define the term *additive effects.*

26. **C** In the present case, the response elicited by combined drugs (8 L of urine) is equal to the combined responses of the individual drugs (5 L + 3 L). When this occurs, the drug–drug interaction is referred to as additive. In other words, the effect of the two drugs used together is the sum of their individual effects.

    A, B, D, E See correct answer explanation.

Learning objective: Identify the response time to activation of steroid receptors.

27. **E** Drugs that activate nuclear receptors to affect transcription usually have a relatively long response time following receptor activation. These drugs regulate gene transcription, which in turn causes an increase or decrease of synthesis of specific proteins. This is consistent with the observation that there is a time lag of hours or days between drug administration and the therapeutic effect of these drugs.

   B–E See correct answer explanation.

Learning objective: Identify the drug with the highest affinity for the receptor from a graph of multiple log dose–response curves.

28. **A** Affinity is defined as the tendency of a drug to bind to its receptor. For drugs acting on the same receptors, affinity is directly proportional to the potency of the drug. From the graph it can be seen that drug P is the most potent and therefore has the greatest affinity for the receptor.

   B–E See correct answer explanation.

Learning objective: Define the term *inverse agonist.*

29. **C** Although most receptors are activated only when an agonist molecule is bound, it has been shown that some receptors can show an appreciable level of activation (called constitutive activation) even when no ligand is present. Examples include receptors for gamma-aminobutyric acid (GABA), cannabinoids, and serotonin. Drugs acting on these receptors are

   - Defined as *agonists* if they increase the level of constitutive activation (e.g., drug Y)
   - Defined as *inverse agonists* if they decrease the level of constitutive activation (e.g., drug X)

- Defined as *antagonists* if they do not change the level of constitutive activation but can antagonize the effects of both agonists and inverse agonists (e.g., drug Z)

Constitutive activation is a relatively recent discovery and may prove to be of greater pharmacological significance in the future.

   A, B, D, E See correct answer explanation.

Learning objective: Describe the placebo effect of a drug.

30. **E** When a plasma level of a drug administered 1 hour previously is equal to zero, a pharmacological effect of the drug is exceedingly unlikely. Therefore, the pain relief must be due to an effect that is independent from the pharmacological action of the drug and operates through psychological mechanisms (i.e., a placebo effect). Placebo effect is common in drug therapy. It is always present (more or less pronounced) in any drug effect, even for drugs whose efficacy is undisputed. On average, 35% of diseases are favorably influenced by a placebo treatment.

   A–C All these factors would have caused a significant plasma level of the drug.

   D Poor patient compliance cannot explain a good pharmacological effect.

PHARMACODYNAMICS Answer key		
1. C	6. B	11. B
2. C	7. C	12. E
3. D	8. E	13. E
4. C	9. B	14. B
5. E	10. E	15. B
16. D	21. D	26. C
17. B	22. C	27. E
18. B	23. D	28. A
19. C	24. D	29. C
20. D	25. A	30. E

Answers and Explanations: I-3 Adverse Effects of Drugs

Learning objective: Describe the mechanism of adverse side effects of drugs.

1. **C** According to the most accepted definition, a side effect is an unintended but not toxic pharmacological response to a normal therapeutic dose of a drug. Therefore, the adverse effects of the drug in this patient are classic side effects and are a consequence of a drug–receptor interaction. In fact, all antihistamines used for motion sickness have sedative effects that result from activation of central H_1 receptors, as well as anticholinergic effects that are due to blockade of peripheral cholinergic receptors.

   A, B, D, E See correct answer explanation.

Learning objective: Estimate the risk of overdose toxicity, given sufficient data.

2. **E** The risk of overdose toxicity can be estimated from the therapeutic index of a drug, which is the ratio between a harmful dose (lethal, in this case) and an effective dose of that drug (median effective dose, in this case). The lower the therapeutic index, the higher the risk of overdose toxicity. Because the lethal dose is the same for all drugs, the drug with the highest median effective dose will be the drug with the lowest therapeutic index and thus the highest risk of overdose toxicity.

   A–D See correct answer explanation.

Learning objective: Explain the meaning of overdose toxicity of a drug.

3. **A** Bleeding is the major adverse effect of anticoagulants and is a direct consequence of their pharmacological action. It is therefore due to a dose that is too high for that patient (i.e., overdose toxicity). This risk can be decreased by careful control of dosage and close monitoring with appropriate lab tests. Hematuria (microscopic, or less frequently, macroscopic, as in the present case) is usually the first sign of overdosage, but bleeding in the nose, oral pharynx, or intestinal tract is also common.

    B–E See correct answer explanation.

Learning objective: Describe the idiosyncratic reaction to thiopental in a patient with a genetic deficiency of heme biosynthetic pathway enzymes.

4. **C** Barbiturate-induced attacks of acute porphyria in genetically susceptible people are a well-known example of idiosyncratic drug reaction. These patients have a genetic deficiency of heme biosynthetic pathway enzymes. The heme normally functions as a repressor of d-aminolevulinate synthase (ALA synthase), the enzyme that regulates the rate-limiting step in porphyrin biosynthesis. Barbiturates induce the synthesis of cytochrome P-450 in the liver. This leads to an enhanced consumption of heme, which is a component of cytochrome P-450, and the concentration of heme in the liver cells decreases. The lower concentration of heme enhances the synthesis of ALA synthase (derepression), which in turn stimulates the synthesis of porphyrins. These intermediates accumulate, as they cannot be transformed into heme due to the deficiency of an enzyme in the heme biosynthetic pathway.

    Attacks of acute intermittent porphyria can be very serious and (rarely) fatal. The patient's family history is the best indicator of the risk of acute intermittent porphyria.

    A, B, D, E All of these options are unlikely.

Learning objective: Describe the best course of action for a patient under warfarin therapy who becomes pregnant.

5. **C** Warfarin is a teratogenic drug (category D includes drugs with a positive evidence of human prenatal risk). Exposure to warfarin during the first trimester may cause several malformations, including eye anomalies, dwarfism, congenital heart disease, and deafness. Fetal death can also occur. Heparin is a parenteral anticoagulant that is not harmful to the fetus because it is a large molecule (molecular weight 15,000 daltons [D]) and therefore does not cross the placenta. All penicillins are considered safe during pregnancy.

    A This choice is irrational. Patients with artificial heart valves must receive anticoagulant therapy.

    B The teratogenic risk of warfarin extends to the second and third trimesters of pregnancy. Exposure in these periods may cause central nervous system anomalies, including hydrocephalus, mental retardation, seizures, and spasticity. Moreover, when given shortly before delivery, it may cause a hemorrhagic effect in the newborn.

    D See correct answer explanation.

    E Reducing the dose of warfarin could reduce the risk to the fetus (teratogenic effects are also related to the dose of the offending drug) but does not avoid it. Moreover, reducing the dose will most likely reduce the effectiveness of the therapy for the mother.

Learning objective: Compare the therapeutic windows of different drugs, given sufficient data.

6. **B** By definition, the therapeutic window of a drug is the range between the minimum therapeutic dose (or plasma concentration) and the minimum toxic dose (or plasma concentration) of a drug. The wider this range, the higher the probability of therapeutic success. However, because the range is a relative measure, in order to compare therapeutic windows of different drugs, the ratio between the minimum toxic concentration and the minimum therapeutic concentration of each drug needs to be calculated, which means calculating their therapeutic index. A large therapeutic index represents a wide therapeutic window; a small therapeutic index represents a narrow therapeutic window. Therefore, the therapeutic index can be thought of as a way to quantify the therapeutic window of a drug. In this example, drug Q needs a dose 10 times higher than the minimum therapeutic dose in order to show toxicity. For all other drugs, a dose 2 to 4 times higher than the minimum therapeutic dose is enough to cause toxicity.

    A, C–E See correct answer explanation.

Learning objective: Identify the enzyme involved in an idiosyncratic reaction to chloroquine.

7. **B** The genetic polymorphism of glucose-6-phosphate dehydrogenase (G6PD) is pronounced; over 400 mutant forms of the enzyme have been identified. Only some of these mutations cause clinical symptoms because their activity is 1 to 15% of normal. G6PD deficiency is X-linked and is the most common disease-producing enzyme abnormality in humans; more than 200 million people are estimated to carry the trait. The defect is fully expressed in males and affects about 10% of African American males. Diminished G6PD activity impairs the ability to form NADPH, the reduced form of nicotinamide adenine dinucleotide phosphate, which is essential in detoxification of free radicals and peroxides formed within cells. Although the deficiency occurs in all cells, it is more severe in erythrocytes, where the hexose monophosphate provides the only means of generating NADPH. Thus, red blood cells are especially sensitive to factors such as infections, diabetic acidosis, and oxidant drugs that cause oxidative damage of the cell and lead to hemolysis. Commonly used drugs that produce hemolytic anemia in patients with G6PD deficiency are some antimalarials (e.g., primaquine, chloroquine, and quinine), some sulfonamides (e.g., sulfamethoxazole), and some salicylates.

    A, C–E See correct answer explanation.

Learning objective: Identify the antibiotic contraindicated in a patient with a previous serious allergic reaction to sulfa drugs.

8. **A** Because the woman had a serious hypersensitivity to sulfa drugs, any agent having a sulfur atom in its molecule (sulfamethoxazole, in this case) should be avoided, as cross-sensitivity usually occurs in drugs with similar chemical structure.

    B–E See correct answer explanation.

Learning objective: Define the ED_{50} of a drug.

9. **C** By definition, the dose able to elicit a specific response (sleep, in this case) in 50% of individuals receiving the drug is called the median effective dose (ED_{50}).

    A, B, D, E See correct answer explanation.

Learning objective: Describe the fetal phenytoin syndrome.

10. **B** Many first generation anticonvulsant drugs are classified category D or X by the U.S. Food and Drug Administration (FDA). The syndrome exhibited by this newborn baby is called fetal phenytoin syndrome and may include nearly all possible types of malformations. It is now recognized that this syndrome has been linked to other first generation anticonvulsants and occurs in about 4% of the children of epileptic women who receive this therapy during pregnancy. Yet, because uncontrolled generalized seizures during pregnancy can lead to fetal injury and death, treatment with second generation anticonvulsants is generally advisable.

    A Methyldopa is the antihypertensive of choice during pregnancy because very few adverse effects have been reported in neonates exposed to this drug in utero, despite its extensive use.

    C Erythromycin is considered safe during pregnancy (FDA prenatal risk category B).

    D, E These drugs were given during the delivery, so they could not be associated with the malformations of the newborn baby.

Learning objective: Describe the main features of overdose toxicity of a drug.

11. **E** The very high serum creatinine level indicates renal failure. The nocturia reported by the patient is often an early symptom, principally due to a failure to concentrate the urine. Aminoglycoside antibiotics such as gentamicin can cause nephrotoxicity when given at high doses, and the gentamicin serum level points out that the drug had reached a too-high steady-state concentration. The mechanism of aminoglycoside-induced renal failure is complex but seems to be mainly related to a destruction of brush border cells of the renal tubule.

    A, B Certain renal diseases (e.g., tubulointerstitial nephritis) may be caused by drug hypersensitivity, but aminoglycoside antibiotics rarely cause sensitization, and the high gentamicin concentration indicates that overdose toxicity is the most likely drug reaction.

    C, D See correct answer explanation.

Learning objective: Identify the main type II allergic reactions to penicillins.

12. **D** The signs of the patient (skin rash, eosinophiluria) suggest that his disease was caused by an allergic reaction. The most frequent cause of tubulointerstitial nephritis is a type II allergic drug reaction. Allergic tubulointerstitial nephritis is rather common and is the underlying cause of up to 3% of all cases of acute renal failure. The disease can be caused by many different drugs, including antibiotics, diuretics, and nonsteroidal antiinflammatory drugs (NSAIDs), but penicillins are most frequently implicated. Recognition of a drug-related cause is important, because severe renal damage is often preventable and reversible.

    A–C, E See correct answer explanation.

Learning objective: Describe the main type III allergic reactions to drugs.

13. **E** The patient was most likely suffering from serum sickness, a type III allergic reaction to drugs characterized by acute urticaria and angioedema or by morbilliform eruptions, often accompanied by polyarthritis, myalgia, and fever, due to an

excessive formation of immune complexes. The antigen-antibody complex usually precipitates very quickly and, being phagocytosed by macrophages, elicits no reaction. If the antigen is in excess to the antibody, however, the immune complexes may remain soluble in the blood and continue to circulate. Eventually they may deposit on the walls of blood vessels at basement membranes, causing complement activation and local inflammation. Penicillins are typical causative agents of serum sickness.

A–D See correct answer explanation.

Learning objective: Describe the main type IV allergic reactions to drugs.

14. **E** The patient was likely suffering from contact dermatitis, which is an adverse effect common to many drugs given locally. Topical doxepin, which is effective in many cases of pruritus, is especially prone to cause this adverse effect. Contact dermatitis is the most common manifestation of type IV (cell-mediated) allergic reaction. Patients may become allergic to drugs used to treat skin diseases. It takes 6 to 10 days (in the case of strong sensitizers) to years (for weaker sensitizers) for patients to become sensitized. Contact dermatitis may resemble other types of dermatitis, but skin changes and the history of exposure facilitate the diagnosis.

A–D All of these options are unlikely because of the history of exposure and the result of the patch test.

Learning objective: Describe the idiosyncratic drug reactions due to a genetic deficiency of the reduced form of nicotinamide adenine dinucleotide (NADH)–methemoglobin reductase.

15. **C** The patient was most likely suffering from a genetically determined abnormal reaction to sulfamethoxazole. Several drugs, including sulfonamides, some local anesthetics, nitrites, primaquine, and dapsone, can cause methemoglobinemia. Patients with a genetic deficiency of NADH–methemoglobin reductase are especially sensitive to drug-induced methemoglobinemia, because they lack the enzyme that reduces methemoglobin to hemoglobin.

A, B, D, E See correct answer explanation.

Learning objective: Outline the most important determinant of allergic drug reaction.

16. **B** Some drugs cause allergic reactions very rarely, whereas other compounds (obviously not used as drugs) can cause sensitization in all exposed subjects. Therefore, the drug structure is the major determinant of the frequency of an allergic reaction to a drug.

A Even if in some rare occurrences the dose can be a factor predisposing to allergy (i.e., penicillin-induced hemolytic anemia requires high and sustained drug concentrations), the occurrence and the severity of an allergic reaction are not dose-dependent in most cases.

C The bioavailability refers to the fraction of the drug reaching the general circulation. Because allergy is not related to dose, bioavailability is not an important factor for an allergic drug reaction. Moreover, the oral route carries the lowest risk of allergic reaction.

D The genetic pedigree is important for idiosyncratic drug reactions.

E The patient's liver and kidney functions are important factors for drug overdose toxicity.

Learning objective: Describe the appropriate procedure to minimize the risk of an allergic drug reaction.

17. **E** A detailed personal and family history should be the first procedure to undertake in order to minimize the risk of an allergic drug reaction. This should include information about prior allergic and medication encounters, prior exposure to the same or structurally related medications, and the nature and severity of the reaction. This information can alert the physician about certain types of compounds to which the patient is likely to react.

A Giving a small dose is not a safeguard against allergic reaction to a drug because the seriousness of an allergic reaction is not related to the dose given.

B Skin tests are reliable methods for the diagnosis of allergy to β-lactam antibiotics, but they should be performed only after the history has determined the likelihood of an allergic reaction to them.

C Antiallergic medications (corticosteroids, antihistamines, etc.) can be used for the therapy of specific allergic reactions, but they are not effective for prevention of any supposed (and still unknown) hypersensitivity reaction.

D To change the drug the patient is allergic (or is supposed to be allergic) to with another drug belonging to the same chemical class does not decrease the risk of an allergic reaction because cross-sensitivity is very common among different drugs belonging to the same class.

Learning objective: Describe the allergic reaction to methyldopa.

18. **B** The positive Coombs test indicates that the patient was most likely suffering from autoimmune hemolytic anemia. Positive Coombs reaction occurs in up to 30% of patients treated for 3 to 6 months with methyldopa, with hemolytic anemia occurring in 1 to 5% of cases. This is a type II allergic drug reaction. The drug is able to induce the formation of autoantibodies (immunoglobulin G) to red blood cells, thus causing cell lysis. The anemia usually ceases within 3 weeks after withdrawal of the drug, but a Coombs test can remain positive for more than 1 year.

A, C–E See correct answer explanation.

Learning objective: Identify a pseudoallergic reaction to drugs.

19. **D** The signs and symptoms of the patient indicate that he was suffering from a type I–like allergic reaction, but circulating antibodies cannot be detected. In these cases, the reaction is called pseudoallergic, and the clinical symptoms are due to a drug-induced direct formation and/or release of mediators normally involved in allergic reactions.

    A–C, E See correct answer explanation.

Learning objective: Identify an idiosyncratic reaction to drugs.

20. **C** An idiosyncratic reaction is commonly defined as a genetically determined abnormal reaction to a drug. Succinylcholine and mivacurium are neuromuscular blocking drugs that are primarily metabolized by plasma cholinesterase (butyrylcholinesterase). Because of this extensive and rapid metabolism, the action of these drugs is brief. The neuromuscular blockade by these drugs may be exceedingly prolonged in patients who have a genetically abnormal variant of cholinesterase. Also, because this variant is much less efficient than the normal enzyme, it can take 2 to 3 hours for the paralysis to disappear. In this case, the anesthesiologist must continue the general anesthesia and artificial respiration until cessation of the drug effect.

    A, B, D, E These other options are unlikely.

ADVERSE EFFECTS OF DRUGS Answer key							
1.	C	6.	B	11.	E	16.	B
2.	E	7.	B	12.	D	17.	E
3.	A	8.	A	13.	E	18.	B
4.	C	9.	C	14.	E	19.	D
5.	C	10.	B	15.	C	20.	C

II Autonomic Nervous System

Questions: II-1 Introduction to Autonomic Pharmacology

Directions for questions **1–5**

Match each effect with the activation of the appropriate receptor (each lettered option can be selected once, more than once, or not at all).

- **A.** α_1 adrenergic
- **B.** α_2 adrenergic
- **C.** β_1 adrenergic
- **D.** β_2 adrenergic
- **E.** β_3 adrenergic
- **F.** D_1 dopaminergic
- **G.** D_2 dopaminergic
- **H.** M_2 cholinergic
- **I.** M_3 cholinergic
- **J.** Nm cholinergic
- **K.** Nn cholinergic

Difficulty level: Easy

1. Mydriasis

Difficulty level: Easy

2. Increased gluconeogenesis

Difficulty level: Easy

3. Selective dilation of renal vessels

Difficulty level: Easy

4. Constriction of bladder internal sphincter

Difficulty level: Easy

5. Decreased atrioventricular conduction

Difficulty level: Medium

6. A 2.1-kg (4.6-lb) baby boy was born at 34 weeks gestation by vaginal delivery. One hour after birth, the baby appeared hypothermic and lethargic. Apgar scores were low, and blood pressure was 55/35 mm Hg. Lab tests revealed that the newborn had a genetic dopamine β-hydroxylase deficiency. Lab tests would have also shown which of the following results?

- **A.** Very low plasma levels of norepinephrine
- **B.** Very low plasma levels of dopamine
- **C.** High plasma levels of epinephrine
- **D.** High urinary levels of normetanephrine
- **E.** Low urinary levels of homovanillic acid

Difficulty level: Easy

7. A 43-year-old man recently diagnosed with pheochromocytoma (an adrenal gland tumor) started a treatment with a drug that can cause a pronounced decrease in norepinephrine and epinephrine by blocking the first rate-limiting step in catecholamine biosynthesis. Which of the following enzymes was most likely inhibited by the drug?

- **A.** Aromatic L-amino acid decarboxylase
- **B.** Dopamine-β-hydroxylase
- **C.** Tyrosine hydroxylase
- **D.** Phenylethanolamine methyltransferase
- **E.** Monoamine oxidase

Difficulty level: Medium

8. A 14-year-old boy with type 1 diabetes noticed symptoms of palpitations, inward trembling, sweating, hunger, weakness, and nervousness just after his participation in a basketball game. His medication included twice daily injections of insulin. Most of the boy's symptoms likely resulted from increased firing of which of the following neurons?

- **A.** Somatic motor neurons
- **B.** Pyramidal neurons
- **C.** Preganglionic parasympathetic neurons
- **D.** Preganglionic sympathetic neurons
- **E.** Postganglionic parasympathetic neurons

Difficulty level: Easy

9. A 55-year-old woman suffering from postural hypotension started a treatment with an α_1-adrenergic drug. Which of the following is a body site where autonomic receptors are primarily α_1 adrenergic?

- **A.** Bronchial muscle
- **B.** Sphincter muscle of the iris
- **C.** Atrioventricular node
- **D.** Purkinje fibers
- **E.** Skin vessels

Difficulty level: Easy

10. A 24-year-old woman admitted to the hospital after a car accident was diagnosed with neurogenic shock due to a spinal cord injury. An emergency treatment was started that included the administration of norepinephrine. Which of the following expected effects of the drug was most likely mediated by the activation of peripheral postsynaptic β_1 receptors?

   A. Bronchodilation
   B. Uterine relaxation
   C. Increased liver gluconeogenesis
   D. Increased renin secretion
   E. Decreased insulin secretion
   F. Increased sweating of the palms of the hands

Difficulty level: Medium

11. A 28-year-old woman presented to the emergency department with breathing difficulty and increasing swelling of her face, eyes, lips, and tongue. An hour earlier she had received an intramuscular injection of ampicillin to treat acute pharyngitis. A diagnosis of anaphylactic reaction was made, and an intramuscular injection of epinephrine was given. Which of the following expected effects of the drug was most likely mediated by the activation of peripheral postsynaptic α_2 receptors?

   A. Mydriasis
   B. Decreased secretion of insulin
   C. Increased secretion of renin
   D. Constriction of skin vessels
   E. Increased heart rate
   F. Dilation of skeletal muscle vessels

Difficulty level: Hard

12. A new autonomic drug was administered locally in the conjunctival sac of a healthy volunteer. Twenty minutes later, measurement of several eye parameters gave the following results:

Parameter	Before Drug	After Drug
Pupillary diameter (mm)	3.0	3.5
Lens curvature	Normal	Normal
Intraocular pressure (mm Hg)	20	15

Which of the following pairs of receptors did the drug most likely activate?

   A. α_1 and α_2 adrenergic
   B. α_2 and β_2 adrenergic
   C. Nn and Nm cholinergic
   D. M_2 and M_3 cholinergic
   E. β_1 and β_2 adrenergic

Difficulty level: Hard

13. The cardiovascular effects of a new autonomic drug that does not cross the blood–brain barrier were evaluated in a healthy volunteer. The drug was administered intravenously, and the results are presented below:

Parameter	Control	Drug X
Systolic BP (mm Hg)	120	130
Diastolic BP(mm Hg)	80	100
Heart rate (bpm)	70	60

Abbreviations: BP, blood pressure; bpm, beats per minute.

Which of the following receptors did the drug most likely activate?

   A. α_1 adrenergic
   B. β_2 adrenergic
   C. D_1 dopaminergic
   D. M_2 cholinergic
   E. β_1 adrenergic

Difficulty level: Medium

14. A 62-year-old man suffering from postural hypotension started therapy with a drug that selectively activates α_1 receptors. Which of the following postreceptor mechanisms most likely mediated the therapeutic effect of the drug in this patient?

   A. Decreased synthesis of inositol triphosphate (IP_3) and diacylglycerol (DAG)
   B. Increased activation of phospholipase C
   C. Opening of ligand-gated K^+ channels
   D. Blockade of voltage-gated Ca^{2+} channels
   E. Increased synthesis of cyclic guanosine monophosphate (cGMP)

Difficulty level: Hard

15. The cardiovascular effects of a new autonomic drug that does not cross the blood–brain barrier were evaluated in a healthy male volunteer. The drug was administered intravenously, and the results are presented below:

Parameter	Control	Drug
Systolic BP (mm Hg)	120	130
Diastolic BP (mm Hg)	75	55
Heart rate (bpm)	70	115

Abbreviations: BP, blood pressure; bpm, beats per minute.

Which of the following pairs of receptors were most likely activated by the drug?

A. α_1 and α_2 adrenergic
B. α_1 and β_1 adrenergic
C. Nm and Nn cholinergic
D. M_2 and M_3 cholinergic
E. β_1 and β_2 adrenergic

Difficulty level: Hard

16. The bronchial effects of a new alpha-beta agonist that does not cross the blood–brain barrier was studied in laboratory animals. It was found that the drug caused relaxation of bronchiolar smooth muscle. The activation of which of the following pairs of adrenoceptors most likely mediated the effect of the drug?

A. β_2 postsynaptic and α_2 presynaptic
B. β_1 presynaptic and α_1 postsynaptic
C. α_2 postsynaptic and β_3 postsynaptic
D. α_1 presynaptic and β_2 presynaptic
E. β_1 postsynaptic and α_2 presynaptic

Difficulty level: Hard

17. The metabolic effects of a new autonomic drug were studied in laboratory animals. The following results were obtained:

Liver gluconeogenesis: increased

Renin secretion: unaffected

Plasma K^+: decreased

Degranulation of mast cells: inhibited

Lipolysis in fat cells: increased

Which of the following pairs of receptors were most likely activated by the drug?

A. α_1 and β_1
B. β_2 and β_3
C. β_1 and β_2
D. M_3 and β_3
E. M_2 and M_3
F. α_1 and M_2

Difficulty level: Medium

18. A new autonomic drug was administered locally in the conjunctival sac of a healthy volunteer during a phase 1 clinical trial. Twenty minutes later, measurement of several eye parameters gave the following results:

Pupillary diameter: decreased

Lens curvature: increased

Intraocular pressure: decreased

Which of the following receptors did the drug most likely activate?

A. α_1
B. α_2
C. Nm
D. M_3
E. β_2

Difficulty level: Hard

19. A 54-year-old woman complained to her physician of palpitations, dry mouth, blurred vision, and constipation. The woman had a long history of endogenous depression and had recently started a new antidepressant therapy. The patient's symptoms most likely resulted from a blockade of which of the following pairs of receptors?

A. α_1 and α_2
B. α_1 and β_1
C. M_2 and M_3
D. β_1 and β_2
E. Nm and β_2

Difficulty level: Hard

20. A 35-year-old farmer was brought to the emergency department with severe abdominal cramps and vomiting. He reported that he was working in the field with an organophosphate pesticide. The physician observed all of the typical symptoms of acetylcholine excess. Which of the following symptoms of the patient were most likely due to the activation of nicotinic Nm receptors only?

A. Salivation, decreased blood pressure
B. Difficulty in breathing, miosis
C. Diarrhea, sweating
D. Bradycardia, urinary urgency
E. Diplopia, difficulty in swallowing

Questions: II-2 Adrenergic Drugs

Directions for questions **1–5**

Match each adrenergic drug with the appropriate description (each lettered option can be selected once, more than once, or not at all).

A. Albuterol
B. Apraclonidine
C. Cocaine
D. Dextroamphetamine
E. Dobutamine
F. Dopamine
G. Epinephrine
H. Isoproterenol
I. Methyldopa
J. Norepinephrine
K. Phenylephrine
L. Salmeterol

Difficulty level: Easy

1. An α_2 selective adrenoceptor agonist

Difficulty level: Easy

2. A long-acting β_2 selective adrenoceptor agonist

Difficulty level: Easy

3. An indirect-acting adrenergic agent sometimes used as an antihypertensive

Difficulty level: Easy

4. A nonselective β_1 adrenoceptor agonist

Difficulty level: Easy

5. A selective α_1 adrenoceptor agonist

Difficulty level: Medium

6. A 75-year-old-woman, hospitalized for breast cancer, was found unconscious in her bed by a nurse. A diagnosis of cardiac arrest was made, and cardiopulmonary resuscitation was started without success. The electrocardiogram showed that the patient was in asystole. An intracardiac injection of epinephrine was given. Which of the following postreceptor mechanisms most likely mediated the effect of epinephrine on cardiac contractility in this patient?

A. Opening of ligand-gated K⁺ channels
B. Opening of ligand-gated Na⁺ channels
C. Activation of phospholipase C
D. Activation of phospholipase A₂
E. Activation of adenylyl cyclase

Difficulty level: Medium

7. A 35-year-old man was admitted to the hospital following a car accident, and a blood transfusion was started. A few minutes later, he complained of nausea and pruritus and developed dyspnea with audible wheezing. His skin was mottled and cold, heart rate was 120 bpm, and blood pressure fell to 80/40 mm Hg. An intramuscular injection of epinephrine was given. Which of the following actions of the drug most likely contributed to its therapeutic efficacy in this patient?

A. Increased glycogenolysis
B. β_2 receptor–mediated vasodilation
C. Stimulation of platelet aggregation
D. Inhibition of insulin secretion
E. Inhibition of mast cell degranulation
F. Stimulation of eicosanoid biosynthesis

Difficulty level: Medium

8. A 34-year-old woman was at the dentist for an endodontic procedure. Before starting the procedure, the dentist injected a solution of lidocaine plus epinephrine near the tooth in order to provide local anesthesia. The epinephrine-induced increased duration of the lidocaine effect was most likely mediated by the activation of which of the following adrenoceptors?

A. β_1
B. β_2
C. β_3
D. α_1
E. α_2

Difficulty level: Hard

9. A 51-year-old man was admitted to the coronary care unit with a diagnosis of myocardial infarction. Two hours later, he developed ventricular fibrillation and was defibrillated immediately, but without success. Cardiopulmonary resuscitation (CPR) was started, and two additional shocks were given at a higher energy, but the patient remained unresponsive. At this time a bolus of intravenous epinephrine was given, while continuing the CPR. Which of the following receptor actions of the drug best describes the rationale for adding epinephrine in this setting?

A. α_1 receptor–mediated vasoconstriction
B. β_2 receptor–mediated vasodilation
C. β_2 receptor–mediated increase in cardiac contractility
D. β_1 receptor–mediated increase in renin secretion
E. β_2 receptor–mediated bronchodilation

Difficulty level: Medium

10. A 60-year-old man hospitalized following a myocardial infarction showed a pronounced decrease in blood pressure and urine output 2 hours after the admission. A diagnosis of cardiogenic shock was made, and an emergency therapy was started. An adrenergic drug with both direct and indirect actions was given by intravenous infusion. Which of the following drugs fitting this profile would be appropriate for the patient?

A. Dopamine
B. Norepinephrine
C. Isoproterenol
D. Dobutamine
E. Phenylephrine

Difficulty level: Hard

11. A new autonomic drug that does not enter the brain was given intravenously to healthy volunteers in a phase 1 clinical trial. The results are presented below:

Parameter	Control	Peak Drug Effect
Systolic BP (mm Hg)	125	145
Diastolic BP(mm Hg)	75	95
Heart rate (bpm)	70	51
Cardiac output (L/min)	5.5	5.1
Ejection fraction (%)	60	75

Abbreviations: BP, blood pressure; bpm, beats per minute.

Which of the following drugs does the new agent most resemble?

A. Dobutamine
B. Epinephrine
C. Isoproterenol
D. Norepinephrine
E. Phenylephrine
F. Propranolol

Difficulty level: Easy

12. A 54-year-old man was about to receive local anesthesia before a tooth extraction. One year ago the patient underwent an episode of ventricular fibrillation that was successfully treated with electrical cardioversion. The dentist decided to avoid a local anesthesia with epinephrine because the patient was especially at risk of which of the following drug-induced adverse effects?

A. Cerebral hemorrhage
B. Nausea and vomiting
C. Pulmonary edema
D. Ventricular tachycardia
E. Hyperglycemia

Difficulty level: Hard

13. A 43-year-old man was brought to the emergency room following a car accident. He received an infiltration of a local anesthetic around a skin wound in preparation for suturing. A few minutes later, the man appeared flushed and complained of difficulty breathing. Blood pressure was 90/50 mm Hg, heart rate 92 bpm. Chest auscultation revealed restrictive air flow and stridor. An injection of epinephrine was given. Which of the following actions most likely contributed to the therapeutic efficacy of the drug in the patient's disorder?

A. Antagonism of histamine effects on the heart
B. Antagonism of bradykinin effects on skeletal muscle vessels
C. Antagonism of leukotriene effects on the respiratory system
D. Activation of α_1 receptors on bronchial muscles
E. Activation of β_2 receptors on lung vessels
F. Activation of α_2 receptors on platelets

Difficulty level: Medium

14. A 16-year-old girl was treated topically with eye drops during a routine ophthalmoscopic examination. After 15 minutes, the ophthalmologist measured an increase in pupillary diameter with negligible changes in lens curvature and intraocular pressure. Which of the following drugs was most likely administered to the patient?

A. Phenylephrine
B. Timolol
C. Acetylcholine
D. Apraclonidine
E. Epinephrine

Difficulty level: Easy

15. A 15-year-old boy suffering from asthma routinely self-administered albuterol through a metered-dose inhaler. Which of the following actions most likely contributed to the therapeutic efficacy of the drug in the patient's disorder?

A. Increased microvascular permeability
B. Decreased bronchial secretions
C. Release of histamine from mast cells
D. Increased residual respiratory volume
E. Increased mucociliary clearance

Difficulty level: Hard

16. A new autonomic drug that does not enter the brain was given intravenously to healthy volunteers in a phase 1 clinical trial. The cardiovascular effects are presented below:

Parameter	Control	Peak Drug Effect
Systolic BP (mm Hg)	125	145
Diastolic BP (mm Hg)	75	95
Heart rate (bpm)	70	58
Cardiac output (L/min)	5	4.5
Ejection fraction (%)	60	60

Abbreviations: BP, blood pressure; bpm, beats per minute.

Which of the following drugs does the new agent most resemble?

A. Dobutamine
B. Epinephrine
C. Isoproterenol
D. Norepinephrine
E. Phenylephrine

Difficulty level: Medium

17. A 72-year-old man suffering from prostatic hyperplasia complained to his physician that he had increased difficulty and pain in voiding his bladder. The patient had had been taking an over-the-counter oral nasal decongestant for 3 days because of an annoying common cold. Which of the following drugs most likely contributed to his dysuria?

A. Albuterol
B. Phenylephrine
C. Clonidine
D. Norepinephrine
E. Dopamine
F. Salmeterol

Difficulty level: Easy

18. A 65-year-old woman suffering from open-angle glaucoma was prescribed a treatment regimen that included apraclonidine eye drops. Which of the following actions on aqueous humor most likely mediated the therapeutic effect of the drug in the patient's disease?

A. Increased outflow through the Schlemm canal
B. Decreased production by the trabecular meshwork
C. Increased outflow through the uveoscleral route
D. Decreased production by eye vessel constriction
E. Decreased production by the ciliary epithelium

Difficulty level: Hard

19. A 57-year-old homeless alcoholic man was brought to the hospital by the police, who had found him lying on a sidewalk. Physical examination showed clear signs of alcohol withdrawal. Therapy was started that included clonidine. Which of the following best explains the most likely mechanism of action of clonidine in this patient?

A. Decreased central sympathetic outflow
B. Activation of peripheral α_1 receptors
C. Decreased central parasympathetic outflow
D. Activation of peripheral α_2 receptors
E. Blockade of α receptors on the tractus solitarius
F. Blockade of α receptors on the locus ceruleus

Difficulty level: Medium

20. A 7-year-old girl recently diagnosed with persistent asthma started treatment with inhaled albuterol "as needed." Which of the following adverse effects was most likely to occur during the therapy?

A. Atrioventricular block
B. Restlessness
C. Sleepiness
D. Postural hypotension
E. Ventricular tachycardia

Difficulty level: Medium.

21. A 52-year-old woman suffering from severe bronchial asthma was recently diagnosed with open-angle glaucoma. An appropriate local therapy was prescribed. Which of the following drugs most likely would be included in the glaucoma treatment of this patient?

A. Carbachol
B. Epinephrine
C. Propranolol
D. Pilocarpine
E. Timolol

Difficulty level: Medium

22. A 33-year-old man was brought to the emergency room after a car accident. Upon admission, the patient was lucid but completely paralyzed, with loss of all sensation and reflex activity below the thorax. Vital signs were blood pressure 80/40 mm Hg, heart rate 42 bpm, respirations 36/min. A preliminary diagnosis of spinal shock, due to spinal cord injury, was made, and an intravenous infusion of an appropriate drug was started. Which of the following drugs was most likely administered?

A. Isoproterenol
B. Clonidine
C. Norepinephrine
D. Albuterol
E. Salmeterol

Difficulty level: Hard

23. The cardiovascular effects of a new autonomic drug that does not cross the blood–brain barrier were evaluated in a healthy male volunteer. The drug was administered intravenously, and the results are presented below:

Parameter	Control	Peak Drug Effect
Mean BP (mm Hg)	90	80
Heart rate (bpm)	70	110
Cardiac output (L/min)	5.5	6.5
Ejection fraction (%)	60	80

Abbreviations: BP, blood pressure; bpm, beat per minute.

Which of the following drugs does the new agent most resemble?

A. Albuterol
B. Cocaine
C. Isoproterenol
D. Norepinephrine
E. Phenylephrine

Difficulty level: Medium

24. A 51-year-old man received an intravenous infusion of isoproterenol at the conclusion of heart transplant surgery. Which of the following actions most likely occurred a few minutes after the start of the infusion?

A. Stimulation of renin secretion
B. Inhibition of insulin release
C. Increased total peripheral resistance.
D. Reflex tachycardia
E. Stimulation of platelet aggregation

Difficulty level: Medium

25. A 34-year-old man was brought to the emergency room with a gunshot wound to the abdomen. External blood loss and internal hemorrhage were significant, and he was anxious and disoriented. On examination, his skin was pale and cool, pulse was thready at 130 bpm, blood pressure was 80/70 mm Hg, and respiration was shallow with a rate of 30 breaths/min. The first appropriate therapeutic intervention in this patient would have been an intravenous infusion of which of the following agents?

A. Norepinephrine
B. Epinephrine
C. Dobutamine
D. Isotonic saline
E. Dopamine
F. Isoproterenol

Difficulty level: Hard

26. A 53-year-old man was brought to the emergency department after suffering crushing substernal pain for the past hour. Vital signs on admission were blood pressure 88/50, pulse 115 bpm, respirations 30/min. Further exams led to the diagnosis of cardiogenic shock due to myocardial infarction, and therapy was started that included an intravenous infusion of an appropriate drug. Which of the following molecular actions most likely mediated the therapeutic effectiveness of the drug in this patient?

A. Activation of phospholipase A_2
B. Increased synthesis of inositol triphosphate (IP_3) and diacylglycerol (DAG)
C. Increased synthesis of cyclic adenosine monophosphate (cAMP)
D. Increased synthesis of cyclic guanosine monophosphate (cGMP)
E. Opening of ligand-gated Na^+ channels
F. Opening of ligand-gated K^+ channels

Difficulty level: Medium

27. A 25-year-old healthy male volunteer received an intravenous infusion of a new drug in a phase 1 clinical trial. It was found that the drug causes an increase in cardiac contractility, a slight increase in heart rate, and no major changes or a decrease in systemic vascular resistance. Which of the following drugs does the new agent most resemble?

A. Phenylephrine
B. Norepinephrine
C. Isoproterenol
D. Epinephrine
E. Dobutamine

Difficulty level: Hard

28. A 58-year-old man became confused and disoriented 5 days after he underwent surgery to remove necrotic bowel tissue. Physical findings were high fever (103°F, 39.4°C), blood pressure 90/50 mm Hg, pulse 130 bpm, respirations 30/min. Pertinent lab values were partial pressure of arterial carbon dioxide (P_aCO_2) 30 mm Hg (normal 33–45 mm Hg), bicarbonate (HCO^{3-}) 18 mEq/L (normal 22–28 mEq/L), serum pH 7.31, white blood cell count (WBC) 22,000 cells/mm³. Arterial and pulmonary artery catheters were inserted, revealing a cardiac output of 6 L/min and a pronounced decrease of systemic vascular resistance. Fluid therapy was initiated, but 1 hour later mean blood pressure was still 60 mm Hg. An intravenous infusion of an appropriate drug was started. Which of the following drugs was most likely administered?

  A. Isoproterenol
  B. Epinephrine
  C. Norepinephrine
  D. Albuterol
  E. Clonidine

Difficulty level: Easy

29. A 13-year-old girl with mild persistent allergic asthma started a treatment that included an inhaled bronchodilator "as needed." A drug with which of the following mechanisms of action would be most appropriate for this patient's inhaler?

  A. Blockade of α_1 adrenoreceptors
  B. Blockade of M_2 cholinergic receptors
  C. Activation of β_2 adrenoreceptors
  D. Activation of H_1 histamine receptors
  E. Activation of leukotriene receptors
  F. Blockade of Nm cholinergic receptors

Difficulty level: Medium

30. A 42-year-old woman complained to her physician of tremors, muscle cramping, palpitations, and anxiety. The woman, who was recently diagnosed with severe bronchial asthma, had started an appropriate therapy 2 weeks earlier. Which of the following drugs most likely caused the patient's symptoms?

  A. Isoproterenol
  B. Salmeterol
  C. Propranolol
  D. Dobutamine
  E. Prazosin

Difficulty level: Easy

31. A 16-year-old male snorted cocaine for the first time at a party. A few minutes later he felt euphoric, and friends noted that his pupils were dilated. Which of the following molecular actions most likely mediated the mydriasis?

  A. Inhibition of monoamine oxidase A
  B. Blockade of α_2 receptors in sympathetic terminals
  C. Inhibition of norepinephrine reuptake into sympathetic terminals
  D. Stimulation of epinephrine release from adrenal medulla
  E. Stimulation of norepinephrine release from sympathetic terminals

Difficulty level: Hard

32. A 41-year-old man presented to the clinic complaining of an impairment in his ability to voluntarily raise his left eyelid. Physical examination showed miosis, ptosis, flushed facial skin, and loss of sweating over the left side of the face. Further exams led to the diagnosis of Horner syndrome. To determine the site of the autonomic lesion, a hydroxyamphetamine solution was instilled into the conjunctival sac of the left eye. A few minutes later, mydriasis was observed. The physician correctly concluded that there was a localized lesion in which of the following nervous structures?

  A. Preganglionic sympathetic nerves innervating the face
  B. Postganglionic sympathetic nerves innervating the face
  C. Preganglionic parasympathetic nerves innervating the face
  D. Postganglionic parasympathetic nerves innervating the face

Difficulty level: Medium

33. A 37-year-old man was admitted to the hospital after a work accident. An admitting diagnosis of spinal cord injury was made, and emergency therapy was initiated, which included the intravenous infusion of a low dose of dopamine. Which of the following effects of the drug were most likely mediated by the activation of dopamine D_1 receptors?

  A. Increased diuresis
  B. Nausea and vomiting
  C. Constriction of skin vessels
  D. Increased heart rate
  E. Increased stroke volume

Difficulty level: Medium

34. A 46-year-old woman admitted to the hospital with the presumptive diagnosis of septic shock was given emergency therapy. The treatment included an adrenergic drug that can decrease total peripheral resistance at lower doses and can increase it at higher doses. Which of the following drugs was most likely administered?

A. Norepinephrine
B. Albuterol
C. Isoproterenol
D. Dobutamine
E. Phenylephrine
F. Dopamine

Difficulty level: Hard

35. A 51-year-old patient suffering from postural hypotension was admitted to the hospital for evaluation. A tyramine infusion did not raise the blood pressure, whereas a very small dose of norepinephrine caused a large, transient elevation of blood pressure. These results would suggest a degeneration of which of the following nervous structures?

A. Postganglionic sympathetic neurons
B. Preganglionic sympathetic neurons
C. Postganglionic parasympathetic neurons
D. Preganglionic parasympathetic nerves neurons
E. Medulla oblongata

Difficulty level: Easy

36. A 47-year-old woman suffering from postmenopausal hot flashes tried different drugs with little success. Her physician decided to try another drug that decreases the release of norepinephrine from adrenergic nerve terminals. Which of the following drugs was most likely prescribed?

A. Prazosin
B. Clonidine
C. Albuterol
D. Isoproterenol
E. Labetalol

Difficulty level: Hard

37. A 48-year-old woman suffering from lupus erythematosus was admitted to the hospital because of severe muscle weakness. Pertinent laboratory data on admission were K^+ 7.9 mEq/L, creatinine 5 mg/dL, blood urea nitrogen (BUN) 60 mg/dL. An electrocardiogram (ECG) revealed increased PR intervals and widened QRS complexes. Insulin with dextrose was given intravenously to reduce the high potassium level. Another drug was also given because it has an additive effect with insulin in decreasing serum potassium. Which of the following drugs was most likely administered?

A. Phenylephrine
B. Albuterol
C. Clonidine
D. Isoproterenol
E. Epinephrine
F. Dobutamine

Difficulty level: Medium

38. A 35-year-old woman was admitted to the emergency department because of dyspnea, generalized itching, and swelling of the lips, eyelids, and tongue. The symptoms started a few minutes after an intramuscular (IM) injection of a vaccine. An appropriate therapy was started, which included an IM injection of epinephrine. Which of the following expected effects of the drug were most likely mediated by activation of β_2 adrenoceptors?

A. Inhibition of insulin release
B. Skin vasoconstriction
C. Mydriasis
D. Contraction of the bladder sphincter
E. Increased glycogenolysis

Difficulty level: Medium

39. An intravenous injection of drug X was given to a laboratory animal before and after the administration of atropine, and the heart rate was recorded. The results are depicted below:

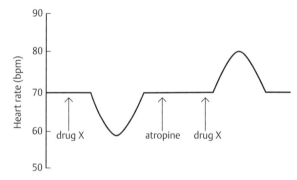

Which of the following drugs was most likely drug X?

A. Epinephrine
B. Norepinephrine
C. Prazosin
D. Albuterol
E. Isoproterenol
F. Dobutamine

Difficulty level: Medium

40. A 43-year-old woman was in the emergency department for the treatment of shock due to spinal trauma. Despite fluid therapy, she was still hypotensive (80/50 mm Hg) and tachycardic (125 bpm). An intravenous infusion of norepinephrine was started, and a few minutes later the blood pressure was 120/85 mm Hg, and the heart rate decreased to 85 bpm. Which of the following actions best explains the drug-induced decrease of heart rate in this patient?

A. Activation of cardiac β_2 receptors
B. Decreased firing rate of vagal neurons
C. Increased firing rate of aortic baroreceptors
D. Activation of cardiac α_2 autoreceptors
E. Decreased firing rate of carotid chemoreceptors

Questions: II-3 Antiadrenergic Drugs

Directions for questions **1–5**

Match each antiadrenergic drug with the appropriate description (each lettered option can be selected once, more than once, or not at all).

- **A.** Atenolol
- **B.** Esmolol
- **C.** Metyrosine
- **D.** Phenoxybenzamine
- **E.** Pindolol
- **F.** Propranolol
- **G.** Sotalol
- **H.** Tamsulosin
- **I.** Timolol

Difficulty level: Easy

1. This drug is a partial agonist at β_1 and β_2 receptors.

Difficulty level: Easy

2. This drug is a selective β_1 antagonist frequently used for the chronic treatment of atrial fibrillation.

Difficulty level: Easy

3. This drug is a β-blocker that can also block potassium channels.

Difficulty level: Easy

4. This drug is frequently used in the treatment of prostatic hyperplasia.

Difficulty level: Easy

5. This drug is sometimes given in cardiovascular emergencies by intravenous infusion because of its extremely short half-life.

Difficulty level: Hard

6. A 25-year-old man complained to his physician of painful erection and impaired ejaculation during intercourse. Three weeks earlier, he had been diagnosed with Raynaud disease and had started an appropriate therapy. A drug with which of the following mechanisms of actions most likely caused the patient's symptoms?

- **A.** β_2-receptor blockade
- **B.** M_3-receptor activation
- **C.** β_1-receptor blockade
- **D.** α_2-receptor activation
- **E.** α_1-receptor blockade
- **F.** Nm-receptor activation

Difficulty level: Medium

7. Phenoxybenzamine was given to rats during a lab experiment. Which of the following sets of effects most likely occurred after treatment?

	Firing Rates of Carotid Baroreceptors	Cardiac Contractility	Cardiac Rate
A	↓	↑	↑
B	↑	↑	↓
C	↑	↓	↑
D	↓	↑	↓
E	↓	↓	↓

Difficulty level: Medium

8. A 51-year-old man, recently diagnosed with pheochromocytoma, was scheduled for surgery to remove the tumor. One week before surgery, phenoxybenzamine was prescribed. Which of the following actions most likely mediated the therapeutic effect of the drug in the patient's disease?

- **A.** Decreased peripheral vascular resistance
- **B.** Increased cardiac output
- **C.** Decreased epinephrine release from the adrenal medulla
- **D.** Increased heart rate
- **E.** Decreased firing from the vasomotor center

Difficulty level: Medium

9. A 58-year-old man complained to his physician of weakness, drowsiness, dizziness, and palpitations. He was recently diagnosed with bladder obstruction due to benign prostatic hyperplasia and had been taking a drug for 2 weeks. Which of the following drugs most likely caused the patient's symptoms?

- **A.** Bethanechol
- **B.** Tamsulosin
- **C.** Propranolol
- **D.** Flutamide
- **E.** Albuterol
- **F.** Phenylephrine

Difficulty level: Medium

10. A 28-year-old woman presented to the outpatient clinic with a 5-day history of left hand and arm pain. She noted that the fingers of her left hand became cold and somewhat blue, especially when exposed to cold. Physical examination showed that the patient's extremities had appropriate sensation. When her hands were placed in cold water, several white splotches appeared, and tingling was felt in the hands.

Which of the following drugs would be appropriate to treat the patient's disorder?

A. Neostigmine
B. Propranolol
C. Prazosin
D. Clonidine
E. Phenylephrine

Difficulty level: Easy

11. A 64-year-old woman, recently diagnosed with open-angle glaucoma, started a topical therapy with timolol and apraclonidine. Which of the following was the most likely site of action of both drugs?

A. Ciliary muscle
B. Uveoscleral vessels
C. Conjunctival vessels
D. Ciliary epithelium
E. Retinal vessels
F. Schlemm canal

Difficulty level: Hard

12. A 22-year-old man was admitted to the hospital for evaluation of a faint systolic murmur and an unusual electrocardiogram reading. After clinical and lab evaluation, a diagnosis of hypertrophic cardiomyopathy was made, and propranolol was prescribed. Which of the following actions most likely contributed to the therapeutic efficacy of the drug in the patient's disease?

A. Decreased renin secretion
B. Increased duration of diastole
C. Blockade of an abnormal pacemaker
D. Decreased ejection fraction
E. Coronary vasodilation

Difficulty level: Medium

13. A new autonomic drug was tested in a healthy volunteer. The man was treated with saline or with the drug, under resting or exercise conditions. His heart rate was measured in both conditions. The results were the following:

	Heart Rate (bpm)	
	Saline	Drug
Resting	70	68
Exercise	150	80

To which of the following drug classes did the tested drug most likely belong?

A. Beta adrenoceptor blockers
B. Cholinergic agonists
C. Cholinergic antagonists
D. Ganglionic blockers
E. Alpha-1 adrenoceptor blockers

Difficulty level: Medium

14. A 58-year-old man recently diagnosed with exertional angina started treatment with atenolol. Which of the following cardiovascular parameters was most likely decreased in this patient?

A. End-systolic volume
B. Ventricular ejection time
C. Cardiac ejection fraction
D. End-diastolic volume
E. Venous tone

Difficulty level: Medium

15. A 57-year-old, woman recently diagnosed with open-angle glaucoma, started treatment with timolol eye drops. Which of the following sets of effects most likely occurred shortly after the administration of the drug?

	Pupillary Diameter	Lens Curvature	Intraocular Pressure
A	+	−	0
B	0	0	−
C	+	0	−
D	0	+	0
E	−	0	+

+ = increased
− = decreased
0 = negligible effect

Difficulty level: Medium

16. Propranolol was given by intramuscular injection to several dogs during a lab experiment. One hour later, each dog received a different autonomic drug, and the effects of that drug were recorded. Which of the following drug-induced effects was most likely best counteracted by propranolol pretreatment?

A. Isoproterenol-induced hyperglycemia
B. Nicotine-induced decrease in skin blood flow
C. Norepinephrine-induced reflex bradycardia
D. Phenylephrine-induced mydriasis
E. Pilocarpine-induced contraction of bronchial muscle

17. A new drug was studied in laboratory animals. Epinephrine was given either alone or after the administration of the new drug X. Some plasma values were then recorded, as reported in the table below:

	Epinephrine Alone	Epinephrine after Drug X
Renin (mU/L)	250	70
Blood glucose (mg/dL)	160	155

Which of the following drugs did the new agent most resemble?

A. Albuterol
B. Timolol
C. Atenolol
D. Atropine
E. Propranolol
F. Prazosin

18. A 44-year-old man who had been suffering from migraine for 3 months complained to his physician that his migraine attacks were effectively aborted by sumatriptan, but they were not reduced in frequency. The physician decided to start a treatment to reduce the frequency of attacks and chose propranolol as the initial agent. Which of the following pairs of adverse effects would be expected to be most likely during the first days of therapy?

A. Postural hypotension and fainting
B. Palpitations and flushing
C. Impairment of far vision and photophobia
D. Insomnia and nightmares
E. Severe constipation and gastroesophageal reflux

19. A 42-year-old man came to the clinic for a follow-up visit 2 months after being diagnosed with essential hypertension. Therapy with propranolol and hydrochlorotiazide was started at the time of diagnosis. His blood pressure remained poorly controlled, and he admitted he had been taking the pills only once in a while, because of a disturbing adverse effect. Which of the following was most likely the effect mentioned by the patient?

A. Palpitations
B. Sexual dysfunction
C. Migraine headache
D. Tremor
E. Anginal pain

20. A 47-year-old man who had been suffering from diabetes for 10 years was admitted to the hospital following a myocardial infarction. He was discharged 10 days later with a postdischarge therapy that included atenolol. The patient was instructed to monitor his blood glucose level carefully for both hyper- and hypoglycemia after the drug was initiated. Which of the following statements about atenolol best explains the reason for glucose monitoring?

A. It can dangerously increase blood sugar levels.
B. It can blunt some symptoms of hypoglycemia.
C. It can increase insulin secretion.
D. It can impair lipid metabolism.
E. It decreases renin release.

21. A 57-year-old woman was discharged from the hospital after an acute myocardial infarction. The woman had been suffering from mild seasonal asthma for 15 years. Her postdischarge therapy included atenolol, one tablet daily. Which of the following was the most likely rationale behind prescribing atenolol to this patient?

A. It can counteract pulmonary vasoconstriction.
B. It blocks β_1 adrenoceptors only.
C. It has antiinflammatory effects in asthmatics.
D. It can block pulmonary α adrenoceptors.
E. It has an intermediate half-life (about 6 hours).

22. A 47-year-old man was diagnosed with benign prostatic hyperplasia. Surgical ablation of the prostate was contraindicated, and a drug suitable for the treatment of the patient's impaired bladder emptying was prescribed. Which of the following molecular actions most likely contributed to the therapeutic effect of that drug in the patient's disease?

A. Decreased blood flow in prostatic vessels
B. Relaxation of prostate capsule
C. Relaxation of the detrusor muscle
D. Decreased systemic blood pressure
E. Decreased diuresis

23. A 25-year-old man complained to his physician of a fine, slow tremor of the hands elicited by performing skilled acts. The patient noticed that the tremor was getting worse, especially when he felt tense and anxious. Medical history showed that the patient's father had a similar symptom. Neurologic examination of the patient was unremarkable. A preliminary diagnosis was made, and a therapy was prescribed. Which of the following drugs would be appropriate for this patient?

A. Prazosin
B. Clonidine
C. Albuterol
D. Physostigmine
E. Propranolol

Difficulty level: Hard

24. A 31-year-old man was brought to the emergency department after the police found him shouting and acting irrationally in the street. The man admitted that for the past few hours he had been using amphetamines that he had obtained from a new dealer. He was agitated and anxious and exhibited psychotic behavior. Vital signs were blood pressure 230/150 mm Hg, heart rate 160 bpm, respirations 20/min. An emergency therapy was started, and the patient was treated with intravenous diazepam, but 30 minutes later his blood pressure was still 210/130. Which of the following pairs of drugs would be appropriate to include in the patient's treatment at this time?

A. Phentolamine followed by propranolol
B. Phenoxybenzamine followed by esmolol
C. Metyrosine followed by neostigmine
D. Bethanechol followed by phenylephrine
E. Clonidine followed by albuterol

Difficulty level: Medium

25. A 57-year-old alcoholic man with liver cirrhosis was admitted to the intensive care unit with a 2-week history of intermittent melena. Esophagoscopy revealed three chains of large varices in the lower esophagus with signs of recent bleeding. An appropriate treatment was performed that included a drug aimed at reducing the portal pressure. Which of the following drugs was most likely given?

A. Albuterol
B. Propranolol
C. Methyldopa
D. Clonidine
E. Prazosin

Difficulty level: Medium

26. A 51-year-old woman presented to the clinic with a 1-month history of palpitations, insomnia, nervousness, fatigue, diarrhea, and heat intolerance. The physical examination revealed hyperreflexia, lid lag, and mild tremor. Vital signs were blood pressure 160/60, heart rate 95 bpm. Which of the following drugs was most likely appropriately included in the therapeutic management of this patient?

A. Albuterol
B. Propranolol
C. Labetalol
D. Prazosin
E. Phenoxybenzamine

Difficulty level: Hard

27. A 32-year-old man complained to his physician that he felt anxious and tense. History revealed that he was a musician and had to give an important piano concert that evening. The physician told the patient that he was suffering from performance anxiety and prescribed a drug to be taken 2 hours before the performance. Which of the following drugs was most likely prescribed?

A. Diazepam
B. Propranolol
C. Fluoxetine
D. Venlafaxine
E. Buspirone

Difficulty level: Easy

28. A 65-year-old man, recently diagnosed with prostatic hyperplasia, started treatment with prazosin, one tablet daily. Which of the following adverse effects would be most likely to occur during the first days of therapy?

A. Mydriasis
B. Impaired micturition
C. Pale and cold skin
D. Bronchoconstriction
E. Postural hypotension

Difficulty level: Easy

29. A 44-year-old woman suffering from open-angle glaucoma had been receiving topical timolol for 3 months. The disease was well controlled, and the treatment stopped the progression of optic nerve damage. Which of the following molecular actions most likely mediated the therapeutic efficacy of the drug in the patient's disease?

A. Opening of ligand-gated K^+ channels
B. Increased synthesis of diacylglycerol (DAG)
C. Decreased synthesis of cyclic guanosine monophosphate (cGMP)
D. Decreased activity of adenylate cyclase
E. Increased synthesis of tyrosine kinase
F. Opening of ligand-gated Na^+ channels

Difficulty level: Easy

30. A 33-year-old man recently diagnosed with pheochromocytoma was scheduled for surgery. The week before the operation he received a treatment with a drug that acts by decreasing catecholamine biosynthesis. Which of the following drugs was most likely administered?

A. Phenoxybenzamine
B. Propranolol
C. Metyrosine
D. Dexamethasone
E. Levothyroxine

Questions: II-4 Cholinergic Drugs

Directions for questions **1–5**

Match each cholinergic drug with the appropriate description (each lettered option can be selected once, more than once, or not at all).

- **A.** Acetylcholine
- **B.** Bethanechol
- **C.** Carbachol
- **D.** Donepezil
- **E.** Edrophonium
- **F.** Muscarine
- **G.** Neostigmine
- **H.** Parathion
- **I.** Pilocarpine
- **J.** Pralidoxime
- **K.** Physostigmine

Difficulty level: Easy

1. Inhibition of cholinesterases by this drug is very short (2–10 minutes).

Difficulty level: Easy

2. This drug can inhibit cholinesterases equally well in the periphery as in the central nervous system.

Difficulty level: Easy

3. This compound can be absorbed effectively through the intact skin.

Difficulty level: Easy

4. This drug is able to regenerate cholinesterases blocked by organophosphates.

Difficulty level: Easy

5. This drug can inhibit cholinesterases and directly activate Nm cholinergic receptors.

Difficulty level: Medium

6. A new autonomic drug was given intravenously to dogs during a lab experiment. It was found that the drug was able to increase cholinergic transmission in both the peripheral and central nervous systems. Which of the following drugs does the new agent most resemble?

- **A.** Acetylcholine
- **B.** Carbachol
- **C.** Bethanechol
- **D.** Neostigmine
- **E.** Physostigmine

Difficulty level: Hard

7. A 62-year-old man suffering from open-angle glaucoma underwent ocular surgery for canaloplasty. Before the operation, the ophthalmologist instilled a few drops of carbachol in the conjunctival sac. Which of the following anatomical structures represents the primary site of action of the drug in this patient?

- **A.** Ganglionic neurons
- **B.** Ciliary muscle
- **C.** Lens
- **D.** Radial muscle of the iris
- **E.** Brainstem

Difficulty level: Hard

8. A 51-year-old diabetic woman presented to the emergency room with severe ocular pain and redness, decreased vision, colored halos, and nausea and vomiting. Ophthalmoscopy revealed anterior chamber inflammation, and tonometry measured an intraocular pressure of 48 mm Hg in the right eye (normal 10–20 mm Hg). A diagnosis of an acute glaucoma attack was made, and two drugs were instilled in the conjunctival sac. Another drug was given by the same route 15 minutes later. Which of the following three drugs were most likely administered?

- **A.** Timolol, apraclonidine, and pilocarpine
- **B.** Homatropine, carbachol, and timolol
- **C.** Scopolamine, dorzolamide, and phenylephrine
- **D.** Homatropine, carbachol, and dorzolamide
- **E.** Prazosin, physostigmine, and mannitol

Difficulty level: Medium

9. A 62-year-old woman had no bowel movements 4 days after surgery to remove a colon cancer. A diagnosis of adynamic ileus was made, and an intramuscular injection of neostigmine was given. The activation of which of the following pairs of receptors most likely mediated the therapeutic effect of the drug in the patient's disorder?

- **A.** Nm and M_2 cholinergic
- **B.** Nn and M_3 cholinergic
- **C.** β_2 adrenergic and M_3 cholinergic
- **D.** β_2 adrenergic and Nn cholinergic
- **E.** Nn cholinergic and α_1 adrenergic
- **F.** Nm cholinergic and α_1 adrenergic

Difficulty level: Easy

10. A 74-year-old man complained to his physician of memory impairment that had worsened over the past 2 months. He also reported that he had increasing difficulty in recognizing familiar objects and in planning everyday activities such as shopping. Physical examination revealed no neurologic deficits, but the man performed very poorly in the Folstein Mini-Mental Status Exam. Donepezil was prescribed. Which of the following molecular mechanisms most likely mediated the therapeutic effect of the drug in the patient's disease?

   A. Inhibition of norepinephrine reuptake
   B. Stimulation of norepinephrine release
   C. Blockade of nicotinic neuronal receptors
   D. Inhibition of cholinesterase
   E. Blockade of muscarinic M_1 receptors
   F. Inhibition of choline acetyltransferase

Difficulty level: Medium

11. A 71-year-old man suffering from myasthenia gravis was admitted to the hospital for evaluation. His therapy included neostigmine, three tablets daily. It was found that the patient had a slow heart rate (46 bpm), which the physician thought was related to neostigmine therapy. Which of the following molecular mechanisms most likely mediated this adverse effect of the drug?

   A. Opening of ligand-gated K^+ channels
   B. Opening of voltage-gated Na^+ channels
   C. Increased synthesis of inositol triphosphate (IP_3) and diacylglycerol (DAG)
   D. Opening of ligand-gated Ca^{2+} channels
   E. Increased synthesis of adenylyl cyclase

Difficulty level: Medium

12. A 67-year-old woman suffering from glaucoma underwent trabeculectomy, a surgical procedure to remove part of the trabecular meshwork of the eye. Before the operation, the ophthalmologist instilled a few drops of pilocarpine in the conjunctival sac. Which of the following sets of effects most likely occurred shortly after the administration of the drug?

	Pupillary Diameter	Lens Curvature	Ocular Pressure
A	0	0	−
B	−	+	−
C	+	0	0
D	+	0	−
E	+	−	+

+ = increased
− = decreased
0 = negligible effect

Difficulty level: Medium

13. A 79-year-old female resident of a nursing home was recently diagnosed with urinary overflow incontinence due to an atonic bladder, and a treatment with bethanechol was prescribed. Which of the following actions most likely mediated the therapeutic effectiveness of the drug in the patient's disorder?

   A. Increased bladder sphincter tone
   B. Decreased ureteral peristalsis
   C. Decreased compliance of the bladder
   D. Decreased diuresis
   E. Increased tone of the bladder trigone

Difficulty level: Hard

14. A 58-year-old woman with a long history of depression was brought to the emergency department with vomiting, urinary incontinence, profuse salivation, cold sweat, rapid and irregular pulse, tachypnea, and mental confusion. She admitted attempting suicide by ingesting several tablets found in her husband's bureau drawer. Soon after admission, the woman experienced a tonic-clonic seizure. Which of the following drugs most likely caused the patient's poisoning?

   A. Clonidine
   B. Scopolamine
   C. Nicotine
   D. Bethanechol
   E. Neostigmine

Difficulty level: Medium

15. A 65-year-old man suffering from open-angle glaucoma had been receiving several drugs over the past 6 months, but the control of intraocular pressure proved inadequate. The ophthalmologist decided to add a drug and prescribed echothiophate. Which of the following actions most likely mediated the therapeutic effect of echothiophate in the patient's disease?

   A. Contraction of the radial muscle of the iris
   B. Contraction of the sphincter of the iris
   C. Decreased production of aqueous humor
   D. Dilation of the episcleral venous plexus
   E. Dilation of retinal vessels
   F. Contraction of the ciliary muscle

Difficulty level: Easy

16. A 49-year-old farmer came to the emergency department complaining of blurred vision, nausea, and painful muscle contractions in his legs. He said the symptoms started soon after coming in from his soybean field. The attending physician appropriately administered pralidoxime intravenously soon after the man arrived. An agent from which of the following drug classes most likely caused the patient's symptoms?

A. Adrenergic antagonists
B. Carbamates
C. Cholinergic antagonists
D. Organophosphates
E. Alcohols

Difficulty level: Medium

17. A 41-year-old man was brought to the emergency department because of severe vomiting and diarrhea that started about 1 hour after a meal. The patient showed profuse salivation, lacrimation, and wheezing. His skin was moist, and his pupils were miotic. Skeletal muscle movements were normal. Blood pressure was 80/50 mm Hg, pulse 46 bpm. Poisoning of this patient was most likely due to which of the following agents?

A. Muscarine-containing mushrooms
B. Nicotine-containing insecticide
C. Organophosphate-containing insecticide
D. Atropine-containing mushrooms
E. Carbamate-containing insecticide

Difficulty level: Easy

18. A 61-year-old man complained to his physician of brow ache, difficulty with far vision, and problems seeing in dim light. The man had a long history of open-angle glaucoma. One month earlier, he had changed his ophthalmic medication. Which of the following was most likely his new drug?

A. Pilocarpine
B. Timolol
C. Apraclonidine
D. Epinephrine
E. Phenylephrine
F. Neostigmine

Difficulty level: Easy

19. A 64-year-old man, recently diagnosed with myasthenia gravis, started treatment with neostigmine. Which of the following adverse effects would be most likely in this patient?

A. Mydriasis
B. Constipation
C. Overflow incontinence
D. Sialorrhea
E. Near vision impairment

Difficulty level: Medium

20. A 63-year-old woman underwent a total hysterectomy to remove a uterine leiomyoma. General anesthesia was induced with thiopental sodium, maintained with halothane and nitrous oxide, and supplemented with tubocurarine. Which of the following drugs did the patient most likely receive after the operation to reverse the skeletal muscle paralysis?

A. Physostigmine
B. Edrophonium
C. Neostigmine
D. Bethanechol
E. Pralidoxime

Difficulty level: Medium

21. A 74-year-old man with a long history of type 2 diabetes complained to his physician of difficult urination. Further examination led to the diagnosis of a disorder, and treatment with bethanechol improved the symptoms. Which of the following was most likely the patient's disorder?

A. Prostatic hyperplasia
B. Impaired diuresis
C. Detrusor hyperreflexia
D. Neurogenic atony of the bladder
E. Urinary tract infection

Difficulty level: Medium

22. A 47-year-old man was admitted to the emergency department because of extreme muscle weakness, ptosis, diplopia, and difficulty in swallowing, speaking, and breathing. The man, recently diagnosed with severe myasthenia gravis, had been receiving neostigmine for the past 3 months. Which of the following responses to 2 mg of intravenous edrophonium would indicate a cholinergic crisis?

A. No fasciculations, increased muscle strength
B. Fasciculations, decreased muscle strength
C. No fasciculations, no change in muscle strength
D. No fasciculations, decreased muscle strength
E. Fasciculations, increased muscle strength

Difficulty level: Hard

23. A 60-year-old male patient presented for routine ophthalmic examination. Tonometry measured an intraocular pressure of 28 mm Hg in both eyes (normal 10–20 mm Hg). The patient had been suffering from complete atrioventricular

(AV) block for 2 years. The ophthalmologist prescribed appropriate eye drops. Which of the following drugs was most likely included in the treatment?

A. Timolol
B. Prazosin
C. Isoproterenol
D. Pilocarpine
E. Albuterol
F. Homatropine

Difficulty level: Medium

24. A 3-year-old boy was rushed to the emergency department with mental confusion, restlessness, incoherence, and hallucinatory behavior. His mother stated that the child had eaten several black berries of a wild plant while playing with friends in the woods. Physical examination revealed mydriasis; dry, hot, and scarlet skin; and a distended abdomen with no bowel sounds. Vital signs were temperature 104.5°F (40.3°C), heart rate 145 bpm, blood pressure 105/60 mm Hg. Which of the following drugs would antagonize most of the symptoms exhibited by the patient?

A. Neostigmine
B. Albuterol
C. Physostigmine
D. Epinephrine
E. Prazosin
F. Phenylephrine

Difficulty level: Medium

25. A high dose of nicotine was administered intravenously to dogs in a laboratory experiment. An initial increase in blood pressure was soon followed by a profound decrease of blood pressure. Which of the following molecular mechanisms most likely mediated the decrease in blood pressure?

A. Long-lasting activation of nicotinic neuronal receptors
B. Long-lasting blockade of muscarinic M_2 receptors
C. Long-lasting blockade of muscarinic M_1 receptors
D. Prevention of acetylcholine release from presynaptic terminals
E. Prevention of catecholamine release from chromaffin cells

Difficulty level: Easy

26. A 55-year-old woman presented to a clinic because of a gradual onset of a scratchy sensation on both eyes and extreme dryness of the mouth and lips. Lab tests showed elevated levels of antibodies against gamma globulin. A diagnosis of Sjögren syndrome was made, and a drug was prescribed to relieve the patient's xerostomia. Which of the following drugs was most likely administered?

A. Acetylcholine
B. Phenylephrine
C. Prazosin
D. Donepezil
E. Pilocarpine

Difficulty level: Hard

27. A 59-year-old man underwent surgery to remove a colon carcinoma. Three days after surgery, he developed fever (103°F, 39.4°C), abdominal distention, and vomiting. Palpation showed tenderness over the entire abdomen, and auscultation revealed no bowel sounds. Which of the following therapeutic measures would be absolutely contraindicated in this case?

A. Parenteral administration of an antipyretic
B. Nasogastric intubation and suction
C. Parenteral antibiotic therapy
D. Subcutaneous administration of neostigmine
E. Intravenous administration of fluid and electrolytes

Difficulty level: Medium

28. A 6-year-old boy, on vacation with his parents in Mexico, was brought unconscious to the emergency department. His parents reported that the boy had eaten an apple bought from a local vendor 2 hours earlier. Physical examination showed that the boy was salivating profusely and was incontinent with regard to both urine and feces. He had pinpoint pupils, moist skin, and shallow respiration. A diagnosis was made, and two appropriate drugs were administered intravenously. Which of the following pairs of drugs were most likely given?

A. Physostigmine and atropine
B. Physostigmine and pralidoxime
C. Physostigmine and propranolol
D. Pralidoxime and propranolol
E. Atropine and propranolol
F. Atropine and pralidoxime

Difficulty level: Easy

29. A 13-year-old boy started smoking his first cigarette. Which of the following effects was most likely elicited by nicotine soon after smoking?

A. Bronchodilation
B. Dilation of the skin and splanchnic vessels
C. Increased epinephrine secretion from the adrenal medulla
D. Inhibition of gastrointestinal secretions
E. Relaxation of the detrusor muscle

Difficulty level: Easy

30. A 12-year-old girl started smoking her first cigarette. A few minutes later, she had two episodes of nausea and vomiting. Activation of receptors located in which of the following sites most likely mediated this adverse effect of nicotine?

A. Sympathetic ganglia
B. Chemoreceptor trigger zone
C. Locus ceruleus
D. Adrenal medulla
E. Vestibular nuclei

Questions: II-5 Anticholinergic Drugs

Directions for questions **1–5**

Match each antimuscarinic or ganglionic drug with the appropriate description (each lettered option can be selected once, more than once, or not at all).

A. Atropine
B. Benztropine
C. Darifenacin
D. Glycopyrrolate
E. Homatropine
F. Ipratropium
G. Mecamylamine
H. Scopolamine

Difficulty level: Easy

1. This drug is currently used in bronchospastic disorders.

Difficulty level: Easy

2. This drug almost exclusively blocks muscarinic M_3 receptors.

Difficulty level: Easy

3. This drug is mainly used in parkinsonism.

Difficulty level: Easy

4. This drug can block only nicotinic neuronal receptors.

Difficulty level: Easy

5. This drug is used almost exclusively to diagnose or treat eye disorders.

Difficulty level: Medium

6. A 25-year-old man experienced severe motion sickness whenever he traveled by air or sea. He felt much better after using a transdermal patch to apply a drug before traveling. Blockade of which of the following receptors most likely mediated the therapeutic effect of the drug in the patient's disorder?

A. H_1 histaminergic
B. β_2 adrenergic
C. D_2 dopaminergic
D. 5-HT_3 serotoninergic
E. M_1 cholinergic
F. Nn cholinergic

Difficulty level: Medium

7. A 33-year-old woman suffering from irritable bowel syndrome was prescribed glycopyrrolate. Blockade of which of the following pairs of receptors most likely mediated the therapeutic effect of the drug in the patient's disease?

A. β_2 and Nm
B. M_2 and Nn
C. M_3 and Nn
D. α_1 and M_2
E. M_1 and M_3

Difficulty level: Hard

8. A 62-year-old woman who was on vacation in Guatemala presented to the local hospital with nausea, vomiting, and profuse, watery diarrhea. The symptoms had appeared after eating raw oysters. She was prescribed atropine, which relieved her diarrhea. Which of the following molecular actions most likely mediated the therapeutic effect of atropine in the patient's disorder?

A. Inhibition of histamine secretion by gastric cells
B. Decreased cytosolic Ca^{2+} in smooth muscle cells
C. Opening of Na^+ channels in smooth muscle cells
D. Increased firing discharge of the vagus nerve
E. Activation of presynaptic cholinergic autoreceptors

Difficulty level: Hard

9. A 42-year old man was hospitalized with the admitting diagnosis of myocardial infarction. Vital signs were blood pressure 100/60 mm Hg, heart rate 40 bpm, respirations 12/min. The bradycardia disappeared after an intramuscular injection of atropine. The increased heart rate was most likely due to counteraction by atropine of which of the following acetylcholine-induced actions?

A. Release of nitric oxide
B. Opening of K^+ channels in sinoatrial node
C. Decrease in cardiac contractility
D. Opening of Na^+ channels in ganglionic neurons
E. Activation of cardiac presynaptic autoreceptors

Difficulty level: Medium

10. A 5-year-old girl who was on vacation in Venezuela with her parents was admitted to the local hospital with fever (103.7°F, 39.8°C), mental confusion, restlessness, and hallucinatory behavior. History revealed that the girl had eaten some honey bought from a local vendor. Physical examination revealed mydriasis; dry, hot, and red skin; and a distended abdomen. A diagnosis of atropine poisoning was made, and an appropriate therapy was started. Which of the following molecular actions most likely contributed to the atropine-induced hyperthermia in this patient?

A. Skin vasoconstriction
B. Blockade of prostaglandin synthesis in the hypothalamus
C. Uncoupling of oxidative phosphorylation in skeletal muscle
D. Blockade of muscarinic receptors in the hypothalamus
E. Blockade of muscarinic receptors of sweat glands

Difficulty level: Medium

11. A 54-year-old man, recently diagnosed with chronic obstructive pulmonary disease, started a therapy with ipratropium bromide using a metered-dose inhaler. Which of the following statements best explains why drugs from the ipratropium class are the only antimuscarinic drugs used to treat bronchospastic disorders?

A. They are more potent than other antimuscarinic drugs.
B. They have an oral bioavailability higher than that of other antimuscarinic drugs.
C. They have excellent inhalatory bioavailability.
D. They have negligible effects on bronchial secretions and mucociliary clearance.
E. They have negligible effects on the central nervous system.

Difficulty level: Medium

12. A 25-year-old man went to his ophthalmologist's office for a routine visit. He received one drop of homatropine in the conjunctival sac to prepare the eye for examination. Which of the following sets of effects did the drug most likely cause in the patient's eye, a few minutes after the administration?

	Pupillary Diameter	Lens Curvature	Intraocular Pressure
A	+	−	−
B	+	0	
C	0	−	0
D	−	0	−
E	+	−	+

+ = increased
− = decreased
0 = negligible effect

Difficulty level: Medium

13. A 77-year-old woman was found to have elevated intraocular pressure during a routine eye examination. History indicated that she had recently been taking several antimuscarinic medications to treat her bladder hyperreflexia. The ophthalmologist told her that he believed the increased intraocular pressure was an adverse effect of those medications. Which of the following ocular actions most likely mediated this adverse effect?

A. Relaxation of the ciliary muscle
B. Increased aqueous humor production
C. Dilation of ciliary body vessels
D. Relaxation of the radial muscle of the iris
E. Decreased episcleral aqueous humor outflow
F. Relaxation of the tarsal muscle

Difficulty level: Easy

14. An 85-year-old male resident of a nursing facility complained of frequent urinary urges that often resulted in urine leakage. Darifenacin was prescribed to manage the patient's incontinence. Which of the following actions most likely mediate the therapeutic effect of the drug?

A. Decreased bladder internal sphincter tone
B. Relaxation of the prostate capsule
C. Contraction of the detrusor muscle
D. Decreased diuresis
E. Increased compliance of the bladder

Difficulty level: Medium

15. A 77-year-old man suffering from chronic obstructive pulmonary disease had been taking ipratropium by inhalation. Shortly after inadvertently spraying the medication on his face, which of the following effects did the patient most likely experience?

A. Urge incontinence
B. Drowsiness
C. Salivation
D. Atrioventricular (AV) block
E. Difficulty in near vision
F. Hallucinations

Difficulty level: Medium

16. An 8-year-old boy was in an ophthalmologist's office for the first time and received ophthalmic drops of a drug to prepare his eyes for measurement of refractive errors. A half hour later, he showed mental confusion, restlessness, incoherence, and hallucinatory behavior. His pulse rate was 120 bpm. Which of the following drugs most likely caused the patient's adverse effects?

    A. Phenylephrine
    B. Epinephrine
    C. Atropine
    D. Timolol
    E. Pilocarpine

Difficulty level: Hard

17. A 73-year-old man with atrial fibrillation presented to the clinic because of dizziness, palpitations, dyspnea, and an urgent need to urinate. The man was on vacation in Mexico, and the symptoms started 1 hour after taking an over-the-counter preparation bought at a local pharmacy to treat diarrhea. Which of the following drugs most likely caused the patient's symptoms?

    A. Phenylephrine
    B. Epinephrine
    C. Atropine
    D. Propranolol
    E. Albuterol

Difficulty level: Hard

18. A 23-year-old man was admitted to the emergency department with palpitations, restlessness, and hallucinatory behavior. He admitted that he was a heroin addict and that 1 hour earlier, he had self-injected his usual dose of "smack," bought from a new vendor. Physical examination showed a distressed man with the following signs:

    Blood pressure: 160/80 mm Hg

    Pulse 135

    Pupils: dilated

    Skin: hot and dry

    Bowel sounds: decreased

    Which of the following drugs most likely caused the patient's signs and symptoms?

    A. Nicotine
    B. Bethanechol
    C. Scopolamine
    D. Pralidoxime
    E. Neostigmine

Difficulty level: Medium

19. A 67-year-old man recently diagnosed with benign prostatic hyperplasia was scheduled for surgery. Which of the following drug classes would be absolutely contraindicated in this patient?

    A. Alpha-1 blockers
    B. Antimuscarinics
    C. Beta blockers
    D. Alpha-2 agonists
    E. Beta-1 agonists

Difficulty level: Medium

20. A 55-year-old woman was admitted to the hospital with shallow breathing, wheezing, profuse rhinorrhea, lacrimation, ocular pain, and diminished vision. She reported that the symptoms started when she was in her garden spraying flowers with an insecticide containing carbaryl, a reversible cholinesterase inhibitor. Which of the following drugs would be appropriate to treat this patient's disorder?

    A. Pralidoxime
    B. Terbutaline
    C. Epinephrine
    D. Glycopyrrolate
    E. Atropine

Difficulty level: Easy

21. A 64-year-old man complained to his physician of a recent onset of diarrhea. The physician believed the diarrhea was related to aspirin and misoprostol that the patient had started taking 1 week earlier for the treatment of joint pain due to osteoarthritis. Which of the following drugs would be most appropriate to treat the patient's diarrhea?

    A. Phenylephrine
    B. Ipratropium
    C. Propranolol
    D. Glycopyrrolate
    E. Prazosin
    F. Donepezil

Difficulty level: Easy

22. A 63-year-old man underwent surgery to remove a laryngeal carcinoma. Before surgery, the anesthesiologist administered a drug intramuscularly to decrease bronchial secretions and to prevent bradycardia due to manipulation of the vagus nerve. Which of the following drugs would be most appropriate in this situation?

    A. Ipratropium
    B. Dopamine
    C. Atropine
    D. Isoproterenol
    E. Epinephrine

Difficulty level: Hard

23. A 44-year-old man collapsed at work and was found to be unresponsive. When the paramedics arrived, he had ventricular fibrillation and was cardioverted successfully. He was admitted to the coronary unit, but shortly thereafter he developed asystole. Cardiopulmonary resuscitation was started, and escalating doses of epinephrine were given without success. Which of the following drugs would be most appropriately administered at this point?

   A. Neostigmine
   B. Norepinephrine
   C. Dopamine
   D. Atropine
   E. Ipratropium

Difficulty level: Medium

24. In a laboratory experiment, a mecamylamine pretreatment was given intramuscularly to several dogs. One hour later, each dog received an autonomic drug, and the effect of that drug was recorded. Which of the following expected drug-induced effects was most likely best counteracted by mecamylamine pretreatment?

   A. Neostigmine-induced increase in intestinal peristalsis
   B. Nicotine-induced contraction of skeletal muscle
   C. Norepinephrine-induced bradycardia
   D. Epinephrine-induced tachycardia
   E. Propranolol-induced hypotension

Difficulty level: Easy

25. A 43-year-old man came to the hospital for a radiologic examination of the colon. Before starting the exam, he received an intramuscular injection of scopolamine to relax the intestine. Which of the following adverse effects did the patient most likely experience a few minutes after the administration?

   A. Salivation
   B. Abdominal pain
   C. Palpitations
   D. Painful erection
   E. Urge urinary incontinence

Difficulty level: Easy

26. Atropine was given intramuscularly to several dogs during a lab experiment. One hour later each dog received an intramuscular injection of an autonomic drug, and the effects of that drug were recorded. Which of the following expected drug-induced effects was most likely best antagonized by atropine pretreatment?

   A. Physostigmine-induced sweating
   B. Epinephrine-induced hypertension
   C. Nicotine-induced skin vasoconstriction
   D. Prazosin-induced reflex tachycardia
   E. Glycopyrrolate-induced bronchodilation

Difficulty level: Easy

27. A 23-year-old man complained to his physician of photophobia and difficulty in reading the newspaper. A few days earlier, the man had started using a nasal spray of ipratropium to manage profuse rhinorrhea associated with a cold. Which of the following molecular actions most likely mediated the adverse effects of the drug?

   A. Blockade of M_3 muscarinic receptors
   B. Activation of M_3 muscarinic receptors
   C. Blockade of β_2 adrenoceptors
   D. Activation of β_2 adrenoceptors
   E. Blockade of α_1 adrenoceptors
   F. Activation of α_1 adrenoceptors

Difficulty level: Easy

28. A 55-year-old man was admitted to the coronary unit following a myocardial infarction. Four hours after admission, the electrocardiogram indicated bradycardia that disappeared after an intramuscular injection of atropine. Which of the following actions most likely mediated the therapeutic effect of atropine in the patient's disorder?

   A. Dilation of capacitance vessels
   B. Increased heart contractility
   C. Decreased blood pressure
   D. Increased atrioventricular (AV) conduction
   E. Constriction of resistance vessels
   F. Increased heart refractoriness

Difficulty level: Medium

29. A 25-year-old woman complained to her physician of excessive axillary sweating and a sweaty forehead, primarily when she was anxious or excited. The woman stated that the symptom were very disturbing and asked for a treatment. The physician prescribed glycopyrrolate cream, to apply to the affected areas. Blockade of which of the following receptors most likely mediated the therapeutic effect of the drug in the patient's disorder?

   A. β_2 adrenergic
   B. Nn cholinergic
   C. D_1 dopaminergic
   D. α_2 adrenergic
   E. M_3 muscarinic

Difficulty level: Easy

30. In a clinical experimental setting, a 33-year-old healthy man received an intramuscular injection of a ganglionic blocker with a fast onset of action. A few minutes after the injection, which of the following heart rates, in beats per minute (bpm), was most likely observed in the man?

A. 70
B. 50
C. 100
D. 130
E. 150

Answers and Explanations: II-1 Introduction to Autonomic Pharmacology

Questions 1–5

1. **A**
2. **D**
3. **F**
4. **A**
5. **H**

Learning objective: Describe the metabolism of catecholamines.

6. **A** Dopamine β-hydroxylase is the enzyme that catalyzes the conversion of dopamine into norepinephrine. Because the enzyme is lacking, plasma levels of norepinephrine will be very low.

B Plasma levels of dopamine would be high, not low.

C Epinephrine is synthesized from norepinephrine in the adrenal medulla. Because plasma levels of norepinephrine are low, plasma levels of epinephrine will also be low, not high.

D Normetanephrine is a urinary metabolite of norepinephrine. Because plasma levels of norepinephrine are low, normetanephrine will also be low, not high.

E Homovanillic acid is the main urinary metabolite of dopamine. Because plasma levels of dopamine are high, homovanillic acid will also be high, not low.

Learning objective: Identify the enzyme that controls the rate-limiting step in norepinephrine biosynthesis.

7. **C** The hydroxylation of tyrosine to dopa is the rate-limiting step in norepinephrine biosynthesis and is catalyzed by the enzyme tyrosine hydroxylase. The inhibition of this enzyme will therefore cause a big reduction in biosynthesis of the final product.

A Aromatic L-amino acid decarboxylase transforms dopa into dopamine.

B Dopamine-β-hydroxylase transforms dopamine into norepinephrine.

D Phenylethanolamine methyltransferase transforms norepinephrine into epinephrine.

E Monoamine oxidase transforms norepinephrine and epinephrine into dihydroxymandelic acid and dopamine into dihydroxyphenylacetic acid.

Learning objective: Explain the autonomic activation that follows hypoglycemia.

8. **D** The described symptoms are most likely due to sympathetic activation that occurs any time significant hypoglycemia is present. In insulin-dependent diabetics, hypoglycemia is common after physical exercise that increases sugar metabolism, as in the present case. Sympathetic activation includes an increased firing of preganglionic sympathetic neurons, which in turn will increase firing in postganglionic sympathetic neurons and epinephrine secretion from the adrenal medulla.

A–C, E These neurons are not involved in sympathetic activation.

Learning objective: Identify the vessels where autonomic receptors are primarily α_1 adrenergic.

9. **E** The vascular system has both α_1 and β_2 receptors. Alpha-1 receptors predominate in the vessels of the skin and the gastrointestinal and genitourinary systems. Beta-2 receptors predominate in the vessels of skeletal muscle and liver. Parasympathetic receptors are not widely represented in the vascular system.

A Autonomic receptors in the bronchial muscle are primarily M_3 and β_2.

B Autonomic receptors in the sphincter muscle of the iris are primarily M_3.

C Autonomic receptors in the atrioventricular node are primarily M_2 and β_1.

D Autonomic receptors in Purkinje fibers are primarily β_1.

Learning objective: Describe the effects of the activation of peripheral postsynaptic β_1 receptors.

10. **D** Beta-1 receptors are abundant in juxtaglomerular cells, and the activation of these receptors increases renin secretion.

A Bronchodilation is due mainly to activation of bronchial β_2 receptors.

B Uterine relaxation is due mainly to activation of uterine β_2 receptors.

C Increased liver gluconeogenesis is due mainly to activation of liver β_2 receptors.

E Decreased insulin secretion is due mainly to activation of pancreas α_2 receptors.

F Increased sweating of the palms of the hands is due mainly to activation of the palms' α_1 receptors.

Learning objective: Describe the effects of the activation of pancreatic α_2 receptors.

11. **B** Activation of α_2 receptors located on pancreatic β cells inhibits insulin secretion. This is one of the actions that contribute to the final hyperglycemic effect of epinephrine.

A, D These effects are due to activation of α_1, not α_2, receptors.

C, E These effects are due to activation of β_1 receptors.

F This effect is due to activation of β_2 receptors.

Learning objective: Describe the effects of the activation of α_1 and α_2 receptors on the eye.

12. **A** Pupillary diameter can be increased either by the activation of α_1 receptors (which contracts the radial muscle of the iris) or by the blockade of M_3 receptors (which relaxes the sphincter muscle of the iris). The question asks for an activation of a receptor, so the α_1 receptor must be involved. Intraocular pressure can be decreased by a decreased production or by an increased outflow of aqueous humor. A decreased production can follow either the activation of α_2 receptors or the blockade of β_2 receptors. The question asks for an activation of a receptor, so the α_2 receptor must be involved.

B Beta-2 receptor activation would cause an increased production of aqueous humor and therefore would increase, not decrease, the intraocular pressure.

C Activation of Nn receptors would cause an increase in sympathetic as well as parasympathetic firing. Because in the eye the parasympathetic system is predominant, this would lead to an activation of M_3 receptors in the ciliary muscle, which would increase the lens curvature and an activation of the iris sphincter muscle, which would decrease, not increase, the pupillary diameter. Activation of Nm receptors causes the contraction of skeletal muscles only and therefore can affect the extrinsic, not the intrinsic, eye muscles.

D See answer explanation for item C.

E See answer explanation for item B.

Learning objective: Describe the effects of activation of α_1 receptors of the cardiovascular system.

13. **A** Activation of α_1 receptors contracts vascular smooth muscle. This will increase the systolic blood pressure (which is dependent on both cardiac output and total peripheral resistance [TPR]), as well as diastolic blood pressure (which is dependent mainly on TPR). The increase in mean blood pressure causes an activation of the baroreceptor reflex, which in turn will decrease the heart rate.

B Activation of β_2 receptors would cause a decrease, not an increase, of TPR, because β_2 receptors are abundant in skeletal muscle vessels, and approximately one half of the body weight is skeletal muscle.

C Activation of D_1 receptors would cause a dilation of splanchnic and renal vessels; therefore, the diastolic blood pressure would decrease, not increase.

D Activation of M_2 receptors would decrease the heart contractility and rate, which in turn would decrease cardiac output. Therefore, the systolic blood pressure would decrease, not increase.

E Activation of β_1 receptors would increase, not decrease, the heart rate.

Learning objective: Describe the postreceptor mechanisms of α_1 receptor activation.

14. **B** Alpha-1 receptor activation may initiate several postreceptor mechanisms, depending on the tissue where the receptors are located. Among these, one of the most common is the activation of phospholipase C, which in turn results in the generation of two second messengers, IP_3 and DAG. IP_3 stimulates the release of calcium from endoplasmic stores. DAG is a potent activator of protein kinase C, which in turn increases intracellular Ca^{2+}. The final effect is therefore increased Ca^{2+} availability, which enhances smooth muscle contraction.

A The synthesis of IP_3 and DAG is actually increased, not decreased, by α_1 receptor activation (see correct answer explanation).

C Alpha-1 receptors are mainly excitatory, so the opening of K^+ channels (which would lead to a hyperpolarization of the membrane) is unlikely. In fact, they can close K^+ channels.

D Blockade of voltage-gated Ca^{2+} channels is the mechanism of action of Ca^{2+} channel blockers

E Increased synthesis of cGMP is the postreceptor mechanism triggered by beta-, not by alpha-, receptor activation.

Learning objective: Describe the effects of activation of β_1 and β_2 receptors

15. **E** The activation of β_1 receptors increases cardiac contractility and rate, thus increasing cardiac output, which in turn increases systolic blood pressure. The activation of β_2 receptors causes peripheral vasodilation, thus decreasing the diastolic blood pressure. The mean blood pressure (diastolic plus one third of pulse pressure [the difference between the systolic and diastolic pressure readings]) of the volunteer was 90 mm Hg under control conditions and 80 mm Hg after the drug administration. The decreased blood pressure activated the baroreceptor reflex, causing reflex tachycardia. Moreover, the activation of both β_1 and β_2 receptors also caused a direct increase in heart rate, so the final effect was a pronounced tachycardia.

    A–D Activation of none of these pairs of receptors can explain the cardiovascular actions of the autonomic drug under study.

Learning objective: Identify the autonomic receptors that mediate the relaxation of bronchial smooth muscle.

16. **A** Alpha-beta agonists induce relaxation of most smooth muscles both directly, by activating postsynaptic β_2 receptors, and indirectly, by activating presynaptic α_2 receptors on cholinergic terminals, which in turn inhibit acetylcholine release.

    B–E See correct answer explanation.

Learning objective: Describe the effect of the activation of β_2 and β_3 receptors.

17. **B** Activation of β_2 receptors increases liver gluconeogenesis, inhibits degranulation of mast cells, and decreases plasma K^+ (because of increased K^+ uptake by skeletal muscle). Activation of β_3 receptors in fat cells increases lipolysis with enhanced release of free fatty acids into the blood.

    C Beta-1 receptor activation is not involved, as the secretion of renin is unaffected.

    A, D–F These pairs of receptors can mediate some, but not all, of the effects listed.

Learning objective: Describe the effects of the activation of M_3 receptors on the eye.

18. **D** Pupillary diameter and lens curvature are mainly under the control of the parasympathetic nervous system. Activation of M_3 receptors on the iris sphincter muscle causes contraction of the muscle, decreasing pupillary diameter. Activation of M_3 receptors on ciliary muscle causes contraction of the muscle, which leads to (1) relaxation of the zonula fibers, which in turn increases the lens curvature, and (2) opening the pores of the trabecular meshwork, which increases the outflow of the aqueous humor, decreasing the intraocular pressure.

    A Activation of α_1 receptors would contract the iris radial muscle, causing an increase, not a decrease, in pupillary diameter.

    B Activation of α_2 receptors would decrease the production of the aqueous humor. This would lead to a decrease in intraocular pressure, but pupil diameter and lens curvature would not be affected.

    C Activation of Nm receptors would cause the contraction of skeletal muscles only and therefore would affect the extrinsic, not the intrinsic, eye muscles.

    E Activation of β_2 receptors would cause relaxation, not contraction, of ciliary muscle.

Learning objective: Describe the effects of activation of M_2 and M_3 receptors.

19. **C** The new drug the woman was taking was most likely amitriptyline, an antidepressant medication with pronounced antimuscarinic effects. Palpitations are due to blockade of M_2 receptors, whereas dry mouth, blurred vision, and constipation are due to blockade of M_3 receptors.

    A, B, D, E Blockade of these pairs of receptors would not cause the symptoms reported by the patient.

Learning objective: Describe the effects of activation of nicotinic Nm receptors.

20. **E** Nm receptors are found only in the motor end plate; therefore, the symptoms must refer to skeletal muscles. When Nm receptors are activated by acetylcholine, the ion channel opens, allowing Na^+ to enter the cell. The end-plate membrane becomes depolarized; this depolarization is called end-plate potential. If its amplitude reaches the threshold for excitation, voltage-gated Na^+ channels open, generating

an action potential that propagates the depolarization and causes the contraction of the skeletal muscle. The end-plate depolarization is short-lasting, as acetylcholine is rapidly metabolized. However, when an excessive amount of acetylcholine causes a persistent activation of Nm receptors, a loss of electrical excitability of the muscle cells occurs. The main reason for this loss is that, even if the membrane is still depolarized because of the activation of Nm receptors, voltage-sensitive Na^+ channels become inactivated and therefore not able to open in response to a brief depolarizing stimulus. This loss of electrical excitability in the presence of a depolarized membrane is called depolarization blockade. The main consequence of this block in skeletal muscle cells is the paralysis of the muscle. It should be noted that this paralysis

is not due to the blockade of Nm receptors but to the persistent activation of those receptors. When the paralysis involves the extrinsic muscles of the eye, diplopia results. The paralysis of the striated muscles of the pharynx causes difficulty in swallowing.

A–D All of these effects are due to the activation of muscarinic receptors.

INTRODUCTION TO AUTONOMIC PHARMACOLOGY Answer key							
1.	A	6.	A	11.	B	16.	A
2.	D	7.	C	12.	A	17.	B
3.	F	8.	D	13.	A	18.	D
4.	A	9.	E	14.	B	19.	C
5.	H	10.	D	15.	E	20.	E

Answers and Explanations: II-2 Adrenergic Drugs

Questions 1–5

1. **B**
2. **L**
3. **I**
4. **H**
5. **K**

Learning objective: Describe the postreceptor mechanism that mediates the therapeutic effect of epinephrine in cardiac arrest.

6. **E** Epinephrine effects on the heart are due to the activation of β_1 and β_2 receptors. The postreceptor mechanism common to all β receptor activation is the stimulation of adenylyl cyclase, which in turn increases the amount of cyclic adenosine monophosphate (cAMP) in target tissues.

  A This postreceptor mechanism is triggered by the activation of M_2 receptors.

  B This postreceptor mechanism is triggered by the activation of nicotinic receptors.

  C This postreceptor mechanism is triggered by the activation α_1 and M_3 receptors.

  D This postreceptor mechanism is triggered by the activation of α_1 receptors.

Learning objective: Describe the actions that mediate the therapeutic effect of epinephrine in allergic reactions.

7. **E** The symptoms and signs of the patient suggest that he had an acute anaphylactic reaction, which sometimes occurs following a blood transfusion. One of the useful actions of epinephrine in this disorder is the β_2 receptor–mediated inhibition of degranulation of mast cells, which prevents the release of histamine and other inflammatory mediators.

  A–D, F All these actions of epinephrine contribute little, if any, to the therapeutic efficacy of the drug in anaphylaxis.

Learning objective: Identify the adrenoceptors that mediate the effect of epinephrine to increase the duration of the local anesthetic effect of lidocaine when the two drugs are given concomitantly.

8. **D** Epinephrine is often used together with local anesthetics to prolong the action of the anesthetic. This increased duration is due to the epinephrine-induced vasoconstriction (mediated by α_1 receptor activation), which localizes the anesthetic at the desired site, thus slowing down its systemic distribution.

  A–C, E See correct answer explanation.

Learning objective: Explain the action that mediates the therapeutic effect of epinephrine in cardiac arrest.

9. **A** The most appropriate management of cardiac arrest induced by ventricular fibrillation is a 200-joule defibrillation. Additional shocks at higher energy should be given in case of initial failure. If ventricular fibrillation persists, the American Heart Association indicates that epinephrine should be administered. Most likely the two major mechanisms through which epinephrine increases blood flow to the brain and heart during CPR are the following:

- It prevents carotid arterial collapse at the thoracic inlet. Collapse results from high extravascular intrathoracic pressure coupled with low intravascular pressure and loss of arteriolar tone. By constricting arterial vessels (an α_1 action) and by increasing venous return, epinephrine increases the aortic diastolic pressure during closed chest compression.
- Preferential reduction of blood flow to the renal and splanchnic beds, due to α_1 receptor action, facilitates the distribution of the limited cardiac output to the cerebral and coronary circulation during external cardiac massage. Because cerebral blood vessels are relatively insensitive to the vasoconstricting effect of α agonists, perfusion of the brain is increased.

It seems, therefore, that the main beneficial effects of epinephrine in cardiac arrest are related to its α_1 receptor activation.

It is worthwhile to note that, unlike what happens under normal conditions, epinephrine increases total peripheral resistance in people with cardiac arrest. During cardiac arrest, there is a complete loss of arteriolar tone; therefore, β_2-mediated vasodilation cannot occur, whereas the α_1-mediated vasoconstriction is still operative.

Additional beneficial effects of epinephrine that are primarily related to β_1 receptor activation are changing a fine ventricular fibrillation into a coarse one, which is more susceptible to electrical defibrillation, and stimulating spontaneous ventricular contraction in case of asystole.

Because the benefits of epinephrine are mainly due to α_1-mediated vasoconstriction, norepinephrine could also be used. In fact a large preclinical trial failed to identify any difference in survival following treatment with norepinephrine or standard doses of epinephrine. Other vasoconstricting agents have been evaluated. Recently, vasopressin has been tested, with promising results.

The fact that epinephrine is still the agent of choice in cardiac arrest is likely related to the long experience achieved with this drug, as well as to the additional benefits listed above. For example, epinephrine activates both β_1 and β_2 receptors; therefore, it is likely more effective than norepinephrine in stimulating spontaneous contraction of the heart during asystole.

B The β_2 receptor–mediated vasodilation would be counterproductive, but it does not occur in cardiac arrest (see correct answer explanation).

C This action of the drug could add a benefit (see correct answer explanation), but it is mainly related to β_1 receptor activation (the increase in cardiac contractility due to β_2 receptor activation is minor). In any case, the main epinephrine mechanism is most likely the α_1 receptor–mediated vasoconstriction.

D, E The beneficial effects of epinephrine-induced increase in renin secretion and of epinephrine-induced bronchodilation are, at the most, only marginal.

Learning objective: Describe the direct and indirect mechanisms of action of dopamine.

10. **A** Dopamine is a mixed-acting adrenergic drug that can directly activate α, β, and dopamine receptors. It can also increase the release of norepinephrine from adrenergic terminals.

B–E All of these drugs are adrenergic agonists (i.e., direct-acting adrenergic agents).

Learning objective: Describe the cardiovascular effects of norepinephrine.

11. **D** The investigational drug causes a parallel increase in both systolic and diastolic pressure and a concomitant decrease in heart rate. This pattern suggests that the decrease in heart rate is due to a reflex vagal discharge. Drugs that cause this effect must be vasoconstricting agents (e.g., norepinephrine and phenylephrine) devoid of vasodilating activity. In this case, however, stroke volume is substantially increased (stroke volume = cardiac output/heart rate, 78.6–100 mL). Phenylephrine would increase the stroke volume only slightly (if venous constriction causes an increase in venous return) or not at all, as it has no β-adrenergic activity. Moreover the ejection fraction is increased, which confirms that the drug does increase cardiac contractility. (The ejection fraction is the ratio of the stroke volume to the end diastolic volume. Remember that the only way to increase the ejection fraction is to increase cardiac contractility).

A–C Dobutamine, epinephrine, and isoproterenol would increase, not decrease, the cardiac output of the heart.

E See correct answer explanation.

F Propranolol would decrease, not increase, the ejection fraction of the heart.

Learning objective: Describe the cardiac adverse effects of epinephrine in patients at risk.

12. **D** Epinephrine can cause several cardiovascular adverse effects, including angina, hypertension, and cardiac arrhythmias, and is therefore contraindicated in patients at risk.

Because the patient had an episode of ventricular fibrillation, he was at high risk of ventricular arrhythmias.

A–C, E These are adverse effects of epinephrine but are less likely in this patient because he did not have specific risk factors for these effects.

Learning objective: Relate the therapeutic efficacy of epinephrine to its mechanism of action.

13. **C** The symptoms and signs of the patient indicate that he was most likely suffering from an acute anaphylactic reaction to the injected local anesthetic. The strong bronchoconstriction of an anaphylactic reaction is known to be caused by both histamine and leukotrienes, but today leukotrienes (once known as the slow-reacting substance of anaphylaxis) are thought to be the main bronchoconstricting agents. Epinephrine, a first-line agent for anaphylaxis, works as a functional antagonist of the mediators of the disorder. It counteracts the histamine-mediated vasodilation by activating α_1 receptors and counteracts the leukotriene-mediated bronchoconstriction by activating β_2 receptors. Epinephrine also inhibits the release of mediators from basophils and mast cells by activating β_2 receptors.

A Histamine effects on the heart are weak and are mainly excitatory. Epinephrine would enhance, not antagonize, histamine effects on the heart.

B Bradykinin has generalized vasodilating activity. Epinephrine would enhance, not antagonize, bradykinins effect on skeletal muscle vessels by activating β_2 receptors.

D Alpha-1 receptors are not located in bronchial smooth muscles.

E Activation of β_2 receptors in bronchial vessels would cause vasodilation, which would be detrimental by diminishing the ventilation/perfusion ratio.

F Epinephrine activation of α_2 receptors on platelets promotes platelet aggregation, but this effect has negligible relevance in the therapy of anaphylaxis.

Learning objective: Describe the effect of phenylephrine given topically in the eye.

14. **A** Phenylephrine is a selective α_1 agonist frequently used to facilitate the examination of the retina. The drug causes mydriasis by contracting the radial muscle of the iris, which receives only sympathetic innervation. Because M_3, α_2, and β_2 receptors are not activated, lens curvature and intraocular pressure are not affected.

B–E Each of these drugs, given locally, would affect the intraocular pressure.

Learning objective: Describe the pharmacological actions of albuterol.

15. **E** Albuterol is a β_2-selective agonist. Activation of β_2 receptors in the respiratory tract increases mucociliary clearance, thus improving the flow of the coat of mucus toward the pharynx.

A–C Beta-2 receptor agonists actually decrease microvascular permeability, increase bronchial secretion, and prevent the release of histamine from mast cells. All these actions are useful in treating bronchospastic disorders.

D Residual respiratory volume is not significantly affected in normal individuals but is actually decreased in asthmatic patients.

Learning objective: Describe the cardiovascular effects of phenylephrine.

16. **E** The drug causes a parallel increase in both systolic and diastolic pressure and a concomitant decrease in heart rate. This pattern suggests that the decrease in heart rate is due to a reflex vagal discharge. Drugs that cause this effect must be vasoconstricting agents (e.g., norepinephrine and phenylephrine) devoid of vasodilating activity. In this case, however, the stroke volume has increased only slightly (stroke volume [SV] = cardiac output/heart rate; therefore, control SV = 5/70 = 71.4 mL; SV after drug = 4.5/58 = 77.6 mL), and the ejection fraction has not changed. Norepinephrine would substantially increase the stroke volume and the ejection fraction, as it has β-adrenergic activity (remember that the only way to increase the ejection fraction is to increase the contractility of the heart).

A–D See correct answer explanation.

Learning objective: Describe the main adverse effects of phenylephrine.

17. **B** Phenylephrine is used as a nasal decongestant both topically and orally even though its effectiveness is controversial. When taken orally, it can reach the general circulation and activate α_1 receptors of the internal sphincter of the bladder. This in turn leads to sphincter constriction, thus causing difficulty in voiding, especially in men suffering from prostatic hyperplasia, as in this case.

A, C–F These drug are not used as nasal decongestants.

Learning objective: Explain the reason for the therapeutic use of apraclonidine in glaucoma.

18. **E** Apraclonidine is a selective α_2 agonist that can decrease the production of aqueous humor by the ciliary epithelium. The aqueous humor of the eye is produced by the epithelial cells of the ciliary body and is under the control of α_2 and β receptors (mainly β_2) located on these cells. Activation of α_2 receptors decreases the production, whereas activation of β receptors increases the production.

A–D See correct answer explanation.

Learning objective: Explain the mechanism of the therapeutic effect of clonidine in alcohol withdrawal.

19. **A** Clonidine is often used to decrease the symptoms of sympathetic activation, which are prominent during withdrawal from many sedative drugs, including alcohol and opioids. Many of those symptoms are due to an increased firing from the locus ceruleus, a brain nucleus with a very high concentration of α receptors. By activating α_2 presynaptic receptors, clonidine decreases the central sympathetic outflow, antagonizing the increased firing of the locus ceruleus.

     B, D Clonidine activates peripheral adrenoceptors only when very high doses are given.

     C Clonidine increases, not decreases, central parasympathetic outflow.

     E, F Clonidine activates, not blocks, these receptors.

Learning objective: Describe the adverse effects of albuterol.

20. **B** Restlessness and anxiety are common adverse effects of β_2 adrenoceptor agonists. They occur in 10 to 20% of children receiving inhalatory therapy. This points out that β agonists are mainly excitatory drugs in the central nervous system. In fact, toxic doses usually cause convulsions.

     A Beta-2 receptor activation increases atrioventricular (AV) conduction, so AV block is unlikely.

     C Beta-2 receptor activation actually causes insomnia.

     D Hypotension can rarely occur with β_2 agonists, but postural hypotension is unlikely, as the baroreceptor reflex is not affected.

     E Arrhythmias can occur with β_2 agonists, but ventricular tachycardia is rare.

Learning objective: Describe the therapy of open-angle glaucoma in a patient with a concomitant disease.

21. **B** Epinephrine is sometimes used in open-angle glaucoma because it decreases aqueous humor production by activating α_2 receptors in the ciliary epithelium, and it also increases aqueous humor outflow through the uveoscleral route.

     A, C–E All of these drugs are effective in open-angle glaucoma but are contraindicated in this case because of severe asthma. In fact, even when given topically, β-blockers and cholinergic agonists can increase the risk of bronchospastic disorders from systemic absorption via the nasolacrimal system.

Learning objective: Describe the therapeutic uses of norepinephrine.

22. **C** The shock due to the spinal cord injury is vasodilatory (also called neurogenic or distributive shock), which occurs because the injured sympathetic nervous system fails to maintain the arteriolar tone. Drugs with α_1-adrenergic activity such as norepinephrine, phenylephrine, and dopamine are used to restore the arteriolar tone, thus counteracting the decreased blood pressure.

     A, B, D These drugs are devoid of α_1-adrenergic activity.

     E Salmeterol is an antiadrenergic drug.

Learning objective: Describe the cardiovascular effects of isoproterenol.

23. **C** The drug causes a substantial increase in heart rate, cardiac output, and ejection fraction and a concomitant decrease in mean blood pressure. An increase in ejection fraction indicates that the contractility of the heart is increased. The fact that mean blood pressure is decreased despite the increased cardiac output indicates that the drug must decrease total peripheral resistance (TPR). The two listed drugs that can decrease TPR are isoproterenol and albuterol. However, because albuterol is a selective β_2 agonist, it would have caused a decrease in TPR and a reflex increase in the heart rate, but the ejection fraction would have been minimally affected.

     A, B, D, E See correct answer explanation.

Learning objective: Describe the pharmacological actions of isoproterenol.

24. **A** Isoproterenol is often used in the operating room after heart transplant, because contractility and sinus node function of the new heart are temporarily impaired to varying degrees, based on the condition of the donor heart, quality of preservation, and so on. Isoproterenol is a nonselective β agonist (i.e., it activates all β receptors). Activation of β_1 receptors in the juxtaglomerular cells of the macula densa stimulates renin secretion.

     B Activation of β_2 receptors in the pancreas actually increases insulin release.

     C Activation of β_2 receptors in the vessels causes vasodilation, which in turn decreases, not increases, total peripheral resistance.

     D Isoproterenol causes tachycardia, which is, in a normal person, both direct (due to activation of cardiac β receptors) and reflex (due to drug-induced peripheral vasodilation). In this patient, however, the new heart is denervated, so reflex tachycardia cannot occur.

     E This effect is mediated by the activation of α_2 receptors. Isoproterenol has no activity on α receptors.

Learning objective: Describe the first therapeutic intervention for a patient with hypovolemic shock.

25. **D** The symptoms and signs of the patient indicate that he was most likely suffering from hypovolemic shock due to the extensive hemorrhage. The most important therapeutic intervention in hypovolemic shock is the infusion of

intravenous fluids. Crystalloids (isotonic solutions that contain either normal saline or saline equivalents) or colloid solutions (which contain large oncotically active molecules, e.g., albumin and carbohydrates) can be given. The choice between the two remains controversial, but normal isotonic saline is extensively used.

A Norepinephrine is used in neurogenic shock.

B Epinephrine is the first-line agent in anaphylactic shock.

C Dobutamine is used in cardiogenic shock.

E Dopamine is used in neurogenic and cardiogenic shock

F Isoproterenol is contraindicated in any type of shock.

Learning objective: Describe the postreceptor mechanism of drugs used to treat cardiogenic shock.

26. **C** The therapy of cardiogenic shock requires a rapid-acting inotropic drug to increase myocardial contractility and cardiac output. Dobutamine and dopamine are the two drugs most frequently used. In both cases, the therapeutic efficacy is mediated mainly by the direct (dobutamine) or indirect and direct (dopamine) activation of β_1 receptors, which in turn increase the synthesis of cAMP.

A, B, D–F See correct answer explanation.

Learning objective: Describe the cardiovascular effects of dobutamine.

27. **E** Dobutamine is a selective β agonist that activates mainly β_1 receptors. This should cause an increase of all the parameters of heart activity, but for unknown reasons, frequency and automaticity are increased only slightly. Affinity of dobutamine for α_1 and β_2 receptors is slight (high doses are needed); moreover, the consequences of this activation on the vessel caliber can balance each other. This can explain why there are no major changes or a decrease (when the β_2-mediated vasodilation overrides the α_1-mediated vasoconstriction) in total peripheral resistance.

A–D All of these drugs cause substantial changes in heart rate and systemic vascular resistance.

Learning objective: Describe the therapeutic uses of norepinephrine.

28. **C** The signs and symptoms of the patient strongly suggest the diagnosis of septic shock. Signs consistent with this diagnosis are the high fever, high WBC, hypotension, tachycardia, elevated cardiac output, and low systemic vascular resistance. Septic shock is a vasodilatory shock (vasodilation may be partly due to the vasodilatory effects of endotoxins or other chemical mediators). In this kind of shock, even if cardiac output is increased, it is inadequate to maintain a blood pressure that will perfuse the essential organs in the face of a decreased systemic peripheral resistance. In fact, the patient has metabolic acidosis, indicating anaerobic metabolism and lactic acidosis. Even if fluid administration is still the mainstay therapy in septic shock, recent evidence suggests that early aggressive vasopressor support may be the key to a positive outcome. Dopamine is frequently the initial pharmacological agent chosen for the treatment, but when the systemic vascular resistance is very low, as in this case, norepinephrine was found to be superior to dopamine.

A, B, D, E All of these drugs tend to decrease the systemic vascular resistance and are therefore not indicated in this case.

Learning objective: Explain the mechanism of action of antiasthmatic β agonists.

29. **C** According to the Expert Panel Report of the National Institutes of Health, all patients with asthma should receive a short-acting β_2 agonist on an "as needed" basis. Therefore, the most appropriate drug for this patient's inhaler would be a drug like albuterol.

B Activation of M_2 receptors in nonvascular smooth muscle can cause smooth muscle contraction. Therefore, blockade of M_2 receptors (with an anticholinergic drug, e.g., ipratropium) could cause a bronchodilating effect. However, anticholinergics are less effective than β_2 agonists in asthma, and the bronchoconstricting action of M_2 receptors is less effective than that of M_3 receptors.

A, D–F See correct answer explanation.

Learning objective: Describe the adverse effects of salmeterol.

30. **B** Beta-2 agonists administered by inhalation are first-line drugs for asthma. Tremor is the most frequent adverse effect of β_2 agonists (in up to 40% of patients). It likely occurs because β_2-receptor activation accelerates the sequestration of cytosolic Ca^{2+} (by opening Ca^{2+} channels in the sarcoplasmic reticulum of skeletal muscle) and increases discharge in muscle spindles. Anxiety is the second most frequent adverse effect of these drugs (in up to 20% of patients). Palpitations can occur in up to 10% of patients and are related to the cardiac effects of these drugs (β_2 specificity is never absolute; moreover, β_2-receptor activation also increases heart contractility and rate). Muscle cramping is likely a consequence of hypokalemia (β_2 agonists stimulate Na/K^+ ATPase, thus facilitating K^+ entry into cells), as K^+ is needed for vasodilation in the skeletal muscle.

A Isoproterenol can cause the pattern of adverse effects reported by the patient but is very rarely used today in asthmatic patients.

C–E These drugs are not used to treat asthmatic patients.

Learning objective: Explain the main mechanism of action of cocaine.

31. **C** Cocaine is an indirect-acting adrenergic drug that blocks catecholamine uptake in both the central and peripheral nervous systems. Therefore, the adrenergic actions of cocaine are due to the increased availability of norepinephrine in the synaptic cleft.

    A, B, D, E All of these listed mechanisms can increase the availability of norepinephrine or epinephrine, but these are not mechanisms of action of cocaine.

Learning objective: Describe the diagnostic uses of cholinergic drugs.

32. **A** Horner syndrome results when the cervical sympathetic pathway running from the hypothalamus to the eye is disrupted. The lesion causes vasodilation (loss of α_1 receptor–mediated vascular tone), ptosis (loss of α_1 receptor–mediated contraction of the superior tarsal muscle), miosis (loss of the α_1 receptor–mediated dilation of the pupil), and anhidrosis (loss of sympathetic cholinergic firing to the sweat glands). The use of adrenergic drugs can help to determine if the lesion is pre- or postganglionic. Hydroxyamphetamine is an indirect-acting adrenergic drug that stimulates the release of norepinephrine from adrenergic nerve endings. Because mydriasis was observed, the postganglionic neuron is intact and therefore able to release norepinephrine. Damage to the postganglionic neuron would results in less or no norepinephrine being released, and mydriasis would be incomplete or absent. The conclusion is that the lesion must be on the preganglionic neuron.

    B See correct answer explanation.

    C, D A lesion of either pre- or postganglionic parasympathetic nerves would cause a completely different clinical picture (mydriasis, no ptosis, etc.).

Learning objective: Describe the mechanism of dopamine-induced diuresis.

33. **A** Activation of D_1 receptors in the kidney causes vasodilation and inhibition of Na^+ reabsorption by the proximal tubule. Both actions contribute to the increased diuresis that can occur with low doses of dopamine.

    B This effect occurs with high dose of dopamine, which activiates D_2 receptions in the area postrema.

    C–E These effects occur with an intermediate dose of dopamine, which still activates D_1 receptors, but also activates β_1 receptors and release of norepinephrine from nerve terminals.

Learning objective: Describe the pharmacological effects of dopamine.

34. **F** Dopamine decreases total peripheral resistance (TPR) at low doses by selectively activating D_1 receptors (mainly in mesenteric and renal beds). At higher doses, dopamine can also activate α receptors and increase norepinephrine release from adrenergic terminals. The α-mediated vasoconstriction overrides the vasodilating effects on the kidney, and TPR increases.

    A, E Norepinephrine and phenylephrine have only vasoconstricting effects mediated by activation of α_1 receptors.

    B, C Albuterol and isoproterenol have only vasodilating effects mediated by the activation of β_2 receptors.

    D Dobutamine has negligible effects on TPR.

Learning objective: Describe the diagnostic uses of tyramine.

35. **A** Tyramine is a normal by-product of tyrosine metabolism in the body and is also found in high concentration in fermented food. It is normally inactive when ingested, because of a very large first-pass effect (metabolism by hepatic monoamine oxidase [MAO]). If administered parenterally, it has an indirect sympathomimetic action due to the release of stored catecholamines. This is the basis of the tyramine test, sometimes used clinically for the diagnosis of some autonomic nervous system (ANS) diseases.

    In this case, the patient is most likely affected by pure autonomic failure, a rare degenerative disorder of the ANS presenting in middle to late life. In this disease, there is a degeneration of postganglionic sympathetic neurons, which can explain the postural hypotension. An intravenous injection of tyramine normally causes an elevation of blood pressure due to the release of stored catecholamines. In this case, however, the elevation did not occur because catecholamines had been lost from the nerve endings. On the contrary, an intravenous injection of epinephrine caused a big elevation in blood pressure, as epinephrine directly activates adrenoceptors. Moreover, these receptors were upregulated, due to a decreased availability of the neurotransmitter (denervation supersensitivity).

    B A lesion of the preganglionic sympathetic nerve would have caused orthostatic hypotension, but tyramine would have caused hypertension, as the postganglionic adrenergic neurons were intact.

    C, D In case of a lesion of either pre- or postganglionic parasympathetic nerves, tyramine would have been effective.

    E Lesions of the sympathetic pathways in the medulla oblongata would have caused symptoms similar to those due to lesions of the preganglionic sympathetic nerves. In this case, tyramine would have been effective.

Learning objective: Describe the pharmacological action of clonidine.

36. **B** Hot flashes are symptomatic of a disorder in thermoregulation due to the complex hormonal changes that accompany estrogen withdrawal. Several chemical mediators are thought to be involved, including norepinephrine, epinephrine, serotonin, and prostaglandins. Clonidine is sometimes used to treat hot flashes, even if it is not a first-line agent for that disorder. In fact, it is less effective compared to other nonhormonal therapies (gabapentin, venlafaxine, and fluoxetine). By activating presynaptic α_2 receptors, clonidine causes a decrease of norepinephrine release from adrenergic terminals. However, how this mechanism decreases hot flashes is still unknown.

   A, C–E These drugs do not activate α_2 receptors.

Learning objective: Identify the drugs used to treat hyperkalemia.

37. **B** This patient's lab data indicate that she is suffering from renal failure, which frequently leads to hyperkalemia. Hyperkalemia with ECG changes requires emergency treatment. The therapy includes

   - Agents that antagonize the cardiac effects of hyperkalemia (e.g., calcium, which counteracts the depolarizing effect of hyperkalemia)
   - Drugs that shift K^+ from the extracellular to the intracellular space (e.g., insulin and β_2 agonists)
   - Drugs that enhance K^+ elimination (e.g., ion-exchange resins that bind K^+ in the bowel lumen)

   Albuterol is the only drug in the list that has one of these effects (β_2 agonist) without other actions that would be deleterious in this patient.

   A, C, F Phenylephrine, clonidine, and dobutamine do not affect K^+ concentration.

   D, E Isoproterenol and epinephrine can cause hypokalemia, but they are not used therapeutically for this purpose because of many other unwanted effects.

Learning objective: Relate the effects of epinephrine to the activation of specific receptors.

38. **E** Activation of β_2 receptors by epinephrine increases cyclic adenosine monophosphate (cAMP), which in turn activates the cAMP-dependent protein kinase A. This enzyme activates a cascade of enzymes that promote glycogen degradation.

   A This action is mediated by activation of α_2 receptors.

   B–D These actions are mediated by activation of α_1 receptors.

Learning objective: Explain the reversal of norepinephrine effect on heart rate by atropine.

39. **B** The drug causes a decrease in heart rate that is reversed by a pretreatment with atropine. This suggests that the bradycardia is caused by a reflex vagal discharge. Norepinephrine is the only listed drug that causes a vagal reflex bradycardia strong enough to overcome its own direct tachycardic effect. When the reflex vagal discharge is blocked by atropine, the direct tachycardic effect of norepinephrine becomes evident.

   A, C–F See correct answer explanation.

Learning objective: Explain the reason for the decrease in heart rate caused by an intravenous injection of norepinephrine.

40. **C** Norepinephrine usually causes a reflex bradycardia in patients with intact innervation of the heart for the following reason: the increase in blood pressure due to activation of α_1 receptors activates baroreceptors located in the carotid sinus and aortic arch (baroreceptors are stretch receptors). This increases the firing rate to the nucleus of the tractus solitarius in the medulla, which in turn increases its firing to the vagal motor neurons (dorsal motor neuron and nucleus ambiguus). When this vagal excitation is strong enough, it can overcome the norepinephrine-induced tachycardia due to activation of cardiac β receptors; therefore, bradycardia ensues.

   A, B These actions would cause an increase, not a decrease, in heart rate.

   D Activation of α_2 autoreceptors causes a decrease of norepinephrine release, but this is not the main mechanism of norepinephrine-induced bradycardia.

   E Decreased firing rate of carotid chemoreceptors occurs only in severe pathologic conditions and would cause an increase, not a decrease, in heart rate.

ADRENERGIC DRUGS Answer key							
1.	B	6.	E	11.	D	16.	E
2.	L	7.	E	12.	D	17.	B
3.	I	8.	D	13.	C	18.	E
4.	H	9.	A	14.	A	19.	A
5.	K	10.	A	15.	E	20.	B
21.	B	26.	C	31.	C	36.	B
22.	C	27.	E	32.	A	37.	B
23.	C	28.	C	33.	A	38.	E
24.	A	29.	C	34.	F	39.	B
25.	D	30.	B	35.	A	40.	C

Answers and Explanations: II-3 Antiadrenergic Drugs

Questions 1–5

1. **E**
2. **A**
3. **G**
4. **H**
5. **B**

Learning objective: Explain the mechanism of impaired ejaculation caused by α_1 antagonists.

6. **E** Vasospasm in the fingers, which is the most common sign of Raynaud disease, is treated by a vasodilator, usually a calcium channel blocker, such as nifedipine, or an α_1 antagonist, such as prazosin. The patient most likely received prazosin because he complained of impaired ejaculation. The increased firing of the sympathetic nervous system that occurs during sex activates α_1 receptors located on the vas deferens and prostate capsule. The contraction of smooth muscles of these organs puts the semen into the urethra, thus causing ejaculation. Prazosin blocks α_1 adrenoceptors, so ejaculation is impaired.

A–D, F See correct answer explanation.

Learning objective: Describe the pharmacological effects of phenoxybenzamine.

7. **A** Phenoxybenzamine is a nonselective α-adrenergic blocker. The blockade of α_1 adrenoceptors causes peripheral vasodilation, which in turn decreases the blood pressure. A reduction in blood pressure decreases the firing rate of carotid baroreceptors. Because the baroreceptor discharge increases the vagal outflow to the heart, a decreased firing rate will have the opposite effect; that is, it will increase the sympathetic outflow, causing tachycardia and increased cardiac contractility.

B–E See correct answer explanation.

Learning objective: Identify the action mediating the therapeutic effect of phenoxybenzamine.

8. **A** Phenoxybenzamine is a nonselective α antagonist frequently used in pheochromocytoma both in the preoperative management of the disease and to handle inoperable or metastatic cases. By blocking α_1 receptors, the drug decreases peripheral vascular resistance, thus counteracting the hypertension that is a prominent symptom of the tumor.

B, D These are actions of phenoxybenzamine, but they mediate unwanted effects, not the therapeutic effect of the drug.

C By blocking α_2 presynaptic receptors, phenoxybenzamine actually increases, not decreases, epinephrine release from the adrenal medulla.

E Alpha-2 agonists reduce firing from the vasomotor center, so an α_2 antagonist such as phenoxybenzamine would increase, not decrease, firing from the vasomotor center.

Learning objective: Describe the main adverse effects of tamsulosin.

9. **B** Tamsulosin is a selective α_1 antagonist frequently used to counteract bladder obstruction due to prostatic hyperplasia. Fatigue, sleepiness, and dizziness are common adverse effects most likely related to the drug-induced hypotension. Palpitations are infrequently reported and are most likely related to the reflex tachycardia triggered by the drug-induced vasodilation.

D Flutamide is an androgen receptor blocker that is used in patients with prostatic hyperplasia. However, it does not cause the symptoms reported by the patient.

A, C, E, F These drugs are not used for prostatic hyperplasia.

Learning objective: Describe the therapeutic uses of prazosin.

10. **C** The patient's signs and symptoms suggest the diagnosis of Raynaud disease. In this disease, which is idiopathic and is most common in young women, the threshold for vasospastic response is lowered by local cold or anything that activates the sympathetic outflow or the release of catecholamines. By blocking α_1 receptors, prazosin is often helpful in reducing vasospastic episodes.

A, B, D, E There is no rationale for the use of any of these drugs in Raynaud disease.

Learning objective: Identify the site of action of apraclonidine and timolol in open-angle glaucoma.

11. **D** Open-angle glaucoma is characterized in most cases by increased intraocular pressure, which in turn is due to an excessive amount of aqueous humor in the anterior chamber of the eye. Pharmacological therapy for this disease aims to decrease this volume, either by lowering aqueous humor production or by increasing aqueous humor outflow. In the eye, aqueous humor is manufactured by the cells of ciliary epithelium and is under the control of both β adrenoceptors (which increase the production) and α_2 adrenoceptors (which decrease the production). Production of aqueous humor can be reduced either by drugs that block β receptors (e.g., timolol) or by drugs that activate α_2 receptors (e.g., apraclonidine). The site of action of both drugs is the ciliary epithelium.

A–C, E, F See correct answer explanation.

Learning objective: Explain the mechanism of action of β-blocker in hypertrophic cardiomyopathy.

12. **B** In hypertrophic cardiomyopathy, the stiff, noncompliant ventricle resists diastolic filling. This can cause insufficient end-diastolic volume and therefore diastolic failure. Beta-blockers slow the heart rate, which allows an increased duration of diastole and thus more complete diastolic filling. They also decrease myocardial contractility, which increases ventricle compliance.

A, C, D All of these effects can be caused by propranolol, but they do not mediate the efficacy of the drug in hypertrophic cardiomyopathy.

E Propranolol causes coronary vasoconstriction, not vasodilation. The effect is due primarily to the decrease in cardiac contractility and, to a lesser extent, to the blockade of β_2 receptor–mediated vasodilation.

Learning objective: Describe the cardiovascular actions of β-blockers.

13. **A** The actions of a β-blocker on the cardiovascular system are much more pronounced when sympathetic tone is high. Therefore, under resting conditions, the drug-induced decrease of heart rate is minimal, whereas it is pronounced during exercise, when the sympathetic tone is high.

B A cholinergic agonist would cause a more pronounced decrease of the heart rate under resting conditions, because it further increases the parasympathetic activity that is already predominant under resting conditions.

C–E All of these drugs tend to increase the heart rate under resting conditions.

Learning objective: Describe the cardiovascular effects of atenolol.

14. **C** Atenolol is a selective β adrenoceptor blocker. By blocking β_1 receptors, atenolol decreases cardiac contractility. The best index of cardiac contractility is the ejection fraction, which is the fraction of the end-diastolic volume that is ejected during systole (remember that stroke volume is not the best index of cardiac contractility, as it also depends on preload).

A, D Because contractility is decreased, these volumes are actually increased, not decreased.

B Beta-blockers actually increase ventricular ejection time.

E Venous tone (which is mainly dependent on α_1-receptor activation) is minimally affected by β-blockers.

Learning objective: Describe the ocular effects of timolol.

15. **B** Beta-blockers decrease aqueous humor production by blocking β receptors in the ciliary epithelium. The consequent reduction in intraocular pressure usually can be detected within 30 minutes after a single dose. Beta-blockers have negligible effects on pupillary diameter (which is under the control of M_3 receptors on the sphincter muscle of the iris and of α_1 receptors on the radial muscle of the iris) and on lens curvature (which is mainly under the control of M_3 receptors on the ciliary muscle).

A, C–E See correct answer explanation.

Learning objective: Describe the interactions between propranolol and isoproterenol.

16. **A** Isoproterenol-induced hyperglycemia is mainly due to β_2 receptor–mediated gluconeogenesis and glycogenolysis. Because of this, it can be effectively counteracted by propranolol, which blocks β_2 receptors. None of the other listed actions can be antagonized by propranolol, because they are not mediated by activation of β receptors.

B Nicotine-induced activation of Nn receptors in ganglia increases the firing of postganglionic sympathetic nerves, which in turn causes skin vasoconstriction by activating α_1 receptors.

C Norepinephrine-induced reflex bradycardia is mediated by the activation of M_2 cardiac receptors. Moreover, propranolol itself can cause bradycardia.

D Phenylephrine-induced mydriasis is mediated by the activation of α_1 receptors.

E Pilocarpine-induced contraction of bronchial musculature is mediated by the activation of M_3 receptors. Moreover, propranolol itself can cause bronchoconstriction.

Learning objective: Describe the pharmacological effects of atenolol.

17. **C** The new drug completely antagonizes the epinephrine-induced increase in renin (which is mediated by β_1 receptor activation) but does not antagonize the epinephrine-induced hyperglycemia (which is due to several actions, including β_2 adrenoceptor–mediated glycogenolysis). Therefore, the drug must be a selective β blocker, such as atenolol.

A, D, F Albuterol, atropine, and prazosin cannot antagonize either of the epinephrine-induced effects.

B, E Timolol and propranolol are nonselective β–blockers, so they would antagonize both effects of epinephrine.

Learning objective: Describe the adverse effects of propranolol on the central nervous system.

18. **D** Propranolol is a first-line agent for migraine prophylaxis, and a large number of studies support its effectiveness. Adverse effects of propranolol include insomnia, vivid dreams, and nightmares (in up to 5% of patients). The mechanism underlying these central effects is still uncertain, but propranolol is a highly lipophilic drug and concentrates in the brain.

    A Beta-blockers do not cause postural hypotension, as the preload and the baroreceptor reflex are not affected by these drugs.

    B Beta-blockers decrease the heart rate and have anti-arrhythmic properties, so palpitations are unlikely. Beta-blockers block β adrenoceptor–mediated vasodilation, so flushing is also unlikely.

    C Beta-blockers have no significant effect on eye accommodation and do not cause mydriasis, so impairment of far vision and photophobia are unlikely.

    E Beta-blockers commonly cause diarrhea, which is likely related to the blockade of β_2 receptors in the gut and do not cause gastroesophageal reflux. Even if constipation can occur with some β-blockers, it is uncommon and never severe.

Learning objective: Describe the main adverse effects of β-blocker/diuretic combination.

19. **B** Beta-blockers can cause dose-related sexual dysfunction, which is more frequent when diuretics are given concomitantly, as in this case. The dysfunction includes erectile problems, decreased libido, and anorgasmia. The mechanism underlying these effects is still uncertain but probably related to the hypotensive effect and to central effects.

    A, C–E All of these disorders are generally relieved, not caused, by β-blockers.

Learning objective: Explain why β-blockers are relatively contraindicated in a diabetic patient.

20. **B** Historically, the presence of diabetes was a contraindication for β-blockade, due to the adverse effects on insulin release and blunting of hypoglycemia-associated tachycardia. However, diabetics comprise a large portion of infarct patients, and many studies have found that patients treated with β-blockers following myocardial infarction experience a 30 to 35% reduction in mortality. Therefore, β-blockers can be given to diabetic patients, but they must carefully control their sugar levels. In fact, hypoglycemia-associated tachycardia can be blunted by β-blockers, depriving the patient of an important diagnostic sign.

    A Beta-2 blockers occasionally can increase sugar levels by blocking β_2-mediated increase in insulin secretion, but this effect is mild and is not shared by selective β_1-blockers, such as atenolol.

    C Beta-2 blockers can decrease, not increase, insulin secretion.

    D, E Beta-blockers have these effects, but this is not the reason why diabetic patients receiving β-blockers must carefully control their sugar levels.

Learning objective: Explain the rationale of prescribing selective β_1-blockers in asthmatics.

21. **B** Beta-blockers are usually contraindicated in asthmatics because of their bronchoconstricting activity due to blockade of bronchial β_2 receptors. However, they are first-line therapy after a myocardial infarction, as they substantially decrease morbidity and mortality. In deciding whether to attempt to use β-blockers in asthmatic patients with previous MI, weighing the risk versus benefit is imperative. In this case, asthma was mild and intermittent, so one could make a case for cautiously administering a β-blocker. A selective antagonist such as atenolol was a rational choice, as blockade of β_2 receptors is negligible at therapeutic doses. However, caution must be used, because at higher doses selectivity may be lost.

    A By decreasing renin secretion, β-blockers can counteract pulmonary vasoconstriction, but this is not the reason for the choice of selective agents in asthmatics.

    C, D Atenolol does not have these effects.

    E Atenolol has a half-life of about 6 hours, but this is not the reason for the choice of the drug in an asthmatic patient.

Learning objective: Explain the mechanism of action of α_1-blockers in the treatment of impaired bladder emptying.

22. **B** The patient most likely received a selective α_1 antagonist. These drugs (prazosin, tamsulosin, etc.) are first-line agents for the treatment of impaired bladder emptying in prostatic hyperplasia. By blocking α_1 receptors, they relax the prostate capsule and the internal sphincter of the bladder, which have plentiful α_1 receptors, allowing a better urine flow.

    A By blocking vascular α_1 receptors, α_1 antagonists would increase, not decrease, blood flow.

    C The detrusor muscle is mainly under the control of the parasympathetic system.

    D Alpha-1 antagonists decrease blood pressure, but this is not the reason for their therapeutic effect in prostatic hyperplasia.

    E Alpha-1 antagonists have negligible effects on diuresis.

Learning objective: Describe the therapeutic uses of propranolol.

23. **E** The patient was most likely suffering from benign essential tremor, a disorder that is often inherited (autosomal dominant in 50% of cases), as in this case. Propranolol (and other nonselective β-blockers) is effective in treating the disorder. The mechanism of this therapeutic effect is still uncertain, but it seems related to blockade of the β_2 receptor–mediated increase in sequestration of cytosolic Ca^{2+} and enhanced discharge of muscle spindles.

    A–D None of these drugs are of value for the treatment of essential tremor.

Learning objective: Describe the therapeutic uses of α- and β-blockers in amphetamine poisoning.

24. **A** The patient's history and symptoms point out that he was most likely suffering from amphetamine poisoning. Most symptoms, including hypertension, can be managed with generous titration of benzodiazepines. If sedation fails to reduce blood pressure, a cardiovascular treatment is needed, as in this case. Amphetamines stimulate norepinephrine release from adrenergic terminals, increasing norepinephrine availability in the synaptic cleft. Therefore, both α- and β blockers can be used to effectively counteract norepinephrine-induced activation of α and β receptors. Parenteral α-blockers, such as phentolamine (or vasodilators, e.g., nitroprusside and nitroglycerin), must be given first. When the blood pressure is back to normal limits, a β-blocker is usually administered to control tachyarrhythmias that are frequent when circulating levels of catecholamines are high.

    B This drug combination could antagonize norepinephrine effects, but phenoxybenzamine is an irreversible antagonist with a very long duration of action and is not available for parenteral use. It is therefore not suitable for an emergency treatment.

    C–E These drugs cannot antagonize norepinephrine effects.

Learning objective: Describe the therapeutic uses of β-blockers in esophageal varices.

25. **B** The creation of arteriovenous anastomoses, which occurs in cirrhosis, allows the perfusion pressure of the hepatic artery to be partly transmitted into the portal vein. Therefore, arteriovenous anastomoses are a primary cause of portal hypertension in cirrhosis. Because the esophageal veins are tributaries of the portal vein, portal hypertension causes the esophageal veins to dilate and become varicose. By blocking β_2 receptors (particularly abundant in the liver vascular bed), liver arterial vessels are constricted, and the pressure transmitted into the portal vein decreases.

A Activation of β_2 receptors by albuterol would worsen the varices by increasing the portal pressure.

C–E Methyldopa, clonidine, and prazosin can reduce the systemic blood pressure, but they have unpredictable effects on the perfusion pressure of liver arterial vessels.

Learning objective: Describe the therapeutic use of propranolol in hyperthyroidism.

26. **B** The symptoms and signs of this patient indicate that the woman was most likely suffering from hyperthyroidism. In addition to the specific therapy (antithyroid drugs and radioiodine), the treatment of this disease almost always includes the administration of β-blockers that rapidly decrease the nervousness, palpitations, heat intolerance, tremors, and hypertension, most likely because many of these signs and symptoms are due to sympathetic overactivity. Propranolol is the drug of choice.

    A, C–E All of these drugs are contraindicated in hyperthyroidism, as they can further decrease the diastolic blood pressure, which is abnormally low in this disease.

Learning objective: Describe the therapeutic uses of β-blockers.

27. **B** Beta-blockers are effective in treating nongeneralized social phobias involving performance-related situations, although they are not approved by the U.S. Food and Drug Administration for this purpose. They are often used by musicians and have been called "the musicians' underground drug." The antianxiety effect of β-blockers in situational anxiety seems to be related to their blocking of norepinephrine effects, thus reducing physical symptoms of anxiety (palpitation, tremor, and blushing). In fact, even β-blockers that do not cross the blood–brain barrier are effective in performance anxiety.

    A Benzodiazepines such as diazepam are effective antianxiety agents but are not indicated in this situation, as they can have depressive effects on the central nervous system that could negatively affect the performance.

    C, D Selective serotonin reuptake inhibitors (e.g., fluoxetine) and serotonin-norepinephrine reuptake inhibitors (e.g., venlaflaxine) are currently first-line agents for anxiety disorders, but they are not indicated in this situation, as effects occur gradually over several days.

    E Buspirone is an effective anxiolytic agent, but its initial effects are observed after 7 to 10 days of therapy.

Learning objective: Describe the main adverse effects of prazosin.

28. **E** Postural hypotension is a common adverse effect of α_1 antagonists such as prazosin, especially during the first days of therapy. The effect is due to an impairment of baroreceptor reflex, as the α_1 blockade hinders the vasoconstriction that normally occurs when the body assumes a standing position.

    A Blockade of α_1 receptors in the radial muscle of the iris would cause miosis, not mydriasis.

    B Micturition is facilitated, not impaired, when an α_1-blocker is administered to a man with prostatic hyperplasia.

    C The blockade of α_1 receptors in skin vessels would cause red and hot, not pale and cold, skin.

    D Bronchoconstriction is caused by blockade of β_2, not α_1, receptors.

Learning objective: Explain the molecular mechanism of action of timolol.

29. **D** Timolol is a nonselective β-receptor blocker. Activation of all β receptors increases the synthesis of cyclic adenosine monophosphate (cAMP) through increased activity of the adenylate cyclase enzyme. By blocking these receptors, all β-blockers do the opposite (i.e., the activity of adenylate cyclase is decreased).

    A–C, E, F See correct answer explanation.

Learning objective: Explain the mechanism of action of metyrosine.

30. **C** Metyrosine inhibits the enzyme tyrosine hydroxylase, which catalyzes the hydroxylation of tyrosine to dopa. This is the rate-limiting step in catecholamine biosynthesis, and the inhibition of the enzyme can cause up to a 70% decrease of catecholamine content in adrenergic terminals. The only therapeutic use of this drug is for the short-term management of patients with pheochromocytoma who are awaiting surgery or for long-term management of malignant pheochromocytoma when surgery is contraindicated.

    A, B, D, E See correct answer explanation.

ANTIADRENERGIC DRUGS Answer key		
1. E	6. E	11. D
2. A	7. A	12. B
3. G	8. A	13. A
4. H	9. B	14. C
5. B	10. C	15. B
16. A	21. B	26. B
17. C	22. B	27. B
18. D	23. E	28. E
19. B	24. A	29. D
20. B	25. B	30. C

Answers and Explanations: II-4 Cholinergic Drugs

Questions 1–5

1. **E**
2. **K**
3. **H**
4. **J**
5. **G**

Learning objective: Describe the mechanism of action of physostigmine.

6. **E** To increase cholinergic transmission in the central nervous system, the drug must activate (directly or indirectly) central acetylcholine receptors. Physostigmine is an anticholinesterase drug that is able to cross the blood–brain barrier. The increased acetylcholine availability in the central nervous system accounts for the increased cholinergic transmission.

    A–D These drugs do not affect cholinergic transmission in the central nervous system because they very poorly cross the blood–brain barrier.

Learning objective: Identify the sites of action of carbachol given locally in the conjunctival sac.

7. **B** Carbachol is used in ocular surgery to decrease the intraocular pressure by increasing the outflow of the aqueous humor. The drug can activate both muscarinic and nicotinic neuronal receptors located on the body of autonomic ganglia. However, when the drug is given locally, it can reach the ciliary muscle but cannot reach the ciliary ganglion that is located on the posterior orbit. Therefore, the primary site of action of the drug given locally in the conjunctival sac is the ciliary muscle. Activation of muscarinic M_3 receptors leads to the contraction of the ciliary muscle, which in turn causes the opening of trabecular meshwork, thus increasing the outflow of the aqueous humor.

    C, D The lens and the radial muscle of the iris are devoid of Nn and M_3 receptors.

    A, E See correct answer explanation.

Learning objective: Identify the drugs used in an acute glaucoma attack.

8. **A** An acute glaucoma attack is usually the first symptom of acute angle-closure glaucoma, a disease associated with a closed anterior chamber angle. When this occurs, intraocular pressure rises, because the obstruction of the peripheral iris prevents the normal drainage of aqueous humor from the eye. An acute glaucoma attack is a medical emergency because vision can be lost quickly. Aqueous humor production must be decreased. Therefore, a topical β-blocker (e.g., timolol) and an α_2 agonist (e.g., apraclonidine) are immediately administered. Then pilocarpine is given to increase aqueous humor outflow (cholinergic drugs alone are generally ineffective when the intraocular pressure is more than 40 mm Hg).

    B–D Homatropine and scopolamine are contraindicated in angle-closure glaucoma because they induce mydriasis, which increases the risk of closing the anterior chamber.

    E Prazosin is ineffective in glaucoma. Mannitol is not given topically, but intravenously, and is used to lower the intraocular pressure only if the response to the first treatment is inadequate.

Learning objective: Identify the receptors mediating the neostigmine-induced increase in bowel movements.

9. **B** Neostigmine is a reversible cholinesterase inhibitor sometimes used to increase smooth muscle activity in adynamic ileus or atony of the urinary bladder. The drug increases the availability of acetylcholine at cholinergic terminals, which in turn activates both the nicotinic neuronal receptors on parasympathetic ganglia and the muscarinic M_3 receptors on smooth muscle.

    A, C–F See correct answer explanation.

Learning objective: Explain the mechanism of action of donepezil in Alzheimer disease.

10. **D** The patient's symptoms and the results of the Mini-Mental Status Exam indicate that he was most likely in the early stages of Alzheimer disease (AD). To date, no drugs are available that can halt or reverse the progression of the disease, but drugs are approved for the treatment of memory deficit associated with AD. Acetylcholine is significantly reduced in AD, and drugs that can increase its levels in the brain have shown moderate success in slowing the progression of the disease. Donepezil selectively inhibits cholinesterase in the central nervous system with less effect on cholinesterase in peripheral tissues.

    A–C, E, F See correct answer explanation.

Learning objective: Explain the molecular mechanism of neostigmine-induced bradycardia.

11. **A** By inhibiting cholinesterase, neostigmine increases acetylcholine availability in the synaptic cleft of cholinergic fibers. This can increase the activity of both sympathetic and parasympathetic ganglia supplying the heart and can activate muscarinic M_2 receptors, which are the most abundant acetylcholine receptors in the sinoatrial (SA), atrium, and atrioventricular (AV) nodes. This activation in turn opens acetylcholine-sensitive K^+ channels, increasing the hyperpolarization of SA and AV cardiac fibers. The final result is a negative chronotropic and dromotropic effect.

    B–E See correct answer explanation.

Learning objective: Describe the pharmacological effects of pilocarpine on the eye.

12. **B** Pilocarpine is a muscarinic agonist. The drug-induced activation of M_3 receptors causes contraction of the sphincter muscle of the iris (decreasing pupillary diameter) and contraction of the ciliary muscle (increasing lens curvature). Ocular pressure is decreased because the contraction of the ciliary muscle opens the pores of the trabecular meshwork, facilitating the outflow of aqueous humor into the Schlemm canal.

    A, C–E See correct answer explanation.

Learning objective: Describe the pharmacological action of bethanechol.

13. **C** Overflow incontinence occurs when the weight of urine in a distended bladder overcomes outlet resistance. It results from an anatomical outlet obstruction or an atonic bladder, as in this case. Bethanechol is a cholinergic agonist that primarily activates muscarinic M_3 receptors. This activation causes a contraction of the detrusor muscle of the bladder; therefore, the amount of bladder space that can be filled (i.e., the distensibility of the bladder, or its compliance) is decreased

    A, B, E Activation of M_3 receptors causes effects opposite to those described

    D Diuresis refers to the production of urine by the kidney. Bethanechol does not affect diuresis.

Learning objective: Describe the pharmacological actions of nicotine.

14. **C** The history of the patient, together with her symptoms and signs, is consistent with the diagnosis of nicotine poisoning, likely due to lozenge tablets used by her husband to quit smoking. Nicotine causes a rapid activation of both the sympathetic and parasympathetic nervous systems, as well as stimulation of different areas of the brain. Signs in this patient due to parasympathetic activation are vomiting, urinary incontinence, and profuse salivation. Signs of sympathetic activation are cold sweat (sweat glands are stimulated and skin vessels constricted) and rapid and irregular pulse (activation of nicotinic neuronal [Nn] receptors releases epinephrine from adrenal medulla). Central stimulation accounts for the mental confusion and the tonic-clonic seizure.

    A Clonidine does not cause most of the symptoms exhibited by the patient.

    B Scopolamine is used for the prevention of motion sickness. The drug is a muscarinic antagonist; therefore, the symptoms of overdose would be the opposite of those exhibited by the patient.

    D Bethanechol is a muscarinic agonist. Symptoms of overdose would be limited to parasympathetic activation.

    E Neostigmine is a cholinesterase inhibitor. Many symptoms of poisoning by cholinesterase inhibitors are similar to those of nicotine overdose (both drugs can activate, directly or indirectly, nicotinic receptors). However, in the case of neostigmine poisoning, central effects would be minimal, as the amount of drug crossing the blood–brain barrier is negligible.

Learning objective: Describe the ocular actions of echothiophate.

15. **F** When control of glaucoma is not achieved with standard pharmacotherapy, anticholinesterase agents may be prescribed as a last topical therapy option. Echothiophate is an irreversible cholinesterase inhibitor. When given locally in the subconjunctival sac, it increases the availability of acetylcholine at cholinergic synapses. By activating muscarinic M_3 receptors, acetylcholine contracts the ciliary muscle, which in turn opens the trabecular meshwork and Schlemm canal, increasing the outflow of aqueous humor. In this way, the intraocular pressure is decreased. Being an irreversible inhibitor, the drug has a long duration of action that affords good control of glaucoma.

    A, C–E Acetylcholine does not cause these effects.

    B By activating M_3 receptors, acetylcholine can contract the sphincter of the iris, but this action has negligible effects on the intraocular pressure.

Learning objective: Describe the poisoning by organophosphate insecticides.

16. **D** The history and the patient's symptoms and signs indicate that he was most likely suffering from organophosphate poisoning. Serious poisoning from organophosphate pesticides is rare today because of enforced occupational health and safety standards, but mild poisoning is still surprisingly common.

    A, C, E Poisoning by these drugs does not cause the symptoms and signs shown by the patient.

    B Symptoms of poisoning from carbamates, which are reversible cholinesterase inhibitors, are usually indistinguishable from those caused by organophosphates. However, in case of poisoning from reversible cholinesterase inhibitors, pralidoxime is useless (and can also be dangerous). The fact that the attending physician administered pralidoxime indicates that he or she was sure, from the patient's information, that an organophosphate was the culprit drug.

Learning objective: Describe the signs and symptoms of muscarine poisoning.

17. **A** The patient's signs and symptoms are consistent with the diagnosis of muscarine poisoning. High concentrations of muscarine are present in various species of *Inocybe* and *Clitocybe* mushrooms. The symptoms of muscarine intoxication start within 1 hour after the ingestion and are all attributable to activation of muscarinic receptors.

    B Nicotine poisoning results from the activation, and later the blockade, of nicotinic neuronal (Nn) and nicotinic muscular (Nm) receptors. Activation of Nn receptors in ganglia and adrenal medulla causes increased sympathetic firing and increased release of norepinephrine. Early signs include cold sweat, rapid and irregular pulse, and hypertension, followed by hypotension and collapse. Moreover, the activation of Nm receptors at the motor end plate would cause muscle paralysis due to depolarization blockade, which is absent in this patient.

    C Poisoning by organophosphates causes symptoms due to activation of muscarinic receptors; in addition, there are symptoms due to activation of nicotinic receptors (i.e., skeletal muscle paralysis due to depolarization blockade).

    D Some mushroom species contain atropine. The symptoms of atropine poisoning are due to blockade of muscarinic receptors and are the opposite of those exhibited by the patient.

    E Carbamate insecticides are reversible cholinesterase inhibitors. Symptoms of poisoning by these agents are the same as the symptoms of poisoning by organophosphates.

Learning objective: Describe the ocular adverse effects of pilocarpine.

18. **A** Pilocarpine is a cholinergic agonist that activates only muscarinic M_1, M_2, and M_3 receptors (activation of nicotinic receptors is negligible). Activation of M_3 receptors in the ciliary muscle causes cyclospasm, which in turn increases the lens curvature. The eye is accommodated for near vision, and far vision becomes difficult. Activation of M_3 receptors in the sphincter muscle of the iris causes miosis, which impairs vision in poor light.

   B, C Timolol and apraclonidine decrease the production of aqueous humor but have a negligible effect on accommodation.

   D, E Epinephrine and phenylephrine activate α_1 receptors in the radial muscle of the iris. This would cause mydriasis, which would favor, not impair, vision in poor light.

   F Neostigmine is a cholinesterase inhibitor that could have caused effects similar to those of pilocarpine. However, it has been approved only for the treatment of myasthenia gravis and some gastrointestinal and urologic problems. It is not used to treat glaucoma.

Learning objective: Describe the main adverse effects of neostigmine.

19. **D** Neostigmine is a cholinesterase inhibitor and therefore increases the availability of acetylcholine at all cholinergic synapses, eliciting muscarinic effects, mainly in the gastrointestinal tract.

   A–C, E By increasing acetylcholine availability, neostigmine causes effects opposite to those listed.

Learning objective: Describe the therapeutic uses of neostigmine.

20. **C** Reversible cholinesterase inhibitors such as neostigmine can reverse the paralysis induced by nondepolarizing neuromuscular blocking drugs such as tubocurarine. Tubocurarine blocks nicotinic muscular (Nm) receptors at the motor end plate, whereas acetylcholine activates these receptors. The two drugs competitively antagonize each other, and the increased availability of acetylcholine brought about by cholinesterase inhibitors can therefore reverse the muscle paralysis induced by tubocurarine. This antagonism is exploited clinically, and reversible cholinesterase inhibitors are often used to speed recovery from the neuromuscular blockade remaining after completion of surgery. Neostigmine is the preferred drug, as it does not enter the brain and is therefore free of central adverse effects.

   A Physostigmine is not indicated because it can cross the blood–brain barrier.

   B Edrophonium is not indicated because it has a very short duration of action (its half-life is 1 to 10 minutes).

   D, E Bethanechol and pralidoxime do not act at Nm receptors.

Learning objective: Describe the therapeutic uses of bethanechol.

21. **D** The fact that bethanechol was able to improve the patient's symptoms points out that he suffered from overflow incontinence due to an acontractile bladder. Neurogenic atony of the bladder is common in diabetic neuropathy and was most likely the cause of the patient's disorder. By activating muscarinic M_3 receptors, bethanechol causes increased detrusor muscle contractility, which can facilitate voiding of the bladder.

   A Prostatic hyperplasia can cause overflow incontinence due to urethral stricture, but bethanechol is contraindicated in any case of overflow incontinence due to urethral obstruction, as the increased detrusor contractility cannot overcome the obstruction, thus causing painful bladder spasms.

   B Diuresis refers to the production of urine by the kidney. A drug acting on the bladder has nothing to do with urine production.

   C, E Bethanechol is contraindicated, not indicated, in these conditions, as the activity of the detrusor muscle is already increased.

Learning objective: Describe the use of edrophonium to diagnose a cholinergic crisis.

22. **B** Myasthenic patients under treatment with cholinesterase inhibitors may exhibit decreased muscle strength because of an excessive concentration of acetylcholine that causes depolarization blockade of the motor end plate. This is referred to as a cholinergic crisis. These patients may also exhibit decreased muscle strength because of a sudden exacerbation of the disease. This is called a myasthenic crisis. Edrophonium can be used to distinguish between the two syndromes. In fact, in cases of cholinergic crisis, edrophonium administration will produce no relief or worsen the syndrome. (a decrease in muscle strength), whereas in cases of myasthenic crisis, the drug will improve the syndrome (an increase in muscle strength). Moreover, an edrophonium-induced decrease of muscle strength is accompanied by fasciculations (brief muscle contractions before the paralysis), as acetylcholine briefly activates nicotinic receptors, whereas an increase in muscle strength is not accompanied by fasciculations.

   A, C–E See correct answer explanation.

Learning objective: Describe the therapeutic uses of pilocarpine in glaucoma.

23. **D** The patient was most likely suffering from open-angle glaucoma. Pilocarpine historically was the initial treatment of choice, but today it is used only as an alternative therapy when other drugs are contraindicated, as in this case (see answer explanations below).

    A Beta-blockers are first-line therapy for glaucoma but are contraindicated in this case because of the AV block. In fact, systemic effects can occur even after a topical administration, especially in the elderly, secondary to inadvertent overdose due to poor administration technique. In patients with complete AV block, the heart rate is maintained by a rhythm that is driven by a ventricular pacemaker and is about 50 bpm. By blocking β receptors in the ventricle, a β-blocker can reduce this barely sufficient heart rate, causing heart failure. Pilocarpine is not dangerous because in a patient with a complete AV block, the AV conduction is, by definition, already completely blocked, and the parasympathetic control of the ventricle is negligible, due to lack of innervation.

    B, C, E These drugs are not used for treating glaucoma.

Learning objective: Describe the therapeutic uses of physostigmine.

24. **C** The patient's symptoms, signs, and history indicate that he was most likely poisoned by black berries of deadly nightshade (*Atropa belladonna*), a plant containing antimuscarinic alkaloids (mainly atropine and scopolamine). Antimuscarinic syndrome is due to competitive blockade of muscarinic receptors all over the body. Physostigmine is an anticholinesterase inhibitor that can cross the blood–brain barrier, increasing the availability of acetylcholine both in the central nervous system and in the periphery. Although theoretically a cholinesterase inhibitor would be the ideal therapy for antimuscarinic poisoning, physostigmine can have dangerous central nervous system effects. Therefore, it is used only in patients with dangerous hyperthermia or severe tachycardia, as in this case.

    A Neostigmine, a quaternary ammonium compound, is a cholinesterase inhibitor that cannot cross the blood–brain barrier and therefore is unable to counteract the central effects of atropine and scopolamine.

    B, D–F These drugs interact with the adrenergic system and are therefore useless, or even dangerous, in antimuscarinic poisoning.

Learning objective: Explain the mechanism of hypotension that occurs after the hypertensive effect induced by nicotine.

25. **A** Prolonged activation of nicotinic receptors causes a persistent depolarization of the postjunctional cell membrane that prevents the return to the resting state. Because it is the change in the resting potential that triggers the action potential, the depolarized membrane is resistant to further depolarization, and neuronal transmission is blocked (depolarization blockade). Impairment of neuronal transmission in sympathetic ganglia decreases the sympathetic tone, thus causing a decrease in blood pressure.

    B, C Blockade of ganglionic M_2 and M_1 receptors would prevent the production of inhibitory postsynaptic potential and early slow excitatory postsynaptic potential. These potentials are not involved in the production of the action potential.

    D, E Nicotine does not prevent acetylcholine or catecholamine release.

Learning objective: Describe the therapeutic uses of pilocarpine.

26. **E** Sjögren syndrome is a diffuse connective tissue disease in which lymphocytes infiltrate mucosal and other tissues. Lymphocytic infiltration in salivary glands causes gland atrophy. Saliva diminishes, resulting in extreme dryness of the mouth and lips. If glands are not severely atrophied, pilocarpine can be used to stimulate salivary production.

    A Acetylcholine is not used for systemic therapy because of its very short duration of action.

    B–D Phenylephrine, prazosin, and donepezil have little effect on salivary production.

Learning objective: Describe the absolute contraindications of neostigmine.

27. **D** The patient's signs and symptoms suggest the diagnosis of adynamic ileus due to intraperitoneal infection (see the high-grade fever). Ileus means paralysis of the gut. When this paralysis is due only to a lack of autonomic neurotransmission (as in most cases of postoperative ileus), a drug such as neostigmine, which increases the levels of acetylcholine, can help to restore the motor activity of the gut. On the other hand, when the paralysis is due to obstruction or inflammation of the gut, cholinergic drugs are absolutely contraindicated, as an increase in gut motility in these conditions can exacerbate the inflammation and lead to perforation of the intestine.

    A–C, E All of these therapeutic measures are indicated, not contraindicated, in case of ileus due to intraperitoneal infection.

Learning objective: Describe the therapy of organophosphate poisoning.

28. **F** The patient's symptoms and signs indicate that he was most likely poisoned by an organophosphate insecticide. The use of these pesticides is now banned or restricted in many countries, but they are still commonly used in underdeveloped countries. The two first-line agents for this poisoning are atropine and a cholinesterase reactivator such as pralidoxime. Atropine is essential to counteract muscarinic

effects on the central nervous system, as pralidoxime does not appreciably cross the blood–brain barrier.

A–E See correct answer explanation.

Learning objective: Describe the pharmacological actions of nicotine.

29. **C** By activating nicotinic neuronal receptors, nicotine increases the release of epinephrine from chromaffin cells of the adrenal medulla, which is the only peripheral organ able to synthesize epinephrine.

A, B, D, E Nicotine causes effects opposite to those listed

Learning objective: Explain the mechanism of the emetic action of nicotine.

30. **B** Nicotine can directly stimulate the chemoreceptor trigger zone, and this seems to be the main mechanism of nicotine-induced nausea and vomiting. Additional mechanisms involve the afferent stimulation of the vomiting center by sensory receptors present in the tongue and lungs.

A, C, D Nicotine can act on these sites, but they are not involved in the mechanism of nausea and vomiting.

E Nicotine does not interfere significantly with vestibular function.

CHOLINERGIC DRUGS Answer key					
1.	E	6.	E	11.	A
2.	K	7.	B	12.	B
3.	H	8.	A	13.	C
4.	J	9.	B	14.	C
5.	G	10.	D	15.	F
16.	D	21.	D	26.	E
17.	A	22.	B	27.	D
18.	A	23.	D	28.	F
19.	D	24.	C	29.	C
20.	C	25.	A	30.	B

Answers and Explanations: II-5 Anticholinergic Drugs

Questions 1–5

1. **F**
2. **C**
3. **B**
4. **G**
5. **E**

Learning objective: Identify the receptors that mediate the antiemetic action of scopolamine.

6. **E** The drug used by the patient was most likely scopolamine, the only anti–motion sickness drug that can be applied to the skin via a transdermal patch. Antimuscarinic drugs are used in certain vestibular disorders, including motion sickness and Meniere disease. Their main mechanism of action is most likely related to blockade of muscarinic M_1 receptors located in the vestibular nuclei, in the chemoreceptor trigger zone, and in the solitary tract nucleus. This blockade decreases firing from these regions to the vomiting center, so nausea and vomiting are prevented.

A–D See correct answer explanation.

Learning objective: Explain the molecular mechanism of action of antimuscarinic quaternary ammonium compounds.

7. **C** Glycopyrrolate is a quaternary ammonium antimuscarinic drug. Drugs of this type relax the intestinal smooth muscle and are sometimes given to patients with irritable bowel syndrome during periods of diarrhea, in order to relieve the hyperactivity of the gut. Quaternary ammonium antimuscarinic drugs mainly block muscarinic receptors but also exhibit a significant blocking activity on ganglionic Nn receptors. Both the blockade of M_3 receptors in the gastrointestinal smooth muscle and the blockade of the Nn receptors in the ganglia of the myenteric and submucosal plexus likely contribute to the relaxation of the smooth muscle.

A, B, D, E See correct answer explanation.

Learning objective: Explain the postreceptor mechanism mediating the antidiarrheal effect of atropine.

8. **B** The history and symptoms of the patient indicate that she was most likely suffering from traveler's diarrhea, a gastroenteritis that is usually caused by bacteria endemic to local water. Atropine is still a component of many over-the-counter antidiarrheal preparations available outside the United States. Diarrhea is mediated, at least in part, by an increased activity of the parasympathetic nervous system. By activating M_3 receptors, acetylcholine increases the synthesis of inositol triphosphate/diacylglycerol (IP_3/DAG), which in turn increases the amount of Ca^{2+} available for muscle contraction. By blocking M_3 receptors in the gut, atropine prevents this increase and thus relieves the diarrhea.

A, C, D Atropine does not have these effects.

E Atropine can block presynaptic M_2 receptors, but this action would increase the release of acetylcholine, which would worsen, not relieve, the diarrhea.

Learning objective: Explain the postreceptor mechanism that mediates atropine-induced increase in heart rate.

9. **B** By activating M_2 receptors, acetylcholine opens K^+ channels in the sinoatrial (SA) node. This increases the outward K^+ current, and the membrane becomes hyperpolarized. The result is a decrease in firing rate of the SA node. By blocking M_2 receptors, antimuscarinic drugs counteract the acetylcholine-induced opening of K^+ channels in the SA node. The firing rate of the SA node is increased, causing an increase in heart rate.

   A Acetylcholine-induced release of nitric oxide causes vasodilation, which could lead to reflex tachycardia. By counteracting this action, antimuscarinic drugs would decrease, not increase, the heart rate.

   C Antimuscarinic drugs can counteract acetylcholine-induced decrease in cardiac contractility, but this has nothing to do with the increase in heart rate.

   D Acetylcholine-induced opening of Na^+ channels in ganglionic neurons is mediated by the activation of Nn receptors. Antimuscarinic drugs have weak or negligible blocking activity on these receptors.

   E The blockade of presynaptic autoreceptors increases the release of acetylcholine from cholinergic terminals. This would decrease, not increase, the heart rate.

Learning objective: Explain the mechanism of atropine-induced hyperthermia.

10. **E** Atropine poisoning can occur from honey made from the pollen of plants from the nightshade family. Several cases have been reported in the literature. By blocking M_3 receptors on sweat glands, atropine can reduce sweating enough to raise the body temperature. This occurs primarily in children, because they are especially susceptible to the toxic effects of antimuscarinic drugs.

   A Toxic doses of antimuscarinic drugs cause skin vasodilation.

   B Antimuscarinic drugs do not affect prostaglandin synthesis. Moreover, blockade of prostaglandin synthesis in the hypothalamus has an antipyretic, not a fever-inducing, effect.

   C Uncoupling oxidative phosphorylation in skeletal muscle can cause fever, but this is not an action of antimuscarinic drugs. Uncoupling can be caused by high doses of certain chemicals, such as dinitrophenol and salicylates.

   D The receptors involved in temperature regulation by the hypothalamic thermostatic center are still unknown.

Learning objective: Explain why ipratropium and tiotropium are the only antimuscarinic drugs used to treat bronchospastic disorders.

11. **D** In the past, antimuscarinic drugs were used to treat bronchospastic disorder. However, it was realized that most antimuscarinic drugs reduce the volume of bronchial secretions, which then become thick. This viscous material is difficult to remove from the respiratory tree and can dangerously obstruct airflow. Moreover, the reduced bronchial secretions in turn decrease mucociliary clearance, an important function for the cleaning of the bronchial tree. Therefore, these drugs (except ipratropium and tiotropium) have become contraindicated in respiratory disorders. Ipratropium, for unknown reasons, has negligible effects on bronchial secretions and mucociliary clearance. Thus, its anticholinergic properties can be safely exploited in the treatment of bronchospastic disease.

   A Potency, or the inverse of the dose needed to get a predetermined effect, is almost never the reason for the choice of a specific drug.

   B These drugs are given only by the inhalatory route, so oral bioavailability is not an issue. Moreover, the oral bioavailability is very low, as these drugs are quaternary ammonium compounds and therefore cannot cross lipid membranes.

   C By definition, bioavailability is the fraction of drug reaching the general circulation. When given by inhalatory route, the fraction of ipratropium reaching the general circulation is negligible.

   E Central effects of these drugs are negligible (the drugs are poorly absorbed), but this is not the reason why these drugs are the preferred antimuscarinic agents to treat bronchospastic disorders.

Learning objective: Describe the ocular effects of homatropine.

12. **E** Homatropine is an antimuscarinic drug that blocks M_3 receptors in the sphincter muscle of the iris and in the ciliary muscle. The relaxation of the sphincter muscle of the iris increases pupillary diameter, thus facilitating the eye fundus inspection. The relaxation of the muscle stretches the zonula fibers, which in turn pull the lens capsule and decrease lens curvature. The relaxation of the ciliary muscle also tends to close the spaces of the trabecular meshwork, decreasing aqueous humor outflow, which in turn causes an increase in intraocular pressure.

   A–D See correct answer explanation.

Learning objective: Describe the ocular actions of antimuscarinic drugs.

13. **A** Antimuscarinic drugs relax the ciliary muscle. This action compresses the trabecular meshwork and Schlemm canal, decreasing the outflow of aqueous humor. The final effect is increased intraocular pressure.

    B Aqueous humor production is primarily under the control of the sympathetic nervous system.

    C Vessel tone is primarily under the control of the sympathetic nervous system.

    D The radial muscle of the iris is primarily under the control of the sympathetic nervous system.

    E Episcleral aqueous humor outflow is primarily under the control of prostaglandins.

    F The tarsal is a palpebral smooth muscle and has nothing to do with the control of intraocular pressure.

Learning objective: Describe the pharmacological actions of darifenacin.

14. **E** The patient's symptoms indicate that he was suffering from urge incontinence, the most common form of urinary incontinence affecting the elderly. Darifenacin is a selective M_3 antagonist. By blocking M_3 receptors, the drug relaxes the smooth muscle of the bladder, so the compliance (i.e., a measure of the ease with which a hollow internal organ may be distended) of the bladder is increased.

    A Decreased tone of the internal sphincter of the bladder is mediated by blockade of α_1 adrenoceptors.

    B Relaxation of the prostate capsule is mediated by blockade of α_1 adrenoceptors.

    C Contraction of the detrusor muscle is mediated by activation of M_3 receptors.

    D Diuresis is not under the control of M_3 receptors.

Learning objective: Describe the ocular actions of ipratropium.

15. **E** Ipratropium is a quaternary ammonium antimuscarinic drug. By blocking M_3 receptors in the ciliary muscle, it causes cycloplegia with loss of accommodation for near vision.

    A Systemic effects are unlikely with local administration of the drug. Moreover, urge incontinence is due to contraction of the detrusor muscle. By blocking M_3 receptors, antimuscarinic drugs would cause relaxation, not contraction, of the detrusor muscle.

    B, F Quaternary ammonium antimuscarinic drugs do not cross the blood–brain barrier, so these effects are unlikely.

    C By blocking M_3 receptors, antimuscarinic drugs would cause xerostomia, not salivation.

    D Systemic effects are unlikely with a local administration of the drug. Moreover, by blocking M_2 receptors in the heart, antimuscarinic drugs would increase AV conduction, so AV block is unlikely.

Learning objective: Describe the effects of an overdose of atropine in children.

16. **C** Antimuscarinic drugs are sometime used to prepare the eye for measurement of refractive errors. Even if atropine is administered topically, it can pass into the nasolacrimal duct and be absorbed from the nasal mucosa. Children are especially sensitive to the effects of antimuscarinic drugs and may exhibit the classic central and cardiovascular symptoms of atropine overdose, as in this case.

    A, B Phenylephrine and epinephrine can also be absorbed from the nasal mucosa and could transiently increase the heart rate, but they do not cause central effects, as they do not enter the brain.

    D, E Timolol and pilocarpine would cause a decrease, not an increase, in heart rate.

Learning objective: Describe the adverse effects of atropine.

17. **C** Atropine is still a component of many over-the-counter antidiarrheal preparations available outside the United States. By blocking M_2 receptors in the heart, atropine increases atrioventricular conduction. In a patient with atrial fibrillation, this increase can cause tachycardia (more impulses originating in the atrium can reach the ventricle), which in turn stimulates the release of atrial natriuretic peptide. This explains the patient's urgent need to urinate. It is interesting to note that atropine will increase the urge to urinate while inhibiting the ability to do so. The urge to urinate is due to the increased diuresis that in turn increases filling of the bladder. The consequent increased firing from stretch receptors ascends the spinal cord to the periaqueductal gray, where it projects both to the pontine micturition center and to the cerebrum. At the same time, the anticholinergic activity of atropine tends to relax the detrusor, thus inhibiting the ability to urinate.

    A, B, D, E None of these drugs are used to relieve diarrhea.

Learning objective: Describe the symptoms and signs of scopolamine poisoning.

18. **C** The patient's signs and symptoms indicate he was most likely poisoned by scopolamine, a drug frequently used to "cut" heroin. Epidemics of poisoning caused by heroin adulterated with scopolamine have occurred in New York and the eastern United States. The most frequent symptoms of antimuscarinic poisoning are tachycardia, mild hypertension, dilated pupils, dry and hot skin, and diminished or absent bowel sounds.

    A, B, D, E See correct answer explanation.

Learning objective: Explain the main contraindication of antimuscarinic drugs.

19. **B** Antimuscarinic drugs relax the detrusor muscle, so voiding of the bladder becomes more difficult. This can be especially dangerous in patients with prostatic hyperplasia who already have difficulty in micturition, due to prostate-induced narrowing of the urethra. In these patients, antimuscarinic drugs can precipitate acute urinary retention.

   A Alpha-1 antagonists such as prazosin are actually indicated in prostatic hyperplasia, as they relax the internal sphincter of the bladder.

   C Beta-blockers tend to contract the smooth muscle, as they block β_2 receptor–mediated relaxation. However, these drugs have little influence on nonvascular smooth muscles, which are mainly under parasympathetic control.

   D Alpha-2 agonists activate α_2 receptors, which are mainly presynaptic. This activation in turn can decrease the release of norepinephrine, thereby decreasing the contractility of the internal sphincter of the bladder.

   E Beta-1 agonists do not affect the contractility of smooth muscle.

Learning objective: Describe the therapeutic uses of atropine.

20. **E** Atropine is always used to treat poisoning by cholinesterase inhibitors, because it is able to counteract both the central and peripheral symptoms of acetylcholine excess.

   A Pralidoxime rapidly regenerates the phosphorylated acetylcholinesterase and therefore is useful for the treatment of poisoning due to organophosphates (irreversible cholinesterase inhibitors). However, the drug is contraindicated when poisoning is due to reversible cholinesterase inhibitors, as in this case. In fact, pralidoxime is not able to regenerate the acetylcholinesterase blocked by carbamates; it also has weak anticholinesterase activity.

   B, C Sympathomimetic drugs such as terbutaline and epinephrine are useless in the treatment of poisoning by cholinesterase inhibitors.

   D Glycopyrrolate is a quaternary ammonium antimuscarinic drug. Therefore, it would not be able to counteract the central effects of acetylcholine excess because it does not cross the blood–brain barrier very well.

Learning objective: Describe the therapeutic uses of glycopyrrolate.

21. **D** Antimuscarinic drugs are currently used to treat diarrhea from various causes, including drug-induced diarrhea, as in this case. Quaternary ammonium compounds, such as glycopyrrolate, are sometimes preferred for two reasons:

- There is a clinical impression that they have a relatively greater effect on gastrointestinal activity. This has been attributed to the fact that they can also block nicotinic receptors in parasympathetic ganglia of myenteric and submucosal plexus.
- Because their oral bioavailability is low, when given orally, their effects are mainly limited to the gastrointestinal wall (where they are, initially, more concentrated).

   B Ipratropium is an antimuscarinic quaternary ammonium compound but is given only by the inhalatory route for bronchospastic disorders.

   A, C, E Sympathetic agonists and antagonists have little effect on the gastrointestinal system and are not used to treat diarrhea.

   F Donepezil is a cholinesterase inhibitor and therefore would be contraindicated in this case of diarrhea.

Learning objective: Describe the therapeutic uses of atropine.

22. **C** Atropine is sometimes used to prevent vagal reflexes when surgery is performed near the location of the vagus nerve, as in this case.

   A Ipratropium is an antimuscarinic drug, but it is used only by inhalation for bronchospastic disease.

   B, D, E Dopamine, isoproterenol, and epinephrine can increase the heart rate, but atropine is much more effective when bradycardia is due to parasympathetic activation.

Learning objective: Describe the therapeutic uses of atropine.

23. **D** Asystole is the complete electrocardiographic absence of electrical activity. Its development usually indicates a prolonged cardiac arrest and carries a very grave prognosis.

   In the treatment of asystole, epinephrine is the initial agent of choice to generate a rhythm. Because enhanced parasympathetic tone, possibly also due to chest compression, may play a role in inhibiting supraventricular and ventricular pacemakers, anticholinergic drugs may be beneficial, and atropine is usually tried when epinephrine fails.

   A Neostigmine increases cholinergic activity and is therefore absolutely contraindicated in this setting.

   B, C When epinephrine does not work, the choice of other sympathomimetic drugs, such as norepinephrine and dopamine, is irrational.

   E Ipratropium is an anticholinergic agent but is used only by inhalation for bronchospastic disorders.

Learning objective: Describe the interactions between mecamylamine and other autonomic drugs.

24. **C** Norepinephrine increases the mean blood pressure. This increase causes a stimulation of aortic baroreceptors, which activates the baroreceptor reflex. The increased vagal discharge overcomes the direct effect of norepinephrine on the heart rate (an increase due to the activation of β_1 receptors), so the final effect is a decrease in heart rate. Ganglionic blockers such as mecamylamine impair the baroreceptor reflex, thereby abolishing bradycardia.

    A Neostigmine is a cholinesterase inhibitor that increases the availability of acetylcholine at every cholinergic synapse. Acetylcholine activates M_3 receptors in the gut and Nn receptors in the autonomic ganglia. Both actions contribute to the increase in intestinal peristalsis. A ganglionic blocker can prevent the activation of Nn receptors but has no effect on the activation of M_3 receptors. Therefore, peristalsis will be decreased but not completely abolished.

    B Nicotine-induced contraction of skeletal muscle is due to activation of Nm receptors. Ganglionic blockers have negligible activity on these receptors.

    D Epinephrine-induced tachycardia is due to the activation of cardiac β_1 and β_2 receptors. A ganglionic blocker cannot block these receptors.

    E Ganglionic blockers actually cause hypotension by blocking the sympathetic discharge to the vessels. Therefore, the propranolol-induced hypotension is in fact enhanced, not prevented.

Learning objective: Describe the adverse effects of antimuscarinic drugs.

25. **C** By blocking M_2 receptors, antimuscarinic drugs decrease the vagal control to the heart, which is mainly on sinoatrial and atrioventricular nodes. This can lead to an increased heart rate that in turn can cause a conscious awareness of the heart beating (i.e., palpitations).

    A, B, D, E By blocking muscarinic receptors, atropine tends to cause effects opposite to those listed.

Learning objective: Describe the interactions between atropine and other autonomic drugs.

26. **A** Physostigmine is a cholinesterase inhibitor, and therefore it can increase the availability of acetylcholine at cholinergic neuroeffector junctions. Activation of M_3 receptors in sweat glands promotes sweating. By blocking M_3 receptors, atropine can counteract this action.

    B Epinephrine increase blood pressure by activating α_1 and β_1 receptors. These receptors are not affected by atropine.

    C Nicotine can cause skin vasoconstriction by activating Nn receptors in sympathetic ganglia. Atropine has negligible effects on Nn receptors.

D Prazosin can cause reflex tachycardia by blocking α_1 receptors, which in turn decreases the blood pressure. Atropine actually can cause tachycardia and therefore can increase, not counteract, the action of prazosin.

    E Glycopyrrolate induces bronchodilation by blocking M_3 and Nn receptors. Atropine can block M_3 receptors and therefore can increase, not counteract, the action of glycopyrrolate.

Learning objective: Explain the molecular mechanism of action of ipratropium on the eye.

27. **A** Ipratropium nasal spray is approved by the U.S. Food and Drug Administration for the management of rhinorrhea from various causes. When given by this route, the drug can cause antimuscarinic effects on the eye. The blockade of M_3 receptors on the sphincter muscle of the iris causes mydriasis, which in turn can lead to photophobia, whereas the blockade of M_3 receptors in the ciliary muscle causes cycloplegia, which in turn leads to impairment of near vision.

    B Ipratropium blocks, not activates, M_3 receptors.

    C–F Ipratropium has no effect on adrenoceptors.

Learning objective: Describe the pharmacological action that contributes to atropine-induced increase in heart rate.

28. **D** Bradycardia that occurs after a myocardial infarction is often due to an AV block, which often results from increased parasympathetic tone and usually responds to atropine. Sometimes the block resolves spontaneously, but atropine is given when the heart rate is too low for sufficient cardiac output.

    A–C, E, F See correct answer explanation.

Learning objective: Explain the molecular mechanism of action of glycopyrrolate given topically to manage hyperhidrosis.

29. **E** Glycopyrrolate is a quaternary antimuscarinic drug sometimes used locally to counteract excessive sweating. The drug blocks M_3 receptors located in the sweat glands, thus relieving hyperhidrosis. However, relief is incomplete at best, likely because apocrine rather than exocrine glands are usually involved in the excessive sweating, and the autonomic control of apocrine glands seems adrenergic rather than cholinergic.

    A, C, D These receptors do not mediate sweating.

    B Glycopyrrolate can block Nn receptors in autonomic ganglia. This action can contribute to the final effect of relieving excessive sweating when the drug is given parenterally. However, when given locally, the drug can reach the sweat glands located in the dermis but not the sympathetic ganglia located on the spinal cord.

Learning objective: Describe the action of ganglionic blockers on heart rate.

30. **C** Ganglionic blocking drugs block Nn receptors on both sympathetic and parasympathetic ganglia. Therefore, the heart is no longer under autonomic control and goes back to its intrinsic rate, which is approximately 100 bpm.

   A, B, D, E See correct answer explanation.

CHOLINERGIC DRUGS
Answer key

1.	F	6.	E	11.	D
2.	C	7.	C	12.	E
3.	B	8.	B	13.	A
4.	G	9.	B	14.	E
5.	E	10.	E	15.	E
16.	C	21.	D	26.	A
17.	C	22.	C	27.	A
18.	C	23.	D	28.	D
19.	B	24.	C	29.	E
20.	E	25.	C	30.	C

III Central Nervous System

Questions: III-1 Introduction to Central Nervous System Pharmacology

Difficulty level: Easy

1. A 3-year-old boy was brought to the emergency department after eating some black berries from a plant in the woods. Physical examination showed a disoriented and hallucinating patient with dilated pupils, dry mouth, red and dry skin, and body temperature of 103.4°F (39.7°C). Vital signs were blood pressure 90/50 mm Hg, pulse 122 bpm, respirations 24/min. The central and peripheral symptoms of this patient were most likely mediated by the blockade of which of the following receptors?

   A. Noradrenergic
   B. Nicotinic
   C. Muscarinic
   D. Dopaminergic
   E. Serotonergic
   F. GABAergic
   G. Glutamatergic

Difficulty level: Hard

2. A 33-year-old man who was a heavy smoker started a medically assisted program to quit smoking. Therapy included the administration of an agonist at α_2 presynaptic receptors that acts mainly on noradrenergic neurons in the brain. Which of the following brain regions was most likely involved in the therapeutic effect of the drug in this patient?

   A. Nucleus basalis of Meynert
   B. Central raphe nucleus
   C. Locus ceruleus
   D. Substantia nigra
   E. Amygdala
   F. Nucleus tractus solitarius

Difficulty level: Medium

3. A 46-year-old woman complained to her physician of daytime sleepiness. One day earlier, she had started taking an antihistamine for allergic rhinitis. The physician explained that drowsiness was most likely due to inhibition of the action of histaminergic neurons in the brain. Which of the following brain regions was most likely involved in the adverse effect of this drug?

   A. Nucleus tractus solitarius
   B. Caudatum
   C. Hippocampus
   D. Nucleus basalis of Meynert
   E. Amygdala
   F. Ventral posterior hypothalamus

Difficulty level: Medium

4. A 51-year-old man suffering from episodic leg cramps started a treatment with a drug that activates $GABA_B$ receptors both in the brain and in the spinal cord. This activation most likely opened which of the following ion channels?

   A. K^+
   B. Cl^-
   C. Ca^{2+}
   D. Mg^{++}
   E. Na^+

Difficulty level: Easy

5. A 54-year-old woman suffering from initial insomnia was prescribed a hypnotic drug that increases the activity of a major neurotransmitter system in the brain. Which of the following neurotransmitter systems was most likely involved in the therapeutic action of that drug?

   A. Cholinergic
   B. Noradrenergic
   C. Glutamatergic
   D. GABAergic
   E. Dopaminergic
   F. Endorphinergic

Difficulty level: Medium

6. A 54-year-old woman was admitted unconscious to the emergency department after a car accident. After physical and lab exams, a diagnosis of brain injury was made. It is known that in brain injury, a rapid and large increase of Ca^{2+} influx into damaged neurons can contribute significantly to neuronal death (a process called excitotoxicity). Activation of which of the following brain receptors most likely caused this metabolic derangement in the patient?

   A. Presynaptic α_2 adrenoceptors
   B. Postsynaptic α_2 adrenoceptors
   C. Presynaptic NMDA receptors
   D. Postsynaptic NMDA receptors
   E. Presynaptic GABA receptors
   F. Postsynaptic GABA receptors

Difficulty level: Easy

7. A 35-year-old woman was admitted to a psychiatric hospital for evaluation. She reported episodic feelings of sadness since adolescence, but she had noticed a gradual worsening in her mood over the past 3 weeks. She had depressed mood most of the day, had lost interest in any leisure activity, and had difficulty sleeping, poor appetite, low energy, feelings of guilt, and recurrent thoughts of death. Which of the following pairs of neurotransmitters were most likely involved in the patient's disorder?

A. Glutamate and serotonin
B. Norepinephrine and glutamate
C. Glutamate and acetylcholine
D. Serotonin and acetylcholine
E. Serotonin and norepinephrine
F. Acetylcholine and norepinephrine

Difficulty level: Easy

8. A 63-year-old woman recently diagnosed with generalized anxiety disorder started a treatment with a drug that increases serotonin availability in the synaptic cleft. Which of the following enzymes is the rate-limiting step in serotonin biosynthesis?

A. Tyrosine hydroxylase
B. Dopamine-ß-hydroxylase
C. Tryptophan hydroxylase
D. Choline acetyl transferase
E. L-amino acid decarboxylase

Difficulty level: Easy

9. A 26-year-old man with a long history of polydrug abuse stated that he felt an intense euphoric sensation every time he self-administered any illicit drug. Which of the following items correctly pairs the neurotransmitter and the central nervous system site most likely involved in the rewarding effect of abused drugs?

A. GABA–amygdala
B. Acetylcholine–nucleus basalis of Meynert
C. Histamine–nucleus accumbens
D. Dopamine–basal ganglia
E. Serotonin–raphe nuclei
F. Dopamine–nucleus accumbens
G. Serotonin–amygdala

Difficulty level: Easy

10. The pharmacological activity of five new central nervous system (CNS) drugs (P, Q, R, S, and T) was studied in laboratory animals. All drugs were able to change the availability of specific CNS neurotransmitters in the synaptic cleft. The results are reported in the table below.

Drug	Norepinephrine	Acetylcholine	GABA	Serotonin
P	+	0	+	+
Q	– –	++	0	++
R	0	0	+++	+
S	+++	–	–	+++
T	0	+++	0	0

+ = increased availability
– = decreased availability
0 = negligible effect
Abbreviation: GABA, gamma-aminobutyric acid.

Which of the following drugs is likely to be most effective in the treatment of Alzheimer disease?

A. Drug P
B. Drug Q
C. Drug R
D. Drug S
E. Drug T

Difficulty level: Easy

11. A 32-year-old woman was brought to the emergency department because of a generalized tonic-clonic seizure. Her husband stated that his wife had been suffering from epilepsy since childhood, but the seizures were only partially controlled by medication. Which of the following pairs of neurotransmitters are thought to be most involved in seizure disorders?

A. GABA and serotonin
B. GABA and glutamate
C. GABA and acetylcholine
D. Serotonin and glutamate
E. Serotonin and acetylcholine
F. Acetylcholine and glutamate

Difficulty level: Medium

12. A 34-year-old female patient in a psychiatric hospital had been standing immobile for several hours with one of her arms stretched upward. The patient was mute, unresponsive, and did not appear aware of her surroundings. When placed in another awkward posture, the patient maintained that posture for a long time without apparent distress. Which of the following neurotransmitters has been consistently implicated in the patient's syndrome?

A. Norepinephrine
B. Acetylcholine
C. Histamine
D. Dopamine
E. GABA

Difficulty level: Medium

13. The pharmacological activity of five new central nervous system drugs (P, Q, R, S, and T) was studied in laboratory

animals. All drugs were able to change the availability of specific central nervous system neurotransmitters in the synaptic cleft. The results are reported in the table below.

Drug	Dopamine	Acetylcholine	GABA	Serotonin
P	+++	+++	0	- - -
Q	- -	++	0	+
R	+++	- -	0	0
S	+	0	+++	+++
T	+	+++	+	-

+ = increased availability
− = decreased availability
0 = negligible effect
Abbreviation: GABA, gamma-aminobutyric acid.

Which of the drugs would be most effective in the treatment of Parkinson disease?

A. Drug P
B. Drug Q
C. Drug R
D. Drug S
E. Drug T

Difficulty level: Easy

14. A 71-year-old man recently diagnosed with Alzheimer disease started a therapy with a drug that acts mainly on the central cholinergic system. Which of the following brain regions was most likely involved in the therapeutic effect of the drug in this patient?

A. Nucleus basalis of Meynert
B. Central raphe nucleus
C. Locus ceruleus
D. Substantia nigra
E. Amygdala
F. Nucleus tractus solitarius

Difficulty level: Easy

15. A 41-year-old woman was admitted to the psychiatric hospital because of a 1-year history of apprehension and worry. She had been feeling tense most of the time, was often irritable, and found it hard to concentrate because of her constant distress. After psychiatric examination, a diagnosis of generalized anxiety disorder was made, and a therapy was prescribed that included a drug with pronounced anxiolytic activity. Which of the following neurophysiological actions most likely mediated the therapeutic effect of that drug?

A. Increased serotonergic transmission
B. Decreased serotonergic transmission
C. Increased dopaminergic transmission
D. Decreased dopaminergic transmission
E. Increased glutamatergic transmission
F. Decreased glutamatergic transmission

Difficulty level: Easy

16. A 32-year-old man who had been injured in a car accident 1 month earlier presented to the hospital for a follow-up visit. Neurologic examination disclosed slowness of intentional movements and spasticity. A diagnosis of upper motor neuron syndrome due to damage of pyramidal motor neurons was made. Which of the following neurotransmitters was most likely involved in the patient's syndrome?

A. Norepinephrine
B. Glutamate
C. Acetylcholine
D. Dopamine
E. GABA

Difficulty level: Medium

17. A 24-year-old woman presented to a psychiatrist complaining of a distressing behavior. For the past several months she experienced an irresistible urge to check that everything was in a certain order at home and found it hard to get out of the house because she needed, again and again, to verify that the door was locked. She admitted her urge was irrational, but she was unable to control it. After psychiatric examination, a diagnosis was made, and a drug was prescribed. Which of the following neurotransmitters has been most consistently implicated in the patient's disorder?

A. Acetylcholine
B. Norepinephrine
C. GABA
D. Serotonin
E. Glutamate
F. Histamine

Difficulty level: Easy

18. A 44-year-old man was admitted unconscious to the emergency department. Shortly after admission, he had a tonic-clonic seizure. Further exams led to the diagnosis of status epilepticus, and he was treated with a drug that increased the activity of a central neurotransmitter able to generate only inhibitory postsynaptic potentials (IPSPs) by increasing Cl^- or K^+ conductance. Which of the following neurotransmitters was most likely affected by the drug treatment?

A. Glutamate
B. Acetylcholine
C. Norepinephrine
D. GABA
E. Dopamine

19. A 37-year-old man recently diagnosed with partial seizures started a treatment with a drug that is thought to act by blocking *N*-methyl-D-aspartate (NMDA) receptors in the brain. Which of the following central systems was most likely affected by that drug?

   A. Noradrenergic
   B. Cholinergic
   C. Histaminergic
   D. Dopaminergic
   E. Serotonergic
   F. GABAergic
   G. Glutamatergic

20. A 36-year-old man was brought to the emergency department after a serious car accident. He began to experience severe pain throughout his body. Which of the following triplets of neurotransmitters most likely acted in the central nervous system to decrease pain signaling in this patient?

   A. Norepinephrine, GABA, glutamate
   B. Glutamate, norepinephrine, opioid peptides
   C. Histamine, acetylcholine, GABA
   D. Histamine, acetylcholine, opioid peptides
   E. Glutamate, GABA, serotonin
   F. Opioid peptides, norepinephrine, serotonin

Questions: III-2 Sedative and Hypnotic Drugs

Directions for questions **1–6**

Match each sedative-hypnotic drug with the appropriate description (each lettered option can be selected once, more than once, or not at all).

   A. Alprazolam
   B. Buspirone
   C. Clonazepam
   D. Flumazenil
   E. Flunitrazepam
   F. Lorazepam
   G. Midazolam
   H. Phenobarbital
   I. Thiopental
   J. Zolpidem

1. A partial agonist at serotonin (5-hydroxytryptamine, 5-HT) 5-HT$_{1A}$ receptors

2. A competitive antagonist at benzodiazepine receptors

3. A hypnotic drug with negligible effects on sleep architecture and stages

4. The barbiturate most frequently used to induce general anesthesia

5. A benzodiazepine with a very short half-life (about 2 hours)

6. An anxiolytic drug with negligible abuse liability

7. A 42-year-old man recently diagnosed with generalized anxiety disorder had started a treatment with sertraline, but the drug caused some sexual dysfunction, and the psychiatrist decided to switch to a short course of alprazolam. Which of the following molecular actions on neuronal membranes most likely mediated the therapeutic effect of alprazolam in the patient's disorder?

   A. Decreased outward Na$^+$ current
   B. Increased inward Cl$^-$ current
   C. Decreased outward K$^+$ current
   D. Increased inward Ca^{2+} current
   E. Increased inward H current

8. A 63-year-old woman was referred to a psychiatrist because of easy fatigue, worry, irritability, and difficulty concentrating. These symptoms had been present almost continuously during the daytime since she retired from her job as a schoolteacher 1 month ago. She told the doctor that those symptoms were unbearable and that she wanted to die. A preliminary diagnosis of severe generalized anxiety disorder was made, and a treatment with sertraline and diazepam was prescribed. Which of the following adverse effects were most likely to occur during the first days of therapy?

   A. Excitement and irritability
   B. Mental confusion and anterograde amnesia
   C. Excessive sedation and drowsiness
   D. Respiratory depression and apnea
   E. Disturbing dreams and early awakening

Difficulty level: Medium

9. A 36-year-old man was referred to a psychiatrist because of irritability, worrying thoughts, palpitations, dry mouth, and insomnia of 1-month duration. The man had a past history of alcohol abuse, but he was able to quit 1 year ago after psychological counseling and drug therapy. Recently, he suffered from erectile dysfunction, treated with sildenafil. A provisional diagnosis of generalized anxiety disorder was made, and cognitive behavioral therapy with a drug treatment was prescribed. Which of the following drugs would be most appropriate for this patient?

A. Diazepam
B. Fluoxetine
C. Lorazepam
D. Haloperidol
E. Lithium
F. Buspirone

Difficulty level: Easy

10. A 75-year-old woman was undergoing cystoscopy for a suspected papilloma of the bladder. Before the procedure, the anesthesiologist administered alprazolam to induce conscious sedation and to avoid situational anxiety. When the cystoscopy was over, flumazenil was administered. Which of the following terms best defines the mode of action of this drug?

A. Full agonist
B. Functional antagonist
C. Partial agonist
D. Inverse agonist
E. Competitive antagonist

Difficulty level: Easy

11. A 44-year-old man complained to his physician of being tired, irritable, and tense, with frequent stomach upset and diarrhea. The man denied past or present use of any illicit drugs or alcohol. Past medical history of the patient was significant for peptic ulcer, presently treated with omeprazole, and for myasthenia gravis, presently treated with neostigmine. After further clinical assessment, a diagnosis of generalized anxiety disorder was made, and an appropriate therapy was prescribed. Which of the following drugs would be relatively contraindicated for this patient?

A. Venlafaxine
B. Buspirone
C. Paroxetine
D. Diazepam
E. Sertraline

Difficulty level: Easy

12. A 63-year-old woman complained to her physician of difficulty in falling asleep. She denied nocturnal insomnia or early awaking. The doctor prescribed ramelteon, one tablet at bedtime. Which of the following molecular actions most likely mediated the therapeutic effect of the drug?

A. Activation of $GABA_B$ receptors
B. Blockade of α_1 receptors
C. Activation of melatonin receptors
D. Blockade of glutamate receptors
E. Activation of serotonin 5-HT_3 receptors

Difficulty level: Easy

13. A 58-year-old man was admitted to the hospital for a laparoscopic hernia repair. General anesthesia was induced by intravenous diazepam, and the patient lost consciousness in about 1 minute. He regained consciousness about 35 minutes later. Knowing that the half-life of diazepam is about 40 hours, which of the following items best explains the short action of the drug?

A. Rapid metabolism of the drug within the central nervous system
B. Rapid excretion of the drug by the kidneys
C. Redistribution of the drug from central nervous system to other tissues
D. Biotransformation of the drug into inactive metabolites
E. Development of a rapid tolerance to drug effects

Difficulty level: Easy

14. A 43-year-old man suffering from rectal bleeding was admitted to the hospital for a colonoscopy. An intravenous injection of diazepam was given before the procedure to induce a conscious sedation. Which of the following symptoms did the patient most likely experience upon recovery from sedation?

A. Nausea and vomiting
B. Increased respiratory rate
C. Anterograde amnesia
D. Limb muscle spasms
E. Delusional thoughts

Difficulty level: Easy

15. A 34-year-old man exhibited severe agitation, fearfulness, and apprehension upon recovery from surgery to remove a colon cancer. He was given an intravenous injection of a drug that acts by making the resting membrane potentials of short interneurons in several brain areas more negative. Which of the following drugs was most likely administered?

A. Trazodone
B. Haloperidol
C. Thiopental
D. Alprazolam
E. Buspirone
F. Imipramine

Difficulty level: Easy

16. A 16-year-old girl brought by ambulance to the emergency department was diagnosed with status epilepticus and was given an intravenous injection of a drug that binds to the α subunit of the GABA$_A$ receptor complex. Which of the following drugs was most likely administered?

A. Lorazepam
B. Zolpidem
C. Flumazenil
D. Phenytoin
E. Valproic acid

Difficulty level: Medium

17. A 67-year-old woman suffering from primary insomnia had started treatment with zolpidem, but the drug was withdrawn because she developed conjunctivitis, apparently due to a hypersensitivity reaction to the drug. Her physician prescribed behavioral therapy and a short course of temazepam, one tablet at bedtime. Which of the following was most likely an action of the drug on the patient's sleep architecture?

A. Decreased number of rapid eye movement (REM) sleep cycles
B. Decreased latency of sleep onset
C. Increased duration of slow-wave sleep
D. Increased duration of stage 1 sleep
E. Decreased duration of stage 2 sleep

Difficulty level: Medium

18. An 82-year-old man was brought to his physician by his son, who reported that his father appeared oversedated, spending the whole day dozing. Further questioning revealed that the man had for some time been taking a "sleeping pill" given to him by a friend, but he did not remember the name of the drug. Which of the following drugs most likely caused the patient's disorder?

A. Zolpidem
B. Temazepam
C. Ramelteon
D. Chlorpromazine
E. Buspirone
F. Phenobarbital

Difficulty level: Easy

19. A 78-year-old man was admitted to the hospital because of a broken leg. His wife reported that he was walking in the dining room when he suddenly lost his balance and fell down. The man had been suffering from atrial fibrillation, insomnia, hypertension, and anxiety. The patient's medications on admission were atenolol, warfarin, diazepam, losartan, and hydrochlorothiazide. Which of these drugs was most likely to have contributed to the patient's accident?

A. Atenolol
B. Warfarin
C. Diazepam
D. Losartan
E. Hydrochlorothiazide

Difficulty level: Easy

20. A 45-year-old man had been suffering from a central nervous system disorder for many years. Recently, a barbiturate was added to his pharmacotherapy. Which of the following central nervous system effects was most likely elicited by that drug?

A. Antidepressant
B. Antiparkinson
C. Antipsychotic
D. Anticonvulsant
E. Analgesic

Difficulty level: Medium

21. A 66-year-old man who had been a heavy smoker for 30 years was undergoing bronchoscopy for suspected bronchogenic carcinoma. Before starting the intervention, the anesthesiologist administered a drug to prevent situational anxiety and to provide anterograde amnesia of the procedure. Which of the following drugs would be appropriate for this patient?

A. Buspirone
B. Chlorpromazine
C. Zolpidem
D. Oxazepam
E. Haloperidol

Difficulty level: Easy

22. A 37-year-old man was brought unconscious to the emergency department. His roommate stated that the man had been very depressed for the last few days and that he had

been drinking whiskey all day. The roommate also said he found an empty, unlabeled drug bottle next to him on the bed. Which of the following drugs most likely contributed to the patient's intoxication?

A. Buspirone
B. Diazepam
C. Venlafaxine
D. Fluoxetine
E. Lithium

Difficulty level: Medium

23. A 61-year-old obese man complained of difficulty in falling asleep and asked his physician for a sleeping pill. The man had been recently diagnosed with obstructive sleep apnea, most likely due to obesity. Which of the following drugs would be contraindicated for this patient?

A. Temazepam
B. Acetazolamide
C. Imipramine
D. Medroxyprogesterone
E. Protriptyline

Difficulty level: Easy

24. A 26-year-old woman, suffering from cerebral palsy and seizures secondary to head injury, was seen in a clinic for a scheduled visit. She was spastic and unable to walk. Medical history indicated that for the month prior to the visit, her seizures had not been well controlled. Which of the following drugs would be appropriate to improve her seizure control and muscle spasms?

A. Buspirone
B. Lithium
C. Donepezil
D. Haloperidol
E. Fluoxetine
F. Diazepam

Difficulty level: Medium

25. A 32-year-old man complained to his physician of attacks of intense terror while he was asleep, such as feeling crushed. He often woke up screaming but without remembering any specific dream. He also felt worried and restless from time to time during the day. Which of the following drugs would be most likely to provide a short-term decrease in the patient's symptoms?

A. Lithium
B. Temazepam
C. Haloperidol
D. Imipramine
E. Phenobarbital

Difficulty level: Medium

26. A 34-year-old woman visited a psychiatrist because of overwhelming panic symptoms that occurred "out of the blue." She felt light-headed, dizzy, and feared losing control or going crazy. She also felt nausea, a lump in her throat, shortness of breath, and palpitations. These symptoms lasted about 30 minutes. The woman had two of these attacks the previous month. Two days ago she had started a treatment with sertraline prescribed by her family physician, but yesterday she suffered another attack. After further clinical assessment, a preliminary diagnosis was made, and the psychiatrist decided to prescribe a drug in addition to sertraline. Which of the following would be an appropriate additional drug for the patient at this time?

A. Aripiprazole
B. Thiopental
C. Buspirone
D. Alprazolam
E. Eszopiclone

Difficulty level: Easy

27. A 56-year-old homeless alcoholic man was brought to the emergency department by police, who found him wandering in the street. The man was nauseated, tremulous, and hallucinating. He stated he was out of money and unable to buy his usual daily amount of whiskey. Which of the following would be an appropriate drug to treat the acute alcohol withdrawal of this patient?

A. Naltrexone
B. Imipramine
C. Haloperidol
D. Buspirone
E. Ethanol
F. Diazepam

Difficulty level: Easy

28. A 57-year-old man complained to his physician that he had difficulty in falling asleep. He was a schoolteacher and needed a good night's sleep to perform effectively during the day. Zolpidem was prescribed, one tablet at bedtime. The prescribed drug most likely caused which of the following effects on ion conductance of central nervous system neurons?

A. Decreased Na^+ conductance
B. Increased Cl^- conductance
C. Decreased K^+ conductance
D. Decreased Ca^{2+} conductance
E. Increased K^+ conductance

Difficulty level: Medium

29. A 49-year-old woman complained to her physician that she could get to sleep when she went to bed but woke up several times during the night and never felt refreshed in the morning. The woman had no medical problems and took no medications. Which of the following drugs would be most appropriate for this patient?

   A. Flunitrazepam
   B. Buspirone
   C. Eszopiclone
   D. Fluoxetine
   E. Haloperidol
   F. Imipramine

Difficulty level: Medium

30. A 43-year-old man was brought to the emergency department after a car accident. He showed only minor injuries but was very anxious and excited. The patient had a history of epilepsy and had been stabilized on phenobarbital for several years. The attending physician administered a sedative drug intravenously. Several minutes later the patient became cyanotic and apneic, and his blood pressure was 100/55 mm Hg. Which of the following drugs most likely caused these adverse effects?

   A. Buspirone
   B. Haloperidol
   C. Diazepam
   D. Fluoxetine
   E. Thiopental
   F. Chlorpromazine

Questions: III-3 General Anesthetics

Directions for questions **1–5**

Match each general anesthetic with the appropriate description (each lettered option can be selected once, more than once, or not at all).

   A. Halothane
   B. Sevoflurane
   C. Nitrous oxide
   D. Thiopental
   E. Propofol
   F. Etomidate
   G. Ketamine
   H. Midazolam
   I. Fentanyl

Difficulty level: Easy

1. A halogenated anesthetic that causes fast induction and recovery

Difficulty level: Easy

2. A drug that can trigger an attack of acute porphyria in at-risk patients

Difficulty level: Easy

3. This drug has the highest incidence of postanesthetic nausea and vomiting.

Difficulty level: Easy

4. This inhaled anesthetic substantially reduces the required concentration of other inhaled anesthetics given concomitantly.

Difficulty level: Easy

5. A drug that can cause a cataleptic state called dissociative anesthesia

Difficulty level: Medium

6. Five new potential inhalational anesthetics (P, Q, R, S, and T) were tested in laboratory animals. Some pharmacological parameters of each drug are recorded in the table below:

Drug	MAC	Induction
P	5.5	Slow
Q	45.2	Fast
R	12.7	Fast
S	0.9	Slow
T	3.2	Fast

Abbreviation: MAC, minimum alveolar concentration.

Which of the following drugs has the highest potency?

   A. Drug P
   B. Drug Q
   C. Drug R
   D. Drug S
   E. Drug T

Difficulty level: Easy

7. A 59-year-old man underwent surgery to repair an inguinal hernia. Lorazepam was administered as preanesthetic medication. General anesthesia was induced by propofol and maintained with halothane and nitrous oxide. Ondansetron was also given to prevent vomiting. Fifteen minutes after starting the operation, the electrocardiogram monitor showed ventricular tachycardia. Which of the drugs most likely caused this adverse effect?

A. Lorazepam
B. Propofol
C. Nitrous oxide
D. Halothane
E. Ondansetron

Difficulty level: Easy

8. A 32-year-old man was admitted to the hospital for reduction of a dislocated shoulder. Sedation with diazepam was supplemented with a 30% concentration of nitrous oxide. Which of the following effects most likely occurred after nitrous oxide administration?

A. Excellent skeletal muscle relaxation
B. Very pronounced analgesia
C. Rapidly achieved unconsciousness
D. Sharp decrease in blood pressure
E. Profound respiratory depression

Difficulty level: Hard

9. A 64-year-old man underwent surgery for prostate cancer. An intravenous injection of thiopental was administered, and the patient lost consciousness in about 10 seconds. Which of the following was most likely the major mechanism of action mediating the anesthetic effect of this drug?

A. Increased affinity of GABA for $GABA_A$ receptors
B. Enhancement of β-carboline affinity for $GABA_A$ receptors
C. Blockade of NMDA glutamate receptors in the central nervous system
D. Enhancement of Cl^- channel opening in the absence of GABA
E. Activation of $GABA_B$ receptors on presynaptic terminals

Difficulty level: Easy

10. A 34-year-old woman was admitted to the day surgery center for strabismus surgery. This surgery is considered highly emetogenic due to a stimulation of the vomiting center during the operative manipulation of extraocular muscles. Which of the following anesthetics would be most appropriate for this patient?

A. Ketamine
B. Halothane
C. Fentanyl
D. Propofol
E. Thiopental

Difficulty level: Easy

11. A 52-year-old woman underwent hysterectomy to remove an endometrial carcinoma. Anesthesia was induced with thiopental and maintained with nitrous oxide and halothane. Which of the following reasons best explains why another anesthetic, in this case halothane, was added to nitrous oxide?

A. To achieve a more complete analgesia
B. To maintain unconsciousness and muscle relaxation
C. To prevent sensitization of the myocardium to catecholamines
D. To prevent anesthesia-induced respiratory depression
E. To prevent postanesthetic nausea and vomiting

Difficulty level: Easy

12. A 12-year-old boy was admitted to the hospital with the admitting diagnosis of acute appendicitis. Family history of the patient indicated that his father underwent surgery a few years earlier and suffered a serious disorder just after the beginning of general anesthesia. Further analysis indicated that the disorder was an inherited autosomal dominant disease. Because of this, the anesthesiologist avoided the use of halogenated anesthetics in this boy. Which of the following was most likely the disorder suffered by the patient's father?

A. Acute intermittent porphyria
B. Malignant hyperthermia
C. Acute hepatitis
D. Hemolytic anemia
E. Myasthenia gravis

Difficulty level: Easy

13. A 43-year-old man underwent surgery to remove a prostatic cancer. Sevoflurane was used for general anesthesia. The drug has a minimum alveolar concentration (MAC) of 2%. Which of the following best describes the MAC of an inhalational anesthetic?

A. The blood/gas partition coefficient of the anesthetic
B. The concentration of anesthetic needed for short surgery
C. The ED_{50} on a conventional quantal dose–response curve
D. The maximal efficacy of the anesthetic
E. The concentration of anesthetic in the inspired air

14. A 48-year-old woman underwent surgery to remove a uterine myoma. General anesthesia was induced with propofol and maintained by sevoflurane and nitrous oxide. The blockade of which of the following receptors most likely mediated the effectiveness of nitrous oxide in this patient?

    A. Nm cholinergic
    B. Alpha-1 adrenergic
    C. NMDA glutamatergic
    D. GABAergic
    E. 5-HT$_3$ serotonergic

15. A 44-year-old woman underwent surgery because of a prolapsed intervertebral disk. General anesthesia was induced with propofol and maintained with sevoflurane. When administration of sevoflurane was discontinued, the patient regained consciousness in a few minutes. Which of the following statements best explains why anesthetic recovery is so rapid when sevoflurane administration is stopped?

    A. It redistributed rapidly to the lipid tissue.
    B. It is rapidly metabolized.
    C. It has a low minimum alveolar concentration (MAC) value.
    D. It has a low blood/gas partition coefficient.
    E. It distributes mainly into the cerebral cortex.

16. A 63-year-old woman underwent surgery to remove a vulvar cancer. The patient was a heavy smoker and had been suffering from chronic obstructive pulmonary disease for 20 years. General anesthesia was induced with propofol and maintained with isoflurane. Which of the following effects most likely occurred during surgery?

    A. Decreased cardiac output
    B. Increased ventilatory response to carbon dioxide
    C. Bronchodilation
    D. Increased skeletal muscle tone
    E. Increased uterine tone

17. A 55-year-old man suffering from chronic heart failure underwent an exploratory laparotomy because of an abdominal swelling. The anesthesia protocol included a drug that causes rapid induction, a very rapid rate of recovery, and minimal changes in cardiovascular and respiratory functions. Which of the following drugs was most likely administered?

    A. Halothane
    B. Ketamine
    C. Propofol
    D. Thiopental
    E. Etomidate

18. A 4-year-old girl who had been suffering from severe asthma for 6 months was scheduled for a short suture procedure that was anticipated to take approximately 10 minutes. She was brought to the operating room by her parents and was in distress over parting from them and afraid of the doctors. Which of the following drugs would be appropriate for providing sedation and analgesia for this girl?

    A. Ketamine
    B. Thiopental
    C. Fentanyl
    D. Halothane
    E. Sevoflurane

19. A 52-year-old man underwent liver biopsy for a suspected liver cancer. Conscious sedation was induced with a drug combination that has the advantage of being reversible by the administration of specific receptor antagonists. Which of the following pairs of drugs was most likely administered?

    A. Fentanyl and thiopental
    B. Fentanyl and midazolam
    C. Fentanyl and ketamine
    D. Thiopental and midazolam
    E. Thiopental and ketamine

20. A 57-year-old man was undergoing surgery to remove a kidney carcinoma. The anesthesia was induced with propofol, maintained with halothane, and supplemented by succinylcholine. A few minutes into the operation, the patient exhibited a fever of 104°F (40°C), skeletal muscle contracture, and profuse diaphoresis. His blood pressure dropped to 80/50 mm Hg, and the heart rate was 125 bpm. Which of the following molecular actions best explains the signs and symptoms of the patient?

    A. Excessive release of acetylcholine from motor neuron terminals
    B. Opening of K^+ channels in the skeletal muscle membrane
    C. Excessive release of Ca^{2+} from the sarcoplasmic reticulum
    D. Blockade of Ca^{2+} channel in the skeletal muscle membrane
    E. Opening of Cl^- channels in the motor end plate

Difficulty level: Easy

21. A 60-year-old man was about to undergo surgery to remove a prostate cancer. The man had been suffering from ischemic heart disease for 2 years. The anesthesiologist decided to use nitrous oxide and another general anesthetic that causes a pronounced increase in coronary blood flow with concomitant decrease in myocardial oxygen consumption and negligible effects on cardiac output. Which of the following anesthetics was most likely given with nitrous oxide for anesthesia maintenance?

A. Halothane
B. Etomidate
C. Propofol
D. Isoflurane
E. Sevoflurane

Difficulty level: Easy

22. A 68-year-old hospitalized woman developed general malaise, fever (100.7°F. 38.2°C), nausea and vomiting, jaundice, and a skin rash. The woman had undergone surgery 4 days earlier to remove a uterine myoma. Emergency lab exams showed the following pertinent results: aspartate aminotransferase 240 U/L, alkaline phosphatase 380 U/L. The patient's condition rapidly deteriorated, and coma ensued. Which of the following drugs most likely caused the patient's syndrome?

A. Sevoflurane
B. Halothane
C. Nitrous oxide
D. Thiopental
E. Fentanyl
F. Isoflurane

Difficulty level: Medium

23. A 22-year-old woman was about to undergo surgery to remove a mandibular cancer. The anesthesiologist had decided to use nitrous oxide and sevoflurane for anesthesia maintenance. Which of the following would be the minimum alveolar concentration of both drugs needed to provide an appropriate general anesthesia in this patient?

A. Nitrous oxide 0.2; sevoflurane 0.3
B. Nitrous oxide 0.7; sevoflurane 0.6
C. Nitrous oxide 0.4; sevoflurane 0.1
D. Nitrous oxide 1.0; sevoflurane 1.6
E. Nitrous oxide 1.0; sevoflurane 0.7

Difficulty level: Easy

24. A 43-year-old woman underwent dilation and curettage for abnormal vaginal bleeding. General anesthesia was performed with thiopental. The patient lost consciousness in about 10 seconds and regained it 15 minutes later. Which

of the following reasons best explains why general anesthesia induced by a standard dose of thiopental lasts 5 to 15 minutes?

A. Slow distribution of the drug into the central nervous system (CNS)
B. Fast elimination of the drug from the body
C. Redistribution of the drug into peripheral tissues
D. Rapid biotransformation of the drug by the brain
E. Poor diffusion of the drug into the central neurons

Difficulty level: Medium

25. A 29-year-old woman was admitted to the hospital for dilation and curettage after a spontaneous abortion. General anesthesia was induced by propofol. Which of the following drugs would be most appropriately co-injected with propofol?

A. Thiopental
B. Etomidate
C. Paroxetine
D. Lidocaine
E. Diazepam

Difficulty level: Medium

26. An 80-year-old woman underwent surgery to remove a bladder cancer. Medical history indicated that she had been suffering from gastrointestinal reflux disease presently treated with omeprazole. General anesthesia was maintained with nitrous oxide and sevoflurane. In this patient, the sum of the minimum alveolar concentration (MAC) of the two inhalational anesthetics needed to obtain surgical anesthesia turned out to be 0.7 MAC. In most patients this total is 1.3 MAC. Which of the following variables most likely caused the decrease in MAC in this case?

A. The cancer of the patient
B. The use of two anesthetics
C. The age of the patient
D. The addition of nitrous oxide
E. The use of omeprazole

Difficulty level: Easy

27. A 46-year-old man recently diagnosed with pheochromocytoma was scheduled for surgery to remove the tumor. He had normal pulmonary and renal function, but his blood catecholamine levels were substantially elevated. Which of the following drugs would be contraindicated for inclusion in his anesthetic protocol?

A. Halothane
B. Fentanyl
C. Lorazepam
D. Thiopental
E. Nitrous oxide

Difficulty level: Easy

28. A 62-year-old man was about to undergo surgery to repair a small bowel closed loop obstruction. Which of the following general anesthetics would be contraindicated in this patient?

    A. Halothane
    B. Nitrous oxide
    C. Thiopental
    D. Propofol
    E. Sevoflurane
    F. Enflurane

Difficulty level: Easy

29. A 61-year-old woman underwent colonoscopy because of rectal bleeding. The woman was very afraid of the procedure and asked for a general anesthesia. Because she had been suffering from exertional angina for 7 years, etomidate was chosen for anesthesia. Which of the following adverse effects would be most likely to occur in this patient during the postanesthetic period?

    A. Nausea and vomiting
    B. Delusions
    C. Pronounced respiratory depression
    D. Hypertension
    E. Decreased cardiac output

Difficulty level: Medium

30. A 49-year-old man underwent emergency surgery because of multiple fractures due to a car accident. Because the patient was experiencing severe pain, fentanyl was given before surgery. General anesthesia was induced by propofol and maintained by nitrous oxide and isoflurane. Cisatracurium was added to ensure a complete muscle relaxation. After the operation, the anesthesiologist administered oxygen for five minutes before disconnecting the face mask. The procedure was performed to prevent an adverse effect of which of the following drugs?

    A. Isoflurane
    B. Propofol
    C. Fentanyl
    D. Nitrous oxide
    E. Cisatracurium

Questions: III-4 Local Anesthetics

Directions for questions **1–3**

Match each local anesthetic with the appropriate description (each lettered option can be selected once, more than once, or not at all).

    A. Benzocaine
    B. Bupivacaine
    C. Cocaine
    D. Lidocaine
    E. Prilocaine
    F. Procaine
    G. Tetracaine

Difficulty level: Easy

1. An ester-type local anesthetic with a short duration of action

Difficulty level: Easy

2. The most cardiotoxic local anesthetic

Difficulty level: Easy

3. An amide-type local anesthetic with a long duration of action

Difficulty level: Easy

4. A 27-year-old woman underwent a minor suture procedure for a skin cut on her right leg. A local anesthetic was injected around the wound to provide regional anesthesia. Blockade of which of the following ion channels most likely mediated the pharmacological effect of the drug in the patient?

    A. Inactivated, voltage-gated Na^+ channels
    B. Resting, voltage-gated K^+ channels
    C. Activated, ligand-gated Ca^{2+} channels
    D. Inactivated, ligand-gated K^+ channels
    E. Resting, ligand-gated Na^+ channels
    F. Activated, voltage-gated Ca^{2+} channels

Difficulty level: Easy

5. A 43-year-old man underwent an emergency minor arm repair procedure after a car accident. A standard dose of lidocaine was administered near the brachial plexus for peripheral nerve block. Fifteen minutes later, the anesthesia was still incomplete, and another dose of lidocaine was administered. Which of the following adverse effects would most likely occur after the administration?

    A. Ventricular tachycardia
    B. Abdominal colic
    C. Drowsiness
    D. Convulsions
    E. Hypertensive crisis

Difficulty level: Medium

6. A 53-year-old man was brought to the emergency department after suffering a hand injury that required immediate surgery. Local anesthesia was performed by brachial plexus block. The surgeon estimated that the procedure should last about 3 hours. Which of the following local anesthetics would be most appropriate for this patient?

   A. Prilocaine
   B. Procaine
   C. Tetracaine
   D. Benzocaine
   E. Cocaine

Difficulty level: Medium

7. A 62-year-old man was undergoing surgery to remove a hyperplastic prostate. Spinal anesthesia was performed with lidocaine. The pK_a of lidocaine is about 7.8. What fraction of the drug was most likely lipid soluble in the patient's cerebrospinal fluid (pH = 7.3)?

   A. 10%
   B. 24%
   C. 50%
   D. 76%
   E. 90%

Difficulty level: Easy

8. A new potential local anesthetic drug was studied in the laboratory using an isolated nerve fiber preparation. Which of the following nerve properties most likely increased when the drug was applied to the nerve fiber?

   A. Rate of rise of the action potential
   B. Amplitude of the action potential
   C. Refractory period of the nerve
   D. Conduction velocity of the nerve
   E. Resting potential of the nerve membrane

Difficulty level: Easy

9. A 2-year-old girl was brought to the emergency department after cutting herself with a kitchen knife a few minutes earlier. The fingers were bleeding. Examination revealed two clean wounds on the middle and ring fingers of the right hand. The doctor decided to suture the wounds under local anesthesia using lidocaine without epinephrine. Epinephrine was avoided to prevent which of the following possible complications?

   A. Wound infection
   B. Ischemic gangrene
   C. Excessive bleeding
   D. Delayed wound repair
   E. Systemic toxicity

Difficulty level: Medium

10. The action of a new potential local anesthetic was studied on different isolated nerve fiber preparations. Membrane potential and conduction velocity of those fibers are reported below:

Nerve Fiber	Membrane Potential (mV)	Conduction Velocity (m/sec)
P	−90	9
Q	−82	25
R	−45	2
S	−60	15
T	−55	50

Which of the nerve fibers was likely to be most sensitive to the action of the new drug?

   A. Fiber P
   B. Fiber Q
   C. Fiber R
   D. Fiber S
   E. Fiber T

Difficulty level: Easy

11. A 46-year-old man was in the dentist's office for a dental extraction. A local anesthetic was injected near the mandibular nerve. Which of the following physiological functions was most likely the last to be blocked in that patient?

   A. Motor function
   B. Pain sensation
   C. Muscle tone
   D. Touch sensation
   E. Vasomotor function

Difficulty level: Easy

12. A 55-year-old diabetic man was admitted to the emergency department with fever (101.5°F, 38.6°C) and abdominal pain. Physical examination disclosed a superficial abscess on the right side of the abdomen. A local anesthetic was injected around the abscess in preparation for surgery. Which of the following tissue properties most likely account for the slower onset of local anesthetic action in infected tissues?

   A. High levels of drug-metabolizing enzymes
   B. Low vessel density
   C. Higher extracellular K^+
   D. High levels of para-aminobenzoic acid
   E. Lower extracelluar pH

Difficulty level: Medium

13. A 4-day-old boy was brought to the emergency department with bluish discoloration of the lips and extremities. He was born full term, had no perinatal problems, and weighed 3.5 kg (7.7 lb). Medical history of the baby disclosed that he had undergone a circumcision procedure with local anesthesia the previous day, and cyanosis had begun 1.5 hours after the procedure. Lab results showed methemoglobinemia. Which of the following drugs was most likely used for local anesthesia?

A. Lidocaine
B. Benzocaine
C. Bupivacaine
D. Prilocaine
E. Tetracaine

Difficulty level: Easy

14. A 59-year-old man was admitted to the emergency department with extensive burns on his arms and thorax. Pertinent plasma levels on admission were K$^+$ 6.3 mEq/L, Ca 13.0 mg/dL, creatinine 2.8 mg/dL, blood urea nitrogen (BUN) 35 mg/dL. An emergency treatment was started that included the administration of a topical local anesthetic on the burned area. Which of the following molecular events most likely made the nerve membrane more sensitive to the action of the local anesthetic in this patient?

A. Increased extracellular concentration of Ca^{2+}
B. Increased extracellular concentration Na$^+$
C. Decreased extracellular concentration of Cl$^-$
D. Increased extracellular concentration of K$^+$
E. Increased extracellular concentration of Mg^{2+}

Difficulty level: Medium

15. A 45-year-old woman was undergoing surgery to remove an extensive lipoma in her right arm. Her medical history was significant for long-term, severe chronic obstructive pulmonary disease (COPD) due to heavy smoking. Local anesthesia with a peripheral nerve block was planned. Which of the following local anesthetics would be contraindicated in this patient?

A. Prilocaine
B. Procaine
C. Tetracaine
D. Lidocaine
E. Bupivacaine

Difficulty level: Easy

16. A 60-year-old man was scheduled for a lithotripsy to shatter a bladder stone. Lumbar epidural anesthesia was selected for the procedure. The anticipated duration of the procedure was about 20 minutes. Which of the following local anesthetics would be most appropriate for this patient?

A. Cocaine
B. Benzocaine
C. Bupivacaine
D. Tetracaine
E. Lidocaine

Difficulty level: Medium

17. A 28-year-old pregnant woman who was near term decided to have the delivery under spinal anesthesia. The patient's past history included an anaphylactic reaction 3 years earlier, apparently due to a sun screen containing para-aminobenzoic acid (PABA). Which of the following local anesthetics would be appropriate for this patient?

A. Procaine
B. Tetracaine
C. Lidocaine
D. Benzocaine
E. Cocaine

Difficulty level: Medium

18. A 56-year-old woman, who had been suffering from atrial fibrillation for 3 years, was in the dentist's office for the application of an implant. The dentist was about to initiate local anesthesia by injecting a local anesthetic close to the mandibular nerve. Which of the following local anesthetic preparations would be most appropriate for this patient?

A. Lidocaine alone
B. Lidocaine plus epinephrine
C. Bupivacaine plus epinephrine
D. Benzocaine plus epinephrine
E. Benzocaine alone

Difficulty level: Easy

19. A 16-year-old boy complained of burning pain due to multiple superficial skin abrasions after a motorcycle accident. A local anesthetic was applied topically to the abraded areas. Which of the following local anesthetics would be most appropriate for this patient?

A. Benzocaine
B. Procaine
C. Cocaine
D. Prilocaine
E. Bupivacaine

Difficulty level: Medium

20. A 44-year-old woman got a scratch on her arm while working at home. She put a cream containing a local anesthetic on the wounded area. It is known that on the body, local anesthetics can exist either as the uncharged base (non-ionized form) or as a cation (ionized form). The ionized form most likely mediated which of the following properties of the drug?

A. Tissue redistribution
B. Liver biotransformation
C. Blood–brain crossing
D. Receptor binding
E. Half-life

Difficulty level: Easy

21. A 56-year-old woman was about to undergo emergency minor skin suturing after an accidental self-injury with a

knife. The woman was agitated and firmly refused any injection procedure. Examination of the wound showed a long superficial cut of the skin with extensive bleeding. The anesthesiologist chose to apply a solution of a topical anesthetic that could also cause local vasoconstriction. Which of the following drugs was most likely administered?

A. Cocaine
B. Prilocaine
C. Bupivacaine
D. Tetracaine
E. Lidocaine

Questions: III-5 Skeletal Muscle Relaxants

Directions for questions **1–4**

Match each skeletal muscle relaxant with the appropriate description (each lettered option can be selected once, more than once, or not at all).

A. Tubocurarine
B. Cisatracurium
C. Mivacurium
D. Succinylcholine
E. Dantrolene
F. Gabapentin
G. Diazepam
H. Tizanidine
I. Baclofen

Difficulty level: Easy

1. An antagonist at Nn acetylcholine receptors in autonomic ganglia

Difficulty level: Easy

2. An agonist at Nm acetylcholine receptors

Difficulty level: Easy

3. Primarily an agonist at α_2 receptors located in the spinal cord.

Difficulty level: Easy

4. An anticonvulsant agent that can reduce spasticity in patients with multiple sclerosis

Difficulty level: Easy

5. A 63-year-old man underwent abdominal surgery for prostate cancer. General anesthesia was supplemented with tubocurarine. Which of the following anatomical structures most likely represents the main site of action of the drug for this clinical application?

A. Ganglionic neuron membranes
B. Adrenal medulla
C. Postjunctional folds of motor end plates
D. Autonomic cholinergic nerve terminals
E. Spinal motor neuron membranes
F. Skeletal muscle cell membranes

Difficulty level: Easy

6. A 38-year-old patient was admitted to the emergency department with extensive soft tissue burns. He was semiconscious and was artificially ventilated. His uncoordinated respiratory movements were interfering with the mechanical ventilation. Which of the following drugs would most likely be effective to decrease the patient's spontaneous breathing?

A. Diazepam
B. Vecuronium
C. Botulinum toxin
D. Dantrolene
E. Baclofen
F. Tizanidine

Difficulty level: Easy

7. A 57-year-old woman was admitted semiconscious to the emergency department after an accident at home. Artificial ventilation was needed, and a drug was given to facilitate intubation. This drug has the shortest duration of action among skeletal muscle relaxants. Which of the following drugs was most likely administered?

A. Succinylcholine
B. Cisatracurium
C. Dantrolene
D. Vecuronium
E. Tubocurarine
F. Tizanidine

Difficulty level: Hard

8. A 49-year-old man diagnosed with inguinal hernia was prepared for surgery. Shortly after the initiation of general anesthesia with halothane and succinylcholine, the patient developed muscle rigidity, tachycardia, labile blood pressure, profuse diaphoresis, and high fever (104.2°F, 40.1°C). The anesthesia was discontinued at once, and a drug was administered by rapid intravenous push. Which of the following was most likely the mechanism of action of the administered drug?

   A. Activation of $GABA_B$ receptors in the spinal cord
   B. Blockade of excitatory neurotransmitter release in the brain
   C. Blockade of Ca^{2+} channels in the skeletal muscle membrane
   D. Blockade of Ca^{2+} channels in the sarcoplasmic reticulum
   E. Increased K^+ conductance in the skeletal muscle membrane

Difficulty level: Easy

9. A 22-year-old man suffering from strabismus started treatment with local injections of botulinum toxin into the extrinsic ocular muscles. Which of the following structures was most likely the site of the therapeutic action of the drug?

   A. Nicotinic muscular receptors
   B. Somatic nerve terminals
   C. Muscarinic receptors
   D. Autonomic nerve terminals
   E. Nicotinic neuronal receptors

Difficulty level: Easy

10. A 73-year-old man underwent thoracic surgery to remove a lung cancer. General anesthesia was supplemented with vecuronium. Which of the following molecular actions most likely mediated the muscle relaxant effect of this drug?

   A. Stimulation of plasma cholinesterase
   B. Long-lasting activation of postsynaptic Nm receptors
   C. Competitive blockade of postsynaptic Nm receptors
   D. Blockade of action potential of the motor nerves
   E. Blockade of Ca^{2+} release from the sarcoplasmic reticulum
   F. Competitive blockade of Nn receptors in the brain

Difficulty level: Medium

11. A 61-year-old man underwent surgery for prostate cancer. The anesthesia was induced by thiopental and maintained by halothane and nitrous oxide. Vecuronium was added to ensure adequate muscle relaxation. Which of the following was most likely the sequence of the paralysis of skeletal muscles induced by vecuronium in this patient?

   A. Eye extrinsic muscles, limb muscles, diaphragm
   B. Limb muscles, diaphragm, eye extrinsic muscles
   C. Diaphragm, eye extrinsic muscles, limb muscles
   D. Diaphragm, limb muscles, eye extrinsic muscles
   E. Limb muscles, eye extrinsic muscles, diaphragm

Difficulty level: Easy

12. A 59-year-old woman was undergoing surgery for breast cancer. General anesthesia was supplemented with a nondepolarizing neuromuscular blocker that has a short duration of action and is metabolized by plasma pseudocholinesterase. Which of the following drugs was most likely administered?

   A. Succinylcholine
   B. Tubocurarine
   C. Vecuronium
   D. Mivacurium
   E. Cisatracurium

Difficulty level: Easy

13. A 74-year-old man underwent abdominal surgery to remove a colon carcinoma. The patient had severely impaired hepatic and renal function, and the anesthesiologist decided to supplement general anesthesia with a muscle relaxant that is inactivated primarily by a form of spontaneous breakdown (also known as Hoffmann elimination). Which of the following drugs was most likely given?

   A. Succinylcholine
   B. Dantrolene
   C. Tubocurarine
   D. Cisatracurium
   E. Mivacurium

Difficulty level: Medium

14. A 65-year-old woman underwent hysterectomy for endometrial carcinoma. The general anesthesia protocol included sodium thiopental, isoflurane, nitrous oxide, and tubocurarine. The anesthesiologist also administered another drug to counteract tubocurarine-induced hypotension. To which of the following classes did this drug most likely belong?

   A. β_1 agonists
   B. D_1 antagonists
   C. Muscarinic agonists
   D. Cholinesterase inhibitors
   E. H_1 antagonists

Difficulty level: Easy

15. A 66-year-old woman was brought to the emergency department following a car accident. Surgery was needed to repair a badly damaged leg. Medications of the patient on admission were gentamicin and darifenacin for urinary tract

infection, timolol and latanoprost for glaucoma, and lovastatin for hypercholesterolemia. General anesthesia was induced by thiopental sodium, maintained by isoflurane and nitrous oxide, and supplemented by vecuronium. Which of the following of the patient's medications most likely enhanced the action of vecuronium?

A. Gentamicin
B. Darifenacin
C. Timolol
D. Latanoprost
E. Lovastatin

Difficulty level: Easy

16. A 44-year-old man brought to the emergency department after a car accident required intubation and mechanical ventilation. The patient's history was significant for a genetic deficiency of plasma cholinesterase. A muscle relaxant was administered intravenously. Which of the following muscle relaxants would be contraindicated in this patient?

A. Tubocurarine
B. Cisatracurium
C. Baclofen
D. Mivacurium
E. Vecuronium
F. Tizanidine

Difficulty level: Medium

17. A 56-year-old woman was undergoing major surgery to remove a breast carcinoma. The woman, who was a heavy smoker, had been suffering from chronic obstructive pulmonary disease for 15 years. A drug was administered preoperatively, and the anesthesia was supplemented with a skeletal muscle relaxant. Which of the following drugs would be contraindicated for this patient?

A. Tubocurarine
B. Glycopyrrolate
C. Clonidine
D. Vecuronium
E. Cisatracurium

Difficulty level: Hard

18. A 49-year-old woman required intubation and mechanical ventilation for management of respiratory failure due to severe emphysema. The patient was agitated, attempting to sit up in bed and reach for the endotracheal tube. Lorazepam was given intravenously (IV) for sedation, and the patient got drowsy, but motor restlessness was only marginally improved. An IV muscle relaxant was given. The patient relaxed as paralysis developed, but 5 minutes later her heart rate was 160 bpm. Which of the following drugs most likely caused this adverse effect?

A. Botulinum toxin
B. Dantrolene
C. Succinylcholine
D. Tubocurarine
E. Cisatracurium

Difficulty level: Easy

19. A 57-year-old woman underwent surgery for breast cancer. General anesthesia was induced by thiopental, maintained by sevoflurane and nitrous oxide, and supplemented with a muscle relaxant that causes a long lasting activation of Nm receptors. Which of the following drugs was most likely administered?

A. Succinylcholine
B. Cisatracurium
C. Tubocurarine
D. Mivacurium
E. Vecuronium
F. Baclofen

Difficulty level: Easy

20. A 48-year-old woman underwent heart surgery for placement of an artificial valve. Anesthesia was induced by thiopental, and a muscle relaxant was then given intravenously to facilitate intubation. Soon after the administration of the drug, the patient exhibited transient muscle fasciculations that progressed to generalized paralysis within 1 minute. Which of the following muscle relaxants was most likely given?

A. Cisatracurium
B. Succinylcholine
C. Dantrolene
D. Vecuronium
E. Tubocurarine
F. Tizanidine

Difficulty level: Easy

21. A 10-year-old boy diagnosed with hereditary spastic paraparesis 2 years ago was treated with several spasmolytic drugs with limited success. Recently, the neurologist prescribed another spasmolytic agent that acts as an α_2-receptor agonist in the spinal cord. Which of the following drugs was most likely prescribed?

A. Diazepam
B. Baclofen
C. Dantrolene
D. Mivacurium
E. Tizanidine

Difficulty level: Easy

22. A 54-year-old man who had been suffering from amyotrophic lateral sclerosis for 1 year complained of generalized muscle spasms. His physician prescribed diazepam to reduce spasticity. Which of the following statements best explains the mechanism of the spasmolytic effect of diazepam in this patient?

    A. Blockade of calcium release from the sarcoplasmic reticulum
    B. Blockade of acetylcholine release from motor nerves
    C. Depolarization blockade of Nm receptors
    D. Facilitation of $GABA_A$ actions in the spinal cord
    E. Activation of $GABA_B$ receptors in the spinal cord

Difficulty level: Easy

23. A 67-year-old woman required intubation and mechanical ventilation for management of respiratory failure. Vecuronium was given intravenously to reduce chest wall resistance and ineffective spontaneous ventilation. Which of the following membrane potentials was most likely blocked by vecuronium in this patient?

    A. Action potential of motor nerve
    B. Miniature end-plate potential
    C. Resting potential of smooth muscle
    D. Action potential of cardiac muscle
    E. Action potential of corticospinal tract

Difficulty level: Hard

24. A 40-year-old woman, admitted to the emergency department after a car collision, had multiple surgeries to repair her injuries and was placed on mechanical ventilation to assist respiration. On day 13 she was scheduled for a transesophageal electrocardiogram (ECG) and was given a muscle relaxant intravenously to facilitate the procedure. Soon afterward, the patient suffered cardiac arrest, and cardiopulmonary resuscitation was performed successfully. The serum potassium levels recorded just before the arrest peaked at 7.3 mEq/L. Which of the following muscle relaxants most likely caused the cardiac arrest?

    A. Cisatracurium
    B. Vecuronium
    C. Tubocurarine
    D. Dantrolene
    E. Succinylcholine

Difficulty level: Easy

25. A 40-year-old woman underwent surgery for ovarian cancer. She received atropine, loratadine, and morphine as preanesthetic medication. The anesthesia was then performed with thiopental, sevoflurane, nitrous oxide, and succinylcholine.

A few minutes later, the patient developed muscle fasciculations, trismus, rigidity, tachycardia, and hypotension, and her body temperature rose to 103.8°F (39.8°C). Which of the following drugs most likely caused the patient's syndrome?

    A. Atropine
    B. Morphine
    C. Loratadine
    D. Succinylcholine
    E. Thiopental
    F. Nitrous oxide

Difficulty level: Easy

26. A 43-year-old man complained of generalized muscle soreness upon recovering from surgery to remove prostate cancer. General anesthesia had been performed with thiopental, halothane, and a skeletal muscle relaxant. Which of the following muscle relaxants most likely caused the patient's complaint?

    A. Tubocurarine
    B. Cisatracurium
    C. Succinylcholine
    D. Dantrolene
    E. Diazepam

Difficulty level: Easy

27. A 34-year-old woman suffering from hemifacial spasms started treatment with botulinum toxin injected directly into the abnormally contracting muscles. Which of the following molecular actions most likely mediated the therapeutic effect of the drug in the patient's disorder?

    A. Long-lasting activation of Nm acetylcholine receptors
    B. Inhibition of acetylcholine storage into synaptic vesicles
    C. Inhibition of choline acetyltransferase
    D. Inhibition of acetylcholine exocytosis from cholinergic terminals
    E. Stimulation of acetylcholinesterase
    F. Opening of Ca^{2+} channels in cholinergic terminals

Difficulty level: Easy

28. A 64-year-old woman complained to her physician of involuntary blinking and closing of the eyes. She noticed that the eyelid spasm was made worse by fatigue and anxiety. Further exams led to the diagnosis of benign essential blepharospasm, and a treatment with local injections of botulinum toxin was prescribed. Which of the following adverse effects was most likely to occur in this patient?

    A. Retinal detachment
    B. Visual hallucinations
    C. Visual loss
    D. Eyelid ptosis
    E. Limb muscle paralysis

Difficulty level: Easy

29. A 41-year-old man suffering from amyotrophic lateral sclerosis presented to his physician with muscle fasciculations, limb spasticity, hyperactive deep tendon reflexes, and extensor plantar reflexes. Baclofen was prescribed to reduce spasticity and cramps. Which of the following actions most likely mediated the therapeutic effect of the drug in the patient's disease?

A. Activation of $GABA_B$ receptors in the spinal cord
B. Blockade of Nm receptors of motor end plates
C. Increased substance P release in the spinal cord
D. Blockade of Ca^{2+} channels in skeletal muscle membranes
E. Increased K^+ conductance in skeletal muscle membranes

Difficulty level: Easy

30. A 48-year-old man presented to his physician complaining of intermittent limb muscle spasms. The patient was referred to the neurologic clinic, where the diagnosis of stiff man syndrome was made. A pharmacotherapy was prescribed to improve his muscle spasms. Which of the following drugs would be most appropriate for this patient?

A. Phenobarbital
B. Baclofen
C. Tubocurarine
D. Succinylcholine
E. Chlorpromazine
F. Mivacurium

Difficulty level: Medium

31. A 62-year-old woman underwent surgery to remove an ovarian cancer. General anesthesia was induced by thiopental, maintained by sevoflurane and nitrous oxide, and supplemented by vecuronium, which is currently one of the most commonly used skeletal muscle relaxants during surgery. Which of the following is a primary advantage of vecuronium over tubocurarine?

A. A very short duration of action (less than 5 minutes)
B. Negligible effects on histamine release
C. No fasciculations before paralysis
D. Lack of effects on the central nervous system
E. Induction of complete anterograde amnesia

Difficulty level: Easy

32. A 79-year-old man underwent surgery to remove a stomach cancer. Pertinent laboratory results before surgery were creatinine 3.5 mg/dL (normal 0.6–1.2 mg/dL), alanine aminotransferase 25 U/L (normal 8–20 U/L), urea nitrogen 65 mg/dL (normal 7–18 mg/dL). Diazepam was given the night before surgery. The general anesthesia was induced by propofol, maintained by sevoflurane and nitrous oxide, and supplemented by cisatracurium. Which of the following was most likely the primary reason for the use of cisatracurium instead of tubocurarine in this patient?

A. Liver insufficiency
B. Advanced age
C. Propofol induction
D. Renal insufficiency
E. Diazepam administration

Questions: III-6 Antiseizure Drugs

Directions for questions **1–3**

For each numbered item select the one lettered option that is most closely associated with it (each lettered option can be selected once, more than once, or not at all).

A. Acetazolamide
B. Carbamazepine
C. Ethosuximide
D. Felbamate
E. Gabapentin
F. Lamotrigine
G. Levetiracetam
H. Phenytoin
I. Tiagabine
J. Topiramate
K. Valproic acid
L. Zonisamide

Difficulty level: Easy

1. This drug is effective in all forms of epilepsy in all age groups.

Difficulty level: Easy

2. This drug binds selectively to a synaptic vesicular protein, altering the synaptic release of glutamate and gamma-aminobutyric acid (GABA).

Difficulty level: Easy

3. This drug inhibits gamma-aminobutyric acid (GABA) reuptake in both neurons and glia, enhancing GABAergic transmission.

Difficulty level: Easy

4. A 28-year-old man was brought to the emergency department because of a generalized tonic-clonic seizure. History showed that the man had been suffering from epilepsy since childhood, but the seizures were only partially controlled by medication. Which of the following pairs of neurotransmitters are thought to be mainly involved in seizure disorders?

   A. Gamma-aminobutyric acid (GABA) and serotonin
   B. Serotonin and acetylcholine
   C. GABA and acetylcholine
   D. Serotonin and glutamate
   E. GABA and glutamate
   F. Acetylcholine and glutamate

Difficulty level: Easy

5. A 37-year-old woman was at a routine neurology clinic visit. The woman had a long history of refractory grand mal epilepsy. She was being treated with several drugs, but with poor results. The neurologist decided to prescribe phenytoin. Blockade of which of the following types of ion channels is most likely to mediate the therapeutic efficacy of the drug in the patient's disease?

   A. Na⁺ channels in the resting state
   B. Na⁺ channels that open and close at high frequency
   C. Na⁺ channels that open and close at low frequency
   D. K⁺ channels in a resting state
   E. K⁺ channels that open and close at high frequency
   F. K⁺ channels that open and close at low frequency

Difficulty level: Easy

6. A 32-year-old woman complained to her physician that two breakthrough seizures occurred last week. One month earlier the woman was diagnosed with simple partial seizure and started treatment with an antiepileptic drug. The physician increased the dose of the drug, thinking that the decreased effect was most likely because the drug is a potent enzyme inducer and can induce its own metabolism. Which of the following drugs did the patient most likely take?

   A. Valproic acid
   B. Carbamazepine
   C. Lamotrigine
   D. Ethosuximide
   E. Clonazepam

Difficulty level: Easy

7. A 45-year-old man recently diagnosed with partial seizures came to his neurologist's office for a routine visit. The man had been receiving an antiseizure drug for the past 3 months. An electroencephalogram showed left temporal sharp waves, and the neurologist decided to add lamotrigine to the patient's

regimen. A relatively low dose of lamotrigine was prescribed because the drug the patient was already taking can inhibit the metabolism of lamotrigine. Which of the following was most likely that drug?

   A. Phenytoin
   B. Phenobarbital
   C. Levetiracetam
   D. Clonazepam
   E. Valproic acid
   F. Gabapentin

Difficulty level: Easy

8. A 47-year-old woman complained to her physician of blurred and double vision. She had been suffering from a central nervous system disorder and had been receiving a drug treatment for 6 months. Physical examination showed mild hirsutism, broadening of her lips and nose, and thickening and bleeding of her gums. Which of the following drugs most likely caused these adverse effects?

   A. Lithium
   B. Fluphenazine
   C. Fluoxetine
   D. Diazepam
   E. Valproic acid
   F. Gabapentin
   G. Phenytoin

Difficulty level: Medium

9. A 26-year-old woman discovered she was unexpectedly pregnant. She had been regularly taking an oral contraceptive medication for several years. Two months earlier, she was diagnosed with complex partial seizures and started the prescribed therapy. Which of the following drugs was she most likely taking?

   A. Lamotrigine
   B. Valproic acid
   C. Clonazepam
   D. Gabapentin
   E. Levetiracetam
   F. Carbamazepine

Difficulty level: Easy

10. A 41-year-old man was admitted to the hospital after he suffered a seizure with loss of consciousness while at home. Two weeks earlier, the man was involved in a car accident and had suffered from a closed head injury. A neurologic examination and an electroencephalogram led to the discovery of an epileptic focus in the patient's temporal lobe. The neurologist ordered an anticonvulsant drug that most likely acts with multiple mechanisms, including blockade of *N*-methyl-D-aspartate (NMDA) receptor–mediated excitation, blockade

of T-type Ca^{2+} channels in thalamic neurons, and increased gamma-aminobutyric acid (GABA) content in the brain. Which of the following drugs was most likely prescribed?

A. Valproic acid
B. Gabapentin
C. Tiagabine
D. Levetiracetam
E. Ethosuximide
F. Clonazepam

Difficulty level: Easy

11. A 12-year-old boy who was recently diagnosed with absence seizures started a therapy with ethosuximide. Which of the following molecular actions most likely mediated the therapeutic efficacy of the drug in the patient's disorder?

A. Opening of voltage-gated K^+ channels
B. Blockade of T-type Ca^{2+} channels
C. Blockade of ligand-gated Na^+ channels
D. Activation of $GABA_A$ receptors
E. Blockade of NMDA receptors
F. Activation of $5-HT_1$ receptors

Difficulty level: Medium

12. A 14-month-old baby boy exhibited jerkiness of the upper limbs for a few weeks. The jerks never caused him to fall but were repeated several dozens of times each day, including when falling asleep. An electroencephalogram showed that the jerks were combined in all instances with spike waves, and that there was an increase of jerks and spike waves when he fell asleep. Which of the following drugs would be most appropriate for this boy?

A. Phenytoin
B. Carbamazepine
C. Phenobarbital
D. Valproic acid
E. Gabapentin
F. Acetazolamide

Difficulty level: Medium

13. A 54-year-old woman with a previously well-controlled seizure disorder was brought to the hospital because of recurrent, generalized tonic-clonic seizures. The patient was intubated and mechanically ventilated. She was treated with intravenous diazepam and fosphenytoin but continued to exhibit intermittent seizures and did not regain consciousness between them. A diagnosis of refractory status epilepticus was made. A large dose of which of the following drugs would be appropriate to add to the patient's therapy at this time?

A. Levetiracetam
B. Carbamazepine
C. Valproic acid
D. Phenobarbital
E. Clonazepam
F. Zonisamide

Difficulty level: Easy

14. A 36-year-old woman recently diagnosed with simple partial seizures started a therapy with lamotrigine. Which of the following adverse effects is most likely to occur during the therapy?

A. Macrocytic anemia
B. Hallucinations
C. Liver cirrhosis
D. Pancreatitis
E. Lupoid syndrome
F. Erythematous skin rash

Difficulty level: Medium

15. A 35-year-old woman experienced an abrupt onset of unilateral clonic contractions of her finger that progressively involve her hand, then lower and upper arm. History revealed that she had sustained a brain trauma 5 months earlier. She was diagnosed with simple partial seizure, and an appropriate drug was prescribed. A drug with which of the following mechanisms of action would be appropriate for the patient's disease?

A. Blockade of neuromuscular transmission
B. Blockade of inactivated K^+ channels
C. Decreased release of gamma-aminobutyric acid (GABA) from nerve terminals
D. Activation of glutamate receptor in the motor cortex
E. Blockade of inactivated Na^+ channels

Difficulty level: Easy

16. A 39-year-old man diagnosed with tonic-clonic seizures 2 years ago had been receiving a drug that exhibits dose-dependent elimination kinetics. Which of the following drugs did the patient most likely take?

A. Valproic acid
B. Lamotrigine
C. Phenytoin
D. Topiramate
E. Carbamazepine
F. Gabapentin

Difficulty level: Easy

17. A 54-year-old man had been receiving carbamazepine since he was diagnosed with complex partial seizures 5 years earlier. The drug was fully effective in controlling the seizures. Blockade of which of the following molecular targets most likely mediated the therapeutic effect of the drug in the patient's disease?

- **A.** Acetylcholine receptors
- **B.** Glutamate receptors
- **C.** Monoamine receptors
- **D.** Na^+ channels
- **E.** K^+ channels
- **F.** Ca^{2+} channels

Difficulty level: Medium

18. A 53-year-old man suffering from partial seizures had been receiving a high dose of carbamazepine for 6 months. Which of the following dose-related adverse effects most likely occurred during the therapy?

- **A.** Gingival hyperplasia
- **B.** Hallucinations
- **C.** Ataxia
- **D.** Stevens–Johnson syndrome
- **E.** Heart failure
- **F.** Dilutional hyponatremia

Difficulty level: Easy

19. A 13-month-old boy was brought to the hospital after having a generalized tonic-clonic convulsion lasting approximately 4 minutes. The episode occurred in association with an upper respiratory tract infection. On admission his rectal temperature was 103°F (39.4°C). The parents reported that two similar episodes occurred 8 and 3 months ago, always in association with fever. The boy had no history of neurologic abnormality, and all laboratory and neurologic findings were normal. A presumptive diagnosis was made, and measures to reduce his elevated temperature were initiated. The parents were instructed to give a drug rectally to the boy whenever he had fever. Which of the following anticonvulsant drugs would be most appropriate for this boy?

- **A.** Carbamazepine
- **B.** Topiramate
- **C.** Diazepam
- **D.** Ethosuximide
- **E.** Zonisamide
- **F.** Felbamate

Difficulty level: Hard

20. A 35-year-old woman, recently diagnosed with simple partial seizures, started the prescribed therapy. Her past history was unremarkable, but her mother was known to suffer from acute intermittent porphyria. Which of the following anticonvulsant drugs would be appropriate for this patient?

- **A.** Diazepam
- **B.** Ethosuximide
- **C.** Valproic acid
- **D.** Carbamazepine
- **E.** Phenytoin
- **F.** Lamotrigine

Difficulty level: Hard

21. An 81-year-old male resident of a nursing facility recently developed a partial seizure disorder secondary to a stroke. The man had multiple medical problems, including liver cirrhosis, open-angle glaucoma, type 2 diabetes mellitus, and a history of kidney stones. He had been taking multiple medications for these conditions. The neurologist ordered a drug to treat the patient's seizure disorder. Which of the following drugs would be most appropriate for this patient?

- **A.** Levetiracetam
- **B.** Phenytoin
- **C.** Carbamazepine
- **D.** Valproic acid
- **E.** Topiramate
- **F.** Zonisamide

Difficulty level: Medium

22. A 12-year-old boy with a long history of Lennox–Gastaut syndrome was admitted to the neurologic clinic for evaluation. In the past, the boy had been treated with several drugs, but the response to the antiepileptic therapy was rather poor. After a neurologic examination and an electroencephalogram, the neurologist decided to prescribe an antiepileptic drug with a broad spectrum of action, including partial, tonic-clonic, myoclonic, and atonic seizures, as well as infantile spasm and Lennox–Gastaut syndrome. Which of the following drugs was most likely prescribed?

- **A.** Phenobarbital
- **B.** Topiramate
- **C.** Tiagabine
- **D.** Zonisamide
- **E.** Carbamazepine
- **F.** Phenytoin
- **G.** Gabapentin

Difficulty level: Medium

23. A 52-year-old man came to his neurologist's office for a routine visit. Medical history revealed that he had a myocardial infarction 2 years ago and had been suffering from a third-degree atrioventricular block since then. One month earlier, he was diagnosed with simple partial seizures and was prescribed lamotrigine. The seizure attacks were diminished but not completely controlled. The neurologist decided to discontinue lamotrigine and to start another drug. Which of the following drugs would be appropriate for the patient at this time?

A. Ethosuximide

B. Gabapentin

C. Diazepam

D. Acetazolamide

E. Carbamazepine

F. Phenytoin

Difficulty level: Medium

24. A 24-year-old woman with a long history of absence seizures had been successfully managed with valproic acid for the past 5 years. The patient had recently married, and during her last office visit she expressed the desire to start a family. Which of the following drugs would be most appropriate for this patient to substitute for valproic acid therapy?

A. Carbamazepine

B. Clonazepam

C. Phenytoin

D. Ethosuximide

E. Phenobarbital

F. Tiagabine

Difficulty level: Hard

25. A 45-year-old man visited his physician's office for consultation regarding his antimigraine medication. The man had a 1-month history of disabling migraine headaches occurring two or three times weekly. About 70% of his headache attacks had been aborted with one sumatriptan tablet and rest. The patient had also been suffering from idiopathic second-degree atrioventricular block diagnosed 3 years ago and from open-angle glaucoma for 4 years. Which of the following prophylactic therapies would be appropriate for this patient to reduce the frequency of migraine attacks?

A. Atenolol

B. Verapamil

C. Amitriptyline

D. Lamotrigine

E. Valproic acid

F. Felbamate

Difficulty level: Medium

26. A 44-year-old man complained to his physician of burning and tickling in his hands and feet. The man was diagnosed with tonic-clonic seizures 3 years earlier and had been receiving a high dose of an antiseizure drug since then. Physical examination disclosed large inguinal lymph nodes, and reflex testing showed a lack of knee and ankle tendon reflexes. Further lab exams showed megaloblastic anemia. Which of the following drugs most likely caused the patient's signs and symptoms?

A. Gabapentin

B. Lamotrigine

C. Clonazepam

D. Phenytoin

E. Levetiracetam

F. Tiagabine

Difficulty level: Medium

27. A 44-year-old woman complained to her physician of daytime sedation and diplopia. The woman had been suffering from tonic-clonic seizures for 1 year and had been treated with phenytoin. Recently, the neurologist had slightly increased the dose of the drug because the seizures were not completely controlled. The physician told the patient that her symptoms were probably due to overdose toxicity of the drug. Which of the following statements most likely explains the reason for this toxicity?

A. The woman developed hypersensitivity to the drug.

B. The first-pass effect of the drug was unexpectedly high.

C. The volume of distribution of the drug is very low.

D. The clearance of the drug is dose-dependent.

E. The steady state of the drug was reached too quickly.

Difficulty level: Hard

28. A 10-year-old girl was brought to the neurology clinic by her mother, who reported that her daughter had two tonic-clonic seizures in the past 7 days. The girl's teacher had also noted that the girl had four episodes of "staring" in 1 day during this same time period. The girl had a history of absence seizures for which she had been taking ethosuximide for the past 2 months. Which of the following changes in the patient's therapy would be most appropriate at this time?

A. Discontinue ethosuximide and substitute phenobarbital.

B. Discontinue ethosuximide and substitute carbamazepine.

C. Increase ethosuximide dose and add diazepam.

D. Increase ethosuximide dose and add phenobarbital.

E. Discontinue ethosuximide and substitute valproic acid.

Difficulty level: Hard

29. A 15-month-old boy was admitted to the hospital because of repeated episodes of powerful contractions of trunk and limb muscles that lasted 5 to 10 seconds. These episodes occurred in clusters, frequently upon awakening. A brain magnetic resonance image showed agenesis of the corpus callosum. An appropriate diagnosis was made, and a therapy was prescribed. Which of the following drugs would be appropriate for the treatment of this patient?

    A. Carbamazepine
    B. Ethosuximide
    C. Phenytoin
    D. Phenobarbital
    E. Prednisone

Difficulty level: Hard.

30. A 50-year-old man complained of occasional episodes of excruciating unilateral facial pain that arose near the mouth, diffused toward the nostrils and eyes, and seemed to be triggered by eating or talking. The pain lasted about 1 minute. He was referred to a neurologist, who made a presumptive diagnosis and ordered an appropriate treatment. Which of the following drugs would be appropriate for this patient?

    A. Phenobarbital
    B. Clonazepam
    C. Codeine
    D. Diclofenac
    E. Carbamazepine

Difficulty level: Easy

31. A 15-year-old boy was in the neurology clinic for a routine visit. Two months earlier, the boy was diagnosed with absence seizures and started therapy with ethosuximide. He reported that the drug decreased the frequency of his seizures, but he still had some absence attacks from time to time. After further exams, the neurologist decided to add a drug that most likely acts by increasing the carbon dioxide concentration within brain neurons. Which of the following drugs was most likely prescribed?

    A. Ethosuximide
    B. Levetiracetam
    C. Tiagabine
    D. Acetazolamide
    E. Zonisamide
    F. Felbamate

Difficulty level: Easy

32. A 10-year-old girl suffering from Lennox–Gastaut syndrome recently had felbamate added to her current therapy. Which of the following actions on brain receptors most likely mediated the therapeutic effect of the drug in the patient's disorder?

    A. Blockade of $GABA_A$ receptors
    B. Activation of $GABA_B$ receptors
    C. Blockade of $5\text{-}HT_1$ receptors
    D. Activation of AMPA receptors
    E. Blockade of NMDA receptors
    F. Activation of $5\text{-}HT_3$ receptors

Difficulty level: Medium

33. A 64-year-old man was brought to the hospital after two consecutive seizures at home. On admission, he was noted to be only semiconscious, and shortly after his arrival another tonic-clonic seizure began. He was given intravenous lorazepam, and seizure activity ceased 5 minutes after the injection was completed. At this time, which of the following drugs was most likely administered for prolonged control of the patient's seizures?

    A. Levetiracetam
    B. Tiagabine
    C. Ethosuximide
    D. Fosphenytoin
    E. Zonisamide
    F. Felbamate

Difficulty level: Medium

34. A 34-year-old woman complained to her neurologist of a pronounced skin rash. Two weeks earlier, the woman had been diagnosed with simple partial seizure and started treatment with lamotrigine. She reported that apparently the therapy was effective, as she had not suffered any attacks during the treatment. Physical examination showed an extensive erythematous rash over her trunk and abdomen. The neurologist was certain that the adverse effect was drug-related. He decided to substitute the offending drug with another agent that most likely acts by blocking both Na^+ channels and Ca^{2+} channels on brain neurons. Which of the following drugs was most likely prescribed?

    A. Felbamate
    B. Phenobarbital
    C. Clonazepam
    D. Zonisamide
    E. Carbamazepine
    F. Levetiracetam

Difficulty level: Easy

35. A 12-year-old girl was admitted to the hospital because of vomiting, drowsiness, lethargy, and jaundice of 6 hours' duration. The girl had a long history of refractory absence seizure and had been receiving several drugs over the past 2 years. She was presently treated with two antiseizure agents and had no absence seizures for 5 weeks. Physical examination showed a patient in obvious distress with extensive jaundice of the skin and sclera. Significant lab results on admission were alanine aminotransferase 400 U/L (normal 10–40 U/L), total bilirubin 20 mg/dL (normal 0.3–1.0 mg/dL), and ammonia 190 µg/dL (normal for children 36–85 µg). Which of the following drugs most likely caused the patient's signs and symptoms?

A. Ethosuximide
B. Valproic acid
C. Lamotrigine
D. Levetiracetam
E. Zonisamide
F. Clonazepam

Difficulty level: Easy

36. A 6-year-old girl was diagnosed with myoclonic seizures. A brain magnetic resonance image showed no overt neurologic deficit. Her past medical history was negative for epileptic seizures. Which of the following drugs would be appropriate for this patient?

A. Carbamazepine
B. Haloperidol
C. Phenobarbital
D. Phenytoin
E. Fluoxetine
F. Clonazepam

Difficulty level: Easy

37. A 44-year-old woman came to her neurologist for a routine visit. The patient had a long history of poorly controlled simple partial seizures. Two months ago, she started therapy with valproic acid that was only partially effective. The neurologist decided to add to the ongoing therapy a recently approved drug that most likely acts with a novel mechanism of action, a noncompetitive blockade of α-amino-3-hydroxy-5-methylisoxazole-4-propionic acid (AMPA) receptors on brain neurons. Which of the following drugs was most likely prescribed?

A. Ethosuximide
B. Gabapentin
C. Diazepam
D. Perampanel
E. Lamotrigine
F. Carbamazepine

Difficulty level: Easy

38. A 37-year-old man recently diagnosed with generalized seizures started treatment with valproic acid, but 1 month later the frequency of seizures was not significantly reduced. His neurologist decided to add a second-generation antiepileptic drug that blocks voltage-gated Na$^+$ and Ca^{2+} channels and may inhibit the synaptic release of glutamate. Which of the following drugs was most likely prescribed?

A. Gabapentin
B. Lamotrigine
C. Phenobarbital
D. Diazepam
E. Ethosuximide
F. Felbamate

Difficulty level: Medium

39. A 54-year-old man was recently diagnosed with complex partial seizure. The patient had been suffering from atrioventricular block for 1 year and from nephrolithiasis for 3 years. Which of the following antiepileptic drugs would be most appropriate for this patient?

A. Carbamazepine
B. Phenytoin
C. Valproic acid
D. Ethosuximide
E. Zonisamide

Difficulty level: Easy

40. A 45-year-old man was in the neurology clinic for a routine visit. Two months earlier, the man was diagnosed with simple partial seizure and started therapy with lamotrigine. He reported that the drug was able to decrease the frequency of his attacks, but he still had an occasional attack. The neurologist decided to add a drug that acts by opening a certain family of potassium channels on brain neurons. Which of the following drugs was most likely prescribed?

A. Levetiracetam
B. Felbamate
C. Topiramate
D. Perampanel
E. Ezogabine
F. Zonisamide

Questions: III-7 Drugs for Degenerative Disorders of the Central Nervous System

Directions for questions **1–5**

For each numbered item select the one lettered option that is most closely associated with it (each lettered option can be selected once, more than once, or not at all).

- **A.** Amantadine
- **B.** Benztropine
- **C.** Bromocriptine
- **D.** Carbidopa
- **E.** Donepezil
- **F.** Entacapone
- **G.** Levodopa
- **H.** Memantine
- **I.** Selegiline

Difficulty level: Easy

1. A central muscarinic receptor blocker

Difficulty level: Easy

2. A central acetylcholinesterase inhibitor

Difficulty level: Easy

3. An N-methyl-D-aspartate (NMDA) receptor blocker used in Alzheimer disease

Difficulty level: Easy

4. A selective monoamine oxygenase B (MAO B) inhibitor

Difficulty level: Easy

5. A peripheral inhibitor of catechol-O-methyltransferase (COMT)

Difficulty level: Easy

6. A 63-year-old man recently diagnosed with Parkinson disease started treatment with levodopa/carbidopa. Which of the following actions most likely mediated the therapeutic effect of levodopa in the patient's disease?

- **A.** Downregulation of dopaminergic receptors in the striatum
- **B.** Increased synthesis of dopamine in the subthalamic nucleus
- **C.** Increased synthesis of dopamine in the striatum
- **D.** Inhibition of dopa decarboxylase in the striatum
- **E.** Inhibition of catechol-O-methyltransferase in the substantia nigra

Difficulty level: Medium

7. A 79-year-old man who had been suffering from Parkinson disease for 5 years complained of a resting tremor, which presently was one of the most debilitating symptoms of his disease. His therapy with levodopa/carbidopa had resulted in improvement in rigidity, bradykinesia, and posture, as well as improvement in the "on-off" effects, but he had experienced little if any improvement in tremor. Which of the following therapeutic approaches would be appropriate to reduce the patient's tremor?

- **A.** Decrease the dose of carbidopa.
- **B.** Substitute levodopa/carbidopa with pramipexole.
- **C.** Add benztropine to the present drug regimen.
- **D.** Add propranolol to the present drug regimen.
- **E.** Start brief periods of "drug holidays" during therapy.

Difficulty level: Easy

8. A 62-year-old man complained to his physician of facial grimacing, lip smacking, and rocking of the trunk that occurred 1 to 2 hours after taking his prescribed medication. The man, who suffered from Parkinson disease, had been receiving an antiparkinson drug for 3 years. Which of the following drugs most likely caused the adverse effects reported by the patient?

- **A.** Selegiline
- **B.** Levodopa
- **C.** Entacapone
- **D.** Amantadine
- **E.** Benztropine

Difficulty level: Easy

9. A 75-year-old diabetic man with Parkinson disease complained of worsening of his tremor and rigidity in his arms and legs. His Parkinson disease had been responding well to a treatment with levodopa/carbidopa and amantadine, and his diabetes had been controlled by glyburide and metformin. Recently, metoclopramide was prescribed to manage diabetic gastroparesis. Which of the following drugs could have triggered the worsening of symptoms reported by the patient?

- **A.** Glyburide
- **B.** Amantadine
- **C.** Carbidopa
- **D.** Metformin
- **E.** Metoclopramide

Difficulty level: Medium

10. A 53-year-old man complained to his physician of persistent and annoying salivation. The man, recently diagnosed with Parkinson disease, had started treatment with levodopa/carbidopa that significantly improved his motor symptoms. The physician decided to include another drug in the treatment. Which of the following drugs would be appropriate to add to the therapy at this time?

A. Entacapone
B. Selegiline
C. Benztropine
D. Pramipexole
E. Apomorphine

Difficulty level: Hard

11. A 51-year-old woman complained of a resting tremor in her left hand, difficulty in writing, and a distressing sensation of inner restlessness. After careful neurologic examination, a diagnosis was made, and an appropriate therapy was ordered that included a drug acting as a partial agonist at dopamine D_2 receptors in the brain. Which of the following drugs was most likely prescribed?

A. Pramipexole
B. Dopamine
C. Clozapine
D. Levodopa
E. Ergotamine
F. Selegiline

Difficulty level: Medium

12. A 67-year-old man presented to the clinic complaining of vague chest pains and difficulty in breathing. Medical history revealed that the patient had been diagnosed with Parkinson disease 10 years earlier and had been using several antiparkinson drugs since then. Physical examination revealed prominent breath sounds and end-inspiratory crackles, primarily at the lung bases. An x-ray showed extensive honeycombing. A diagnosis of pulmonary fibrosis was made. Which of the following drugs would have been most likely to cause the patient's disorder?

A. Bromocriptine
B. Benztropine
C. Selegiline
D. Amantadine
E. Levodopa
F. Entacapone

Difficulty level: Medium

13. A 54-year-old man complained to his physician of difficulty in writing, because of unsteadiness in his right hand, and of tightness in his arms and legs. These symptoms started about 1 week earlier. Physical examination showed a well-nourished, anxious patient with a notable lack of normal changes in facial expression and with a soft, monotone voice. Tremor was present in his hands, and a festinating gait was noted. A diagnosis was made, and a single-agent pharmacotherapy was prescribed. Which of the following drugs would be appropriate for this patient?

A. Carbidopa
B. Entacapone
C. Benztropine
D. Pramipexole
E. Clonazepam
F. Propranolol

Difficulty level: Easy

14. A 63-year-old woman with Parkinson disease had been maintained on levodopa/carbidopa with adjunctive use of a drug that acts by reducing central dopamine metabolism. Which of the following drugs was most likely the adjunctive drug?

A. Levodopa
B. Pramipexole
C. Selegiline
D. Phenelzine
E. Benztropine

Difficulty level: Medium

15. A 57-year-old woman with Parkinson disease complained that her tremor had gradually worsened over the past 2 weeks. She had been taking a levodopa/carbidopa combination for 6 months. The neurologist decided to add benztropine to the therapeutic regimen, and 2 weeks later the tremor was well controlled. Which of the following actions most likely mediated the reduction in the patient's tremor?

A. Inhibition of levodopa metabolism in the striatum
B. Inhibition of the abnormally high cholinergic tone in the striatum
C. Activation of dopaminergic receptors in the striatum
D. Blockade of β_2 adrenoceptors in skeletal muscle
E. Increased GABAergic activity in the subthalamic nucleus

Difficulty level: Easy

16. A 45-year-old woman complained of blurred vision, dry mouth, palpitations, and constipation. The patient was diagnosed with Parkinson disease 4 months earlier and had been receiving a levodopa/carbidopa combination since then. Recently, her neurologist added a drug to the therapeutic regimen because of an increase in the patient's resting tremor. Which of the following drugs most likely caused the patient's symptoms?

A. Pramipexole
B. Selegiline
C. Levodopa
D. Amantadine
E. Benztropine
F. Carbidopa

Difficulty level: Medium

17. A 53-year-old diabetic woman complained to her physician of a recent appearance of an unpleasant, creeping discomfort in her legs when she was lying down. The sensation urged the woman to move about, and walking relieved her symptoms. She also complained of difficulty falling asleep and interrupted nocturnal sleep. A preliminary diagnosis of restless leg syndrome was made, and a therapy was prescribed. Which of the following drugs would be most appropriate for the patient's disorder?

    A. Haloperidol
    B. Chlorpromazine
    C. Pramipexole
    D. Imipramine
    E. Carbidopa
    F. Entacapone

Difficulty level: Easy

18. A 59-year-old woman had been suffering from Parkinson disease for 4 years. Her disease was well controlled with a therapy that included levodopa/carbidopa. Which of the following actions most likely mediated the therapeutic efficacy of carbidopa in the patient's disease?

    A. Decreased dopamine metabolism in the striatum
    B. Increased active transport of dopamine into the brain
    C. Increased peripheral biotransformation of dopamine
    D. Decreased peripheral biotransformation of levodopa
    E. Decreased levodopa reuptake in the striatum

Difficulty level: Medium

19. A 65-year-old man complained to his physician that recently he felt increasingly confused at times, often had vivid dreams, and sometimes saw strange objects floating in the air. The patient, suffering from Parkinson disease, had been receiving levodopa/carbidopa for 1 year, and his disease was well controlled. Which of the following actions could be implemented to reduce the occurrence of the adverse effects being experienced by the patient?

    A. Substitute levodopa with selegiline.
    B. Substitute levodopa with pramipexole.
    C. Add benztropine to the present regimen.
    D. Add amantadine to the present regimen.
    E. Add clozapine to the present regimen.

Difficulty level: Easy

20. A 78-year-old woman recently diagnosed with Parkinson disease had been receiving levodopa/carbidopa for 3 weeks. Which of the following adverse effects could most likely occur in this patient?

    A. Blurred vision
    B. Diarrhea
    C. Postural hypotension
    D. Bradycardia
    E. Bradykinesia

Difficulty level: Easy

21. A 52-year-old woman with a long history of Parkinson disease had been receiving levodopa/carbidopa. Which of the following adverse effects of levodopa were most likely reduced by adding carbidopa to the treatment?

    A. Visual hallucinations
    B. Cardiac arrhythmias
    C. Nightmares
    D. Dyskinesias
    E. Mood changes

Difficulty level: Medium

22. A 53-year-old woman presented to her physician complaining of a unilateral resting tremor and slowing down of all movements. Her medical history was significant for two schizophrenic episodes in her late 40s that were successfully treated with haloperidol. On examination she showed cogwheel rigidity. A presumptive diagnosis of parkinsonism was made. Which of the following drugs would be contraindicated for this patient?

    A. Amantadine
    B. Carbidopa
    C. Pramipexole
    D. Benztropine
    E. Entacapone

Difficulty level: Medium

23. A 62-year-old woman with Parkinson disease had been receiving levodopa/carbidopa combination therapy. Coadministration of which of the following drugs would most likely increase the availability of levodopa in the patient's brain?

    A. Haloperidol
    B. Entacapone
    C. Benztropine
    D. Pramipexole
    E. Bromocriptine

Difficulty level: Easy

24. A 68-year-old patient was recently diagnosed with Parkinson disease. His medical history included benign prostatic hyperplasia for 2 years and chronic constipation for 5 years. Which of the following antiparkinson drugs would be contraindicated for this patient?

A. Levodopa
B. Benztropine
C. Selegiline
D. Amantadine
E. Pramipexole
F. Entacapone

Difficulty level: Easy

25. A 74-year-old man who had been suffering from Parkinson disease for 4 years complained of a purplish red mottling of the skin that began on his thighs and spread to his lower legs. The eruption appeared 2 weeks after a drug was added to his therapeutic regimen. A diagnosis of livedo reticularis was made. Which of the following drugs most likely caused this skin eruption?

A. Levodopa
B. Carbidopa
C. Selegiline
D. Amantadine
E. Pramipexole
F. Benztropine

Difficulty level: Medium

26. A 63-year-old woman complained to her physician of frequent palpitations. The woman, recently diagnosed with Parkinson disease, had been receiving levodopa/carbidopa for 3 weeks. Subsequent exams led to the diagnosis of sinus tachycardia likely due to the antiparkinson therapy. Which of the following actions most likely mediate the adverse effect reported by the patient?

A. Activation of cardiac dopamine receptors
B. Decreased acetylcholine release from cholinergic terminals
C. Activation of cardiac β receptors
D. Blockade of cardiac M_2 receptors
E. Increased sympathetic firing from the vasomotor center

Difficulty level: Easy

27. A 72-year-old woman recently diagnosed with Alzheimer disease started a pharmacotherapy with donepezil. Which of the following sets of adverse effects most likely occurred during the first days of treatment?

A. Hypertension, palpitations
B. Nausea, vomiting and diarrhea
C. Dry mouth, anhidrosis
D. Drowsiness, lethargy
E. Mydriasis, cycloplegia

Difficulty level: Medium

28. A 74-year-old woman presented to her neurologist complaining of a recent appearance of involuntary, slow movements involving her trunk and lower extremities. The woman, suffering from Parkinson disease, had been receiving levodopa/carbidopa for 3 years. Further exams led to the diagnosis of levodopa-induced dyskinesias. Which of the following drugs could be added to the therapy to decrease the patient's dyskinesias?

A. Selegiline
B. Entacapone
C. Pramipexole
D. Amantadine
E. Phenelzine

Difficulty level: Medium

29. A 78-year-old man had been showing increasing memory impairment and recognition deficits over the past 2 years. Recently, he became disoriented and confused at night. Physical examination revealed an alert person oriented to place with no focal neurologic deficits. His physician prescribed a drug that might help to slow the progression of his symptoms. Which of the following drugs would be appropriate for this patient?

A. Buspirone
B. Diazepam
C. Rivastigmine
D. Haloperidol
E. Physostigmine

Difficulty level: Medium

30. A 64-year-old man with Parkinson disease complained of periods of a few minutes of complete immobility, followed by a sudden switch to involuntary movements, such as twitching, nodding, and jerking. The patient's current medications included levodopa/carbidopa. To reduce these rapid fluctuations, the neurologist reduced the daily dose of levodopa/carbidopa and added a drug. Which of the following drugs was most likely prescribed?

A. Amantadine
B. Benztropine
C. Haloperidol
D. Pramipexole
E. Fluoxetine

Difficulty level: Medium

31. A 48-year-old woman complained to her physician that the drugs she was taking caused a disturbing nausea. Medication presently taken by the patient included omeprazole for heartburn and ciprofloxacin for a urinary tract infection. One week earlier, the woman was diagnosed with Parkinson disease and started an appropriate treatment. The physician advised the patient to take the drug in divided doses immediately after meals and said that the effect should subside in a few days. Which of the following drugs most likely caused the patient's nausea?

A. Carbidopa
B. Benztropine
C. Pramipexole
D. Omeprazole
E. Ciprofloxacin

Questions: III-8 Neuroleptic Drugs

Directions for questions **1–3**

Match each neuroleptic drug with the appropriate description (each lettered option can be selected once, more than once, or not at all).

A. Aripiprazole
B. Chlorpromazine
C. Clozapine
D. Fluphenazine
E. Haloperidol
F. Risperidone
G. Thioridazine
H. Thiotixene

Difficulty level: Easy

1. A drug with high affinity for dopamine D_4 receptors

Difficulty level: Easy

2. A phenothiazine that frequently causes extrapyramidal adverse effects

Difficulty level: Easy

3. A partial agonist at central dopaminergic receptors

Difficulty level: Medium

4. A 44-year-old woman was admitted to the psychiatric hospital for the sixth time since the age of 36. She was confused and threatening, saying that "the voices are back." The woman had been on antipsychotic therapy for several years, but she had stopped her medications 1 month prior to this admission. Physical examination showed abnormal involuntary movements manifested by tongue protrusion, frequent blinking, and continuous writhing of her arms and legs. A drug-induced primary dysfunction in which of the following brain regions was most likely responsible for the patient's syndrome?

A. Frontal cortex
B. Vestibular nuclei
C. Mesolimbic pathway
D. Striatum
E. Tuberoinfundibular pathway
F. Cerebellum

Difficulty level: Easy

5. An 82-year-old man who was a resident in a nursing facility presented with complete urinary retention. The man had a long history of hypertension and prostatic hyperplasia and was currently being treated with hydrochlorothiazide, captopril, and prazosin. Two days earlier, he became agitated and hostile, refused to cooperate, and tried to assault other residents. He received 50 mg of chlorpromazine intramuscularly and a second injection 8 hours later. Which of the following would be the most likely explanation for his urinary retention?

A. Decreased diuresis due to chlorpromazine
B. Chlorpromazine-induced relaxation of the detrusor muscle
C. Decreased diuresis due to captopril
D. Prazosin-induced relaxation of the r internal sphincter of the bladder
E. Prazosin-induced relaxation of the prostate capsule

Difficulty level: Medium

6. A 34-year-old woman recently diagnosed with undifferentiated schizophrenia started treatment with haloperidol. Which of the patient's presenting symptoms was most likely best controlled after 1 week of therapy?

A. Social withdrawal
B. Lack of emotion
C. Low energy
D. Persecutory delusions
E. Affective flattening

Difficulty level: Easy

7. A 30-year-old man complained of dry mouth, constipation, and blurred vision while reading the newspaper. The man, recently diagnosed with a schizoid disorder, had started treatment with clozapine 2 weeks previously. Blockade of which of the following receptors most likely mediated the adverse effects reported by the patient?

A. 5-HT$_2$ serotonergic
B. Alpha-1 adrenergic
C. H$_1$ histaminergic
D. Nm cholinergic
E. M$_3$ cholinergic

Difficulty level: Medium

8. A 23-year-old healthy volunteer received a new potential neuroleptic drug intravenously during a phase I clinical trial. It was known that the drug had significant blocking activity on dopamine D$_2$, histamine H$_1$, and serotonin 5-HT$_{2A}$ receptors. The volunteer was asked about the subjective symptoms he felt during the experiment. Which of the following pairs of mental effects were most likely reported by the subject?

A. Euphoria, increased self-confidence
B. Increased alertness, rapid flow of thought
C. Dysphoria, sleepiness
D. Irritability, restlessness
E. Delusions, perseverations

Difficulty level: Hard

9. A 17-year-old boy presented with brief episodes of protruding tongue, grimacing, and spasmodic torticollis on day 2 after admission to the psychiatric emergency department. The patient was brought there by the police because of assaultive behavior toward his mother. He struck her after a heavy drinking bout because he thought she was about to kill him with a knife. A drug treatment was started to control his assaultive behavior, and he received three intramuscular injections over 24 hours. Which of the following drugs most likely caused the adverse effects reported by the patient?

A. Haloperidol
B. Lorazepam
C. Buspirone
D. The large dose of ethanol
E. Fluoxetine
F. Clozapine

Difficulty level: Hard

10. A 32-year-old woman was brought to the hospital after she was found unconscious in a park on a hot summer day. The woman had been a resident in a psychiatric unit for the past year. She had a history of a chronic mental disorder, but she had recently shown improvement in her target symptoms and enjoyed outside privileges. She had left the ward to go jogging 2 hours before being found in the park. Her rectal temperature was 105°F (40.6°C), and a diagnosis of heat stroke was made. Which of the following drugs most likely contributed to the development of the patient's heat stroke?

A. Amitriptyline
B. Clozapine
C. Buspirone
D. Diazepam
E. Lithium
F. Fluoxetine

Difficulty level: Medium

11. A 42-year-old woman who was resident in a psychiatric hospital for a chronic mental illness had been mute and immobile for the past week. She actively resisted any attempt to be moved. Occasionally, she had brief periods of unprovoked agitated and aggressive behavior. Which of the following drugs should be avoided in this patient?

A. Lorazepam
B. Haloperidol
C. Carbamazepine
D. Olanzapine
E. Dantrolene
F. Valproic acid

Difficulty level: Medium

12. A 28-year-old man found wandering half-dressed in the streets complained of hearing voices cursing him, and his reported thoughts were bizarre. Upon admission to the psychiatric ward, his behavior became disruptive. He refused to cooperate and started verbal assaults that included threats of physical violence. A therapy was planned that include the intravenous injection of a drug. Which of the following drugs was most likely administered?

A. Lithium
B. Imipramine
C. Risperidone
D. Fluoxetine
E. Zolpidem
F. Morphine

Difficulty level: Medium

13. A 39-year-old man, a resident in a psychiatric unit because of disorganized schizophrenia, presented with profound lack of motivation, remarkably blunted affect, paucity of speech, and psychomotor retardation. He had been hospitalized three times since his diagnosis, and had been treated with haloperidol, chlorpromazine, and risperidone but had only a partial response to each medication. Which of the following psychotropic drugs would be most appropriate to try at this stage?

    A. Fluphenazine
    B. Thioridazine
    C. Fluoxetine
    D. Clozapine
    E. Lithium

Difficulty level: Easy

14. A 36-year old man complained to his physician of irritability, apathy, and the appearance of flicking movements of his extremities. He was referred to a neurologic clinic, where a diagnosis of Huntington chorea was made. Which of the following drugs would be most appropriate to suppress, at least partially, his choreic movements and agitated behavior?

    A. Imipramine
    B. Buspirone
    C. Trazodone
    D. Lithium
    E. Triazolam
    F. Haloperidol

Difficulty level: Hard

15. A 37-year-old woman was brought to the hospital after assaulting a neighbor. She presented in an acute psychotic state and struck two of the psychiatric unit staff members. The patient had had generalized tonic-clonic seizures since the age of 22, but she had stopped her antiepileptic therapy 2 months previously because she had been seizure-free for 3 months. Which of the following pairs of drugs would be an appropriate therapeutic regimen for this patient?

    A. Haloperidol and clonazepam
    B. Chlorpromazine and lamotrigine
    C. Clozapine and ethosuximide
    D. Thioridazine and ethosuximide
    E. Fluphenazine and gabapentin
    F. Clozapine and clonazepam

Difficulty level: Medium

16. A 29-year-old man was admitted to the psychiatric hospital in a paranoid and hostile state. He was diagnosed with chronic paranoid schizophrenia at the age of 23 and had been rehospitalized four times in the last 2 years, secondary to medication noncompliance. His medical work-up and urine drug screen were negative. During the last hospitalization, he had been stabilized on fluphenazine without any sign of adverse effects. Which of the following treatment would be appropriate for this patient?

    A. Intramuscular (IM) thioridazine
    B. Oral haloperidol
    C. IM fluphenazine decanoate
    D. Oral risperidone
    E. IM olanzapine
    F. Rectal chlorpromazine

Difficulty level: Medium

17. A 35-year-old man was admitted to a psychiatric hospital following a failed suicide attempt. He had a history of multiple drug abuse and was in jail for 2 months after wounding a relative. The psychiatric interview disclosed a patient with persecutory delusions, auditory hallucinations, remarkably flat affect, and social withdrawal. A presumptive diagnosis was made, and a therapy was prescribed. Which of the following drugs would be most appropriate for this patient?

    A. Amitriptyline
    B. Lorazepam
    C. Fluoxetine
    D. Lithium
    E. Clozapine
    F. Thioridazine

Difficulty level: Easy

18. A 60-year-old man complained to his physician of obstinate constipation. The man, recently diagnosed with a schizoaffective disorder, had started treatment with olanzapine. Blockade of which of the following pairs of receptors most likely mediated the adverse effect of the drug?

    A. Nicotinic and dopaminergic
    B. GABAergic and muscarinic
    C. Nicotinic and α_1
    D. Dopaminergic and α_1
    E. Muscarinic and serotonergic

Difficulty level: Medium

19. A 28-year-old man recently diagnosed with paranoid schizophrenia started treatment with aripiprazole. The therapeutic effect of this drug was most likely mediated by decreased dopaminergic transmission in which of the following brain structures?

A. Tuberoinfundibular pathway
B. Locus ceruleus
C. Mesolimbic mesocortical pathway
D. Nigrostriatal pathway
E. Nucleus basalis of Meynert

Difficulty level: Medium

20. A 24-year-old woman complained to her physician of amenorrhea of 2 months' duration and of a white discharge from her breasts during the past week. The woman had been on haloperidol and paroxetine for 3 months to treat a schizoaffective disorder. She was medication-compliant, and her illness was well controlled. Which of the following mechanisms was most likely responsible for the patient's symptoms?

A. Blockade of dopamine receptors in the hypothalamus
B. Increased serotonin availability in the pituitary
C. Increased serotonin availability in the striatum
D. Blockade of dopamine receptors in the pituitary
E. Blockade of adrencoceptors in the locus ceruleus

Difficulty level: Medium

21. A 34-year-old man, recently diagnosed with paranoid schizophrenia, became increasingly restless, was unable to sit or lie down for more than few minutes, and stated that he wanted "to jump out of my skin." Two weeks earlier, the patient had started therapy with fluphenazine. Which of the following drug-induced adverse effects did the patient most likely exhibit?

A. Acute dystonia
B. Complex partial seizure
C. Parkinsonism
D. Akathisia
E. Catalonia
F. Tardive dyskinesia

Difficulty level: Easy

22. A 27-year-old man complained to his physician of feeling "real slow" and of a bilateral hand tremor that improved when he picked up his coffee cup. The man, suffering from paranoid schizophrenia, was currently treated in an outpatient program. Physical examination showed cogwheel rigidity in both arms, stooped posture, and a shuffling gait. Which of the following drugs most likely caused these adverse effects?

A. Clozapine
B. Haloperidol
C. Metoclopramide
D. Olanzapine
E. Aripiprazole

Difficulty level: Hard

23. A 78-year-old man was admitted to the hospital with multiple fractures after falling at home. Two days after admission, his behavior changed. He accused the staff of torturing him. He was not able to recall why he was admitted to the hospital, was disoriented to time and place, and tried to pull out his intravenous line. His son reported that his father was fine before the accident. Which of the following drugs would be most appropriate to treat the acute symptoms in this patient?

A. Clozapine
B. Haloperidol
C. Diazepam
D. Lithium
E. Trazodone
F. Paroxetine

Difficulty level: Medium

24. A 33-year-old woman was brought to the emergency department with increased agitation and confusion. Physical examination revealed a temperature of 104°F (40°C), pulse of 125 bpm, labile blood pressure, profuse diaphoresis, sialorrhea, and muscle rigidity. The woman, recently diagnosed with schizophrenia, had started a therapy a few days previously. Which of the following drugs most likely caused the patient's syndrome?

A. Imipramine
B. Temazepam
C. Haloperidol
D. Fluoxetine
E. Lithium
F. Venlafaxine

Difficulty level: Medium

25. A 62-year-old schizophrenic woman was hospitalized because of palpitations and light-headedness of 2 hours' duration. Physical examination showed a patient in moderate distress with the following vital signs: blood pressure 110/85 mm Hg, heart rate 158 bpm, respiration 20 breaths/min. An electrocardiogram disclosed polymorphic ventricular tachycardia. Upon questioning, the patient admitted she had recently increased the dosage of her prescribed psychotropic drug because of her augmenting agitation. Which of the following drugs most likely caused the patient's symptoms and signs?

A. Trazodone
B. Thioridazine
C. Amitriptyline
D. Paroxetine
E. Lithium
F. Lorazepam

Difficulty level: Easy

26. A 51-year-old woman, a resident in a psychiatric unit, complained about feeling dizzy to the point of fainting upon standing up rapidly. The patient was hospitalized because over the past 3 months she had become increasingly agitated and afraid. She was convinced that people near her house were devils, plotting about stealing her money and cutting her throat. The patient started a psychotropic medication 2 weeks previously. Which of the following drugs most likely caused the patient's symptoms?

   A. Haloperidol
   B. Risperidone
   C. Amitriptyline
   D. Buspirone
   E. Lithium
   F. Trazodone

Difficulty level: Medium

27. A 34-year-old man complained to his physician that during intercourse, erection was difficult to achieve, and ejaculation was delayed. The man, recently diagnosed with paranoid schizophrenia, was treated initially with haloperidol, but he was switched to another drug because of the appearance of symptoms of pseudoparkinsonism. Which of the following drugs most likely caused the patient's symptoms?

   A. Fluphenazine
   B. Amitriptyline
   C. Paroxetine
   D. Thioridazine
   E. Fluoxetine
   F. Trazodone

Difficulty level: Medium

28. A 57-year-old man was admitted to the hospital because he did not urinate for the past 10 hours. The man was diagnosed with chronic undifferentiated schizophrenia 8 years ago and had taken many different antipsychotic drugs since then. Recently, insomnia became a problem, and his psychiatrist decided to change the therapy. One week ago, the man was diagnosed with prostatic hyperplasia and was scheduled for surgery. Which of the following drugs most likely contributed to the patient's acute urinary retention?

   A. Fluphenazine
   B. Haloperidol
   C. Olanzapine
   D. Venlafaxine
   E. Benztropine
   F. Amitriptyline

Difficulty level: Easy

29. A 29-year-old man complained to his psychiatrist of abnormal growth of his breast. The man had been receiving a psychotropic drug for 6 months to treat paranoid schizophrenia. He was medication-compliant, and his illness was well controlled. Which of the following drugs most likely caused the adverse effect reported by the patient?

   A. Clozapine
   B. Amitriptyline
   C. Haloperidol
   D. Venlafaxine
   E. Diazepam
   F. Fluoxetine

Difficulty level: Medium

30. A 41-year-old man was admitted to a psychiatric hospital because of worsening of his psychosis. The man was recently diagnosed with paranoid schizophrenia and had been treated with risperidone and aripiprazole without success. A new treatment was started. One week later, a blood test gave the following results:

   • White blood cell count: 1200/mm^3 (normal 4500–11,000/mm^3)
   • Neutrophils 12% (normal 54–62%)
   • Red blood cell count: 4.3 million/mm^3 (normal 4.0–5.5 million/mm^3)
   • Platelet count: 145,000/mm^3 (normal 150,000–400,000/mm^3)
   • Hemoglobin (Hb): 15 g/dL (normal >12 g/dL)

   Which of the following drugs did the patient most likely receive as the new treatment?

   A. Clozapine
   B. Fluphenazine
   C. Haloperidol
   D. Chlorpromazine
   E. Diazepam
   F. Fluoxetine

Questions: III-9 Drugs for Depressive and Anxiety Disorders

Directions for questions **1–5**

Match each drug with the appropriate description (each lettered option can be selected once, more than once, or not at all).

A. Amitriptyline
B. Bupropion
C. Citalopram
D. Fluoxetine
E. Mirtazapine
F. Phenelzine
G. Selegiline
H. Trazodone
I. Venlafaxine

Difficulty level: Easy

1. A drug with pronounced anticholinergic properties

Difficulty level: Easy

2. A nonselective monoamine oxidase inhibitor

Difficulty level: Easy

3. An active metabolite of this drug has a half-life of about 10 days.

Difficulty level: Easy

4. This drug can prolong the electrocardiogram QT interval.

Difficulty level: Easy

5. A serotonin 5-HT_{2A} presynaptic receptor blocker

Difficulty level: Medium

6. A 43-year-old man recently diagnosed with major depressive disorder started a pharmacotherapy with an antidepressant drug. Which of the following is most likely the common mechanism underlying the therapeutic effectiveness of long-term therapy with most antidepressants drugs?

   A. Inhibition of central monoamine metabolism
   B. Upregulation of central postsynaptic adrenoceptors
   C. Increased expression of brain-derived neurotrophic factor
   D. Decreased hippocampal neurogenesis
   E. Increased glutamatergic transmission

Difficulty level: Medium

7. A 55-year-old man suffering from severe depression was brought to the emergency department after an overdose of an unknown medication. Physical examination showed a lethargic patient with dilated pupils. Vital signs were blood pressure 95/55 mm Hg, heart rate 130 bpm, respirations 10/min. An electrocardiogram (ECG) showed tachycardia with wide QRS complex. Which of the following drugs most likely caused the patient's signs and symptoms?

   A. Sertraline
   B. Lithium
   C. Bupropion
   D. Phenelzine
   E. Amitriptyline
   F. Clonazepam

Difficulty level: Medium

8. A 45-year-old woman complained of dizziness to the point of fainting upon standing. She also felt drowsy for most of the day. The patient had been admitted to a hospital psychiatric unit 2 weeks earlier because of her third episode of major depressive disorder. She had been receiving an antidepressant therapy for the past 10 days. Which of the following drugs most likely caused the patient's symptoms?

   A. Bupropion
   B. Mirtazapine
   C. Amitriptyline
   D. Paroxetine
   E. Venlafaxine
   F. Lithium

Difficulty level: Medium

9. A 48-year-old man recently diagnosed with generalized anxiety disorder started an appropriate therapy with a drug that acts by increasing the availability of both norepinephrine and serotonin in the synaptic cleft of central nervous system neurons. Which of the following drugs was most likely prescribed?

   A. Amitriptyline
   B. Citalopram
   C. Venlafaxine
   D. Lorazepam
   E. Bupropion
   F. Trazodone

Difficulty level: Easy

10. A 33-year-old woman visited a psychiatrist for what she described as a very disturbing problem. The woman, who delivered a healthy boy 1 month earlier, was distraught by recurrent intrusive thoughts about stabbing her baby. After further questioning, the psychiatrist made a preliminary diagnosis and prescribed cognitive behavioral therapy and a pharmacotherapy. A drug with which of the following molecular mechanisms of action would be appropriate for this patient?

    A. Inhibition of monoamine oxidase A
    B. Blockade of serotonergic receptors
    C. Inhibition of serotonin transporter
    D. Blockade of β receptors
    E. Inhibition of norepinephrine transporter

Difficulty level: Hard

11. A 75-year-old woman recently diagnosed with pancreatic cancer was sent by her family physician to a psychiatrist because she complained of significant weight loss, forgetfulness, initial insomnia, and sadness. She also reported that she was discouraged, fearful, and very anxious and that sometimes she experienced sweating with a racing heart. The woman had been suffering from paroxysmal atrial tachycardia for 5 years. Considering the clinical picture and side effect profiles, which of the following would be an appropriate therapeutic regimen for addressing these complaints?

    A. Imipramine and chlorpromazine
    B. Amitriptyline and bupropion
    C. Paroxetine and zaleplon
    D. Haloperidol and buspirone
    E. Fluphenazine and lithium

Difficulty level: Medium

12. A 54-year-old woman complained to her physician of dizziness and vertigo when standing up rapidly. She had a long history of recurrent major depressive disorder and had taken various antidepressant drugs over the past several years. Recently, her psychiatrist decided to prescribe imipramine. Which of the following receptors most likely mediated the adverse effects of the drug in this patient?

    A. Beta-1 adrenergic
    B. 5-HT_3 serotonergic
    C. M_1 cholinergic
    D. Alpha-1 adrenergic
    E. H_1 histaminergic
    F. Nn cholinergic

Difficulty level: Hard

13. A 25-year-old woman visited a psychiatrist because she felt very anxious when she had to eat or drink in public. She acknowledged that her ideas of being watched by others were irrational, but she could not get beyond them. She also realized that alcohol helped her cope with her anxiety, and she had started drinking two or three glasses of brandy every day. After further questioning, a preliminary diagnosis was made, and cognitive behavioral therapy was prescribed, together with a pharmacological treatment. Which of the following drugs would be appropriate for this patient?

    A. Diazepam
    B. Zolpidem
    C. Bupropion
    D. Haloperidol
    E. Paroxetine
    F. Fluphenazine

Difficulty level: Medium

14. A 56-year-old woman with a long history of major depressive disorder was brought unconscious to the emergency department after her husband discovered she had taken several pills of amitriptyline in a suicide attempt. Which of the following symptoms did the patient most likely show?

    A. Bradycardia
    B. Pale skin
    C. Fecal incontinence
    D. Hyperpnea
    E. Hypertension
    F. Mydriasis

Difficulty level: Easy

15. A 52-year-old woman complained to her physician that the drug she was taking caused diarrhea. The woman, recently diagnosed with social anxiety disorder, had started a therapy with paroxetine 2 week earlier. Which of the following molecular actions in the enteric nervous system most likely mediated the adverse effect of this drug?

    A. Blockade of M_3 receptors
    B. Increased serotonergic activity
    C. Activation of $β_2$ receptors
    D. Increased adrenergic activity
    E. Decreased histaminergic activity
    F. Activation of $GABA_A$ receptors

Difficulty level: Medium

16. A 37-year-old man complained to his physician of persistent, intolerable pain in his left leg that started about 2 days earlier. He reported that he had tried several over-the-counter pain medications without success. One month earlier, the

patient underwent the amputation of his left leg following an accident at work. Physical examination revealed that pain could be elicited by a nonnoxious stimulus applied to the region of amputation. The physician made a preliminary diagnosis and prescribed a drug for pain. Which of the following drugs would be appropriate for this patient?

A. Phenobarbital
B. Acetaminophen
C. Clozapine
D. Venlafaxine
E. Diazepam
F. Lithium

Difficulty level: Medium

17. A 41-year-old man recently diagnosed with major depressive disorder complained to his psychiatrist that he felt drowsy for most of the day. The patient had started a treatment with paroxetine 2 months earlier, but his depressive symptoms were minimally improved. One week ago, his psychiatrist decided to shift to another antidepressant and prescribed a drug that acts by increasing the availability of both norepinephrine and serotonin in the synaptic cleft of central nervous system neurons. Which of the following drugs was most likely prescribed?

A. Amitriptyline
B. Trazodone
C. Bupropion
D. Citalopram
E. Sertraline

Difficulty level: Medium

18. A 43-year-old man went to his physician complaining of difficulty in maintaining an erection during intercourse. Past history of the patient was significant for an episode of ventricular tachycardia 1 year earlier. He was recently diagnosed with major depressive disorder and started a drug treatment 2 weeks ago. Which of the following drugs most likely caused the symptom reported by the patient?

A. Lithium
B. Amitriptyline
C. Fluoxetine
D. Chlorpromazine
E. Bupropion
F. Mirtazapine

Difficulty level: Medium

19. A 53-year-old woman with a long history of depression was admitted to the hospital because of agitation, insomnia, and tremors. She had been taking fluoxetine, lorazepam, and mirtazapine for several months. The doses of fluoxetine and mirtazapine had just been increased. Physical examination

showed a confused patient with hyperhidrosis, hyperreflexia, and myoclonus but without focal neurologic deficits. Vital signs were blood pressure 105/60 mm Hg, heart rate 130 bpm, respirations 32/min, body temperature 103.8°F (39.8°C). Qualitative plasma tests for alcohol, opioids, benzodiazepines, and tricyclic antidepressants were negative. An electrocardiogram indicated sinus tachycardia. A brain computed tomography scan was normal. Which of the following disorders most likely caused the patient's signs and symptoms?

A. Selective serotonin reuptake inhibitor (SSRI) discontinuation syndrome
B. Mirtazapine overdose
C. Serotonin syndrome
D. Brain glioblastoma
E. Benzodiazepine abstinence syndrome
F. Cerebral hemorrhage

Difficulty level: Medium

20. A 48-year-old woman visited a psychiatrist because for the past 2 months she had been depressed and was not interested in any of her usual activities, nor did she find anything enjoyable. She was also worried and anxious and felt very sleepy nearly every day. Her medical history was significant for exertional angina for the past 5 years. The psychiatrist made a preliminary diagnosis of major depressive disorder and prescribed cognitive behavioral therapy and a drug treatment. Which of the following drugs would be appropriate for this patient?

A. Amitriptyline
B. Fluoxetine
C. Trazodone
D. Mirtazapine
E. Lithium
F. Haloperidol

Difficulty level: Easy

21. A 34-year-old man suffering from a major depressive disorder had started a therapy with paroxetine, but 1 month later his symptoms were minimally improved, and his psychiatrist decided to add a drug to the treatment. The prescribed drug has a complex molecular mechanism of action that includes a blockade of presynaptic α_2 receptors. Which of the following drugs was most likely given?

A. Amitriptyline
B. Clonidine
C. Bupropion
D. Mirtazapine
E. Venlafaxine
F. Trazodone

Difficulty level: Medium

22. A 61-year-old woman came to her psychiatrist's office for a routine visit. She stated that the drug she was taking improved her depressed mood, but that she was still suffering from sadness and fatigue from time to time and from heavy drowsiness, nearly every day. The woman, recently diagnosed with major depressive disorder, had started fluoxetine 1 month earlier. After further questioning, the psychiatrist decided to add to the therapy a drug that is thought to act by decreasing reuptake of both norepinephrine and dopamine by brain neurons. Which of the following drugs was most likely prescribed?

A. Bupropion
B. Methylphenidate
C. Lamotrigine
D. Aripiprazole
E. Lithium

Difficulty level: Hard

23. A 36-year-old woman presented at an outpatient psychiatric clinic complaining of extreme lethargy and depressed mood more days than not, for the past 5 weeks. On interview she also reported an intense fear of being in confined spaces, and she carefully avoided elevators and traveling by airplane. Her psychiatric history indicated two similar episodes in the past, treated, respectively, with fluoxetine and venlafaxine, but with negligible results. After further questioning, a diagnosis of depression with atypical features was made. A drug was prescribed that acts by inactivating enzymes involved in neurotransmitter metabolism. Which of the following drugs was most likely prescribed?

A. Phenelzine
B. Entacapone
C. Fluoxetine
D. Amitriptyline
E. Citalopram

Difficulty level: Medium

24. A 22-year-old man was sent by his physician to a psychiatrist because of the onset of a distressing and embarrassing behavior. For the previous 3 months, the man had being experiencing an irresistible urge to disinfect any object in his room and to wash his hands again and again. He was disturbed by the unreasonable amount of time spent on such activities, and he acknowledged that his behavior was totally inappropriate, but he felt he could not stop it. He denied any substance abuse or use of medications. The psychiatrist made a preliminary diagnosis and prescribed cognitive behavioral therapy and a drug treatment. Which of the following drugs would be most appropriate for this patient?

A. Amitriptyline
B. Lithium
C. Fluoxetine
D. Haloperidol
E. Diazepam
F. Clozapine

Difficulty level: Easy

25. A 56-year-old man complained to his physician that he felt like he had the flu. He was dizzy, shivering, very irritable, anxious, and nauseated. The man was suffering from a major depressive disorder and had taken paroxetine for 4 months, but 3 days ago he decided to stop the drug, as his depression had been in full remission for the past month. Medical history of the patient was significant for hypertension, presently treated with losartan and hydrochlorothiazide. Which of the following disorders best explains the syndrome reported by the patient?

A. Acute depressive relapse
B. Selective serotonin reuptake inhibitor discontinuation syndrome
C. Poorly controlled hypertension
D. Paroxetine–losartan interaction
E. Serotonin syndrome
F. Paroxetine–hydrochlorotiazide interaction

Difficulty level: Hard

26. A 54-year-old man was admitted to the hospital because of generalized shaking, jerking movements of the limbs, twitching of the jaw, and clenching of the teeth. The patient had been suffering from gastrointestinal reflux disease for 2 years. Four months ago, he was diagnosed with an obsessive-compulsive disorder and started cognitive behavioral therapy and a pharmacological treatment. Three hours before admission, he took a tablet of metoclopramide given to him by a friend to decrease his heartburn. Which of the following drugs most likely interacted with metoclopramide, thus triggering the adverse effects reported by the patient?

A. Amitriptyline
B. Lithium
C. Zolpidem
D. Paroxetine
E. Bupropion
F. Buspirone

Difficulty level: Hard

27. A 25-year-old woman was admitted to the emergency department because of sudden onset of chest pain, difficulty in breathing, dizziness, and nausea. She described feeling "as if my head is going off in space and I am outside my body." She

stated that she had been under extreme stress lately, working too much, and that a similar episode had occurred, "out of the blue," 1 month ago. Physical examination and laboratory analyses revealed no abnormalities. A preliminary diagnosis was made, and an appropriate therapy was prescribed. Which of the following drugs would be appropriate for this patient?

A. Zolpidem
B. Ethosuximide
C. Clozapine
D. Haloperidol
E. Sertraline
F. Pramipexole

Difficulty level: Medium

28. A 17-year-old girl was admitted to an eating disorder clinic with a 3-month history of binge eating and vomiting and purging episodes occurring from twice per week to four times a day. After physical examination and lab tests, psychotherapy and a drug treatment were prescribed. Which of the following drugs would be appropriate for this patient?

A. Fluoxetine
B. Diazepam
C. Phenobarbital
D. Haloperidol
E. Clozapine
F. Lithium

Difficulty level: Medium

29. A 38-year-old man complained to his physician that the drug he was taking was effective in relieving his anxiety but caused a disturbing adverse effect. The patient had been recently diagnosed with a social anxiety disorder and started treatment with venlafaxine 2 weeks ago. Which of the following adverse effects did the patient most likely experience?

A. Obstinate constipation
B. Negligible orgasm during intercourse
C. Urge urinary incontinence
D. Dizziness and vertigo upon standing
E. Dry mouth, most of the day
F. Difficulty in near vision

Difficulty level: Hard

30. A 54-year-old man was admitted to the hospital with severe lower abdominal discomfort and complete inability to urinate for the past 6 hours. The man reported that he needed

to urinate 5 to 7 times during the previous night. Past history of the patient was significant for hypertension, insomnia, and chronic lower back pain, as well as for recently diagnosed depression. Present medications included lovastatin, losartan, hydrochlorothiazide, amitriptyline, and lorazepam. Which of the drugs most likely triggered the patient's anuria?

A. Losartan
B. Lovastatin
C. Hydrochlorotiazide
D. Amitriptyline
E. Lorazepam

Difficulty level: Easy

31. A 67-year-old woman complained to her psychiatrist that the drug she was taking did not improve her depressed mood at all. Three months earlier, the woman had suffered a myocardial infarction, and she had been suffering from a second-degree atrioventricular block since then. Eight days ago, she was diagnosed with a depressive disorder and started an appropriate treatment. The psychiatrist advised the patient to continue the treatment, explaining that the therapeutic effects of the prescribed drug usually take 2 to 3 weeks or more to become evident. Which of the following drugs was the patient most likely taking?

A. Amitriptyline
B. Paroxetine
C. Bupropion
D. Phenelzine
E. Diazepam

Difficulty level: Medium

32. A 21-year-old man was brought semiconscious to the emergency department after he jumped out of a window in a suicide attempt. History revealed that the patient was suffering from Hodgkin lymphoma and had been receiving the third cycle of chemotherapy. One month earlier, he was diagnosed with a depressive disorder and had been taking an appropriate pharmacotherapy since then. Which of the following drugs taken by the patient would be most likely to have increased his risk of suicide?

A. Zolpidem
B. Doxorubicin
C. Bleomycin
D. Vinblastine
E. Fluoxetine
F. Dacarbazine

Questions: III-10 Drugs for Bipolar Disorders

Directions for questions **1–4**

Match each drug used in bipolar disorder with the appropriate description (each lettered option can be selected once, more than once, or not at all).

- **A.** Aripiprazole
- **B.** Carbamazepine
- **C.** Lamotrigine
- **D.** Lithium
- **E.** Quetiapine
- **F.** Risperidone
- **G.** Valproic acid

Difficulty level: Easy

1. A dopaminergic receptor partial agonist effective in bipolar disorders

Difficulty level: Easy

2. This drug can increase the risk of spina bifida in the newborn when given during pregnancy.

Difficulty level: Easy

3. This drug is effective for the treatment of both acute mania and all types of epilepsy.

Difficulty level: Easy

4. The hepatic clearance of this drug is zero.

Difficulty level: Medium

5. A 45-year-old man with a long history of bipolar disorder had been stable on a maintenance lithium treatment for the past year. Which of the following best describes a current working hypothesis about the molecular mechanism of action of lithium?

- **A.** Increased synthesis of adenylyl cyclase
- **B.** Increased synthesis of inositol monophosphatase
- **C.** Increased serotonin reuptake into serotonergic terminals
- **D.** Upregulated β-adrenoceptors
- **E.** Decreased synthesis of inositol triphosphate (IP_3) and diacylglycerol (DAG)
- **F.** Increased glutamatergic activity

Difficulty level: Medium

6. A 68-year-old man was admitted to a psychiatric hospital because of depression, hopelessness about his condition, sleep disturbances, and poor appetite. He had a long history of previous hospitalizations for manic or depressive episodes and had experienced five mood swings in the past year, including episodes of depression and hypomania. Despite adequate plasma levels, he had not responded to lithium. Which of the following drugs would be appropriate for the patient at this time?

- **A.** Haloperidol
- **B.** Bupropion
- **C.** Fluphenazine
- **D.** Quetiapine
- **E.** Diazepam
- **F.** Amitriptyline

Difficulty level: Easy

7. A 34-year-old man was admitted to a psychiatric hospital during an acute manic attack. The man had his first manic attack at the age of 27 and had had three other manic attacks since then. A diagnosis of acute mania was made, and a therapy was prescribed that included a drug that acts by blocking D_2 and 5-HT_2 receptors in the brain. Which of the following drugs was most likely prescribed?

- **A.** Lamotrigine
- **B.** Clomipramine
- **C.** Valproic acid
- **D.** Olanzapine
- **E.** Lithium
- **F.** Trazodone

Difficulty level: Medium

8. A 36-year-old woman complained to her physician that she felt tired, suffered from constipation, and had gained weight in recent weeks. She also complained of feeling cold and of absence of menses during the last 3 months. The woman had been suffering from a bipolar disorder and had been maintained successfully on lithium therapy for 1 year. In addition to lithium, her present medication included cimetidine for duodenal ulcer and loratadine for hay fever. Which of the following was the most likely cause of the patient's symptoms?

- **A.** Lithium-induced hypothyroidism
- **B.** Cimetidine-induced decrease in lithium metabolism
- **C.** Adverse effects of cimetidine
- **D.** Central depressant effects of loratadine
- **E.** Worsening of the disease due to inadequate lithium dosage

Difficulty level: Medium

9. A 57-year-old woman complained to her physician of tremor, polyuria, mental confusion, and speech disturbances. The woman had a diagnosis of bipolar disorder and had been receiving lithium for 7 months. Two weeks ago, she was found to have successive high blood pressure readings, and her physician started an antihypertensive treatment with

hydrochlorothiazide and losartan. Which of the following was most likely the reason for the adverse effects reported by the patient?

A. Thiazide-induced dilutional hypernatremia
B. Decreased renal elimination of lithium
C. Decreased hepatic metabolism of lithium
D. Thiazide-induced hypokalemia
E. Losartan-induced hyperkalemia

Difficulty level: Medium

10. A 30-year-old woman was brought to a psychiatric hospital by her parents because she had been in bed most of the day for the last 2 weeks. The woman was admitted to the hospital 4 months ago because of an acute manic episode and was discharged on valproic acid with a favorable response. On questioning, she said she discontinued her therapy 2 week ago because she felt cured, but now she admitted she was depressed most of the time and wanted to die. The patient was dismissed from the hospital 1 week later with an appropriate maintenance therapy. Which of the following drugs would be appropriate for the patient at this time?

A. Amitriptyline
B. Lorazepam
C. Haloperidol
D. Buspirone
E. Lithium
F. Zolpidem

Difficulty level: Easy

11. A 49-year-old woman visited her physician complaining of a fine hand tremor and of an increasing need to urinate. The woman, recently diagnosed with a psychiatric disorder, had been taking a psychotropic drug for 3 weeks. Physical examination disclosed cystic acne with folliculitis over the trunk and thorax. Which of the following drugs was most likely to have caused the patient's symptoms and signs?

A. Fluoxetine
B. Haloperidol
C. Lithium
D. Fluphenazine
E. Valproic acid
F. Trazodone

Difficulty level: Medium

12. A 49-year-old woman was discharged from a psychiatric hospital after an episode of acute mania. Over the past 2 years, the patient had had five previous hospitalizations for major manic or depressive episodes. Her postdischarge therapy included lithium. How long should the patient continue to take lithium?

A. For 3 months
B. For 6 months
C. For 9 months
D. For 1 year
E. Indefinitely

Difficulty level: Medium

13. A 33-year-old woman suffering from a bipolar disorder had been maintained successfully on lithium therapy. Now she planned to become pregnant. Her psychiatrist decided to stop lithium and to start another medication. Which of the following drugs would be appropriate for this patient?

A. Carbamazepine
B. Valproic acid
C. Quetiapine
D. Haloperidol
E. Clozapine
F. Amitriptyline

Difficulty level: Easy

14. A 57-year-old man complained to his physician that he was always thirsty and had frequent and profuse micturition. The man, recently diagnosed with bipolar disorder, had been receiving lithium for 3 weeks. Which of the following was most likely the cause of the patient's symptoms?

A. Blockade of Na^+ reabsorption in the thick ascending loop of Henle
B. Blockade of vasopressin-induced increase of cAMP in the collecting tubule
C. Increased plasma glucose levels
D. Stimulation of the thirst center in the hypothalamus
E. Blockade of vasopressin secretion from the pituitary

Difficulty level: Medium

15. A 43-year-old woman recently diagnosed with major depressive disorder had started a therapy with sertraline, but 1 month later her condition had not changed appreciably, and her psychiatrist decided to add a second medication (augmentation therapy). He prescribed a drug with multiple mechanisms of action, including an inhibition of glycogen synthase kinase 3. Which of the following drugs was most likely prescribed?

A. Olanzapine
B. Triiodothyronine
C. Bupropion
D. Lamotrigine
E. Buspirone
F. Lithium

Difficulty level: Easy

16. A 55-year-old man suffering from bipolar disorder started a maintenance therapy with lithium. Which of the following adverse effects is most likely to occur during the first days of therapy?

    A. Constipation
    B. Weight loss
    C. Insomnia
    D. Hypertension
    E. Edema

Difficulty level: Hard

17. A 20-year-old man was accompanied to the clinic by his mother, who stated that her son had been exhibiting very unusual behavior over the past few weeks. He was euphoric most of the day, stayed up later and later at night, and frequently awakened his parents shouting and screaming. Recently, he experienced problems at work. Upon arriving at the clinic, he had trouble sitting still or listening and became increasingly irritable throughout the examination. He repeatedly said he heard a voice telling him he had a superpower. Which of the following pairs of drugs would be most helpful for the patient's condition?

    A. Fluoxetine and risperidone
    B. Imipramine and lithium
    C. Fluoxetine and haloperidol
    D. Imipramine and haloperidol
    E. Risperidone and lithium

Difficulty level: Hard

18. A 44-year-old woman reported to her psychiatrist that the prescribed drug improved her feelings, but that she was still somewhat depressed and lethargic almost every day. The woman, recently diagnosed with major depressive disorder, had been taking venlafaxine for 2 months. The psychiatrist decided to add a second drug to the present regimen. Which of the following drugs would be appropriate for the patient at this time?

    A. Amitriptyline
    B. Mirtazapine
    C. Haloperidol
    D. Lithium
    E. Valproic acid
    F. Diazepam

Difficulty level: Easy

19. A 46-year-old man complained to his physician of a fine hand tremor, diarrhea, and frequent need to urinate. The man had

been receiving lithium therapy for 1 month to treat bipolar disorder. Routine lab tests showed normal renal function and a plasma lithium level of 3 mEq/L. Lithium has a volume of distribution of about 45 L and a half-life of about 20 hours. How many hours should the physician withhold lithium in order to reach a safer, yet likely therapeutic level of 0.75 mEq/L?

    A. 10
    B. 20
    C. 30
    D. 40
    E. 80
    F. 100

Difficulty level: Easy

20. A 34-year-old woman who had been treated for an episode of acute mania was no longer overtly manic. However, because she had had past episodes of depression and mania, her psychiatrist decided to institute prophylactic therapy and prescribed a drug that appears to affect primarily the inositol second messenger system. Which of the following drugs was most likely prescribed?

    A. Valproic acid
    B. Aripiprazole
    C. Lamotigrine
    D. Lithium
    E. Quetiapine
    F. Risperidone

Difficulty level: Medium

21. A 63-year-old man complained to his physician that he had a constant, strong desire to drink and had frequent and profuse micturition. The man was otherwise healthy, but 2 months earlier he was diagnosed with a psychiatric disorder and had been taking an appropriate pharmacotherapy since then. Further exams indicated that the patient's daily urine output was about 12 to 15 L. His urine osmolarity was 216 mOsm/kg under control conditions and 225 mOsm/kg after the administration of desmopressin. The physician decreased the dose of the drug the patient was taking for his psychiatric disorder and prescribed another drug to cure the patient's urinary symptoms. Which of the following drugs would be most appropriate to treat the patient's urinary symptoms at this time?

    A. Furosemide
    B. Hydrochlorothiazide
    C. Amiloride
    D. Spironolactone
    E. Conivaptan

Questions: III-11 Drugs for Childhood Behavioral Disorders

Directions for questions **1–3**

Match each drug with the appropriate description (each lettered option can be selected once, more than once, or not at all).

A. Aripiprazole
B. Atomoxetine
C. Bupropion
D. Clonidine
E. Desmopressin
F. Dextroamphetamine
G. Guanfacine
H. Methylphenidate
I. Lisdexamfetamine
J. Risperidone

Difficulty level: Easy

1. An agonist at α_2 and imidazoline receptors

Difficulty level: Easy

2. A partial agonist at central dopaminergic receptors

Difficulty level: Easy

3. A prodrug that is used to treat attention deficit hyperactivity disorder

Difficulty level: Easy

4. An 8-year-old boy recently diagnosed with attention deficit hyperactivity disorder (ADHD) started a treatment with methylphenidate. Which of the following neural pathways most likely represent the main site of therapeutic action of the drug in this child?

A. Tuberoinfundibular
B. Mesolimbic
C. Corticostriatal
D. Mesocortical
E. Spinothalamic

Difficulty level: Easy

5. A 7-year-old boy was taken to the hospital by his mother for a scheduled checkup. The boy, recently diagnosed with attention deficit hyperactivity disorder (ADHD), had started an appropriate pharmacotherapy 2 weeks earlier. The mother reported that the child was able to focus better and was less hyperactive and less impulsive. However, she was concerned because her son frequently exhibited eye blinking, grimacing, and twitching. The physician said that these abnormal movements could be related to the child's therapy. Which of the following drugs might have caused these adverse effects?

A. Fluphenazine
B. Methylphenidate
C. Atomoxetine
D. Ethosuximide
E. Paroxetine

Difficulty level: Easy

6. A 6-year-old boy was in his family physician's office for a scheduled visit. The boy, recently diagnosed with attention deficit hyperactivity disorder (ADHD), had started an appropriate pharmacotherapy 1 week earlier. Vital signs were blood pressure 155/88 mm Hg, heart rate 85 bpm, respirations 16/min. Which of the following drugs most likely caused the patient's high blood pressure?

A. Atomoxetine
B. Norepinephrine
C. Phenylephrine
D. Guanfacine
E. Clonidine

Difficulty level: Medium

7. A 24-year-old woman who had been suffering from depression for 3 years was recently diagnosed with attention deficit hyperactivity disorder (ADHD). Which of the following pairs of drugs would be appropriate for this patient?

A. Bupropion and haloperidol
B. Methylphenidate and sertraline
C. Dextroamphetamine and diazepam
D. Atomoxetine and fluphenazine
E. Guanfacine and lorazepam

Difficulty level: Easy

8. A 12-year-old girl suffering from attention deficit hyperactivity disorder (ADHD) was treated in the past with different drugs with little success. The physician decided to try another drug that is a selective inhibitor of norepinephrine reuptake. Which of the following drugs was most likely prescribed?

A. Cocaine
B. Atomoxetine
C. Methylphenidate
D. Dextroamphetamine
E. Bupropion

Difficulty level: Medium

9. An 8-year-old boy was brought to his pediatrician with complaints of repeated head jerking, blinking, and grimacing for the past 2 months. The boy had never had a tic-free period for more than a few days and recently had started making grunting noises and saying obscenities. Which of the following drugs would be useful to treat the patient's condition?

    A. Fluoxetine
    B. Aripiprazole
    C. Clonazepam
    D. Naltrexone
    E. Imipramine
    F. Lithium

Difficulty level: Easy

10. A 10-year-old boy recently diagnosed with attention deficit hyperactivity disorder (ADHD) started a treatment with dextroamphetamine. The therapy significantly improved the disease, but the parents were concerned because the boy was never hungry. Which of the following was most likely a site of this anorectic action of amphetamines?

    A. Temporal cortex
    B. Putamen
    C. Ventrolateral medulla
    D. Lateral hypothalamus
    E. Amygdala
    F. Locus ceruleus

Difficulty level: Medium

11. A 23-year-old woman presented to her physician complaining that she felt fearful, helpless, and worried almost continuously during the day. She also had difficulty organizing her thoughts and claimed that cognitive concepts were exceedingly difficult to grasp. Past history of the patient indicated that she was a difficult child to manage and often impulsive and unproductive in school. She started smoking at the age of 12 and now smoked two packs of cigarettes daily. She tried to quit smoking several times with no success. The physician suggested trying a drug that was effective in treating both depressive and attention deficit disorders, as well as in smoking cessation. Which of the following drugs was most likely prescribed?

    A. Methylphenidate
    B. Paroxetine
    C. Bupropion
    D. Guanfacine
    E. Amitriptyline

Difficulty level: Medium

12. A 7-year-old boy was brought by his mother to his family pediatrician because he still wet the bed. The boy achieved daytime bladder control by 3 years of age but wet his bed once or twice a week. A conditioning therapy with the aid of a bell and pad alarm, started 2 weeks previously, was only partially effective. The pediatrician ordered a drug to be given by nasal spray. Which of the following drugs was most likely prescribed?

    A. Desmopressin
    B. Imipramine
    C. Atropine
    D. Fluoxetine
    E. Haloperidol
    F. Clonidine

Difficulty level: Medium

13. A 7-year-old boy was referred for psychiatric evaluation because he was unable to sit still in school for more than 1 minute at a time. During story time, he interrupted, wandered around the classroom, or poked his neighbors. After the psychiatric evaluation, a diagnosis was made, and a drug was prescribed that acts by increasing catecholamine release in the central nervous system. Which of the following drugs was most likely prescribed?

    A. Cocaine
    B. Dextroamphetamine
    C. Methylphenidate
    D. Guanfacine
    E. Bupropion

Difficulty level: Easy

14. A 24-year-old man recently diagnosed with attention deficit hyperactivity disorder (ADHD) started behavioral therapy and treatment with methylphenidate. Which of the following adverse effects was the patient most likely to experience during the first week of therapy?

    A. Increased appetite
    B. Growth suppression
    C. Seizures
    D. Insomnia
    E. Hallucinations

Difficulty level: Medium

15. A 12-year-old boy was referred to a psychiatrist because he recently became very irritable and would hit his head on a wall or furniture if the room was too noisy. The boy lived in

a group home and attended a special school program for adolescents with developmental disabilities. He preferred tasks that allowed him to be alone and was described as a distant child who would not participate in group activities. Although he had superior ability in mathematics, he tested in the medium range of mental retardation. The boy had been diagnosed as autistic at age 4. The psychiatrist prescribed a drug to decrease irritability and self-injurious behavior. Which of the following drugs was most likely appropriately prescribed?

A. Fluoxetine
B. Risperidone
C. Atomoxetine
D. Clonidine
E. Bupropion
F. Methylphenidate

Difficulty level: Easy

16. An 11-year-old girl recently diagnosed with attention deficit hyperactivity disorder (ADHD) started treatment with methylphenidate. Which of the following molecular actions on central adrenergic neurons most likely mediated the therapeutic effect of the drug in the patient's disease?

A. Blockade of dopamine reuptake
B. Stimulation of norepinephrine metabolism
C. Blockade of serotonergic receptors
D. Activation of glutamate receptors
E. Blockade of gamma-aminobutyric acid (GABA) receptors

Difficulty level: Easy

17. A 15-year-old girl was recently diagnosed with attention deficit hyperactivity disorder (ADHD). Her physician was concerned about the abuse potential of drugs used for this disorder, as the girl admitted smoking marijuana occasionally with her friends. Which of the following drugs would be most appropriate for this patient?

A. Methylphenidate
B. Paroxetine
C. Dextroamphetamine
D. Alprazolam
E. Atomoxetine
F. Aripiprazole

Difficulty level: Medium

18. An 8-year-old girl was in her physician's office for a follow-up visit regarding her attention deficit hyperactivity disorder (ADHD). She had been treated with two different drugs over the past 6 weeks with little success. The physician decided to stop the ongoing therapy and to start a drug that acts as a central α_2-receptor agonist. Which of the following drugs was most likely prescribed?

A. Dextroamphetamine
B. Methylphenidate
C. Guanfacine
D. Bupropion
E. Epinephrine

Difficulty level: Easy

19. A 6-year-old girl had difficulty sustaining attention in activities at school and at home. She failed to pay close attention to teachers and often made careless mistakes in schoolwork. She repeatedly exhibited hyperactivity and impulsivity. She has had these symptoms since starting kindergarten last year. A treatment with guanfacine was started. Which of the following adverse effects did the patient most likely experience during the first days of therapy?

A. Hypotension
B. Increased appetite
C. Salivation
D. Aggressive behavior
E. Anhidrosis

Difficulty level: Medium

20. An 8-year-old boy who had been suffering from Tourette syndrome for 1 year was recently diagnosed with attention deficit hyperactivity disorder. Which of the following drugs would be appropriate to treat both disorders?

A. Methylphenidate
B. Clonidine
C. Dextroamphetamine
D. Haloperidol
E. Risperidone

Questions: III-12 Opioid Analgesics and Antagonists

Directions for questions **1–5**

For each numbered item select the one lettered option that is most closely associated with it (each lettered option can be selected once, more than once, or not at all).

A. Buprenorphine
B. Codeine
C. Fentanyl
D. Heroin
E. Loperamide
F. Methadone
G. Morphine
H. Naloxone
I. Pentazocine
J. Propoxyphene
K. Tramadol

Difficulty level: Easy

1. A partial agonist at μ (mu) opioid receptors and antagonist at κ (kappa) opioid receptors

Difficulty level: Easy

2. A full opioid agonist with the highest oral bioavailability

Difficulty level: Easy

3. A drug with very weak opioid activity used in the treatment of diarrhea

Difficulty level: Easy

4. A partial agonist at μ (mu) opioid receptors and full agonist at κ (kappa) opioid receptors

Difficulty level: Easy

5. A drug with high affinity but no intrinsic activity at opioid receptors

Difficulty level: Easy

6. A 34-year-old man was admitted to the emergency department because of a sharp abdominal pain for the past 3 hours. Further exams led to the diagnosis of renal colic, and the patient received an intramuscular injection of morphine. Activation of receptors in which of the following brain areas most likely mediated the analgesic effect of the drug in this patient?

A. Edinger–Westphal nucleus
B. Meynert nucleus
C. Nucleus accumbens
D. Periaqueductal gray matter
E. Medial eminence of the hypothalamus

Difficulty level: Easy

7. A 22-year-old pregnant woman was in labor for 12 hours and was experiencing strong and very painful contractions. Epidural administration of morphine was administered for analgesia. Which of the following neuronal areas was most likely the main site of the analgesic action of morphine in this setting?

A. Locus ceruleus
B. Substantia gelatinosa
C. Periaqueductal gray matter
D. Nucleus accumbens
E. Substantia nigra
F. Rostral ventrolateral medulla

Difficulty level: Easy

8. A 58-year-old woman with metastasized breast cancer received an intramuscular injection of morphine for pain, but she suffered nausea and vomiting soon after the injection. Which of the following brain areas was most likely the main site of these adverse effects of morphine?

A. Locus ceruleus
B. Area postrema
C. Median hypothalamic eminence
D. Nucleus accumbens
E. Putamen
F. Rostral ventrolateral medulla

Difficulty level: Easy

9. A 61-year-old woman complained of severe pain a few hours after surgery for renal cancer. An intramuscular injection of morphine was given. Which of the following actions most likely contributed to the analgesic effect of morphine?

A. Activation of brainstem neurons that modulate pain transmission
B. Stimulation of substance P release from nerve terminals in the spinal cord
C. Induction of dissociative feeling and dysphoria
D. Inhibition of adrenergic pathways from the locus ceruleus
E. Inhibition of serotonergic pathways from the raphe nuclei

Difficulty level: Easy

10. A 55-year-old man complained of severe pain after surgery to remove a colon cancer. The physician prescribed a drug that is a partial μ (mu) opioid agonist, more potent than morphine, and whose effects are not readily antagonized by naloxone. Which of the following drugs was most likely administered?

A. Methadone
B. Meperidine
C. Codeine
D. Buprenorphine
E. Fentanyl
F. Loperamide

Difficulty level: Medium

11. A 34-year-old woman was admitted to the emergency department because of multiple fractures sustained in a car accident. The patient complained of severe pain, and an intramuscular injection of morphine was given. Which of the following molecular actions most likely mediated the analgesic effect of the drug in this patient?

A. Opening of Ca^{2+} channels on presynaptic nerve terminals
B. Closing of chloride channels on postsynaptic neurons
C. Stimulation of substance P release from nociceptive nerve terminals
D. Opening of K^+ channels on postsynaptic neurons
E. Closing of Na^+ channels on presynaptic nerve terminals
F. Stimulation of glutamate release from nociceptive nerve terminals

Difficulty level: Easy

12. A 52-year-old man admitted to the emergency department after a myocardial infarction still complained of severe pain after an intravenous injection of nitroglycerin. Intramuscular administration of morphine was given. Which of the following molecular actions most likely mediated the analgesic effect of the drug?

A. Stimulation of release of endogenous opioid peptides
B. Activation of μ (mu) receptors
C. Blockade of κ (kappa) receptors
D. Stimulation of substance P release from nerve terminals
E. Activation of glutamate receptors
F. Blockade of β adrenoceptors

Difficulty level: Medium

13. A 68-year-old man suffering from metastasized neck cancer had a characteristic pinpoint pupil because of subcutaneous infusion of morphine from a portable pump. Stimulation of which of the following brain areas most likely mediated this drug effect?

A. Locus ceruleus
B. Nucleus ambiguus
C. Edinger–Westphal nucleus
D. Area postrema
E. Nucleus accumbens
F. Hippocampus

Difficulty level: Medium

14. A 55-year-old woman suffering from terminal cancer received a spinal morphine infusion from a portable pump. Which of the following was the most likely electrophysiological consequence of the activation of postsynaptic μ (mu) opioid receptors on the pain transmission neurons in the spinal cord?

A. Increased firing of those neurons
B. Production of an excitatory postsynaptic potential
C. Decrease in membrane K^+ conductance
D. Increase in membrane Na^+ conductance
E. Production of an inhibitory postsynaptic potential

Difficulty level: Hard

15. A 51-year-old woman was seen in the emergency department because of strong abdominal pain for the past hour. Physical examination showed a red-headed, pale-skinned woman in obvious distress, with severe pain and tenderness of the right flank. A presumptive diagnosis of renal colic was made, and the patient was given an intramuscular injection of an opioid drug that is a partial agonist at μ (mu) receptors and a full agonist at κ (kappa) receptors. Which of the following drugs was most likely administered?

A. Pentazocine
B. Buprenorphine
C. Codeine
D. Methadone
E. Fentanyl

Difficulty level: Medium

16. A 56-year-old woman suffering from osteoarthritis complained to her physician that the joint pain in her legs and shoulders had worsened and was now unbearable. She had used several drugs in the past, including ketorolac and ibuprofen, with little success. Full doses of acetaminophen were partially effective until recently, but they were no longer effective. Every morning the patient said that she was "really terrified" by the expected pain and asked for an effective analgesic. Her physician decided to add a drug that can also lower the anxiety, fear, and suffering evoked by pain. Which of the following drugs was most likely prescribed?

A. Indomethacin
B. Ketorolac
C. Sertraline
D. Diazepam
E. Venlafaxine
F. Methadone

Difficulty level: Medium

17. A 64-year-old man suffering from advanced heart failure was admitted to the emergency department because of extreme dyspnea over the past hour. After physical examination, a diagnosis of impending pulmonary edema was made, and an appropriate therapy was prescribed that included the intramuscular injection of morphine. Which of the following cardiovascular actions most likely contributed to the therapeutic effect of the drug in the patient's disorder?

   A. Increased systolic pressure
   B. Constriction of the renal vascular bed
   C. Increased heart rate
   D. Peripheral venous dilation
   E. Increased left ventricular end-diastolic pressure

Difficulty level: Easy

18. A 67-year-old woman complained to her physician of obstinate constipation. The woman, who was suffering bone pain from metastatic breast cancer, had started a therapy with morphine 2 weeks previously. Which of the following actions most likely mediated the adverse effect of the drug in this patient?

   A. Decreased anal sphincter tone
   B. Increased colonic tone
   C. Increased intestinal peristalsis
   D. Increased reflex response to rectal distention
   E. Increased softening of feces

Difficulty level: Easy

19. A 39-year-old woman was admitted to the hospital because of gripping and burning abdominal pain that increased over the past 4 hours. The patient was suffering from stage 4 ovarian cancer metastatic to the pelvis. A treatment with sustained release morphine was started. Which of the following effects on the patient's respiratory system would be expected during the first few days of therapy?

   A. Stimulation of the cough reflex
   B. Bronchodilation
   C. Increased vital capacity
   D. Decreased tidal volume
   E. Increased rate of breathing

Difficulty level: Easy

20. A 52-year-old man was in his physician's office for a routine visit. The man, suffering from metastasized stomach cancer, had started a therapy with morphine 3 weeks ago. Which of the following morphine effects was most likely unchanged in the patient after 3 weeks of therapy?

   A. Respiratory depression
   B. Miosis
   C. Analgesia
   D. Sedation
   E. Euphoria
   F. Nausea and vomiting

Difficulty level: Easy

21. A 34-year-old woman complained to her physician of annoying constipation. One week earlier, she had developed a sore throat and a dry, nonproductive cough and was diagnosed with acute bronchitis. A drug treatment was started, and the cough gradually disappeared. Which of the following drugs most likely caused the constipation reported by the patient?

   A. Buprenorphine
   B. Fentanyl
   C. Albuterol
   D. Codeine
   E. Theophylline
   F. Morphine

Difficulty level: Easy

22. A 36-year-old man complained of severe abdominal pain after surgery to remove a kidney stone. An analgesic drug was administered intramuscularly. Shortly after the administration, an itchy weal developed at the injection site, along with generalized pruritus. Which of the following drugs was most likely given to the patient?

   A. Fentanyl
   B. Acetaminophen
   C. Indomethacin
   D. Clonidine
   E. Ibuprofen
   F. Morphine

Difficulty level: Easy

23. A 74-year-old woman was admitted to the emergency department in a stupor from which she could be aroused only briefly by strong and repeated stimulation. The woman had received an intramuscular analgesic drug 2 hours earlier because of several minor abrasions and wounds secondary to a motor accident. Her records showed she was suffering from an anxiety disorder presently treated with diazepam. Which of the following analgesic drugs was most likely given to the patient?

   A. Acetaminophen
   B. Piroxicam
   C. Indomethacin
   D. Morphine
   E. Ketorolac
   F. Aspirin

Difficulty level: Medium

24. A 33-year-old man was admitted to the emergency department because of severe agitation and hallucinatory behavior. He admitted he had been using marijuana (regularly) and LSD (from time to time). Shortly before admission, he self-injected what he believed to be "smack" (heroin) sold on the street. Which of the following opioids did the patient most likely take?

A. Buprenorphine
B. Morphine
C. Pentazocine
D. Fentanyl
E. Methadone

Difficulty level: Easy

25. A 62-year-old woman recovering from surgical repair of multiple fractures was complaining of severe pain. A standard dose of morphine was given intramuscularly. Which of the following adverse effects most likely occurred in this patient?

A. Dysphoria
B. Impairment of far vision
C. Diarrhea
D. Hypertension
E. Dry cough

Difficulty level: Medium

26. A 63-year-old man with terminal prostate cancer developed fever (101.7°F, 38.7°C) followed by severe respiratory depression. For the past week, the patient had been receiving an analgesic medication by transdermal patch because of severe bone pain. Which of the following drugs was most likely administered to the patient?

A. Pentazocine
B. Codeine
C. Fentanyl
D. Ibuprofen
E. Ketorolac
F. Indomethacin

Difficulty level: Easy

27. A 59-year-old woman with metastatic breast cancer complained of increasing bone pain, no longer managed with acetaminophen and codeine. A daily treatment with oral morphine was started. Which of the following drugs should be given concomitantly to prevent one of the most common adverse effects of opioids?

A. Diazepam
B. Fluoxetine
C. Lactulose

D. Propranolol
E. Nifedipine
F. Omeprazole

Difficulty level: Easy

28. A 62-year-old man suffering from metastatic prostate cancer complained of severe bone pain. The physician prescribed methadone. Which of the following was most likely one of the postreceptor mechanisms triggered by this drug?

A. Inhibition of the synthesis of inositol triphosphate/diacylglycerol (IP_3/DAG)
B. Blockade of Ca^{2+} channels on presynaptic nerve terminals
C. Opening of Na^+ channels on neuronal cell membrane
D. Stimulation of adenylyl cyclase activity
E. Inhibition of phospholipase C activity

Difficulty level: Easy

29. A 35-year-old man admitted to the hospital because of a second-degree burn on his left forearm complained of increasing pain. An oral combination of acetaminophen/codeine was administered for pain control. Which of the following statements best explain the reason for using this drug combination?

A. Codeine counteracts acetaminophen-induced hepatotoxicity.
B. Acetaminophen counteracts codeine-induced constipation.
C. The combination does not cause tolerance or dependence.
D. Acetaminophen speeds up the biotransformation of codeine into morphine.
E. The two drugs enhance each other's analgesic effects.

Difficulty level: Medium

30. A 51-year-old woman was admitted to the hospital with severe, intermittent right upper quadrant pain accompanied by nausea, vomiting, and clay-colored stools. Medical history of the patient indicated that she had been suffering from hypothyroidism for 2 years. The admitting diagnosis was biliary colic. Which of the following statements best explains why opioids were relatively contraindicated in this patient?

A. They can cause smooth muscle spasm in the sphincter of Oddi.
B. They are ineffective in patients with hypothyroidism.
C. They increase the risk of hepatotoxicity in patients with liver disease.
D. They are poorly metabolized in patients with liver disease.
E. They can increase the risk of nausea and vomiting.

Difficulty level: Medium

31. A 64-year-old man was brought to the emergency room for an episode of severe and crushing chest pain that radiated to his left arm and jaw. Thus far the pain had not responded to five nitroglycerin sublingual tablets. Other signs and symptoms were consistent with the diagnosis of acute myocardial infarction, and his physician was considering the use of an opioid analgesic. Which of the following opioids would be contraindicated in this patient?

    A. Morphine
    B. Fentanyl
    C. Buprenorphine
    D. Pentazocine
    E. Methadone

Difficulty level: Easy

32. A 47-year-old man complained of severe pain 3 days after surgery to remove a colon cancer. Physical examination and x-ray confirmed the diagnosis of postoperative adynamic ileus. An analgesic treatment was prescribed. Which of the following analgesic drugs would be contraindicated for this patient?

    A. Acetaminophen
    B. Morphine
    C. Ibuprofen
    D. Ketorolac
    E. Indomethacin

Difficulty level: Easy

33. A 74-year-old man was brought to the emergency department with strong pain following a car accident. Vital signs were blood pressure 190/100, pulse 55 bpm, respirations 12/min. Physical examination showed severe head trauma. The patient was currently taking nitroglycerin, lovastatin, and ranitidine. Which of the following analgesic drugs would be contraindicated for this patient?

    A. Indomethacin
    B. Acetaminophen
    C. Aspirin
    D. Morphine
    E. Ketorolac

Difficulty level: Medium

34. A 74-year-old man who had been suffering from occlusive atherosclerotic disease of the legs for 3 months complained that recently his pain had increased and was not relieved by nonsteroidal antiinflammatory drugs (NSAIDs). His physician changed the therapy and prescribed an appropriate treatment.

A few days later, the patient reported that he was feeling much better and that the pain seemed to be still there, but that "it doesn't bother me so much." He also said that he was a little sleepy during the day and had some difficulty in voiding his bladder. Which of the following drugs was most likely prescribed to the patient?

    A. Amitriptyline
    B. Acetaminophen
    C. Haloperidol
    D. Morphine
    E. Diazepam
    F. Ketorolac

Difficulty level: Medium

35. A 65-year-old man with terminal cancer was suffering from continuous pain that had gradually increased in intensity and now was severe and no longer relieved by full therapeutic doses of ketorolac. His physician decided to change the therapy. Which of the following treatments would be most appropriate for this patient?

    A. Naproxen orally (PO), once daily
    B. Morphine intramuscularly (IM), as needed
    C. Tramadol PO, twice daily
    D. Fentanyl IM, as needed
    E. Methadone PO, once daily

Difficulty level: Hard

36. A 34-year-old man, brought to the emergency department after a car collision, was fully conscious and complained of chest pain. He was also agitated, disoriented, moving all his limbs, and aggressive. Physical examination showed hematoma over the right orbit and strong pain on palpation of the 5th to 9th right ribs. Reflexes were grossly intact. A computed tomography (CT) scan was ordered. Which of the following pairs of drugs would be appropriate to induce "conscious sedation" in this patient to complete the CT scan?

    A. Ibuprofen and codeine
    B. Buspirone and meperidine
    C. Zolpidem and morphine
    D. Lorazepam and fentanyl
    E. Diazepam and acetaminophen

Difficulty level: Hard

37. A 44-year-old man complained to his physician of burning pain on his chest, especially when his clothes rubbed against it, and an itchy feeling in the same area. The patient was diagnosed with herpes zoster 3 weeks ago, but the painful rush on his chest disappeared after 8 days. The physician

made a presumptive diagnosis and ordered a drug to allay pain. Which of the following drugs would be appropriate for this patient?

A. Acetaminophen
B. Ethosuximide
C. Diazepam
D. Tramadol
E. Fluoxetine
F. Ibuprofen

Difficulty level: Hard

38. A 44-year-old man who underwent surgery to remove a lung cancer exhibited pronounced shivering upon recovering from surgery. An appropriate therapy was started that included fluid warming and an intravenous injection of a drug. Which of the following drugs was most likely administered?

A. Amitriptyline
B. Indomethacin
C. Fluoxetine
D. Meperidine
E. Atropine

Difficulty level: Medium

39. A baby boy, born after normal delivery, presented with respiratory depression, pinpoint pupils, and low Apgar scores. His mother received two intramuscular injections of an analgesic drug 3 and 2 hours before the delivery because of strong erratic and very painful contractions. Which of the following drugs would be appropriate for the baby at this time?

A. Flumazenil
B. Theophylline
C. Naloxone
D. Caffeine
E. Albuterol
F. Ipratropium

Difficulty level: Medium

40. A 58-year-old woman was about to be discharged from the hospital after a hysterectomy. Her past medical history was significant for duodenal ulcer, which healed 1 year ago after

appropriate therapy. Because the patient still complained of some episodic abdominal pain, a postdischarge analgesic was prescribed. Which of the following drug combinations would be appropriate for this patient?

A. Buprenorphine/ibuprofen
B. Morphine/indomethacin
C. Codeine/acetaminophen
D. Fentanyl/ketorolac
E. Methadone/aspirin

Difficulty level: Medium

41. A 34-year-old heroin addict was determined to "quit the habit" and started a detoxification program supervised by a certified physician. The program included the administration of a buprenorphine/naloxone combination to be given by the sublingual route. Which of the following was most likely the reason for using naloxone in the patient's detoxification program?

A. To counteract buprenorphine-induced respiratory depression
B. To increase the absorption of buprenorphine
C. To prevent buprenorphine overdose
D. To discourage the intravenous abuse of buprenorphine
E. To minimize buprenorphine tolerance

Difficulty level: Easy

42. A 68-year-old woman with breast cancer metastases complained to her physician of a dull bone pain that had been increasing over the past few days. The pain was initially relieved by ibuprofen, but now the drug was unable to control it. The patient described the pain as continuous but moderate. The physician decided to add to ibuprofen a drug whose analgesic effect is most likely due to its conversion to morphine. Which of the following drugs was most likely prescribed?

A. Fentanyl
B. Codeine
C. Buprenorphine
D. Tramadol
E. Pentazocine
F. Meperidine

Questions: III-13 Drugs of Abuse

Directions for questions **1–5**

Match each drug with the appropriate description (each lettered option can be selected once, more than once, or not at all).

- **A.** Amphetamine
- **B.** Buprenorphine
- **C.** Cannabinoids
- **D.** Caffeine
- **E.** Cocaine
- **F.** Ethanol
- **G.** Gamma-hydroxybutyric acid
- **H.** Heroin
- **L.** LSD
- **M.** Methylenedioxymethamphetamine (MDMA)
- **N.** Naloxone
- **O.** Nicotine
- **P.** Phencyclidine

Difficulty level: Easy

1. This drug is sometimes used to decrease alcohol craving in alcoholics.

Difficulty level: Easy

2. This drug acts mainly by increasing the nonvesicular release of dopamine from dopaminergic neurons.

Difficulty level: Easy

3. The elimination of this drug follows mainly zero-order kinetics.

Difficulty level: Easy

4. This drug is used in heroin detoxification programs.

Difficulty level: Easy

5. The central effects of this drug are most likely mediated by the activation of type B gamma-aminobutyric acid ($GABA_B$) receptors.

Difficulty level: Medium

6. A 28-year-old man was brought to the psychiatric clinic by the police after he attempted to assault a woman in the street. The man presented with elevated mood, rapid speech, muscle twitching, and dilated pupils. He kept on scratching himself repeatedly because he stated that "bugs are crawling under my skin." Vital signs were blood pressure 170/105, heart rate 120 bpm, respirations 20 /min. After a short time, stereotyped behavior developed accompanied by paranoid delusions, but the man remained oriented and alert. Which of the following drugs most likely caused the patient's syndrome?

- **A.** Marijuana
- **B.** LSD
- **C.** Cocaine
- **D.** Ethanol
- **E.** Phencyclidine

Difficulty level: Medium

7. A 44-year-old man was a regular user of high doses of cocaine. Which of the following signs and symptoms was most likely prominent in this person, shortly after the administration of the drug?

- **A.** Disorientation in time and space
- **B.** Ravenous appetite
- **C.** Lethargy
- **D.** Stereotyped behavior
- **E.** Increased feeling of fatigue

Difficulty level: Easy

8. The mother of a 16-year-old boy noticed a change in her son's behavior. When he returned home in the evening after meeting with his friends, he was always very hungry, despite having eaten his dinner. He always appeared happy, would find everything amusing, and laughed a lot. Occasionally, his eyes would be rather red. In the morning he was reluctant to go to school and did not appear to care whether he did well or not. A drug with which of the following mechanisms of action was he most likely abusing?

- **A.** Activation of cannabinoid receptors
- **B.** Blockade of norepinephrine reuptake
- **C.** Activation of serotonin receptors
- **D.** Activation of μ (mu) opioid receptors
- **E.** Blockade of dopaminergic receptors

Difficulty level: Easy

9. An 18-year-old girl who had never used recreational drugs joined in smoking multiple marijuana cigarettes at a party. Which of the following signs and symptoms did the girl most likely experience just after smoking?

- **A.** Hypertension
- **B.** Increased heart rate
- **C.** Depressive mood
- **D.** Hyperalgesia
- **E.** Improved memory
- **F.** Pale skin

Difficulty level: Easy

10. A 33-year-old man was in his physician's office because he started to perceive flashes of colors and fleeting movements of strange objects as he entered a dark room. The man, who was an alcoholic and an occasional user of recreational drugs, took two tablets of an illegal drug while at a party 2 months ago. Which of the following syndromes most likely accounted for the patient's symptoms?

A. Phencyclidine withdrawal
B. Heroin withdrawal
C. LSD flashbacks
D. Cocaine-induced schizophrenic episode
E. Amphetamine-induced schizophrenic episode
F. Alcohol withdrawal

Difficulty level: Easy

11. A 42-year-old woman complained to her doctor about increasing anxiety, insomnia, irritability, and severe craving for cigarettes. The patient, who was a two-pack-a-day smoker for 15 years, had recently quit smoking. The physician prescribed a drug that could relieve her symptoms. Which of the following drugs would be most appropriate for this patient?

A. Naloxone
B. Bupropion
C. Bromocriptine
D. Buprenorphine
E. Methyldopa
F. Imipramine

Difficulty level: Easy

12. A 22-year-old man came to the clinic complaining of muscle aches, nausea, and anxiety. He reported that he was a heroin addict and that he had been smoking phencyclidine occasionally for the past 6 months. He was sweating, shaking, and kept yawning. Physical examination revealed hyperventilation, hyperthermia, high blood pressure, and tachycardia. His pupils were dilated, but no nystagmus was observed. Which of the following types of drugs would be most appropriate to provide immediate relief to this patient?

A. 5-HT receptor agonist
B. Mu receptor agonist
C. Glutamate receptor antagonist
D. GABA receptor agonist
E. D_2 receptor antagonist
F. Alpha$_2$ receptor antagonist

Difficulty level: Easy

13. A 38-year-old heroin addict was determined to quit the habit and was admitted to a detoxification clinic. After physical examination and laboratory tests, treatment was started. Sublingual administration of which of the following drugs would be most appropriate for this patient?

A. Diazepam
B. Buprenorphine
C. Naltrexone
D. Phenobarbital
E. Codeine
F. Pentazocine

Difficulty level: Easy

14. A 35-year-old male body builder was brought to the emergency department for treatment of traumatic injuries to his legs as a result of a motor vehicle accident. He was agitated, hyperaggressive, and in a rage. He had been restrained by security guards following an altercation with one of the nurses. He denied use of alcohol or other mood-altering drugs. Physical examination showed a distraught patient with extensive skin acne. Vital signs were within normal limits, and the results of routine drug screen tests for illegal substances were negative. Which of the following drugs was most likely to have caused the patient's behavior?

A. Diazepam
B. Marijuana
C. Heroin
D. Mifepristone
E. Oxandrolone
F. Danazol

Difficulty level: Easy

15. A 17-year-old girl who had never used drugs decided to join in with her friends who were smoking drugged cigarettes. In the first 5 minutes, she experienced euphoria, uncontrollable laughter, depersonalization, and sharpened vision. Her concentration became difficult, and she noticed that her heart was "pounding." Her friends noted reddening of her conjunctiva but no change in pupil diameter. Which of the following drugs most likely caused the girl's symptoms?

A. Phencyclidine
B. Cannabis
C. Cocaine
D. Heroin
E. LSD

Difficulty level: Medium

16. A 40-year-old female alcoholic was admitted to an alcohol rehabilitation center because she was determined to quit the habit. A drug was given to facilitate avoidance from ethanol dependence, based on research suggesting that compulsive alcohol drinking is influenced by opiate receptor activity. Which of the following drugs was most likely administered?

   A. Diazepam
   B. Clonidine
   C. Disulfiram
   D. Naltrexone
   E. Methadone
   F. Buprenorphine

Difficulty level: Medium

17. A 27-year-old man with a recent history of drug abuse presented to the emergency department with violent, shaking chills. He also complained of restlessness, insomnia, nausea, and abdominal cramps and exhibited profuse sweating, rhinorrhea, yawning, and piloerection. He admitted he was out of money and was unable to get the usual supply of the drug he had been using for 3 months. From which of the following drugs was he most likely experiencing withdrawal?

   A. Heroin
   B. Cocaine
   C. Amphetamines
   D. LSD
   E. MDMA
   F. Phencyclidine

Difficulty level: Medium

18. A 28-year-old woman was admitted unconscious to the emergency department. A friend stated that the woman was a polydrug user and that she had self-injected a drug approximately 45 minutes prior to admission. Vital signs were blood pressure 100/50, heart rate 95 bpm, respirations 5/min. Physical examination showed cyanosis and pinpoint pupils. Which of the following drugs did the woman most likely take?

   A. Amphetamine
   B. Heroin
   C. Cocaine
   D. Phencyclidine
   E. Diazepam
   F. LSD

Difficulty level: Easy

19. A 41-year-old man decided to stop smoking cigarettes and asked his family physician about a possible withdrawal syndrome. He had been smoking two packs of cigarettes daily for 24 years. Which of the following are the withdrawal symptoms the man was most likely to experience?

   A. Irritability and restlessness
   B. Asthenia and sleepiness
   C. Euphoria and elation
   D. Tachycardia and hypertension
   E. Decreased appetite and weight loss

Difficulty level: Medium

20. A 53-year-old woman suffered a generalized seizure and was taken to the emergency department. On admission she was extremely anxious and agitated. She reported she had no history of epilepsy. Further questioning revealed that she had a long history of drug abuse, but the day before she decided to quit and ceased taking the abused drug. Withdrawal from which of the following drugs most likely caused the patient's seizure?

   A. LSD
   B. Cannabis
   C. Alprazolam
   D. Heroin
   E. Cocaine
   F. Methamphetamine

Difficulty level: Medium

21. A 48-year-old male alcoholic complained of flushing, nausea, a throbbing headache, and confusion after drinking a glass of wine. The man was taking a drug as part of his rehabilitation treatment for alcoholism. The symptoms of the patient are most likely caused by the accumulation in the body of which of the following substances?

   A. Dopamine
   B. Acetaldehyde
   C. Ethanol
   D. Serotonin
   E. Methanol
   F. Formaldehyde

Difficulty level: Medium

22. A 15-year-old boy was admitted to the hospital in a panicky state, crying and complaining of being seriously ill. The boy, who had never used recreational drugs, had just smoked two drugged cigarettes at a party with his friends. Physical examination showed a confused and fearful patient with fast pulse (120 bpm), reddening of the conjunctiva with no change in pupil diameter, and diffuse tremor. Which of the following drugs did he most likely take?

   A. Amphetamine
   B. Cocaine
   C. Gamma-hydroxybutyric acid
   D. Heroin
   E. Cannabis

Difficulty level: Easy

23. A 50-year-old homeless man was brought to the emergency room by the police, who had found him disoriented and trembling under a bridge. Physical examination and vital signs led to the diagnosis of delirium tremens. Which of the following signs and symptoms did the patient most likely show?

    A. Pinpoint pupils
    B. Profound hypotension
    C. Hypothermia
    D. Skeletal muscle relaxation
    E. Visual hallucinations

Difficulty level: Medium

24. A 48-year-old woman became agitated and visibly tremulous and showed hallucinatory behavior 1 day after being admitted to the hospital for elective surgery. She also accused the doctors and her husband of being unsympathetic and uncaring. Which of the following statements most likely explains the reason for the patient's behavior?

    A. Benzodiazepine medication given before surgery
    B. Depressive episode triggered by the operation
    C. Ethanol withdrawal
    D. Opioid medication given before surgery
    E. Halothane anesthesia used during surgery

Difficulty level: Hard

25. A 30-year-old man with a long history of polydrug abuse came to the emergency department after expectorating a "basin of blood." The patient admitted he was regularly using intravenous heroin and oral amphetamine. He also said he had smoked marijuana, phencyclidine, and crack cocaine just prior to admission. A chest x-ray showed bilateral alveolar infiltrates, and bronchoscopy revealed diffuse alveolar hemorrhage. Which of the drugs he was taking most likely caused the hemorrhage?

    A. Heroin
    B. Phencyclidine
    C. Marijuana
    D. Amphetamine
    E. Crack cocaine

Difficulty level: Easy

26. A 16-year-old girl attended a party with several friends. A drug was covertly slipped into her drink, and a friend then asked her to join him for a walk in the park. A few hours later she was found with a contused face, bruises on her arms, and a torn dress. She stated she was unable to recall what had happened. Which of the following drugs was most likely put into her drink?

    A. LSD
    B. Imipramine
    C. Phenobarbital
    D. Cocaine
    E. Heroin
    F. Gamma-hydroxybutyric acid

Difficulty level: Medium

27. A 46-year-old homeless alcoholic man was brought to the emergency department in a confused and incoherent state. He constantly repeated that he could not see clearly because of "flickering white spots in front of my eyes." He was breathing rapidly, appeared very anxious, and showed marked mydriasis and loss of pupillary reflex. Laboratory exams on admission showed a serum pH of 7.2. Which of the following syndromes most likely caused the patient's signs and symptoms?

    A. Ethanol poisoning
    B. Ethanol withdrawal
    C. Barbiturate poisoning
    D. Opiate withdrawal
    E. Amphetamine withdrawal
    F. Methanol poisoning

Difficulty level: Medium

28. An 18-year-old male patient started smoking marijuana cigarettes 1 month ago. He was healthy and had no previous history of use of recreational drugs. Three years earlier, he was in a psychiatric hospital for 2 months because of a schizoaffective disorder that disappeared after neuroleptic therapy. The patient was at increased risk of which of the following cannabis-induced adverse effects?

    A. Depressive episode
    B. Atrioventricular block
    C. Psychotic episode
    D. Irritable bowel syndrome
    E. Seizures

Difficulty level: Medium

29. A 39-year-old man had been using many recreational drugs over several years. Which of the following drugs taken by this polydrug user is known to be devoid of physical dependence?

    A. Cocaine
    B. Ethanol
    C. LSD
    D. Heroin
    E. Cannabis
    F. Phencyclidine

30. A 27-year-old man with a long history of drug abuse was brought unconscious to the emergency department. Vital signs were blood pressure 190/110 mm Hg, pulse 150 beats/min, rectal temperature 104°F (40°C). Pupils were mydriatic, and his skin was moist and cold. Twenty minutes later he experienced a tonic-clonic seizure, his respiration became shallow, and his systolic blood pressure fell to 50 mm Hg. Shortly afterward he died from cardiovascular collapse and ventricular fibrillation. Which of the following drugs most likely caused the patient's death?

A. Heroin
B. Gamma-hydroxybutyric acid
C. Ketamine
D. LSD
E. Tetrahydrocannabinol
F. Diazepam
G. Cocaine

Difficulty level: Hard

31. A 30-year-old woman came to the emergency department because she felt disassociated from her body, had no sense of her ego boundaries, and found that objects around her were grossly distorted. The woman, who had been a polydrug user for many years, had smoked three drugged cigarettes bought on the street. Physical examination showed blood pressure of 168/100 mm Hg, miosis, vertical and horizontal nystagmus, sweating, and flushed skin. Which of the following is most likely the major mechanism of action of the drug that apparently caused the patient's signs and symptoms?

A. Inhibition of transmitter reuptake at noradrenergic synapses
B. Activation of μ (mu)-type opiate receptors
C. Activation of serotonergic presynaptic receptors
D. Stimulation of the release of monoamines from the synaptic vesicles
E. Blockade of NMDA subtype of glutamate receptors

Difficulty level: Hard

32. A 16-year-old girl started feeling nervous and experienced mild nausea after taking a drug while at a party. One hour later she became hysterical, crying and yelling about being crazy. Two friends took her to the hospital. Physical examination showed mydriasis but no nystagmus, mild tachycardia, blood pressure of 160/98 mm Hg, sweating, and tremor. She appeared very anxious and stated that she had a strong sense that the furniture in the room was alive and that surrounding sounds were colored. Which of the following drugs most likely caused the patient's signs and symptoms?

A. Cocaine
B. Heroin
C. Cannabis
D. Amyl nitrite
E. Phencyclidine
F. LSD

Difficulty level: Medium

33. A 23-year-old man was brought to the emergency department by police for violent, combative behavior. Friends claimed he took some tablets of a recreational drug at a party. The patient appeared agitated, diaphoretic, and disoriented. His blood pressure was 170/100 mm Hg, pulse 130 bpm, and temperature 101°F (about 38°C). His pupils were miotic, unreactive to light, and vertical and horizontal nystagmus was noted. Which of the following drugs most likely caused the patient's signs and symptoms?

A. Cocaine
B. Heroin
C. Phencyclidine
D. LSD
E. Marijuana

Difficulty level: Easy

34. A 3-year-old boy was brought to the emergency department with severe vomiting after having ingested an antifreeze mixture containing ethylene glycol. Vital signs were blood pressure 70/40 (normal at age 3: 100/67), heart rate 115 bpm, respirations 22 breaths/min. Lab tests showed a plasma pH of 7.2 and oxalate crystals in the urine. An intravenous solution of 10% ethanol was given. Which of the following statements best explains the purpose of ethanol treatment in this patient?

A. It combines with ethylene glycol in blood, leading to an inert product.
B. It prevents the absorption of ethylene glycol from the intestines.
C. It retards the oxidation of ethylene glycol to its toxic metabolites.
D. It speeds up the metabolism of ethylene glycol by the liver.
E. It speeds up the elimination of ethylene glycol by the kidneys.

Difficulty level: Medium

35. A 24-year old man, who had started smoking marijuana 5 years ago, had been smoking 5 to 10 marijuana cigarettes daily and occasionally self-injecting pure hashish oil. The man was most likely at increased risk of which of the following adverse events?

A. Death from parenteral injection of hashish oil
B. Death from acute cannabis withdrawal
C. Colon cancer
D. Driving or work accidents
E. Alzheimer disease

Difficulty level: Easy

36. A 32-year-old man was brought to the emergency department after taking a large amount of ecstasy at a rave party. Physical examination showed a confused and agitated patient with profuse sweating, jaw clenching, muscle twitching and rigidity, and temperature of 103.8°F (39.8°C). Vital signs were blood pressure 170/98 mg Hg, pulse 115 bpm, respirations 22/min. Blood analysis showed the presence of methylenedioxymethamphetamine (MDMA). Which of the following neurotransmitters most likely mediated the effects of the drug in this patient?

A. Acetylcholine
B. Serotonin
C. Norepinephrine
D. Gamma-aminobutyric acid (GABA)
E. Glutamate
F. Dopamine

Difficulty level: Easy

37. An 18-year-old male patient who had never previously drunk a large amount of alcohol was brought unconscious to the emergency department after drinking whiskey in a betting game at a party. His alcohol level on admission was 5 mg/mL. The volume of distribution of ethanol is about 45 L. Which of the following (in grams) was most likely the quantity of alcohol present in the patient's body?

A. 100
B. 225
C. 300
D. 355
E. 400
F. 425

Difficulty level: Easy

38. A 24-year-old woman who had never previously used recreational drugs took one tablet of LSD at a party. The central nervous system (CNS) effects of this drug are primarily related to the activation of which of the following receptor types in the CNS?

A. GABAergic
B. Muscarinic
C. Nicotinic
D. Serotoninergic
E. Noradrenergic
F. Glutamatergic

Difficulty level: Medium

39. A 34-year-old man with a long history of drug abuse came to the hospital complaining of severe somnolence, ravenous appetite, headache, depression, and lack of motivation. He said he failed to get a supply of the drug he was used to taking and repeatedly asked the doctor to give him that drug to reduce his symptoms. Withdrawal from which of the following drugs may have caused these symptoms?

A. Heroin
B. Phencyclidine
C. Diazepam
D. Amphetamine
E. Ethanol

Difficulty level: Medium

40. A 55-year-old woman with a long history of severe alcoholism was admitted to the hospital because of deterioration of her general status. Physical examination and lab tests confirmed advanced liver cirrhosis. Which of the following was most likely another disease found in this patient?

A. Stomach cancer
B. Pulmonary emphysema
C. Renal insufficiency
D. Ulcerative colitis
E. Dilated cardiomyopathy
F. Vasospastic angina

Difficulty level: Easy

41. A 57-year-old homeless man was brought to the emergency department by the police, who had found him wandering the streets. The man had a long history of alcoholism; he also abused various inhalants when he did not have money to buy alcohol. He admitted that almost daily over the past 3 months, he had inhaled a drug supplied by a local vendor in cartridges because it was much cheaper than alcohol. Pertinent findings on physical examination included muscle weakness, unsteady gait, vibratory sense loss on lower extremities, and hyperalgesia. Which of the following drugs most likely caused the patient's syndrome?

A. Amyl nitrite
B. Nitrous oxide
C. Propane
D. Helium
E. Isoflurane

Difficulty level: Easy

42. A 10-year-old boy was brought by his mother to their family physician's office because she realized that recently the boy's behavior had changed. Careful inquiry by the physician eventually made the boy admit he had started sniffing some paint thinners and stain removers, following a friend's suggestion. The pattern of effects caused by these inhalants is most similar to that caused by which of the following drugs?

 A. LSD
 B. Cocaine
 C. Morphine
 D. Amphetamine
 E. Ethanol

Difficulty level: Easy

43. A 23-year-old man was found dead at home by his roommate. The roommate said they were at a party the night before and went home at about 3:00 a.m. He also reported that the patient was a drug user and tried different drugs from time to time. Autopsy showed a blood level of morphine substantially lower than the estimated minimum lethal concentration of the drug. The pathologist was quite sure that the death was caused by the concomitant administration of another drug. Which of the following was most likely the other drug involved in the patient's death?

 A. Marijuana
 B. LSD
 C. Ethanol
 D. Amphetamine
 E. Methylphenidate

Difficulty level: Medium

44. A 16-year-old boy was brought by his friends to the emergency department because he felt a general malaise, strong headache, and nausea and asked for medical assistance. History revealed that 6 hours earlier, the boy, who had never previously used recreational drugs, smoked two drugged cigarettes at a party. Physical examination showed an agitated and talkative patient with mydriasis, muscle twitching, and a fine hand tremor. Vital signs were blood pressure 160/95 mm Hg, pulse 115 bpm, respirations 24/min. Which of the following drugs most likely caused the patient's signs and symptoms?

 A. Cocaine
 B. Marijuana
 C. LSD
 D. Amphetamine
 E. Heroin
 F. Ketamine

Answers and Explanations: III-1 Introduction to Central Nervous System Pharmacology

Learning objective: Describe the signs and symptoms mediated by the blockade of cholinergic receptors.

1. **C** Ingestion of plants and berries by children is one of the top reasons for calls to poison control centers. The child most likely ate some black berries from *Atropa belladonna*, a plant common in the woods. The berries contain atropine, an antimuscarinic drug. The boy's symptoms are classic for atropine poisoning.

 A, B, D–G See correct answer explanation.

Learning objective: Identify the brain area that is most likely the main target for the therapeutic effect of clonidine in nicotine withdrawal.

2. **C** Most noradrenergic neurons in the brain are found in the locus ceruleus, a bluish area on each side of the median eminence of the brainstem. The locus ceruleus sends a large number of projections to the amygdala and hippocampus, where norepinephrine release is thought to mediate emotion and memory formation. Another brain region that is rich in

noradrenergic neurons is the lateral tegmental area of the reticular formation. The drug taken by the patient was most likely clonidine. The drug activates presynaptic α_2 receptors located on noradrenergic terminals, which in turn decreases norepinephrine release from those terminals. It seems that this reduction of central adrenergic activity is the basis of the therapeutic effect of the drugs for treatment of withdrawal from addicting drugs, including nicotine and opioids.

 A, B, D–F See correct answer explanation.

Learning objective: Identify the brain area richest in histaminergic neurons.

3. **F** Histamine and antihistamines have long been known to produce significant effects on animal behavior. Biochemical detection of histamine synthesis by neurons and direct cytochemical localization of these neurons have defined the histaminergic system in the central nervous system. Most of these neurons are located in the ventral posterior hypothalamus. They give rise to long ascending and descending tracts that

are typical of the patterns characteristic of other aminergic systems. The central histaminergic system is thought to affect arousal (H_1 antagonists cause drowsiness), attention, feeding, thermoregulation, and vascular dynamics.

A–E See correct answer explanation.

Learning objective: Describe the postreceptor mechanism of activation of $GABA_B$ receptors.

4. **A** The patient was most likely receiving baclofen, a spasmolytic drug that likely acts by activating $GABA_B$ receptors. This activation most likely opens K^+ channels, thus increasing cell membrane stabilization.

B–E See correct answer explanation.

Learning objective: Identify the neurotransmitter involved in the therapeutic action of hypnotic drugs.

5. **D** Most drugs used to relieve insomnia (z-hypnotics, benzodiazepines, etc.) are GABAergic drugs; that is, they increase the activity of GABA, the most abundant inhibitory neurotransmitter in the brain.

A–C, E, F Currently, drugs acting on these neurotransmitter systems are not used to treat insomnia.

Learning objective: Identify the brain receptors that can mediate excitotoxicity.

6. **D** Excitotoxicity is the pathologic process by which nerve cells are damaged and killed by excessive stimulation by neurotransmitters such as glutamate and similar substances. This occurs when receptors for glutamate, such as the *N*-methyl-d-aspartate (NMDA) receptors and α-amino-3-hydroxy-5-methylisoxazole-4-propionic acid (AMPA) receptors, are overactivated. This activation allows high levels of calcium ions to enter the cell. Ca^{2+} influx into cells activates a number of enzymes, including phospholipases, endonucleases, and proteases, which go on to damage cell structures.

A, B, E, F These receptors do not cause excitotoxicity.

C Like most presynaptic receptors, presynaptic NMDA receptors regulate the release of neurotransmitters and do not alter Ca^{2+} influx into the target neurons.

Learning objective: Identify the neurotransmitters most likely involved in the pathogenesis of major depressive disorder.

7. **E** The patient's symptoms indicate that she was most likely suffering from a major depressive disorder. Both the serotonergic and noradrenergic systems are most likely involved in the pathogenesis of major depressive disorder. This conclusion derives mainly from the fact that most currently available antidepressants have their primary action on the central adrenergic and/or the central serotonergic system.

A–D, F See correct answer explanation.

Learning objective: Identify the enzyme that represents the rate-limiting step in serotonin biosynthesis.

8. **C** Serotonin is synthesized by a two-step pathway from the essential amino acid tryptophan. Tryptophan hydroxylase, a mixed function oxidase enzyme, is the rate-limiting step in serotonin biosynthesis. It converts tryptophan into 5-hydroxytryptophan, which is then converted into serotonin by the aromatic L-amino acid decarboxylase, an enzyme widely distributed and with low substrate specificity.

A, B, D, E See correct answer explanation.

Learning objective: Identify the neurotransmitter most likely involved in the rewarding effect of most abused drugs.

9. **F** Acute rewarding effects of most abused drugs are thought to be mediated by an increase in synaptic levels of dopamine in the nucleus accumbens. This nucleus, located within the striatum, seems to play an important role in reward, pleasure, and addiction. Therefore, dopamine is thought to be substantially involved in drug abuse and addiction.

A–E, G See correct answer explanation.

Learning objective: Describe the pharmacological actions of a drug that may be effective in the therapy of Alzheimer disease.

10. **E** The most striking neurochemical disturbance in Alzheimer disease (AD) is a deficiency of acetylcholine. The anatomical basis of the cholinergic deficit is atrophy and degeneration of subcortical cholinergic neurons, particularly those in the basal forebrain (nucleus basalis of Meynert) that provide cholinergic innervation to the cerebral cortex. The selective deficiency of acetylcholine in AD, as well as the observation that central cholinergic antagonists such as atropine can induce a confusional state that bears some resemblance to the dementia of AD, has given rise to the "cholinergic hypothesis," which proposes that a deficiency of acetylcholine is critical in the genesis of the AD symptoms. Although the "cholinergic deficiency syndrome" provides a useful framework, it is important to note that the deficit in AD is far more complex. Nevertheless, drugs causing augmentation of cholinergic transmission are currently the mainstay of AD treatment.

C Recent experimental research points out that in AD there is a deficiency in GABAergic neurotransmission and that increasing GABA availability could improve AD. However, no GABAergic drug has been approved yet for this indication.

A–D See correct answer explanation.

Learning objective: Identify the two neurotransmitters that are thought to be most involved in seizure disorders.

11. **B** Epilepsy is a chronic recurrent disorder of cerebral function that is characterized by repeated seizures. The essence of epilepsy is probably a chronic low seizure threshold that can be due to several mechanisms. A leading proposed mechanism is that the cause of seizures is either the attenuation of pre- and/or postsynaptic inhibition (mainly due to a genetic or postpathologic hypofunction of GABA neurons) or an increased effectiveness of excitatory synapses (mainly due to a genetic or postpathologic hyperfunction of glutamate neurons).

    A, C–F See correct answer explanation.

Learning objective: Identify the neurotransmitter most likely involved in the pathogenesis of catatonic schizophrenia.

12. **D** The patient is most likely suffering from the catatonic subtype of schizophrenia, which is characterized by motor immobility and abnormal posture maintained for a long time (so-called waxy flexibility). A number of theories related to major neurotransmitter systems have been proposed to explain the symptoms of schizophrenia. Of these, the dopamine hypothesis states that the illness results from an excessive dopaminergic activity in mesolimbic and mesocortical pathways. The dopamine hypothesis is the most fully developed and is supported by several lines of evidence, including the fact that most antipsychotic drugs block dopamine D_2 receptors, and there is a very good correlation between clinical potency of these drugs and their in vitro affinity for these receptors. Two other major hypotheses of schizophrenia are the serotonin hypothesis (it is known that alteration in serotonergic functioning affects multiple neurotransmitter systems) and the glutamate hypothesis, which proposes a hypofunctional glutamate system in schizophrenia.

    A–C, E See correct answer explanation.

Learning objective: Describe the pharmacological actions of a drug that may be effective in the therapy of Parkinson disease.

13. **C** Parkinson disease (PD) is characterized by a loss of the neurons in the substantia nigra that provide dopaminergic innervation to the striatum. Most drugs effective in PD can either increase the availability of dopamine or directly activate dopaminergic receptors. Another group of drugs that have a modest antiparkinsonian action are antimuscarinic drugs. In PD, the loss of dopamine-producing neurons results in a loss of the balance that normally exists between acetylcholine and dopamine-mediated neurotransmission. The anticholinergic agents work by blocking excitatory cholinergic striatal interneurons, thereby minimizing the effect of the relative increase in cholinergic sensitivity. Taking into account these findings, a drug able to increase the availability of dopamine and to decrease the availability of acetylcholine should be quite effective in the treatment of PD.

    A, B, D, E See correct answer explanation.

Learning objective: Identify the brain area that is the richest in cholinergic neurons.

14. **A** The primary concentration of cholinergic neuron cell bodies is in the basal nucleus of Meynert, a group of neurons in the substantia innominata of the basal forebrain that have wide projections to the neocortex. These cholinergic neurons have a number of important functions, in particular with respect to memory. A severe neuronal loss in the nucleus of Meynert has been found in Alzheimer disease, in vascular dementia, and in the dementia accompanying Parkinson disease. Occasional involvement is present in other dementing illnesses.

    B–F See correct answer explanation.

Learning objective: Identify the neurophysiological action that most likely mediated the therapeutic effect of drugs used for generalized anxiety disorders.

15. **A** The prescribed drug was most likely a selective serotonin reuptake inhibitor. Drugs of this class are first-line agents for anxiety disorders. Their therapeutic effect is most likely related to their inhibition of the serotonin transporter that mediates the reuptake of serotonin into serotonergic terminals. As a consequence, serotonergic transmission is increased.

    B–F See correct answer explanation.

Learning objective: Identify the neurotransmitter of pyramidal motor neurons.

16. **B** Pyramidal neurons are excitatory projection neurons that use glutamate as the main neurotransmitter. A lesion of these neurons affects glutamatergic transmission to the lower motor neurons.

    A, C–E See correct answer explanation.

Learning objective: Identify the neurotransmitter that most likely mediates obsessive-compulsive disorders.

17. **D** The patient's symptoms indicate that she was most likely suffering from an obsessive-compulsive disorder (OCD) and was prescribed a selective serotonin reuptake inhibitor. A wealth of research has attempted to identify a specific biological explanation for OCD. One leading hypothesis has focused on the role of serotonin (5-hydroxytryptamine, 5-HT) dysfunction, which is supported by the fact that the only effective drug treatments for OCD primarily influence 5-HT transmission. However, the exact role of 5-HT underlying OCD has not been determined.

    A–C, E, F See correct answer explanation.

Learning objective: Identify the central nervous system neurotransmitter that generates only inhibitory postsynaptic potentials.

18. **D** GABA is a neurotransmitter that can generate only IPSPs by activating GABA receptors. GABA$_A$ receptors are ionotropic; their activation opens ligand-activated Cl$^-$ channels, increasing inward Cl$^-$ conductance. GABA$_B$ receptors are metabotropic; their activation opens voltage-gated K$^+$ channels, increasing outward K$^+$ conductance. In both cases, the intracellular environment becomes more negative, thus inducing cell membrane stabilization.

   A–C, E All of these neurotransmitters can activate both excitatory and inhibitory receptors.

Learning objective: Identify the brain transmission system that targets N-methyl-D-aspartate (NMDA) receptors.

19. **G** Glutamate is an important excitatory neurotransmitter in the brain. Glutamate receptors include NMDA and α-amino-3-hydroxy-5-methylisoxazole-4-propionic acid (AMPA) receptors. Drugs such as felbamate that seem to act by blocking these receptors can be used effectively as anticonvulsants.

   A–E These systems are not exclusively excitatory; therefore, drugs affecting these systems are not used as anticonvulsants.

   F The GABAergic system is central inhibitory. Drugs that increase the activity of this system, such as benzodiazepines and barbiturates, are currently used as anticonvulsants.

Learning objective: Identify the main neurotransmitters that act to decrease pain signaling.

20. **F** Opioid peptides, norepinephrine, and serotonin are the three major neurotransmitters that act in the central nervous system (CNS) to decrease pain signaling, thus producing analgesia. Endogenous opioids are released at several CNS sites in response to noxious stimuli, including the spinal cord, the thalamus, and the cortex. Endogenous opioids can also modulate pain transmission indirectly by activating the following pathways that descend from the brainstem to the dorsal horn:

   • A noradrenergic pathway from the locus ceruleus. Norepinephrine released from these projections in the spinal cord activates α$_2$ receptors (the primary receptors for norepinephrine in the CNS) located on nociceptive neurons of the dorsal horn. This activation causes hyperpolarization of the neuron, inhibiting nociceptive transmission.

   • A serotonergic pathway from the raphe nuclei. Serotonin, released from these projections in the spinal cord, activates serotonergic receptors located on nociceptive neurons of the dorsal horn. This activation causes hyperpolarization of neurons, inhibiting nociceptive transmission.

   A–E See correct answer explanation.

INTRODUCTION TO CENTRAL NERVOUS SYSTEM PHARMACOLOGY Answer key			
1. C	6. D	11. B	16. B
2. C	7. E	12. D	17. D
3. F	8. C	13. C	18. D
4. A	9. F	14. A	19. G
5. D	10. E	15. A	20. F

Answers and Explanations: III-2 Sedative and Hypnotic Drugs

Questions 1–6

1. **B**
2. **D**
3. **J**
4. **I**
5. **G**
6. **B**

Learning objective: Explain the benzodiazepine-induced variation in Cl$^-$ current in the GABA$_A$ receptor–chloride ion channel macromolecular complex.

7. **B** Benzodiazepines bind to receptors located at the interface between α and γ subunits of the GABA$_A$ receptor–chloride ion channel macromolecular complex. The binding increases the affinity of the GABA$_A$ receptor for GABA, which in turn causes an increased frequency of chloride channel opening. Because extracellular chloride concentration is about 120 mM, and intracellular chloride concentration is about 20 mM, chloride channel opening will increase inward Cl$^-$ current. This in turn will increase the negative charges inside the cell, causing hyperpolarization of the cell membrane.

   A, C–E Benzodiazepines do not affect these currents. Moreover, all of these actions would cause depolarization, not hyperpolarization, of cell membranes.

Learning objective: Describe the main adverse effects of benzodiazepines.

8. **C** Today selective serotonin reuptake inhibitors (SSRIs) are first-line agents for generalized anxiety disorder, but because they have a slow onset of action, a benzodiazepine is often given concomitantly for the first few days to provide acute relief of symptoms when anxiety is severe and includes a suicide risk (patient wanted to die). Sedation and drowsiness are adverse effects that occur in more than 50% of patients on long- or medium-acting benzodiazepines. They represent an extension of pharmacological effects and are dose-related. Tolerance (at least partial) to these effects usually occurs after 2 to 3 weeks of use. Drowsiness can occur in about 10% of patients taking sertraline.

A These effects are not common (they occur in 2 to 5% of patients taking benzodiazepines).

B, D These effects occur only with high doses of benzodiazepines.

E Benzodiazepines improve the quality of sleep, and early awakening is unlikely with long- and medium-acting compounds. Nightmares with sertraline are exceedingly rare.

Learning objective: Describe the therapeutic uses of buspirone.

9. **F** Buspirone is considered a second-line agent for generalized anxiety disorders because of inconsistent reports of long-term efficacy. However, it can be the appropriate drug in patients who fail other anxiolytic therapies or in patients with a history of substance abuse, as in this case.

A, C Benzodiazepines can cause dependence and therefore are contraindicated in a person with a past history of substance abuse.

B Selective serotonin reuptake inhibitors are drugs of choice for anxiety disorders but are relatively contraindicated in this patient because of the recent episode of sexual dysfunction.

D, E Neuroleptics, such as haloperidol, and lithium have negligible anxiolytic properties.

Learning objective: Describe the mechanism of action of flumazenil.

10. **E** Flumazenil is a competitive benzodiazepine (BDZ) receptor antagonist that can block both the effects of BDZ and those of β-carboline derivatives, the inverse agonists at BDZ receptors. It can also block the effects of z-hypnotics but does not antagonize those of other central nervous system depressants (barbiturates, buspirone, ethanol, etc.). It is used clinically to counteract excessive effects of BDZ, as in this case. Because it can cause several (and sometimes serious) unwanted effects, it is not currently used in case of BDZ poisoning.

A, B, C, D See correct answer explanation.

Learning objective: Describe the main contraindication for benzodiazepines.

11. **D** Because of their muscle relaxant properties, benzodiazepines are relatively contraindicated in myasthenia gravis.

A–C, E All of these agents are first- or second-choice drugs in treating generalized anxiety disorder. They lack muscle relaxant activities and therefore are not contraindicated in myasthenic patients.

Learning objective: Explain the mechanism of action of melatonin.

12. **C** Melatonin receptors are thought to be involved in maintaining circadian rhythms underlying the sleep–wake cycle. Ramelteon, a novel hypnotic drug prescribed specifically for sleep-onset insomnia, is an agonist at melatonin receptors located in the suprachiasmatic nuclei of the brain.

A, B, D, E See correct answer explanation.

Learning objective: Explain the concept of redistribution of benzodiazepines.

13. **C** Redistribution of a drug from its site of action into other tissues or sites is a main factor in terminating drug effect, primarily when a highly lipid-soluble drug that acts on the brain is administered rapidly by intravenous (IV) injection. A good example of this is the use of IV injection of diazepam (a highly lipid-soluble drug) to induce loss of consciousness. Because blood flow to the brain is so high, the drug reaches its maximal concentration in the brain within 1 minute of its IV injection. After the injection is concluded, the plasma concentration falls as diazepam diffuses into other tissues, such as muscle.

A, D Diazepam is extensively metabolized in the liver (not in the brain) to desmethyldiazepam and oxazepam. Both metabolites are active. Therefore, biotransformation cannot explain the short action of the drug.

B The renal excretion of diazepam is about 1%.

E Tolerance can develop to the action of benzodiazepines, but only after a chronic treatment of several days.

Learning objective: Describe benzodiazepine-induced anterograde amnesia.

14. **C** A classical effect of benzodiazepines (mainly when high doses are given to induce conscious sedation) is anterograde amnesia, that is, loss of memory for events occurring during the drug's duration of action. The effect is exploited therapeutically, because the patient cannot remember the unpleasant sensations felt during endoscopic or surgical procedures, as in this case.

A Benzodiazepines have very mild antiemetic properties.

B, D Benzodiazepines tend to cause effects opposite to those listed.

E Delusion and hallucinations are exceedingly rare effects of benzodiazepines.

Learning objective: Explain the molecular mechanism of action of benzodiazepines.

15. **D** The patient most likely received a short-acting benzodiazepine, such as alprazolam, a drug used in the surgical setting for the rapid relief of agitation in postoperative patients. Benzodiazepines increase the frequency of chloride channel opening, thus making the resting membrane potential of GABA interneurons more negative in several brain areas.

    A–C, E, F All of these drugs can cause, directly or indirectly, neuronal membrane hyperpolarization (i.e., more negative resting membrane potential), but they are not used for rapid relief of postsurgical agitation.

Learning objective: Identify the drug that binds to the α_1 subunit of $GABA_A$ receptors.

16. **A** Benzodiazepines (mainly diazepam and lorazepam) are first-line agents for the emergency treatment of status epilepticus. They bind to receptors located at the α subunit of the $GABA_A$ receptor–chloride ion channel macromolecular complex, near the interface between α and γ subunits. $GABA_A$ receptors in different areas of the central nervous system consist of different isoforms containing five different α subunits (α_1, $_{-2}$, $_{-3}$, $_{-4}$, and $_{-5}$). Benzodiazepines can bind to many of these subunits.

    B, C Zolpidem and flumazenil bind to α subunits of GABA receptors, but they are not used as anticonvulsants.

    D, E Phenytoin and valproic acid are used as anticonvulsants, but they do not bind GABA receptor components.

Learning objective: Describe the action of benzodiazepines upon sleep architecture.

17. **B** Benzodiazepines alter sleep architecture and stages. They decrease sleep latency and decrease awakening during the night. All other effects on sleep are opposite to those listed. Benzodiazepines are less frequently used today for insomnia because of the risk of dependence. Experts agree that these drugs should be used at the lowest effective dose for the shortest duration possible.

    A, C–E See correct answer explanation.

Learning objective: Describe the main adverse effects of benzodiazepines.

18. **B** The patient had most likely taken temazepam, a benzodiazepine often used by practicing physicians to treat insomnia. Elderly people are more sensitive to the depressive effects of these drugs, and the daily dose can easily be mistaken, if the drug is taken without strict supervision, as in this case.

    A, C Zolpidem and ramelteon have very short half-lives, so they are less prone to cause daytime sedation.

    D–F Chlorpromazine, buspirone, and phenobarbital are not prescribed as hypnotics.

Learning objective: Explain why a chronic benzodiazepine treatment can increase the risk of fall in the elderly.

19. **C** The link between benzodiazepine use and falls is well documented and may result from balance impairment, sedation, and muscle relaxant effects. Although tolerance can develop to these benzodiazepine actions, elderly people may experience persistent impairment. The chronic use of benzodiazepines is therefore relatively contraindicated in the elderly.

    A, B, D, E These drugs do not increase the risk of fall-related fractures.

Learning objective: Describe the pharmacological effects of barbiturates.

20. **D** The man most likely suffered from epilepsy, and phenobarbital was added to his pharmacotherapy. Phenobarbital is a barbituric acid derivative and is considered a second-line agent in epilepsy. All barbiturates can offset convulsions when given at doses that cause loss of consciousness, but phenobarbital has anticonvulsant properties even in doses that do not affect alertness.

    A–C Barbiturates are devoid of antidepressant, antipsychotic, or antiparkinson properties.

    E Although barbiturates are still included in analgesic combinations, they are devoid of analgesic properties, and they actually may worsen a patient's perception of pain.

Learning objective: Describe the therapeutic uses of benzodiazepines.

21. **D** In addition to the anxiolytic effect, benzodiazepines given at high doses can cause anterograde amnesia, that is, impairment of memory for events occurring after the administration of the drug. This action is particularly useful when the patient has to undergo a disturbing diagnostic procedure, as in this case. Because the intervention is brief, a short-acting benzodiazepine such as oxazepam is most appropriate.

    A Buspirone is an anxiolytic drug, but the effect develops slowly (in 1 to 2 weeks), and anterograde amnesia does not occur.

    B, C, E These drugs cause negligible anxiolytic effects and negligible anterograde amnesia.

Learning objective: Describe the interaction between benzodiazepines and ethanol.

22. **B** Poisoning by benzodiazepines, such as diazepam, is usually not life-threatening but can be very serious when these drugs are combined with alcohol because of the additive depressant effects on the central nervous system.

    A, C–F These drugs do not cause additive sedative effects when given concomitantly with alcohol.

Learning objective: Describe the main contraindication of benzodiazepines.

23. **A** Sleep apnea is a breathing disorder characterized by frequent and prolonged (more than 15 seconds) pauses in breathing that occur during sleep. Typical symptoms of sleep apnea include alteration in sleep pattern with loud snoring, excessive daytime sleepiness, and severe shortness of breath on exertion. In sleep apnea, the sensitivity of the respiratory center to carbon dioxide is decreased. Sedative-hypnotics drugs are generally contraindicated in this disorder, as they further decrease the sensitivity of the respiratory center to hypercapnia.

    B–E All of these drugs have been used in sleep apnea with modest results.

Learning objective: Outline the anticonvulsant and muscle relaxant uses of benzodiazepines.

24. **F** All benzodiazepines have anticonvulsant and muscle relaxant activity. The latter is at least partly related to the enhancement of GABA-induced inhibition of synaptic transmission in the spinal cord, because they are effective in patients with cord transection. Because the condition of the patient is a chronic one, a long-acting benzodiazepine is most appropriate.

    A–E All of these drugs are devoid of muscle relaxant properties.

Learning objective: Describe the hypnotic uses of benzodiazepines.

25. **B** The patient's symptoms indicate that he is suffering from insomnia characterized by difficulty in maintaining sleep during the night because of nightmares. A benzodiazepine hypnotic is preferable in this patient because of the need for anxiolytic effect in addition to hypnotic efficacy. Moreover, benzodiazepines tend to decrease slow-wave sleep that is commonly associated with nightmares. A medium-acting benzodiazepine, such as temazepam, which can maintain sleep throughout the night, would be appropriate for this patient.

    A, C–E These drugs are devoid of hypnotic properties.

Learning objective: Describe the use of benzodiazepines in panic attacks.

26. **D** The patient's symptoms indicate that she was most likely suffering from a panic disorder. A selective serotonin reuptake inhibitor (SSRI), such as sertraline, is an appropriate first-line treatment for most patients with panic disorder. However, patients with severe or distressing symptoms may initially require concurrent benzodiazepine therapy that provides quick relief until the therapeutic effects of the SSRI are evident.

    A–C, E None of these drugs are effective in panic disorders.

Learning objective: Describe the use of benzodiazepines in ethanol withdrawal.

27. **F** The time-honored principle of treating an abstinence syndrome with an agent to which the abused drug induces cross-tolerance holds for ethanol as well. A long-acting benzodiazepine, such as diazepam, is the drug most commonly used in alcohol withdrawal, but a short-acting agent such as oxazepam can be administered every 4 to 6 hours according to the stage and severity of withdrawal. Theoretically, ethanol itself should be effective but is never used because of its short duration of action and its narrow range of safety.

    A–E See correct answer explanation.

Learning objective: Explain the zolpidem-induced increase in Cl^- conductance in the $GABA_A$ receptor–chloride ion channel macromolecular complex.

28. **B** Z-hypnotics (zolpidem, zaleplon, and eszopiclone) bind selectively to the α_1 subunit of the $GABA_A$ receptor–chloride channel complex. This selectivity may account for their relative lack of effect on sleep architecture and stages, as well as for the negligible anxiolytic, anticonvulsant, and muscle relaxant properties. The binding increases the GABA-mediated opening of Cl^- channels, leading to an increase in Cl^- conductance. The enhanced concentration of Cl^- inside the cell causes hyperpolarization of the cell membrane.

    A, C–E See correct answer explanation.

Learning objective: Describe the therapeutic uses of eszopiclone.

29. **C** Nonbenzodiazepines acting on GABA receptors (the so-called Z-hypnotics) are currently preferred to treat insomnia, because they do not alter sleep architecture and stages, do not have significant anxiolytic or anticonvulsant properties, and have a lower risk of dependence compared to the short-acting benzodiazepines. The choice of hypnotic drugs depends on the type of insomnia presented by the patient. When there is difficulty in falling asleep, a short-acting drug is appropriate; when there is difficulty in maintaining sleep during the night, a medium-acting drug such as eszopiclone ($t_{1/2}$ 4–7 h) is appropriate, as in this case.

    A Flunitrazepam is a long-acting benzodiazepine and is therefore not appropriate as a hypnotic because of the risk of daytime sedation and drowsiness.

    B, D–F These drugs have negligible hypnotic activity.

Learning objective: Describe the interaction between barbiturates and benzodiazepines.

30. **C** Benzodiazepines do not cause significant respiratory depression when given alone, but they can do so when they are given with other central nervous system depressants. In this case, the attending physician most likely did not take a detailed history and thus overlooked the antiepileptic therapy of the patient. Because of the interaction between phenobarbital and diazepam, the patient underwent severe respiratory depression.

A, B, D–F These drugs are not used for the rapid relief of acute anxiety symptoms.

SEDATIVE-HYPNOTIC DRUGS Answer key		
1. B	6. B	11. D
2. D	7. B	12. C
3. J	8. C	13. C
4. I	9. F	14. C
5. G	10. E	15. D
16. A	21. D	26. D
17. B	22. B	27. F
18. B	23. A	28. B
19. C	24. F	29. C
20. D	25. B	30. C

Answers and Explanations: III-3 General Anesthetics

Questions 1–5

1. **B**
2. **D**
3. **F**
4. **C**
5. **G**

Learning objective: Explain the meaning of the minimum alveolar concentration of inhalational anesthetics.

6. **D** During general anesthesia, the partial pressure of an anesthetic in the brain equals that in the lung when equilibrium is reached. Therefore, the measurement of the steady-state alveolar concentration of different anesthetics provides a measure of their relative potencies. The minimum alveolar concentration (MAC) is defined as the alveolar concentration of the anesthetic that results in the immobility of 50% of patients when exposed to a supramaximal noxious stimulus. Thus, MAC represents the ED_{50} on a conventional quantal dose–response curve and is therefore a measure of the potency of the inhaled anesthetic: the lower the MAC, the higher the potency. The speed of induction is a pharmacokinetic parameter and can tell us nothing about the potency of a drug (a pharmacodynamic parameter).

A–C, E See correct answer explanation.

Learning objective: Describe the adverse effects of halothane.

7. **D** Halothane can cause cardiac arrhythmias because it increases the automaticity of the heart and sensitizes the heart to catecholamines. Other halogenated anesthetics are less likely to produce cardiac arrhythmias.

A–C, E See correct answer explanation.

Learning objective: Describe the pharmacological effects of nitrous oxide.

8. **B** In subanesthetic concentrations, nitrous oxide can induce a euphoric state accompanied by very good analgesia. For this reason, it is frequently used as an analgesic in minor orthopedic and dental procedures that do not require general anesthesia, as in this case.

A Muscle relaxation with nitrous oxide is negligible.

C Unconsciousness cannot be achieved with nitrous oxide alone even when given at 100% concentration in the inspired air.

D Blood pressure is well maintained by nitrous oxide because the direct depressant effect upon the heart is counteracted by sympathetic stimulation.

E Respiration is minimally affected by nitrous oxide.

Learning objective: Describe the mechanism of action of barbiturates.

9. **D** All barbiturates increase the affinity of GABA for $GABA_A$ receptors, but unlike benzodiazepines, when given at high doses they can enhance Cl^- channel opening in the absence of GABA. Because the dose of thiopental was high enough to lose consciousness, the mechanism of this action was most likely an enhancement of Cl^- channel opening in the absence of GABA.

A–C, E See correct answer explanation.

Learning objective: Explain why propofol is preferred for general anesthesia in patients at high risk of vomiting.

10. **D** Propofol is an intravenous anesthetic with an onset and duration of anesthesia similar to that of thiopental. It is the only anesthetic with antiemetic action, so it is the preferred drug in patients at high risk of nausea and vomiting, as in this case.

A–C, E See correct answer explanation.

Learning objective: Explain why another inhalational anesthetic is added to nitrous oxide to maintain general anesthesia.

11. **B** Unconsciousness, which is usually achieved with thiopental, cannot be maintained with nitrous oxide alone (the drug has a minimum alveolar concentration higher than 100%), and therefore another potent anesthetic is needed. Moreover, nitrous oxide has negligible effects on skeletal muscle tone, so a halogenated anesthetic is given with it most of the time (all halogenated anesthetics cause relaxation of skeletal muscle and enhance the effects of neuromuscular blocking agents).

    A Nitrous oxide–induced analgesia is excellent, even at low concentration of the gas.

    C–E Halothane can cause, not prevent, all of these effects.

Learning objective: Describe anesthetic-induced malignant hyperthermia.

12. **B** In genetically susceptible patients, all halogenated anesthetics can trigger malignant hyperthermia, an autosomal dominant disorder characterized by severe muscle contraction, rapid development of hyperthermia, and a massive increase in metabolic rate. The syndrome is frequently fatal.

    A Acute intermittent porphyria is an idiosyncratic disorder that can be triggered by barbiturates, not by halogenated anesthetics.

    C Acute hepatitis is a rare disease that can be induced by halothane but not by other halogenated anesthetics. Moreover, it is not a genetic disorder.

    D, E These diseases are not genetically determined and are not induced by halogenated anesthetics.

Learning objective: Explain the meaning of the minimum alveolar concentration of inhalational anesthetics

13. **C** The minimum alveolar concentration (MAC) is defined as the concentration of the anesthetic that results in the immobility of 50% of patients when exposed to a supramaximal noxious stimulus. Thus, MAC represents the ED_{50} on a conventional quantal dose–response curve and is therefore a measure of the potency of the inhaled anesthetic.

    A, B, D, E See correct answer explanation.

Learning objective: Explain the mechanism of action of nitrous oxide.

14. **C** Nitrous oxide is a potent and selective inhibitor of NMDA-activated current, suggesting that its depressant effects on the central nervous system are produced via noncompetitive antagonistic activity at NMDA receptors.

    A, B, D, E See correct answer explanation.

Learning objective: Describe the relationship between the blood/gas partition coefficient and the speed of induction and recovery from general anesthesia.

15. **D** Sevoflurane has a blood/gas partition coefficient of 0.69. Halothane, the prototype of halogenated general anesthetics, has a blood/gas partition of 2.4. Because the speed of induction and recovery of anesthesia are inversely proportional to the blood/gas partition coefficient, sevoflurane causes a rapid anesthetic induction and recovery.

    A Redistribution can be a factor that speeds up the recovery from anesthesia, but sevoflurane has low lipid solubility, so redistribution into lipid tissue is minimal.

    B Metabolism of sevoflurane is very low (about 3%).

    C The minimum alveolar concentration (MAC) of an inhalational anesthetic is a measure of the potency of the drug; that is, it is a pharmacodynamic variable. The speed of induction depends on pharmacokinetic variables.

    E Inhalational anesthetics distribute uniformly into the brain. They are not concentrated in a specific region of the brain.

Learning objective: Describe the pharmacological effects of isoflurane.

16. **C** All halogenated anesthetics have bronchodilating properties, which is beneficial in patients with underlying airway problems, as in this case.

    A Cardiac output is minimally affected by isoflurane.

    B, D, E Isoflurane has effects opposite to those listed.

Learning objective: Describe the pharmacological actions of etomidate.

17. **E** Etomidate is an intravenous anesthetic agent that causes anesthetic induction and recovery similar to that of thiopental (about 5 to 10 minutes of unconsciousness with a standard anesthetic dose), but it has minimal actions on cardiovascular and respiratory functions. It is mainly used for induction of anesthesia in patients with serious respiratory or cardiovascular disease, as in this case.

    A Halothane causes a dose-dependent depression of the cardiovascular and respiratory systems.

    B Ketamine produces cardiovascular stimulation by excitation of the sympathetic nervous system.

    C Propofol causes a marked decrease in blood pressure, primarily due to a decrease in total peripheral resistance.

    D Barbiturates such as thiopental are respiratory and circulatory depressants.

Learning objective: Outline the therapeutic uses of ketamine.

18. **A** Ketamine is a general anesthetic that induces a state of sedation, characterized by immobility, profound analgesia, anterograde amnesia, and a strong feeling of dissociation from the environment without complete loss of consciousness. This state has been termed dissociative anesthesia. Because it can provoke postoperative disorientation, perceptual illusions, and vivid dreams, it is not commonly used in general surgery. The drug causes negligible respiratory depression and significant sympathetic stimulation. It is used for short, painful surgical procedures in children (who are less influenced by the mental effects of the drug), especially when they have respiratory problems, as in this case.

B, C Thiopental and fentanyl can cause significant respiratory depression and therefore are not indicated in asthmatic patients.

D, E Generally, halogenated anesthetics such as halothane and sevoflurane are not used for minor surgical procedures.

Learning objective: Describe the drugs used for conscious sedation and have the advantage of being reversible by the administration of specific receptor antagonists.

19. **B** Conscious sedation refers to a drug-induced state of altered consciousness with the following features:

- Consciousness is not lost (the patient can respond to verbal commands).
- A patent airway is maintained (the patient does not have to be ventilated).
- Cardiovascular effects generally are not marked.
- Anxiety is alleviated.
- Pain is relieved.
- Some degree of anterograde amnesia is present.

A wide variety of intravenous anesthetic agents (benzodiazepines, propofol, and opioids) have been used. Benzodiazepines and opioids have the advantage that their effects can be easily reversed by the use of specific receptor antagonists (flumazenil and naloxone, respectively).

A, C–E There are no specific antagonists for thiopental and ketamine.

Learning objective: Describe the pathophysiology of malignant hyperthermia.

20. **C** The signs of the patient strongly suggest that he was suffering from malignant hyperthermia, a rare autosomal dominant disorder that can be triggered by the administration of halogenated anesthetics and/or succinylcholine. The pathogenesis of the disease is thought to involve a mutation in the gene encoding the skeletal muscle ryanodine receptor, a channel responsible for the regulation of Ca^{2+} release from the sarcoplasmic reticulum. This mutation would result in an excessive release of Ca^{2+}, which would be the main cause of the signs and symptoms of malignant hyperthermia.

A, B, D, E None of these actions cause the syndrome exhibited by the patient.

Learning objective: Describe the cardiovascular effects of isoflurane.

21. **D** Isoflurane is a potent coronary vasodilator, simultaneously producing increased coronary blood flow and decreased myocardial oxygen consumption. It is a particularly safe anesthetic to use for patients with ischemic heart disease, as in this case.

A, E Halothane and sevoflurane cause a dose-dependent decrease in cardiac output.

B, C Etomidate and propofol are used for induction, not for maintenance of general anesthesia.

Learning objective: Identify the general anesthetic with the highest risk of toxic hepatitis.

22. **B** The patient's signs and symptoms indicated that she was most likely suffering from fulminant hepatitis. Halothane can produce fulminant hepatic necrosis in a small number of patients (1/10,000). The syndrome typically starts 3 to 5 days after anesthesia and rapidly progresses to hepatic failure. The prognosis is poor (death occurs in about 50% of these patients).The mechanism of hepatotoxicity is still uncertain. The current hypothesis is that some hepatic proteins become trifluoroacetylated by halothane metabolites and initiate an immune response.

A, F The risk of toxic hepatitis with other fluorinated anesthetics is negligible.

C–E Nitrous oxide, thiopental, and fentanyl do not cause liver toxicity.

Learning objective: Describe the additive property of minimum alveolar concentration of inhalational anesthetics.

23. **B** The minimum alveolar concentration (MAC) is defined as the concentration of the anesthetic that results in the immobility of 50% of patients when exposed to a supramaximal noxious stimulus (i.e., surgical skin incision). MAC values of inhalational anesthetics have a very important property: they are roughly additive. Because the alveolar concentration needed to provide surgical anesthesia in most patients is about 1.3 MAC, a 0.7 MAC of nitrous oxide plus 0.6 MAC of sevoflurane will provide an appropriate surgical anesthesia for the patient. This explains why nitrous oxide, which is a very poor aesthetic when given alone, can enhance the effect of all other inhalational anesthetics given concomitantly. Another important consequence of the additive property of MAC is that the anesthetic effects of two inhalational anesthetics are additive, but the adverse effects are not. As nitrous oxide has low toxicity, the mixture of a large MAC fraction of this gas with a small MAC fraction of another inhalational anesthetic can provide surgical anesthesia with adverse effects substantially lower than that of the other anesthetic given alone.

    A, C The sum of these MACs is not enough to ensure an appropriate surgical anesthesia.

    D, E The sum of these MACs is above the 1.3 level needed for surgical anesthesia. This means that the alveolar concentration is too high and can substantially increase the risk of adverse effects. Moreover, because 1 MAC of nitrous oxide is more than 100% of the gas alveolar concentration, nitrous oxide cannot be used at a concentration above 80% (i.e., about 0.8 MAC), as this would limit the delivery of an adequate amount of oxygen.

Learning objective: Explain the reason for the short duration of anesthesia induced by thiopental.

24. **C** Thiopental rapidly diffuses out of the brain and other highly vascularized tissues and is redistributed to muscle, fat, and eventually to all body tissues. This is the principal mechanism limiting anesthetic duration after a single anesthetic dose.

    A, E Actually, thiopental distributes very rapidly into the CNS. Because it is very lipid soluble, diffusion into the CNS neurons is very good.

    B, D Thiopental half-life is about 12 hours, which indicates that the elimination of the drug from the body is slow.

Learning objective: Identify the drug usually administered with propofol to reduce pain on injection.

25. **D** The intravenous injection of propofol is associated with pain, most likely due to its alcohol nature that irritates the vascular endothelium. Three out of five patients experience pain on injection, with one of these patients reporting severe or excruciating pain. As a result, several interventions have been investigated to alleviate the pain associated with propofol injection. The coadministration of several drugs, including opioids, ketamine, and nonsteroidal antiinflammatory drugs, can be effective in reducing pain, but lidocaine, in conjunction with venous occlusion, is thought to be the most effective intervention.

    A–C, E See correct answer explanation.

Learning objective: Describe the main variables that can decrease the minimum alveolar concentration (MAC) of inhalational anesthetics.

26. **C** It is known that MAC can be decreased by several physiological and pharmacological variables, including age, pregnancy, hypothermia, hypercalcemia, hyponatremia, and in the presence of certain drugs (acute alcohol, opioids, benzodiazepines, barbiturates, ketamine, lithium, clonidine, etc.). One of the most striking is the 6% decrease in MAC per decade of age, regardless of volatile anesthetic. It drops to about half by age 80, as in this case.

    A, B, D, E See correct answer explanation.

Learning objective: Identify the general anesthetic that is contraindicated in patients with pheochromocytoma.

27. **A** Halothane can sensitize the myocardium to the arrhythmogenic effect of catecholamines and is therefore contraindicated in patients with high blood catecholamine levels, as in this case.

    B–E None of these drugs cause sensitization of the myocardium to catecholamines.

Learning objective: Identify the general anesthetic that is contraindicated in small bowel closed loop obstruction.

28. **B** In closed loop obstruction, the lumen of the bowel is occluded at two points, thus preventing prograde and retrograde movements of bowel contents. Because nitrous oxide diffuses into the cavity more rapidly than the air (principally nitrogen) diffuses out, the gas can increase the intraluminal pressure of the obstructed bowel loop, thus increasing the risk of gut rupture. Examples of conditions in which nitrous oxide might be hazardous include all the closed cavities filled with air, such as pneumothorax, pulmonary air cysts, and pneumocephalus.

    A, C–E See correct answer explanation.

Learning objective: Describe the main adverse effects of etomidate.

29. **A** Cardiovascular stability is a major advantage of etomidate over barbiturate or propofol and therefore is most suited in patients with coronary disease, as in this case. Etomidate has

the highest incidence of postoperative nausea and vomiting (more than 30% of cases) among the general anesthetics.

B–E Etomidate does not cause delusion and has minimal cardiovascular and respiratory effects.

Learning objective: Explain the mechanism of diffusion hypoxia caused by nitrous oxide.

30. **D** On recovery from anesthesia, the outpouring of large volumes of nitrous oxide can cause an effect called diffusion hypoxia. These volumes may cause hypoxia in two ways. First, they may directly affect oxygenation by displacing oxygen. Second, by diluting alveolar carbon dioxide, they may decrease respiratory drive and hence ventilation. Both of these effects require that large volumes of nitrous oxide be released into the alveoli. Because these large volumes are released only during the first 5 to 10 minutes of recovery, this is the period of greatest concern. An additional reason is that this period may be the time of greatest respiratory

depression. For these reasons, 100% oxygen is often administered for the first 5 to 10 minutes of recovery. This procedure may be particularly indicated when postoperative respiratory depression is anticipated, as in the present case (see the administration of fentanyl).

A–C, E These drugs do not cause diffusion hypoxia.

GENERAL ANESTHETICS Answer Key		
1. B	6. D	11. B
2. D	7. D	12. B
3. F	8. B	13. C
4. C	9. D	14. C
5. G	10. D	15. D
16. C	21. D	26. C
17. E	22. B	27. A
18. A	23. B	28. B
19. B	24. C	29. A
20. C	25. D	30. D

Answers and Explanations: III-4 Local Anesthetics

Questions 1–3

1. **F**
2. **B**
3. **B**

Learning objective: Explain the molecular mechanism of action of local anesthetic.

4. **A** Local anesthetics block voltage-gated Na^+ channels, preventing depolarization of the membrane and blocking conduction of the action potential. The blockade of Na^+ channel is voltage dependent; that is, the affinity of the channel for the local anesthetics is high when the channel is inactivated or activated (i.e., when the membrane potential is less negative) and is low when the channel is in the resting state (i.e., when the membrane potential is more negative). The same rule holds for antiarrhythmic drugs, which act by blocking ion channels.

B–F See correct answer explanation.

Learning objective: Describe the adverse effects of local anesthetics.

5. **C** Drowsiness is the most frequent complaint that results from central nervous system (CNS) actions of local anesthetics and is usually an early sign of a high plasma level of the drug. CNS effects of lidocaine are common when the drug is administered systemically as an antiarrhythmic or when a sufficient concentration of the drug can reach the general circulation after being given locally for local anesthesia, as was most likely in this case.

A, E Lidocaine tends to cause adverse effects opposite to those listed.

B This adverse effect is not caused by lidocaine.

D This adverse effect can occur only after huge plasma levels of lidocaine.

Learning objective: Identify the local anesthetic used for long surgical procedures.

6. **C** The duration of local anesthesia after a standard dose of tetracaine injected near the brachial plexus is about 210 to 240 minutes. The drug is therefore preferred for more lengthy surgical procedures.

A, B The duration of action of these local anesthetics is less than 2 hours.

D, E These drugs are not used for nerve block anesthesia.

Learning objective: Calculate the percentage of the lipid-soluble form of lidocaine in the extracellular fluids, given sufficient data.

7. **B** Because local anesthetics except benzocaine are weak bases, they are mainly ionized when their pK_a is higher than the pH of the body fluids, as in this case. The ratio between the nonionized and the ionized form can be determined using the Henderson-Hasselbalch equation. When the difference between the pK_a and the pH is +0.5, the percentage of the ionized form is 76%; therefore, the percentage of the nonionized, lipid-soluble form will be 24%.

A, C–E See correct answer explanation.

Learning objective: Identify nerve fiber properties altered by local anesthetics.

8. **C** Local anesthetics primarily block inactivated Na⁺ channels, making them take longer to return to the resting state. As long as the channel is blocked, the fiber is refractory to stimulation, so the refractory period of the nerve will increase.

   A, B, D These nerve properties are in fact decreased, not increased, by local anesthetics.

   E Local anesthetics have very low affinity for channels in the resting state, so they have negligible effects on the resting membrane potential of the nerve.

Learning objective: Explain why epinephrine should not be used with local anesthetics when organs supplied by end arteries (fingers, ears, nose, and penis) need to be anesthetized.

9. **B** Epinephrine-containing solutions should not be injected into organs supplied by end arteries (fingers, ears, nose, and penis) because the resulting vasoconstriction can produce ischemia and even gangrene.

   A, D Epinephrine does not affect the risk of wound infection and does not cause delayed wound repair.

   C, E Excessive bleeding and systemic toxicity are in fact prevented by administration of epinephrine.

Learning objective: Identify the factors that increase the affinity of Na⁺ channels for local anesthetics.

10. **C** Local anesthetics act primarily by blocking Na⁺ channels. The blockade is voltage dependent; the less negative the membrane potential, the higher the channel affinity for local anesthetics. In the resting state, Na⁺ channels predominate at more negative membrane potential. These channels have a much lower affinity for local anesthetics than inactivated or activated channels, which predominate at less negative membrane potential. The blockade is also time-dependent (also referred to as frequency dependent); the faster the firing of the nerve, the higher the channel affinity for local anesthetics.

    A, B, D, E See correct answer explanation.

Learning objective: Identify the physiological function blocked last by local anesthetics.

11. **A** Fiber sensitivity to blockade by local anesthetics depends on different factors; for example, sensitivity is inversely related to diameter and conduction velocity. Fibers with smaller diameter and slower conduction velocity are blocked before fibers that have larger diameter and faster conduction velocity. Therefore, type A-alpha fibers, which convey motor function (diameter 12–20 μ, conduction velocity 70–120 m/sec) are blocked last, when a local anesthetic is applied to a nerve.

    B–E See correct answer explanation.

Learning objective: Explain why local anesthesia has a slower onset in infected tissue.

12. **E** Local anesthetics are weak bases; all but benzocaine have a pK_a in the range of about 7.7 to 9.4. Therefore, they are mainly water-soluble at the physiological pH of the extracellular fluid. However, only the small, lipid soluble portion of the drug can cross the nerve membrane. The extracellular fluid of the infected tissues has a lower pH due to the increased concentration of lactic acid. The lipid solubility of the drug will be even lower, and less drug will be available for diffusion into the nerve fibers.

    A–D See correct answer explanation.

Learning objective: Describe the adverse effects of prilocaine.

13. **D** Prilocaine is the only local anesthetic that can cause methemoglobinemia. This effect is not a problem in healthy persons, but the neonate is more sensitive to methemoglobinemia due to decreased resistance of fetal hemoglobin to oxidant stress and immaturity of the enzymes that convert methemoglobin back to the ferrous state.

    A–C, E See correct answer explanation.

Learning objective: Explain why hyperkalemia makes the nerve membrane more sensitive to the action of local anesthetics.

14. **D** According to the Nernst equation, an increase in extracellular K⁺ concentration makes the membrane potential less negative (depolarization) and favors the inactivated state of Na⁺ channels. Because local anesthetics mainly block inactivated Na⁺ channels, increased extracellular concentration of K⁺ makes the nerve membrane more sensitive to the action of local anesthetics. Local increase in extracellular concentration of K⁺ is common in burned tissues because the damaged cells spill their cytosol into the extracellular fluid. Although patients with burns are known to develop hypocalcemia, hypercalcemia has been reported in about 20% of patients with extensive burns.

    A–C, E All of these events cause hyperpolarization of the membrane, which favors the resting state.

Learning objective: Explain why bupivacaine is contraindicated in a patient with chronic obstructive pulmonary disease.

15. **E** Most local anesthetics can block Na⁺ channels in cardiac muscle, thereby depressing automaticity and conduction. At very high doses they can also depress contractility, most likely by blocking Ca²⁺ channels. Bupivacaine is more cardiotoxic than most other local anesthetics, apparently because the drug dissociates much more slowly than other local anesthetics during diastole, so a significant fraction of Na⁺ channels at physiological heart rates remains blocked with bupivacaine at the end of the diastole. Bupivacaine-induced cardiac toxicity is very difficult to treat and is enhanced by

coexisting acidosis and hypoxemia, which are most likely in this case because of COPD.

A–D See correct answer explanation.

Learning objective: Explain the choice of a local anesthetic according to the anticipated duration of a surgical procedure.

16. **E** Epidural anesthesia is administered by injecting local anesthetic into the epidural space and can be performed in the sacral hiatus or in the lumbar, thoracic, or cervical region of the spine. The anesthesia affects only those nerves leaving the spinal cord at the level of injection. Lidocaine is the most frequently used epidural local anesthetic, especially when the surgical procedure is short, as in this case.

A, B Cocaine and benzocaine are not suitable for spinal or epidural anesthesia.

C, D Bupivacaine and tetracaine are used for spinal and epidural anesthesia when the surgical procedure is long. They are not needed in this case because the anticipated duration of the procedure is only about 20 minutes.

Learning objective: Explain the choice of an amide-type local anesthetic for a patient allergic to para-aminobenzoic acid (PABA).

17. **C** Lidocaine is an amide-type local anesthetic that can be employed in almost any application when a local anesthetic of intermediate duration is needed. It is widely used in spinal anesthesia.

A, B, D, E A serious allergic reaction to PABA contraindicates the administration of all ester-type local anesthetics (procaine, tetracaine, benzocaine, and cocaine), as they are esters of PABA. In addition, procaine and benzocaine are not suitable for spinal anesthesia.

Learning objective: Identify the local anesthetic preparation suitable for a patient with a concomitant cardiac disease.

18. **A** Epinephrine is used in local anesthetic preparations to localize the anesthetic at the desired site and to reduce systemic toxicity. However, epinephrine is contraindicated in patients with cardiac arrhythmias. In this patient, a preparation containing the local anesthetic alone is the most rational choice.

B, C See correct answer explanation.

D, E There are no injectable preparations of benzocaine, as this drug is used only for surface anesthesia.

Learning objective: Describe the therapeutic uses of benzocaine.

19. **A** Unlike other local anesthetics, benzocaine has a pK_a of about 2.5; consequently, it is practically insoluble in water. Therefore, the drug cannot be injected, but it can be applied directly to wounded surfaces, where it remains localized for a long time, producing sustained anesthetic action. Because

of this, benzocaine is incorporated into a large number of topical preparations. Other drugs used for topical anesthesia are lidocaine and tetracaine.

B Procaine is used only for infiltration anesthesia because of its slow onset and short duration of action.

C Cocaine is very rarely used today as a local anesthetic, due to its addictive potential. Moreover, cocaine absorption from abraded skin can be significant.

D, E Prilocaine and bupivacaine are not used for topical anesthesia.

Learning objective: Identify the molecular form of a local anesthetic that mediates receptor binding.

20. **D** Local anesthetics are weak bases, and in the body they exist either as the uncharged base (nonionized form) or as a cation (ionized form). Because the nonionized form is lipid soluble, it is important for diffusion through the cell membranes. However, the cationic form is thought to be the one that binds to the receptor site, located on the Na^+ channel near the inner surface of the membrane.

A–C All of these properties are more related to the nonionized form of the drug. In fact, tissue redistribution usually occurs in lipid-rich tissues; liver biotransforms mainly lipid-soluble drugs, and only the lipid-soluble form of the drug can easily cross the blood–brain barrier.

E The half-life of a drug is related to its volume of distribution and its clearance, which in turn depend on many factors, not only on the ionized form of the drug.

Learning objective: Describe the use of cocaine as a local anesthetic agent.

21. **A** The drug used was most likely cocaine, the only local anesthetic that also has a vasoconstricting action, due to its inhibitory effect on norepinephrine reuptake into adrenergic terminals. Cocaine can provide better tolerance of suturing in patients who are unable to tolerate injections, as in this case. However, the drug is very rarely used today as a topical anesthetic because of its toxicity, expense, and federal regulatory issues. Serious toxic effects (e.g., seizures and cardiac arrhythmias) have been described following topical cocaine application, particularly in children.

B–E See correct answer explanation.

LOCAL ANESTHETICS Answer key			
1. F	6. C	11. A	16. E
2. B	7. B	12. E	17. C
3. B	8. C	13. D	18. A
4. A	9. B	14. D	19. A
5. C	10. C	15. E	20. D
			21. A

Answers and Explanations: III-5 Skeletal Muscle Relaxants

Questions 1–4

1. **A**
2. **D**
3. **H**
4. **F**

Learning objective: Identify the site of action of tubocurarine.

5. **C** All neuromuscular blocking agents bind to Nm receptors located on the postjunctional folds of motor end plates, acting there as competitive antagonists (nondepolarizing blockers) or as partial agonists (depolarizing blockers). The blockade of these receptors mediates the clinical effects of these drugs, that is, skeletal muscle paralysis.

A, B, D Tubocurarine can block Nn receptors located on autonomic ganglia, on the adrenal medulla, and on somatic nerve terminals, but these sites do not represent the main site of action of the drug. In fact, the affinity of the drug for these receptors is much lower than the affinity for Nm receptors.

E Spinal motor neurons are located on the anterior horn of the spinal cord, that is, inside the central nervous system (CNS). Curare-like drugs cannot enter the CNS because they do not cross the blood–brain barrier.

F Nm receptors are on motor end plates only. When activated, they open ligand-gated ion channels, causing depolarization of the motor end plate (miniature end-plate potential). Skeletal muscle cell membranes have voltage-gated ion channels that open when the depolarization of the motor end plate reaches the threshold for the propagation of the potential.

Learning objective: Describe the therapeutic uses of nondepolarizing neuromuscular blockers.

6. **B** The patient most likely received vecuronium, a nondepolarizing neuromuscular blocker. These drugs are often used in patients who need mechanical ventilation. They can facilitate intubation and can block voluntary movements that could interfere with mechanical ventilation. Neuromuscular blockers with an intermediate duration of action such as vecuronium (about 30 minutes after a standard therapeutic dose) are often preferred.

A, C–F All of these drugs have skeletal muscle relaxant properties, but they act with different mechanisms of action and are not used to facilitate intubation and decrease spontaneous breathing.

Learning objective: Describe the pharmacokinetics of succinylcholine.

7. **A** The duration of action of succinylcholine is about 8 minutes after a standard therapeutic dose. The reason is that the drug is rapidly hydrolyzed by pseudocholinesterase in plasma and liver. This duration of action is enough to facilitate intubation. When a longer duration of action is needed, the drug is given by intravenous infusion.

B–F See correct answer explanation.

Learning objective: Explain the mechanism of action of dantrolene

8. **D** The clinical picture of the patient suggests the diagnosis of malignant hyperthermia, a rare but potentially life-threatening disorder that can be triggered by a variety of stimuli, including the administration of certain anesthetics (mainly halothane) and neuromuscular blocking agents (mainly succinylcholine). The disorder is related to a hereditary impairment in the ability of the sarcoplasmic reticulum to sequester calcium; therefore, a prolonged release of calcium occurs after the triggering event through sarcoplasmic calcium channels (sometimes called ryanodine receptors). This causes massive muscle contraction, hyperthermia, and lactic acidosis. Dantrolene is a drug of choice in this disorder because it blocks Ca^{2+} channels in the skeletal muscle sarcoplasmic reticulum, thus preventing the massive release of calcium. Cardiac and smooth muscle are minimally affected by dantrolene because they have a different type of Ca^{2+} channel in their sarcoplasmic reticulum.

A–C, E See correct answer explanation.

Learning objective: Identify the site of action of botulinum toxin.

9. **B** Via endocytosis, botulinum toxin enters cholinergic nerve terminals, where it prevents the exocytotic release of acetylcholine, causing paralysis of the skeletal muscles surrounding the site of injection.

A, C, E Botulinum toxin does not bind to cholinergic receptors.

D Botulinum toxin also prevents acetylcholine release from autonomic cholinergic nerve terminals, but this is not the site of the therapeutic action of the drug.

Learning objective: Explain the mechanism of action of vecuronium.

10. **C** Vecuronium is a nondepolarizing neuromuscular blocker. These drugs act as competitive antagonists at Nm receptors, preventing the activation of the receptors by acetylcholine. In this way, they prevent depolarization of skeletal muscle cell membranes and inhibit muscular contraction. Their action can be overcome by increasing the concentration of acetylcholine in the synaptic cleft.

    A, B, D–F Nondepolarizing neuromuscular blockers are devoid of these effects.

Learning objective: Describe the sequence of muscle paralysis induced by vecuronium.

11. **A** The skeletal muscle paralysis induced by nondepolarizing neuromuscular blocking drugs follows a sequence that is related to the innervation of the skeletal muscles. Muscles that are small, rapidly moving, and richly innervated, such as extrinsic eye muscles, small muscles of the face, and pharynx, are affected first. The paralysis of the extrinsic eye muscles causes a lack of parallelism of the visual axes of the eyes that leads to double vision. As a rule, large muscles (e.g., limb muscles) are paralyzed after small muscles. Ultimately, the intercostal muscles and, finally, the diaphragm are paralyzed.

    B–E See correct answer explanation.

Learning objective: Describe the biotransformation of mivacurium.

12. **D** Mivacurium is the only nondepolarizing neuromuscular blocker that is metabolized by plasma pseudocholinesterase. Because of this rapid metabolism, the action of the drug is short.

    A Succinylcholine is metabolized by plasma cholinesterase, but it is a depolarizing, not a nondepolarizing, neuromuscular blocker.

    B, C, E See correct answer explanation.

Learning objective: Explain the use of cisatracurium in patients with impaired hepatic and renal functions.

13. **D** Cisatracurium is a neuromuscular blocking drug that has the unique property of being inactivated primarily by a form of spontaneous breakdown also known as Hoffmann elimination. Because of this, it does not exhibit an increase in half-life in patients with compromised hepatic or renal function, and it is therefore the agent of choice under these conditions, as in the present case.

A, C, E Succinylcholine, dantrolene, and mivacurium are not metabolized by Hoffmann elimination.

B Dantrolene cannot cause skeletal muscle paralysis (unless huge doses are given) and therefore is not used as a skeletal muscle relaxant during surgery.

Learning objective: Describe the interaction between tubocurarine and H_1 antagonists.

14. **E** Tubocurarine-induced hypotension is primarily due to histamine release, and premedication with an antihistamine drug is often used to attenuate this adverse effect.

    A–D Drugs from these classes would increase, not decrease, tubocurarine-induced hypotension.

Learning objective: Describe the interaction between aminoglycoside antibiotics and nondepolarizing neuromuscular blockers.

15. **A** Aminoglycoside antibiotics inhibit acetylcholine release from cholinergic nerves by blocking a specific type of Ca^{2+} channel. Therefore, they enhance the blockade induced by nondepolarizing neuromuscular blockers.

    B–E See correct answer explanation.

Learning objective: Describe the pharmacokinetics of mivacurium.

16. **D** Mivacurium and succinylcholine are two neuromuscular blockers metabolized by plasma cholinesterase. In patients with a genetic deficiency of normal plasma cholinesterase, these drugs can cause apnea for several hours and are therefore contraindicated.

    A–C, E, F See correct answer explanation.

Learning objective: Describe the main contraindication of tubocurarine.

17. **A** Tubocurarine can cause histamine release from mast cells. A prominent effect of histamine is bronchoconstriction. Because of this, tubocurarine should not be used in patients with asthma or chronic obstructive pulmonary disease.

    B Glycopyrrolate is often given as a preoperative medication to prevent effects related to vagal activation (sialorrhea and bradycardia)

    C Clonidine is sometimes given as a preoperative medication because it has sedative properties and potentiates the action of anesthetic agents.

    D, E Vecuronium and cisatracurium, which are nondepolarizing neuromuscular blocking drugs, could be used, as these agents do not release histamine.

Learning objective: Describe the adverse effects of tubocurarine.

18. **D** Agitation is a frequent problem in patients who are intubated and artificially ventilated. Benzodiazepines are useful agents for controlling anxiety and agitation. They also cause anterograde amnesia (a useful property in this setting) but have no analgesic properties. When sedating drugs are not fully effective, a muscle relaxant is added. Tubocurarine is a neuromuscular blocking drug whose action lasts more than 50 minutes after a standard therapeutic dose. It is still sometimes used because of effectiveness and low cost. The tachycardia that can appear after the administration of tubocurarine can be due either to histamine release or to blockade of nicotinic receptors of autonomic ganglia or, most likely, to both.

    A Botulinum toxin is not used to limit movements in an intubated patient. Its actions would last for months.

    B Dantrolene is a spasmolytic drug. It can reduce spasticity but is unable to cause neuromuscular paralysis when given at therapeutic doses. Therefore, it is not used to limit movements in an intubated patient.

    C Succinylcholine can cause stimulation of both nicotinic receptors in autonomic ganglia and cardiac muscarinic receptors. Therefore, it would tend to cause bradycardia, which is only partially counteracted by its slight tendency to cause histamine release.

    E Cisatracurium has no effect on nicotinic receptors of autonomic ganglia and has negligible histamine-releasing properties.

Learning objective: Explain the mechanism of action of succinylcholine.

19. **A** Succinylcholine acts as a cholinergic agonist at Nm receptors. The Na^+ channels open and cause depolarization of the motor end plate, but because the drug is not metabolized as fast as acetylcholine, the activation of Nm receptors is long lasting. This activation causes a brief period of excitation that may elicit transient and repetitive muscle excitation (fasciculations), followed by block of neuromuscular transmission, as the long-lasting depolarization makes the motor end plate unresponsive to subsequent stimuli (depolarization blockade).

    B–F See correct answer explanation.

Learning objective: Describe the adverse effects of succinylcholine.

20. **B** Succinylcholine activates Nm receptors. This can account for the involuntary contraction of a group of muscle fibers, called fasciculations or twitching, that occurs before the muscle paralysis. Nondepolarizing neuromuscular blockers do not activate Nm receptors, so contractions cannot occur before paralysis.

    A, C–F See correct answer explanation.

Learning objective: Explain the mechanism of muscle relaxant action of tizanidine.

21. **E** Tizanidine is a centrally acting α_2-receptor agonist, structurally and pharmacologically related to clonidine. Its spasmolytic activity most likely results from activation of presynaptic α_2 receptors in the spinal cord. This activation decreases the release of excitatory amino acids, which in turn leads to inhibition of spinal motor neurons.

    A–D See correct answer explanation.

Learning objective: Explain the mechanism of the spasmolytic action of benzodiazepines.

22. **D** Benzodiazepines facilitate the action of GABA in the central nervous system by increasing the affinity of $GABA_A$ receptors for GABA. Their action in reducing spasticity, however, seems to be at least partly mediated in the spinal cord, because they are effective also in patients with cord transection.

    A This is the mechanism of action of dantrolene.

    B This is the mechanism of action of botulinum toxin.

    C This is the mechanism of action of succinylcholine.

    E This is the mechanism of action of baclofen.

Learning objective: Describe the action of vecuronium on miniature membrane potential.

23. **B** The formation of miniature end-plate potentials is caused by the release of small quanta of acetylcholine that activate Nm receptors at the motor end plate. By blocking these receptors, vecuronium blocks the formation of this potential.

    A, D, E Neuromuscular blocking drugs have negligible effects on the formation of action potentials in the motor neuron, cardiac muscle, or corticospinal tract.

    C Smooth muscle membrane has no Nm receptors. Therefore, neuromuscular blocking drugs have no direct effects on smooth muscle.

Learning objective: Describe the adverse effects of succinylcholine.

24. **E** Succinylcholine can rapidly release potassium from intracellular sites. In a normally healthy patient, this results in a small, transient hyperkalemia. In patients with extensive soft tissue trauma or burns, cerebral vascular accident, or prolonged stays in an intensive care unit, this hyperkalemia can be much more pronounced when succinylcholine is given at least several days after the underlying condition has become established. The hyperkalemia can be life-threatening, as it can lead to cardiac arrest, as in this case. The cause of succinylcholine-induced hyperkalemia in these patients seems related to upregulation of nicotinic muscular (Nm) receptors on motor end plates. Patients with the aforementioned conditions are deprived of neural influence or activity

because of prolonged immobilization. Such deprivation stimulates the synthesis of new Nm receptors across the muscle membrane. When these receptors are activated by succinylcholine, an action potential occurs, and ion channels open, allowing Na^+ to flow into and K^+ to flow out of the cell. Because succinylcholine is metabolized more slowly than acetylcholine, the receptor activation is more prolonged, causing a larger influx of Na^+ and a vigorous efflux of K^+. When Nm receptors are increased in skeletal muscle, this K^+ efflux can cause life-threatening hyperkalemia.

A–C Nondepolarizing neuromuscular blockers cause blockade, not activation, of Nm receptors. Therefore, they do not induce hyperkalemia.

D Dantrolene has no effect on Nm receptors.

Learning objective: Describe the adverse effects of succinylcholine.

25. **D** The clinical picture of the patient suggests the diagnosis of malignant hyperthermia, a rare but potentially life-threatening disorder triggered by the administration of certain anesthetics and neuromuscular blocking agents. Uncontrolled release of Ca^+ from the sarcoplasmic reticulum of skeletal muscle is the initiating event. Although most cases of malignant hyperthermia arise from the combination of succinylcholine and halogenated hydrocarbon anesthetics (e.g., halothane, isoflurane, and sevoflurane), succinylcholine or anesthetics alone have been reported to precipitate the response. Susceptibility to malignant hyperthermia is an autosomal dominant trait. In the majority of cases, no clinical signs are visible in the absence of anesthetic intervention.

A–C, E, F See correct answer explanation.

Learning objective: Describe the adverse effects of succinylcholine.

26. **C** Myalgias are common postoperative complaints of patients receiving large doses of succinylcholine. The true incidence of myalgias is difficult to establish because of confounding factors, including the type of surgery and positioning during the operation, but has been reported to be up to 20%. The pain is thought to be secondary to the unsynchronized contractions (i.e., fasciculations) of adjacent muscle fibers just before the onset of paralysis. When these fasciculations are strong enough, muscle soreness can result on recovering from anesthesia.

A, B Nondepolarizing muscle relaxants can sometimes cause myalgias upon recovery from muscle paralysis, but the incidence is much lower than that with succinylcholine.

D, E Dantrolene and diazepam are spasmolytic agents. They do not cause muscle paralysis and are not used to induce complete muscle relaxation during general anesthesia.

Learning objective: Explain the mechanism of action of botulinum toxin.

27. **D** Botulinum toxin must get inside the axon terminals to cause paralysis. Following the attachment of the toxin to proteins on the surface of axon terminals, the toxin can be taken into neurons by endocytosis. There it is able to cleave endocytotic vesicles and reach the cytoplasm. The light chain of the toxin has protease activity and proteolytically degrades a specific protein that is required for vesicle fusion that releases acetylcholine from the axon endings. In this way it prevents neurosecretory vesicles from fusing with the nerve synapse plasma membrane and releasing the neurotransmitter.

A–C, E, F See correct answer explanation.

Learning objective: Describe the adverse effects of a local treatment with botulinum toxin.

28. **D** Blepharospasm is spasm of muscles around the eye that causes involuntary blinking and eye closing. It affects women more than men and tends to occur within families. The cause is most often unknown. Injection of botulinum toxin into the eyelid muscle is often the preferred treatment (the effects of each treatment last about 3 months). The most common adverse effect is eyelid ptosis (up to 20% of cases), which represents an unwanted extension of the pharmacological effect.

A–C, E Botulinum toxin is given locally, so the risk of systemic adverse effects is very low.

Learning objective: Describe the mechanism of action of baclofen.

29. **A** Baclofen is an agonist at $GABA_B$ receptors. These are metabotropic transmembrane receptors for GABA that are linked via Gi proteins to potassium channels. Activation of these receptors by baclofen results in increased K^+ conductance, which in turn causes hyperpolarization of presynaptic terminals. This hyperpolarization reduces the release of excitatory transmitters in both the brain and the spinal cord. Baclofen is at least as effective as diazepam in reducing spasticity and is frequently used for this purpose.

B This is the action of nondepolarizing neuromuscular blockers.

C Baclofen can cause blockade of substance P release from spinal cord; this seems to be one of the reasons for its analgesic activity in patients with spasticity.

D, E Baclofen can indirectly block Ca^{2+} channels as a consequence of membrane hyperpolarization and can increase K^+ conductance, but these actions occur in neuronal, not in skeletal muscle, membranes.

Learning objective: Describe the therapeutic uses of baclofen.

30. **B** Stiff man syndrome is a disorder of neuromuscular transmission characterized by the insidious onset of progressive stiffness in the trunk, abdomen, legs, and arms. The cause of the syndrome is unknown, but an autoimmune pathogenesis is suspected. Only symptomatic therapy is available, and central spasmolytic drugs (benzodiazepines and baclofen) consistently relieve the muscle stiffness.

A, C–F See correct answer explanation.

Learning objective: Identify a prominent advantage of vecuronium over tubocurarine.

31. **B** Vecuronium, a steroid-derivative muscle relaxant, is currently commonly used during surgery. Its main advantages over tubocurarine are negligible effects on histamine release and no action on nicotinic neuronal receptors of autonomic ganglia. Moreover, unlike tubocurarine, the drug is mainly eliminated by liver metabolism, which can allow its use in patients with kidney disease.

A The duration of action of vecuronium after a standard therapeutic dose is 20 to 35 minutes.

C, D These actions are absent with both vecuronium and tubocurarine.

E No skeletal muscle relaxants cause anterograde amnesia, as they do not cross the blood–brain barrier.

Learning objective: Explain why cisatracurium is preferred over tubocurarine in patients with renal insufficiency

32. **D** The patient's creatinine and urea nitrogen levels indicate that he was most likely suffering from renal insufficiency. Tubocurarine is mainly eliminated as such by the kidney and is therefore contraindicated in patients with impaired renal function. Cisatracurium is a neuromuscular blocking drug that is inactivated primarily by a form of spontaneous breakdown and does not exhibit an increase in half-life in patients with renal insufficiency.

A The increased alanine aminotransferase levels are too small to suggest hepatic insufficiency.

B Even if cisatracurium could be safer than tubocurarine in elderly patients, this is not the primary reason for the use of cisatracurium in this patient.

C, E There are no adverse interactions between propofol or diazepam and tubocurarine.

SKELETAL MUSCLE RELAXANTS (Answer key)		
1. A	6. B	11. A
2. D	7. A	12. D
3. H	8. D	13. D
4. F	9. B	14. E
5. C	10. C	15. A
16. D	21. E	26. C
17. A	22. D	27. D
18. D	23. B	28. D
19. A	24. E	29. A
20. B	25. D	30. B
		31. B
		32. D

Answers and Explanations: III-6 Antiseizure Drugs

Questions 1–3

1. **K**
2. **G**
3. **I**

Learning objective: Identify the two neurotransmitters most likely involved in the pathogenesis of epilepsy.

4. **E** Epilepsy is a chronic recurrent disorder of cerebral function that may be characterized by repeated seizures. The essence of epilepsy is probably a chronic low seizure threshold that can be due to several mechanisms. A leading theory postulates that the cause of seizures is either the attenuation of pre- and/or postsynaptic inhibition (mainly due to a genetic or pathology-induced hypofunction of GABA neurons) or an increased effectiveness of excitatory synapses (mainly due to a genetic or pathology-induced hyperfunction of glutamate neurons).

A–D, F See correct answer explanation.

Learning objective: Explain the mechanism of action of phenytoin on ion channels.

5. **B** Phenytoin primarily blocks inactivated voltage-gated Na^+ channels. This blockade is frequency-dependent (also called use-dependent). That is, channels that open and close at high frequency are more susceptible to block than channels that open and close at low frequency. This can explain why phenytoin can readily suppress the discharge from an epileptic focus (where the neurons are discharging at high frequency) with negligible effects on normal-firing neurons.

A Na^+ channels that are in a resting state are not significantly affected by antiseizure drugs.

C See correct answer explanation.

D–F Phenytoin has negligible effects on K^+ channels at therapeutic concentrations.

Learning objective: Describe the effect of carbamazepine on the P-450 system.

6. **B** Carbamazepine is a potent enzyme inducer and can induce its own metabolism; this appears to be mediated via its effects on the hepatic CYP3A4 isoenzyme. Onset of enzyme induction is at about 3 days, with maximum effect at about 30 days.

    A, C Valproic acid and lamotrigine are used to treat simple partial seizures but are not inducers of the P-450 system.

    D, E Ethosuximide and clonazepam are not inducers of the P-450 system and are not used to treat simple partial seizures.

Learning objective: Describe the drug interaction between valproic acid and lamotrigine.

7. **E** Valproic acid can inhibit CYP2C9 and glucuronosyltransferase, thus decreasing the biotransformation of many drugs, including lamotrigine, carbamazepine, phenytoin, topiramate, and felbamate.

    A, B Phenytoin and phenobarbital actually can induce P-450 enzymes, thus increasing, not decreasing, the biotransformation of many drugs.

    C, D, F Levetiracetam, clonazepam, and gabapentin do not cause relevant drug–drug interactions.

Learning objective: Describe the adverse effects of phenytoin.

8. **G** The signs of the patient are classical adverse effects of phenytoin. Hirsutism and gingival hyperplasia occur to some degree in most patients. Blurred vision, diplopia, and broadening of the lips and nose are associated in some patients with long-term use of the drug.

    A–F These drugs do not cause the array of adverse effects exhibited by the patient.

Learning objective: Describe the interaction between carbamazepine and oral contraceptives.

9. **F** There have been several reports of reduced efficacy of oral contraceptives in patients receiving various antiseizure drugs. Carbamazepine, phenytoin, phenobarbital, and felbamate have been shown to increase the metabolism of ethinyl estradiol and progestins by inducing microsomal enzymes. This effect is not associated with other anticonvulsant drugs, including lamotrigine, valproic acid, clonazepam, gabapentin, and levetiracetam.

    A–E See correct answer explanation.

Learning objective: Explain the mechanism of action of valproic acid.

10. **A** The mechanisms of action of valproic acid have not been fully established, but they are most likely multiple, including

    - State-dependent blockade of inactivated Na$^+$ channels
    - Blockade of NMDA receptor–mediated excitation
    - Blockade of T-type Ca^{2+} channels in thalamic neurons
    - Increased GABA content in the brain (mechanism is uncertain)
    - Opening K$^+$ channels (at high doses)

    B–F None of these drugs have all of the mechanisms mentioned in the question.

Learning objective: Explain the mechanism of action of ethosuximide.

11. **B** Ethosuximide is a first-line agent for absence seizures. It most likely acts by blocking voltage-gated T-type Ca^{2+} channels in thalamic neurons. These channels are located on the dendrites of relay thalamic neurons, which connect the thalamus to the cortex. When these channels are activated (during sleep or, for unknown reasons, during an absence seizure), the neurons provide an oscillatory firing rate to the cortex, which has a characteristic 3-Hz spike and wave readout on an electroencephalogram. Excitatory input from the cortex in turn activates the thalamic neurons, thus reinitiating the cycle. Therefore, the absence seizure is generated by a self-sustained cycle of activity between the thalamus and the cortex. Drugs such as ethosuximide and valproic acid, which are able to block voltage-sensitive T-type Ca^{2+} channels in the thalamus, are effective in absence seizures.

    A, C–F Therapeutic doses of ethosuximide do not have these actions.

Learning objective: Outline the therapeutic use of valproic acid.

12. **D** The patient was most likely suffering from myoclonic seizures, a type of epilepsy that occurs mainly during childhood. Valproic acid is a first-line agent for myoclonic seizures and can control the symptoms in most cases. Levetiracetam, clonazepam, lamotrigine, ethosuximide, and topiramate also can be effective.

    A–C Phenytoin, carbamazepine, and phenobarbital can actually worsen myoclonic seizures.

    E, F Gabapentin and acetazolamide are not effective in myoclonic seizures.

Learning objective: Outline the therapeutic uses of phenobarbital.

13. **D** Provision of a patent airway and adequate oxygenation are the initial steps in management of status epilepticus. Emergency drugs include benzodiazepines for seizure control. The control may be short-lived, however, requiring intravenous (IV) phenytoin infusion. If refractory status epilepticus continues after initial treatment, additional IV phenobarbital or thiopental may be given, placing the patient in barbiturate coma.

    A–C, E, F These drugs are not used to treat status epilepticus.

Learning objective: Describe the adverse effects of lamotrigine.

14. **F** Lamotrigine causes a generalized erythematous skin rash in about 85% of patients taking the drug. Several antiseizure drugs can cause skin hypersensitivity reactions, but lamotrigine is by far the drug most frequently involved. The rash is usually mild, but severely affected patients may develop Stevens–Johnson syndrome. The incidence of skin rash is higher in children, and some studies suggest that a potentially life-threatening dermatitis can develop in 1 to 2% of pediatric patients.

A–E The risk of these adverse reactions is negligible.

Learning objective: Describe a mechanism of action common to several antiepileptic drugs.

15. **E** A partial seizure results from synchronous, rapid, uncontrolled firing from a group of neurons and a loss of surrounding cell inhibition. Antiseizure drugs act to enhance central nervous system (CNS) inhibition (i.e., by increasing GABAergic activity or by decreasing glutamatergic activity) and prevent the spread of synchronous activity (i.e., by blocking inactivated Na^+ channels, thus increasing the refractory period of nerve fibers). Several antiseizure drugs effective against partial seizures act by blocking inactivated Na^+ channels.

A Antiseizure drugs do not affect neuromuscular transmission.

B–D All of these actions would decrease, not increase, the inhibitory activity of the CNS cells surrounding the rapidly firing neurons.

Learning objective: Describe the main features of the pharmacokinetic of phenytoin.

16. **C** Phenytoin is one of the very few drugs that exhibit first-order elimination kinetics at low doses but switch to zero-order elimination kinetics at higher doses; that is, the elimination kinetics of the drug is dose-dependent. Important consequences of dose-dependent kinetics are

- The clearance and the half-life of the drug are dose-dependent.
- The time taken to reach steady state is also dose-dependent and therefore cannot be predicted.
- A slight increase in dose can have a big effect on plasma levels, leading to toxicity.

A, B, D–F All of these drugs follow first-order elimination kinetics.

Learning objective: Explain the main molecular mechanism of action of carbamazepine.

17. **D** Like phenytoin, carbamazepine causes a voltage- and frequency-dependent blockade of inactivated Na^+ channels.

This is most likely the primary mechanism of action of the drug.

A–C, E, F Carbamazepine interactions with all of these molecular targets have been proposed, but their role in the final therapeutic effect of the drug is still uncertain.

Learning objective: Describe the adverse effects of carbamazepine.

18. **C** Some of the adverse effects of carbamazepine are related to cerebellar-vestibular impairment. The most common dose-related adverse effect of this kind is ataxia (up to 15% of patients).

A This would be an adverse effect of phenytoin. It does not occur with carbamazepine.

B, D–F All these are serious but quite rare adverse effects of carbamazepine.

Learning objective: Outline the antiseizure uses of diazepam.

19. **C** The history of the patient and the lack of neurologic and laboratory findings indicate that he was most likely affected by febrile seizures, which are the most common type of seizures observed in the pediatric population. Anticonvulsant therapy is usually not required if a patient has recovered from an isolated seizure, but a preventive treatment can be appropriate if the patient experiences repeated fever-related seizures, as in this case. Diazepam, given rectally as soon as a febrile illness appears and maintained until the patient is afebrile for 24 hours, can decrease the number of febrile seizures and is considered the agent of choice.

A, B, D–F These drugs are not appropriate for pediatric febrile seizures.

Learning objective: Outline the therapeutic uses of lamotrigine.

20. **F** Lamotrigine is effective in simple partial seizures, as well as in generalized tonic-clonic and absence seizures. It appears to have comparable effectiveness with more traditional anticonvulsant drugs, such as valproic acid, carbamazepine, and phenytoin. The primary mechanism of action of lamotrigine most likely includes a frequency-dependent blockade of voltage-gated Na^+ channels.

C–E Valproic acid, carbamazepine, and phenytoin are first-choice drugs in partial seizures, but they are contraindicated when there is a risk of acute intermittent porphyria, because they can trigger an attack. Because acute intermittent porphyria is an autosomal disorder, it is better to avoid these drugs in patients whose parents are known to suffer from the disease, as in this case.

A, B Diazepam and ethosuximide are not effective in simple partial seizures.

Learning objective: Outline the therapeutic uses of levetiracetam.

21. **A** Levetiracetam is an antiseizure drug approved for partial, tonic-clonic, and myoclonic seizures. The drug appears to be well tolerated and has no significant drug interactions. Several antiseizure drugs are effective in partial seizures. However, in this patient, other drugs are relatively contraindicated (see answer explanations below).

B Phenytoin can decrease insulin secretion.

C Because carbamazepine is a strong inducer of CYP3A4, it could increase the metabolism of several drugs the patient was taking.

D The risk of valproic acid hepatitis is increased in patients with liver disease.

E Topiramate can cause glaucoma.

F Zonisamide can cause kidney stones.

Learning objective: Outline the therapeutic uses of topiramate.

22. **B** Lennox–Gastaut syndrome is a devastating pediatric epilepsy syndrome (onset 1 to 14 years) characterized by multiple types of seizures. Topiramate is a drug with a broad spectrum of action that includes almost all types of epileptic seizures. Recently, it was approved by the U.S. Food and Drug Administration for Lennox–Gastaut syndrome.

A, C–G None of these drugs have a broad spectrum of antiepileptic activity.

Learning objective: Outline the therapeutic uses of gabapentin.

23. **B** Gabapentin is a second-generation antiseizure drug that is used for patients with partial seizures who have failed the initial treatment, as in this case. In general, if the initial drug does not control seizures, a trial with another agent should be attempted before considering a multidrug regimen.

A, C, D Ethosuximide, diazepam, and acetazolamide are not effective in partial seizures.

E, F Carbamazepine and phenytoin are effective in partial seizures. but they are contraindicated in this patient because of atrioventricular block.

Learning objective: Outline the therapeutic uses of ethosuximide.

24. **D** Valproic acid is classified by the U.S. Food and Drug Administration as pregnancy category D because it increases the risk of neural tube defects (up to 20-fold) when given during pregnancy. Ethosuximide is instead classified as pregnancy category C and is a first-line drug for absence seizures.

A–C, E, F These drugs are not effective (and some of them can even be dangerous) in absence seizures.

Learning objective: Outline the therapeutic use of valproic acid.

25. **E** Anticonvulsant medications have emerged as an important therapeutic option for the prevention of migraine headache. Valproic acid is considered a first-line agent, as its efficacy has been demonstrated in several placebo-controlled studies.

Topiramate also has been approved recently for migraine prevention.

A, B Atenolol and verapamil are used for migraine prophylaxis but are contraindicated in this patient because of atrioventricular block.

C Amitriptyline is effective for prevention of both migraine and tension-type headache but is contraindicated in this patient because of glaucoma.

D, F Lamotrigine and felbamate are not effective for migraine prophylaxis.

Learning objective: Describe the adverse effects of phenytoin.

26. **D** The signs and symptoms of the patient indicated that he was most likely suffering from peripheral neuropathy and lymphadenopathy, which are adverse effects of long-term use of phenytoin. Megaloblastic anemia is also an adverse effect of phenytoin because the drug inhibits the enzyme conjugase, located in the brush border of the intestinal mucosa. This enzyme hydrolyzes the glutamate residues of ingested polyglutamates, thus allowing the absorption of monoglutamates. Patients taking chronic high doses of phenytoin can show megaloblastic anemia, lymphoid hyperplasia, and paresthesias. Knee and ankle tendon reflexes are absent in about 18% of these patients, as in this case.

A–C, E, F None of these drugs show the combination of adverse effects exhibited by the patient.

Learning objective: Describe the main features of the pharmacokinetics of phenytoin.

27. **D** Phenytoin elimination is dose-dependent. At very low blood levels, phenytoin metabolism follows a first-order kinetics, but as blood level rises within the therapeutic range, the maximum capacity of the liver to metabolize phenytoin is approached. This means that the elimination of phenytoin is dose-dependent, so the clearance of the drug is dose-dependent. In this situation, even a small increase in dosage may produce a very large increase in phenytoin concentration, thus leading to toxic effects, as in this case.

A The symptoms reported by the patient are not symptoms of a hypersensitivity reaction.

B This would have caused an increased elimination of the drug, making toxicity unlikely.

C The volume of distribution of a drug is not related to drug elimination.

E The level of the steady state, not the time to reach the steady state, is directly related to the toxicity of the drug. Moreover, when a drug follows dose-dependent kinetics, the half-life of the drug is dose-dependent; therefore, the time to reach steady state will be dose-dependent. In fact, with low doses, the steady state of phenytoin is reached in about 4 days. With high doses it may be 4 to 6 weeks before bloods levels are stable.

Learning objective: Outline the therapeutic use of valproic acid.

28. **E** The patient's symptoms indicate that she had a tonic-clonic seizure concomitant with her absence seizure. Because ethosuximide is not active against mixed seizure disorders, the best strategy is to substitute ethosuximide with another drug, such as valproic acid, that is active on both types of seizures.

    A–D See correct answer explanation.

Learning objective: Outline the therapy of infantile spasms.

29. **E** The boy most likely suffered from infantile spasms (also called West syndrome or salaam seizure). They are primarily generalized seizures characterized by sudden flexion of the arm, forward flexion of the trunk, and extension of the legs. Seizures last a few seconds and are repeated many times a day. They occur primarily in the first 3 years of life and are then replaced by other types of seizures. Mental retardation is usually apparent. Most patients have structural brain anomalies on neuroimaging studies, as in this case. Drugs of choice for infantile spasms are adrenocorticotropic hormone (ACTH) and corticosteroids (prednisone, dexamethasone, etc.). ACTH seems more effective, but this subject remains controversial. Alternative drugs include benzodiazepines (clonazepam), valproic acid, and vigabatrin. The therapy of infantile spasms is able to reduce the number of attacks in 40 to 50% of patients, but it rarely reduces the progression of mental retardation.

    A–D These drugs are not effective in infantile spasms.

Learning objective: Outline the therapeutic uses of carbamazepine.

30. **E** The patient's symptoms suggest that he is affected by trigeminal neuralgia, a neuropathy that usually affects only adults, especially the elderly. Carbamazepine is a drug of choice in this disease, and the benefit is often sustained. If the drug is ineffective or produces toxic reactions, other options are phenytoin, baclofen, and amitriptyline.

    A, B These anticonvulsants are not effective against trigeminal neuralgia.

    C, D Trigeminal neuralgia is a form of neuropathic pain. This type of pain is usually resistant to opioids and analgesic-antipyretic drugs.

Learning objective: Describe the anticonvulsant effect of carbonic anhydrase inhibitors.

31. **D** The patient most likely received acetazolamide, the prototype drug of carbonic anhydrase inhibitors. These drugs are rarely used today, but they can be employed, primarily as an add-on therapy, in patients with absence seizures and myoclonic seizures refractory to the main treatment. The mechanism of anticonvulsant activity of carbonic anhydrase inhibitors is not fully understood, but it may depend on a direct inhibition of carbonic anhydrase in the central nervous system. Carbonic anhydrase is a ubiquitous enzyme that catalyzes the first part of the reaction that converts carbon dioxide (CO_2) and water into carbonic acid. By inhibiting this reaction, carbon dioxide tension is increased; the gas can diffuse freely across neuronal cell membranes, inhibiting neuronal transmission.

    A–C, E, F These drugs do not affect the intracellular concentration of CO_2.

Learning objective: Describe the most likely mechanism of action of felbamate.

32. **E** Felbamate is an anticonvulsant drug approved by the U.S. Food and Drug Administration for partial seizures and Lennox–Gastaut syndrome. The drug can cause aplastic anemia and severe hepatitis at unexpectedly high rates and is therefore used only as a third-line drug for refractory cases. Nevertheless, the drug is frequently used in Lennox–Gastaut syndrome, as this type of epilepsy is often resistant to several antiepileptic drugs. The mechanism of anticonvulsant action of felbamate most likely involves the ionotropic NMDA receptors present in the central nervous system. Seizures can be initiated and propagated by stimulation of the NMDA receptors, which results in the opening of an ion channel that is nonselective to cations. Felbamate produces a use-dependent block of NMDA receptors, thereby increasing the seizure threshold and preventing the spread of seizures.

    A Felbamate potentiates, not blocks, $GABA_A$ receptor responses.

    B–D, F Felbamate does not act on these receptors.

Learning objective: Outline the therapeutic uses of fosphenytoin.

33. **D** The patient was most likely suffering from convulsive status epilepticus, a life-threatening neurologic disorder characterized by a prolonged tonic-clonic seizure or by recurrent tonic-clonic seizures without complete recovery of consciousness between attacks, as in this case. The first-line agents for the initial treatment of convulsive status epilepticus are lorazepam and diazepam. Other antiseizure drugs that can be employed for the initial treatment are fosphenytoin (a more soluble prodrug of phenytoin) and phenobarbital. The peak effect of fosphenytoin is usually delayed, so this drug is used only after the initial treatment with diazepam or lorazepam. Phenobarbital may be used in patients who cannot tolerate fosphenytoin or when fosphenytoin is not effective.

    A–C, E, F These drugs are not effective in status epilepticus.

Learning objective: Describe the most likely mechanism of action of zonisamide.

34. **D** The patient was most likely suffering from an allergic reaction to lamotrigine, a drug that frequently can cause an erythematous skin rash. When an antiepileptic drug is effective but causes an intolerable hypersensitivity reaction, it is convenient to substitute the offending drug with another agent

with a different chemical structure but with a similar mechanism of action. Zonisamide, like lamotrigine, blocks both Na^+ channels and Ca^{2+} channels and can be used appropriately in this case. Other antiepileptic drugs whose mechanisms of action most likely include blockade of both Na^+ channels and Ca^{2+} channels are topiramate and valproic acid.

A–C, E, F None of these drugs can block both Na^+ channels and Ca^{2+} channels.

Learning objective: Describe the adverse effects of valproic acid.

35. **B** The signs and symptoms of the patient indicate that she was most likely suffering from acute hepatitis, which is the most serious adverse effect of valproic acid therapy. The disease is rare when valproic acid is given alone, but its occurrence is about 1/6000 when the drug is given with other antiseizure drugs, as in this case. Hepatitis is always serious, often lethal, and can have a fulminant course. The pathologic lesion consists of a microvesicular steatosis without any sign of inflammation. The cause of the disease is unknown but is most likely idiosyncratic.

A, C–F Hepatic dysfunction is unusual with all of these drugs.

Learning objective: Describe the antiseizure use of clonazepam.

36. **F** Myoclonic seizures consist of short episodes of bilateral jerks of a limb, several limbs, or the trunk. Consciousness is not lost (unless a generalized seizure occurs). Myoclonic seizures usually occur during childhood or adolescence (in this case, they are called juvenile myoclonic epilepsy, and they are usually followed by generalized tonic-clonic seizures). Treatment options include valproic acid, clonazepam, and several second-generation drugs (lamotrigine, levetiracetam, topiramate, and zonisamide).

A–E These drugs are not effective (and some of them can be dangerous) in myoclonic seizures.

Learning objective: Explain the mechanism of action of perampanel.

37. **D** Perampanel is the prototype of a new class of antiseizure drugs that act as noncompetitive antagonists of AMPA receptors on brain neurons. These are ionotropic transmembrane receptors that are part of a ligand-gated ion channel, which is permeable mainly to Na^+ and K^+. AMPA receptors mediate fast, excitatory neurotransmission and have a critical role in seizure development and spreading. By blocking these receptors, perampanel can reduce neuronal excitability. The drug has been approved for adjunct treatment of simple partial seizures and is mainly used in poorly controlled partial seizures, as in this case.

A–C, E, F These drugs have no effect on AMPA receptors.

Learning objective: Explain the mechanism of action of lamotrigine.

38. **B** Lamotrigine is a second-generation antiepileptic drug that likely acts with multiple mechanisms, including blockade of voltage-gated Na^+ channels, blockade of voltage-gated Ca^{2+} channels (mainly of L, N, and P types), and inhibition of glutamate release. The drug is commonly added to valproic acid therapy in patients resistant to valproic acid alone, as it has been shown that this is the only combination that can consistently increase the efficacy of the therapy.

A, C–F See correct answer explanation.

Learning objective: Describe the therapeutic use of valproic acid.

39. **C** All current antiepileptic drugs, with the exception of ethosuximide, can be used in the treatment of complex partial seizures. However, in this patient carbamazepine, phenytoin, and zonisamide are contraindicated (see explanations below).

A, B Carbamazepine and phenytoin are contraindicated in case of atrioventricular block because the drug-induced blockade of inactivated Na^+ channels can slow down the heart conduction, exacerbating the disease.

D See correct answer explanation.

E Zonisamide is approved for adjunctive treatment of partial seizures. However, it can cause nephrolithiasis in about 2.5% of patients and is therefore contraindicated in this case.

Learning objective: Explain the mechanism of action of ezogabine.

40. **E** Ezogabine (the drug is called retigabine outside the United States) is the prototype of a new class of antiseizure drugs that act by opening a certain family of K^+ channels on brain neurons. This action hyperpolarizes the neuronal cell membrane, making the neuron less excitable. This mechanism of action is unique among antiepileptic drugs and may hold promise for the treatment of other neurologic conditions, including migraine and neuropathic pain.

A–D, F These drugs have no effect on K^+ channels.

ANTISEIZURE DRUGS Answer key			
1. K	6. B	11. B	16. C
2. G	7. E	12. D	17. D
3. I	8. G	13. D	18. C
4. E	9. F	14. F	19. C
5. B	10. A	15. E	20. F
21. A	26. D	31. D	36. F
22. B	27. D	32. E	37. D
23. B	28. E	33. D	38. B
24. D	29. E	34. D	39. C
25. E	30. E	35. B	40. E

Answers and Explanations: III-7 Drugs for Degenerative Disorders of the Central Nervous System

Questions 1–5

1. **B**
2. **E**
3. **H**
4. **I**
5. **F**

Learning objective: Explain the mechanism of action of levodopa in Parkinson disease.

6. **C** Dopamine cannot cross the blood–brain barrier and therefore has no therapeutic effects in parkinsonism if given into the peripheral circulation. However, levodopa, the immediate precursor of dopamine, is readily carried across the blood–brain barrier by the neutral amino acid transporter. In the brain, levodopa is biotransformed into dopamine within the presynaptic terminals of dopaminergic neurons in the striatum. These neurons are therefore able to release more dopamine, and this balances the loss of dopaminergic neurons, which constitutes the pathologic basis of Parkinson disease.

   A Dopaminergic receptors are upregulated, not downregulated, due to the decreased availability of dopamine in the striatum.

   B Subthalamic neurons are mainly glutamatergic, not dopaminergic.

   D This action would decrease, not increase, the availability of dopamine in basal ganglia.

   E The inhibition of catechol-O-methyltransferase (COMT) would increase the availability of dopamine, but this is an action of COMT inhibitors, not of levodopa.

Learning objective: Describe the treatment of parkinsonian tremor resistant to dopaminergic therapy.

7. **D** Parkinsonian tremor is often less responsive to dopaminergic therapy than other symptoms. Tremor can be worsened by peripheral factors, such as catecholamine release, often in association with stress or anxiety. Propranolol improves parkinsonian tremor in about 50% of patients, so a trial with propranolol can be appropriate for this patient.

   A, B, E All of these procedures would minimally affect the patient's tremor.

   C Anticholinergic drugs can improve tremor but they are usually better avoided in the elderly because of an increased risk of adverse effects.

Learning objective: Describe the adverse effects of levodopa.

8. **B** The adverse effects reported by the patient and the timing of the effects suggest that they are levodopa-induced dyskinesias, which occur in up to 80% of patients receiving the drug for long periods. The development of dyskinesias is dose-related, and dyskinesias are usually associated with peak striatal dopamine levels or when the level of the drug is rising or falling. The exact mechanism of these dyskinesias is not known, but simplistically it can be thought of as too much movement caused by too much striatal dopamine receptor stimulation.

   A, C–E Some of these drugs (selegiline and entacapone) can cause dyskinesias, but they are never used as the sole agent to treat Parkinson disease for long periods.

Learning objective: Describe the main drug interactions with levodopa.

9. **E** The symptoms reported by the patient point out a worsening of his Parkinson disease. Metoclopramide, a prokinetic drug used to treat diabetic gastroparesis, can block dopamine D_2 receptors in the brain, thus leading to a decreased levodopa effect that explains the worsening of parkinsonian symptoms.

   A–D See correct answer explanation.

Learning objective: Describe the clinical use of benztropine in Parkinson disease.

10. **C** Autonomic dysfunction is a prominent feature of Parkinson disease, and postural hypotension, urinary urgency, and sialorrhea are common symptoms. Sialorrhea occurs in up to 55% of patients and responds to anticholinergic drugs such as benztropine.

   A, B, D, E These antiparkinson drugs have minimal effects on sialorrhea.

Learning objective: Explain the mechanism of action of pramipexole.

11. **A** The symptoms of the patient indicate that she was most likely suffering from Parkinson disease. Dopaminergic agonists such as pramipexole are often first-line agents in antiparkinson therapy, especially in younger patients, as their use seems associated with a lower incidence of response fluctuations and dyskinesias that can occur with long-term levodopa therapy.

   B–F These drugs are not dopaminergic agonists.

Learning objective: Describe the adverse effects of bromocriptine.

12. **A** Bromocriptine is an ergot-derived dopamine agonist. Ergot-derived drugs may cause connective tissue proliferation leading to fibrosis in different organs, including pulmonary, pleural, and retroperitoneal fibrosis. The exact mechanism of this adverse effect is still unknown, but bromocriptine is no longer used in Parkinson disease due to this effect.

B–F These drugs do not cause pulmonary fibrosis.

Learning objective: Outline the therapeutic use of pramipexole.

13. **D** The patient presented with signs and symptoms typical of Parkinson disease (PD). The four classic features of PD, that is, tremor, rigidity (tightness in his arms and legs), bradykinesia (lack of normal changes in facial expression), and postural instability (festinating gait), are easily recognized. Pramipexole is a dopamine receptor agonist that is effective when used as monotherapy for mild parkinsonism. Dopaminergic agonist therapy of parkinsonism can be initiated with a dopamine agonist, especially in younger patients, as these drugs have a number of potential advantages over levodopa, including a lower incidence of response fluctuations and dyskinesias.

A–C Currently, carbidopa, entacapone, and benztropine are not used as monotherapy, but only in addition to levodopa therapy.

E, F Clonazepam and propranolol are only used adjunctively to control symptoms such as tremor (propranolol) and myoclonus (clonazepam) that, in a particular patient, are resistant to conventional therapy.

Learning objective: Explain the mechanism of action of selegiline.

14. **C** Two isoenzymes of monoamine oxidase (MAO) metabolize monoamines. MAO-A metabolizes primarily norepinephrine and serotonin, MAO-B metabolizes primarily dopamine and is predominant in the striatum. Selegiline is a selective inhibitor of MAO-B, leading to irreversible inhibition of the enzyme, thus retarding the breakdown of dopamine in the striatum. Because MAO-B is primarily found in the brain, selegiline does not inhibit the peripheral metabolism of dopamine and can be safely taken with levodopa.

A, B, E See correct answer explanation.

D Because phenelzine is a nonselective inhibitor of MAO, it can reduce the metabolism of dopamine. However, it is not used in Parkinson disease because it can lead to hypertensive crises probably due to the peripheral accumulation of norepinephrine.

Learning objective: Explain the mechanism of antiparkinson action of benztropine.

15. **B** In Parkinson disease, the loss of dopaminergic neurons results in a loss of the balance that normally exists between acetylcholine- and dopamine-mediated neurotransmission. Antimuscarinic drugs such as benztropine seem to act by blocking muscarinic receptors in the striatum, thus decreasing the abnormally high cholinergic tone, which results from lack of the inhibitory activity of dopamine. These drugs may improve tremor and rigidity but have little effect on bradykinesia.

A, C–E Antimuscarinic drugs do not have these effects.

Learning objective: Describe the adverse effects of benztropine.

16. **E** The symptoms of the patient are typical adverse effects of antimuscarinic drugs, such as benztropine. These drugs had been used extensively in the past before the discovery of levodopa. Because of their undesirable adverse effect profile and poor efficacy, today they are usually reserved for the treatment of persisting resting tremor, particularly in younger patients, as in this case.

A–D, F None of these drugs cause the set of symptoms reported by the patient.

Learning objective: Outline the pharmacotherapy of restless leg syndrome.

17. **C** Restless leg syndrome is characterized by abnormal motion and sometimes sensations in the legs that interfere with sleep. The disorder can occur in isolation but is more common during pregnancy, chronic renal or liver failure, iron deficiency anemia, or diabetes, as in this case. The cause of the disorder is unclear but may involve abnormalities in dopamine neurotransmission in the central nervous system. Numerous drugs have been used to treat the disorder, but only dopaminergic therapy is specific and is the preferred treatment for restless leg syndrome. Dopamine agonists such as pramipexole have replaced levodopa as a first-line therapy.

A, B, D–F These drugs are not effective in restless leg syndrome.

Learning objective: Explain the mechanism of action of carbidopa in Parkinson disease.

18. **D** Carbidopa is a dopa decarboxylase inhibitor that cannot cross the blood–brain barrier. When levodopa is given in combination with carbidopa, the peripheral metabolism of levodopa is reduced, plasma levels of levodopa are higher, and more levodopa is available to enter the brain. Concomitant administration of levodopa and carbidopa may reduce the daily requirement for levodopa by about 75%.

A–C, E Carbidopa does not cause these actions.

Learning objective: Describe the treatment for levodopa-induced hallucinations.

19. **E** The patient's symptoms are typical mental disturbances caused by levodopa and are more common in patients taking the drug in combination with carbidopa, presumably because higher levels are reached in the brain. Psychotic symptoms including hallucinations often respond to neuroleptic treatment, but classical neuroleptics are not indicated because they may cause marked worsening of parkinsonism, likely through the blockade of D_2 receptors in the striatum. Atypical neuroleptics such as clozapine have negligible blocking activity at D_2 receptors, do not worsen parkinsonism, and are effective in the treatment of levodopa-induced psychotic symptoms.

    A Selegiline has only a minor therapeutic effect on parkinsonism when given alone; therefore, the substitution of levodopa with selegiline most likely would cause a worsening of Parkinson disease.

    B Dopaminergic agonists such as pramipexole can cause mental disturbances very similar to those caused by levodopa, likely because both adverse effects have the same underlying mechanism.

    C, D Mental disturbances can be exacerbated, not alleviated, by concurrent anticholinergic or amantadine therapy.

Learning objective: Describe the adverse effects of levodopa.

20. **C** Postural hypotension is the most common cardiovascular adverse effect of levodopa, especially in the early stage of treatment. Levodopa is a prodrug, and all of its effects are due to dopamine. Postural hypotension is most likely due both to activation of D_1 receptors in the renal and mesenteric vascular bed, which leads to vasodilation, and to activation of D_1 receptors in the proximal tubule, which causes inhibition of tubular sodium reabsorption, thus increasing diuresis. Even if peripheral adverse effects are reduced when carbidopa is given together with levodopa, the risk of postural hypotension is significant, especially in older patients, as in this case.

    A Dopamine has negligible effects on accommodation, so blurred vision is unlikely.

    B Dopamine can activate α_1 adrenoceptors in the gastrointestinal system. Activation of these receptors in the gastrointestinal smooth muscle causes hyperpolarization and relaxation, so diarrhea is unlikely.

    D Dopamine can activate β adrenoceptors in the heart, causing tachycardia, not bradycardia.

    E Dopamine can cause dyskinesias, but bradykinesia is a classic symptom of parkinsonism, which is in fact alleviated, not caused, by levodopa.

Learning objective: Describe the reduction of the peripheral effects of levodopa by adding carbidopa to the treatment.

21. **B** Carbidopa is an inhibitor of dopa decarboxylase that cannot cross the blood–brain barrier. When given with levodopa, it diminishes the peripheral metabolism of levodopa, increasing its availability to enter the central nervous system. Therefore, the needed dose of levodopa can be lowered by about 5-fold, and the peripheral adverse effects of levodopa are consequently reduced.

    A, C–E These are central adverse effects of levodopa. They are not reduced and might even be increased, as more levodopa can enter the brain.

Learning objective: Describe the main contraindications of pramipexole.

22. **C** Dopaminergic drugs, such as pramipexole, levodopa, and amphetamines, etc., are contraindicated, or should be used with caution, in patients with a history of psychosis, as they consistently exacerbate the symptoms of schizophrenic disorders.

    A, B, D–F These drugs are not contraindicated in Parkinson patients with a history of psychosis.

Learning objective: Explain the mechanism of action of entacapone.

23. **B** Entacapone is a peripheral inhibitor of catechol-*O*-methyltransferase (COMT). Substrates of the enzyme are levodopa and catecholamines. In the presence of a decarboxylase inhibitor (e.g., carbidopa), COMT becomes the major metabolizing enzyme for levodopa, which is transformed into 3-*O*-methyldopa in the gut and the liver. By inhibiting the enzyme, entacapone causes the following actions:

    - More levodopa becomes available for active transport into the central nervous system (CNS).
    - Less 3-*O*-methyldopa can compete with levodopa for active transport into the CNS.

    A, C–E These drugs do not alter the amount of levodopa in the patient's brain.

Learning objective: Describe the main contraindications of benztropine.

24. **B** Anticholinergic drugs such as benztropine are sometimes used in Parkinson disease but are contraindicated in case of prostatic hypertrophy, because they decrease the contraction of the detrusor muscle, and in the case of chronic constipation, as they decrease intestinal peristalsis. In addition, they are relatively contraindicated in elderly individuals (see the patient's age) because the risk of their central adverse effects increases with age.

    A, C–F See correct answer explanation.

Learning objective: Describe the adverse effects of amantadine.

25. **D** Livedo reticularis can occur in up to 80% of patients taking amantadine and usually clears within 1 month after drug withdrawal. The disorder is believed to be caused by local release of catecholamines that can cause vasoconstriction.

A–C, E, F These drugs do not cause livedo reticularis.

Learning objective: Explain the mechanism of levodopa-induced cardiac arrhythmias.

26. **C** A variety of cardiac arrhythmias have been described in patients receiving levodopa. Like all levodopa-induced effects, they are due to dopamine that can activate cardiac β_1 and β_2 adrenoceptors. Concomitant administration of carbidopa reduces the likelihood of these effects, but arrhythmias are sometimes reported in patients receiving levodopa/carbidopa, as in this case.

A There are no dopamine receptors in the heart that modulate cardiac rhythm.

B, D, E Dopamine does not cause these actions.

Learning objective: Describe the adverse effects of donepezil.

27. **B** The drugs most frequently used in Alzheimer disease are cholinesterase inhibitors, such as donepezil and rivastigmine. Although these drugs preferentially inhibit acetylcholinesterase in the central nervous system, they can cause most of the adverse effects shared by all cholinergic drugs, which are due to the activation of cholinergic receptors. Effects affecting the gastrointestinal tract (nausea, vomiting, and diarrhea) occur in about 15% of patients taking the drug.

A, C–E These effects are usually caused by antimuscarinic, not cholinergic, drugs.

Learning objective: Outline the therapeutic uses of amantadine.

28. **D** Dyskinesias are frequent adverse effects of long-term therapy with levodopa or dopamine agonists. The effects are dose- and time-dependent; dyskinesias occur in most patients receiving levodopa therapy for long periods of time. Amantadine is useful for suppressing levodopa-induced dyskinesias, and its effect is thought to be due to blockade of *N*-methyl-D-aspartate (NMDA) receptors.

Dyskinesias caused by dopaminergic drugs are different from the movement disorders caused by Parkinson disease where tremor, bradykinesia, and akinesia are the prevalent symptoms. However, it is worth noting that even drugs that block dopamine receptors (i.e., neuroleptics) can cause dyskinesias. Because levodopa-induced dyskinesias may be triggered when the level of the drug is rising or falling, the mechanism of the effect may be related to an unequal distribution of striatal dopamine.

A–C, E These drugs would worsen, not decrease, dyskinesias.

Learning objective: Outline the pharmacotherapy of Alzheimer disease.

29. **C** The man was most likely in the early stages of Alzheimer disease (AD). He displayed several symptoms associated with dementia, including impaired reasoning (recognition deficits), loss of memory, confusion, and disorientation. A major approach to the treatment of AD has involved the attempt to augment the cholinergic function in the brain, because a loss of cholinergic neurons is a prominent feature of the disease. Donepezil, rivastigmine, and galantamine are cholinesterase inhibitors approved for treatment of AD.

A, B, D Sedative and neuroleptic drugs are usually contraindicated in dementias.

E Physostigmine is a cholinesterase inhibitor that can enter the brain but is not used in dementias because of its frequent and often serious adverse effects.

Learning objective: Outline the treatment of the on-off periods of Parkinson disease.

30. **D** The patient is most likely suffering from the on-off phenomenon, in which off periods of marked akinesia alternate over the course of a few hours with on periods of improved mobility and marked dyskinesia. These response fluctuations can be decreased by adjunctive drugs, including dopamine agonists such as pramipexole, catechol-*O*-methyltransferase (COMT) inhibitors such as entacapone, and, in some cases, selegiline.

A–C, E These drugs are not useful to improve response fluctuations.

Learning objective: Describe the adverse effects of pramipexole.

31. **C** Pramipexole is a dopamine D_2 receptor agonist often used as the starting therapy for Parkinson disease, mainly in patients younger than 60. All dopamine D_2 receptor agonists, as well as levodopa, can cause nausea and vomiting. When levodopa is given alone, nausea and vomiting occur in about 80% of cases. Levodopa plus carbidopa, or D_2 receptor agonists, cause nausea and vomiting in about 15 to 25% of cases. The effect is most likely mediated by the activation of D_2 receptors in the chemoreceptor trigger zone and nucleus of the tractus solitarius, two centers located in the brainstem that send signals to the vomiting center. Fortunately, tolerance to the nauseant effects develops in many patients.

A, B, D, E These drugs cause nausea in less than 5% of cases.

DRUGS FOR DEGENERATIVE DISORDERS OF THE CENTRAL NERVOUS SYSTEM Answer key		
1. B	6. C	11. A
2. E	7. D	12. A
3. H	8. B	13. D
4. I	9. E	14. C
5. F	10. C	15. B
16. E	21. B	26. C
17. C	22. C	27. B
18. D	23. B	28. D
19. E	24. B	29. C
20. C	25. D	30. D
		31. C

Answers and Explanations: III-8 Neuroleptic Drugs

Questions 1–3

1. **C**

2. **D**

3. **A**

Learning objective: Describe the site of action of neuroleptics-induced tardive dyskinesia.

4. **D** The many years of antipsychotic therapy and the signs and symptoms of the patient indicate that she was most likely suffering from tardive dyskinesia, an extrapyramidal syndrome caused by long-term neuroleptic treatment. The cause of the syndrome is unknown, but one of the most commonly accepted hypotheses relates the syndrome to a sensitization of dopamine receptors in the caudate–putamen.

  A–C, E, F All of these structures can be involved in the actions of neuroleptics, but the primary dysfunction underlying tardive dyskinesia occurs in the striatum.

Learning objective: Explain the mechanism of chlorpromazine-induced urinary retention.

5. **B** Prostatic hyperplasia is the most common cause of difficulty in urination in aged men. If a drug with antimuscarinic effects, such as chlorpromazine, is given to a man with prostatic hyperplasia, the medication can trigger complete urinary retention due to relaxation of the detrusor muscle of the bladder.

  A Chlorpromazine has no effect on the urine formation.

  C Actually, captopril can increase diuresis by inhibiting aldosterone production.

  D, E These prazosin-induced effects would have facilitated, not hindered, the voiding of the bladder.

Learning objective: Outline the efficacy of neuroleptics against positive symptoms of schizophrenia

6. **D** Positive symptoms of schizophrenia (delusions, hallucinations, disorganized speech, grossly disorganized behavior, etc.)

are usually better controlled by typical neuroleptic drugs than negative symptoms (alogia, avolition, affective flattening, social withdrawal, etc.). It seems that atypical neuroleptics can control negative symptoms better than typical ones.

  A–C, E All of these are negative symptoms of schizophrenia and are less well controlled by a typical neuroleptic like haloperidol.

Learning objective: Explain the mechanism of the autonomic adverse effects of clozapine.

7. **E** Some atypical neuroleptics such as clozapine have significant blocking activity on muscarinic receptors. The patient's symptoms are classic antimuscarinic effects due to clozapine. Blockade of cholinergic M_3 receptors in the salivary glands causes dry mouth, in the intestinal system causes a decrease in peristalsis, and in the ciliary muscles causes a loss of accommodation for near vision.

  A–D See correct answer explanation.

Learning objective: Describe the mental effects of neuroleptics in normally healthy individuals.

8. **C** In normally healthy people, neuroleptics do not cause euphoria, but rather a feeling of unpleasantness and discomfort, that is, dysphoria. Neuroleptic-induced dysphoria can explain, at least in part, why these drugs have no abuse liability. In addition to their antipsychotic effects, several neuroleptics have pronounced sedative properties (likely mediated by the blockade of H_1 and $5\text{-}HT_{2A}$ receptors), which account for the sleepiness induced by these drugs.

  A, B, D These effects would be caused by psychostimulant drugs, such as amphetamines.

  E Neuroleptics decrease delusions and perseverations that are classic psychotic symptoms.

Learning objective: Describe neuroleptic-induced acute dystonia.

9. **A** The patient's assaultive behavior and persecutory delusions suggest that he was most likely suffering from a schizophrenic disorder, for which he received a neuroleptic drug. The neurologic signs of the patient indicated that he suffered from acute dystonia, an extrapyramidal symptom that usually occurs after few days of high-dose neuroleptic therapy. Acute dystonias present with a sudden onset of brief abnormal postures, such as tongue protrusion, oculogyris crisis, torticollis, and unusual positions of the trunk and limbs. The extrapyramidal adverse effects of neuroleptics occur more often with high-potency drugs, such as haloperidol and fluphenazine.

B, D Sedative-hypnotic drugs, such as benzodiazepines and ethanol, have a negligible risk of acute dystonia.

C, E Antidepressants, such as fluoxetine, and anxiolytics, such as buspirone, are not used to sedate an aggressive patient and have a negligible risk of acute dystonia.

F Clozapine, a neuroleptic, has a much lower risk of extrapyramidal adverse effects compared to haloperidol and currently is not used to sedate an aggressive patient.

Learning objective: Describe the neuroleptic-induced impairment of the thermoregulatory function.

10. **B** The ability of the body to thermoregulate is dependent upon an intact hypothalamic thermoregulatory center. High doses of neuroleptics strongly diminish the thermoregulatory function of the hypothalamus. Moreover, clozapine can also interfere peripherally with sweating because of its antimuscarinic properties. The result is poikilothermia, in which the body cannot respond to heat or cold, and patients become hypothermic or hyperthermic, depending on the surrounding temperature. Therefore, in an environment of high temperature, neuroleptics can predispose to heat stroke, especially if the person is exercising, as in this case.

A, C–F None of the other listed drugs cause impairment of the hypothalamic thermoregulatory center at therapeutic doses.

Learning objective: Describe the main contraindication of neuroleptics.

11. **B** The symptoms of the patient indicate that she was most likely suffering from catatonia related to a psychiatric disorder. The use of traditional neuroleptics such as haloperidol is avoided in catatonia because of the possible development of neuroleptic malignant syndrome.

A, C–F All of these drugs have been used successfully in the treatment of catatonia.

Learning objective: Describe the uses of atypical neuroleptics in acute psychotic disorder.

12. **C** The behavior and the symptoms of the patient indicated that he was most likely affected by an acute psychotic disorder. Risperidone is an atypical neuroleptic with sedative properties. Neuroleptics with sedative properties are commonly used intravenously to sedate patients with acute psychosis and aggressive behavior. Atypical neuroleptics are sometimes preferred over older neuroleptics because of lower incidence of extrapyramidal adverse effects.

A, B, D–F These drugs are not used for the acute sedation of an aggressive patient.

Learning objective: Outline the therapeutic uses of clozapine in resistant schizophrenia.

13. **D** The poor response to several neuroleptic drugs and the prevalence of negative symptoms of schizophrenia indicate that the patient is a candidate for clozapine therapy. Clozapine is the only neuroleptic approved by the U.S. Food and Drug Administration for the treatment of resistant schizophrenia.

A, B Because the response to previous therapy was inadequate, it is not useful to try other neuroleptics with activity spectra similar to that of chlorpromazine (i.e., thioridazine) or haloperidol (i.e., fluphenazine).

C, E Fluoxetine and lithium are not effective in treating schizophrenia.

Learning objective: Outline the therapeutic uses of haloperidol in Huntington chorea.

14. **F** Huntington disease is a progressive neurodegenerative genetic disorder that affects muscle coordination and leads to cognitive decline and dementia. The disease seems to result from functional overactivity in dopaminergic nigrostriatal pathways, perhaps because of a deficiency of a neurotransmitter (likely gamma-aminobutyric acid [GABA]) that normally inhibits those pathways. The treatment of the disease is supportive. Choreic movements and agitation can be partially suppressed by neuroleptics such as haloperidol, probably because of their antidopaminergic activity.

A–D These drugs are ineffective in Huntington disease.

E Although the development of chorea seems related to an imbalance of GABA transmission in the basal ganglia (GABA is markedly reduced in basal ganglia of patients with Huntington disease), treatment to supplement GABA activity in the brain has been ineffective.

Learning objective: Outline the therapy of an acute psychotic state in a patient with concomitant tonic-clonic seizures.

15. **B** Neuroleptics are the preferred drugs for the control of acute psychotic patients who exhibit aggressive and violent behavior. Neuroleptics with significant sedative properties, such as chlorpromazine, are usually preferred. Neuroleptics lower the seizure threshold, so epileptic patients are at increased risk of seizures, as in this case. For these patients, a prophylactic treatment is appropriate. Because the patient had tonic-clonic seizures, an anticonvulsant drug effective against grand mal epilepsy (e.g., lamotrigine) is appropriate.

    A, C–F All of the antiseizure drugs in these drug pairs are minimally or not effective in generalized tonic-clonic seizures.

Learning objective: Describe the therapeutic uses of fluphenazine decanoate.

16. **C** The clinical scenario exemplifies a classic case of noncompliance, which is a problem in many diseases but is especially prominent in psychiatric disorders. The patient responded to neuroleptic therapy but relapsed because of noncompliance. Noncompliant psychotic patients are good candidates for depot drug preparations administered by IM injection every 1 to 2 weeks. Neuroleptic depot preparations are available for fluphenazine, haloperidol, and risperidone. Because fluphenazine was effective and well tolerated, there is no need to switch to another neuroleptic.

    A, B, D, E See correct answer explanation.

Learning objective: Outline treatment of acute psychosis in a suicidal patient.

17. **E** The symptoms of the patient indicated that he was most likely suffering from an acute psychotic disorder. Clozapine is not a drug of choice for first-episode patients, but it can be a first-line drug for a patient with a history of suicidality, comorbid substance abuse, and significant negative psychotic symptoms, as in this case.

    A–D, F See correct answer explanation.

Learning objective: Explain the mechanism of olanzapine-induced constipation.

18. **E** Neuroleptics can have significant antimuscarinic and antiserotonergic properties in both the central and autonomic nervous systems. Atypical neuroleptics such as olanzapine can cause a substantial blockade of muscarinic and serotonergic receptors in the gut, which would explain the constipation caused by this drug.

    A–D In all of these items, at least one of the mentioned receptors is minimally involved in gastrointestinal motility.

Learning objective: List the brain structure that most likely mediated the therapeutic effects of neuroleptics.

19. **C** Aripiprazole is an atypical (also called second-generation) neuroleptic drug. The fact that all neuroleptics block dopamine receptors supports the hypothesis that their antipsychotic effect might be mediated by decreased dopaminergic transmission in mesolimbic and mesocortical pathways, two pathways of the brain dopaminergic system involved in cognition, stimulus processing, and motivational behavior.

    A, D These two pathways are dopaminergic, but interference with these pathways seems more related to some of the adverse effects, not to the therapeutic effect of neuroleptics.

    B, E Dopaminergic transmission is scarcely represented in these structures.

Learning objective: Explain the mechanism of neuroleptic-induced hyperprolactinemia.

20. **D** The amenorrhea and galactorrhea are adverse effects of neuroleptics that are related to their blockade of D_2 receptors in the anterior pituitary gland. Dopamine acts as a prolactin-inhibiting factor by activating these receptors in the pituitary. When D_2 receptors are blocked, prolactin secretion increases. High plasma levels of prolactin can result in amenorrhea, galactorrhea, and anovulation in women, and azoospermia, impotence, and gynecomastia can develop in men. All typical neuroleptics can cause the above-mentioned symptoms, whereas atypical neuroleptics are minimally associated with hyperprolactinemia.

    A–C, E See correct answer explanation.

Learning objective: Describe neuroleptic-induced akathisia.

21. **D** Akathisia, or uncontrolled motor restlessness, is one of the dose-dependent extrapyramidal disorders that can be caused by neuroleptics. These disorders occur most frequently with butyrophenones and the piperazine side-chain phenothiazines such as fluphenazine. Akathisia is characterized by subjective feelings of restlessness and objective signs of pacing, rocking, and inability to sit or stand in one place for extended periods of time. The disorder develops within days to weeks after initiating a neuroleptic therapy.

    A, C, F These are other extrapyramidal disorders that can be caused by neuroleptics, but the symptoms are not those exhibited by the patient.

    B Rarely, neuroleptics can cause tonic-clonic seizures but not complex partial seizures.

    E Neuroleptics can relieve catatonic signs of schizophrenic patients.

Learning objective: Describe haloperidol-induced pseudo-parkinsonism.

22. **B** The signs and symptoms of the patient indicate that he was most likely suffering from neuroleptic-induced pseudoparkinsonism. The syndrome is caused by blockade of D_2 receptors in the caudate–putamen and is more likely with neuroleptics that have the highest affinity for D_2 receptors, such as fluphenazine and haloperidol.

    A, D, E These neuroleptics rarely cause pseudoparkinsonism.

    C Metoclopramide can block D_2 receptors but is not used to treat schizophrenia.

Learning objective: Outline the use of neuroleptics in case of delirium.

23. **B** The symptoms of the patient indicate that he was most likely suffering from delirium, a severe neuropsychiatric syndrome with core features of acute onset and fluctuating course, attentional deficits, and generalized severe disorganization of behavior. Neuroleptics are commonly used drugs for delirium, although they are not approved by the U.S. Food and Drug Administration for this syndrome. Those with low anticholinergic activity are more appropriate, especially for older patients. Neuroleptics can lessen agitation and psychotic symptoms, but they do not correct the underlying problem, and, though rarely, they may even exacerbate delirium.

    A Clozapine is not a good choice because of its relevant risk of agranulocytosis and its relevant anticholinergic properties.

    C Benzodiazepines can manage agitation but can worsen confusion and can cause delirium in older people. They are used mainly when delirium is caused by alcohol withdrawal.

    D–F These drugs are not effective for delirium.

Learning objective: Describe the neuroleptic malignant syndrome.

24. **C** The clinical picture is typical of neuroleptic malignant syndrome (NMS), a rare but potentially lethal complication that may present in a sudden, unpredictable fashion. The etiology of NMS is unknown, but a proposed mechanism suggests that a neuroleptic-induced, excessively rapid blockade of dopaminergic receptors in the diencephalon may play a role. It is uncertain whether NMS is a specific entity or a variant of malignant hyperthermia. This latter disorder is most commonly associated with administration of halogenated inhalational anesthetics and depolarizing muscle relaxants. It has a shorter duration (3–5 days) than NMS (5–30 days).

    A, B, E None of these drugs cause NMS or malignant hyperthermia.

D, F Although these drugs are not used to treat schizophrenia, if given in overdose or in combination with other serotonergic drugs, they could cause serotonin syndrome, which has signs and symptoms similar to those of NMS.

Learning objective: Describe the cardiac adverse effects of thioridazine.

25. **B** Because of her disease, the woman was most likely under neuroleptic therapy.

    Neuroleptics (mainly thioridazine and clozapine) can cause ECG changes, including prolongation of QT interval, which can lead to polymorphic ventricular tachycardia. The thioridazine effect on QT interval is dose-related and has led to a black box warning in the product labeling approved by the U.S. Food and Drug Administration.

    A, C, D Trazodone, amitriptyline, and paroxetine can increase the risk of polymorphic ventricular tachycardia under certain conditions, but they are not antipsychotic drugs and currently are not used in schizophrenia.

    E, F Lithium and lorazepam do not cause prolongation of the QT interval.

Learning objective: Describe the postural hypotension induced by atypical neuroleptics.

26. **B** The symptoms of the patient indicate that she was most likely suffering from postural hypotension. Atypical neuroleptics (with the exception of clozapine) have become first-line agents for the treatment of an acute psychotic episode, mainly because of few or no acutely occurring extrapyramidal side effects. Most atypical neuroleptics have significant blocking activity on α_1 receptors, so postural hypotension is a frequent adverse effect, as in this case.

    A Haloperidol is used to treat an acute psychotic episode, but postural hypotension is a rare adverse effect, as it has minimal blocking activity on α_1 receptors.

    C–F These drugs are devoid of antipsychotic properties.

Learning objective: Describe the sexual dysfunction caused by thioridazine.

27. **D** Thioridazine is recognized as the most common cause of neuroleptic-induced sexual dysfunction. Sexual adverse effects, however, have also been reported with other typical and atypical neuroleptics. The cause of neuroleptic-induced sexual dysfunction is related to a number of factors, including hyperprolactinemia (via dopamine blockade), α-adrenergic and muscarinic blockade, and sedative effects.

    A Because haloperidol caused symptoms of pseudoparkinsonism, the prescription of another neuroleptic with a high potential for extrapyramidal side effects is unlikely.

    B, C, E, F All of these drugs can cause sexual dysfunction, but they are devoid of antipsychotic properties and are not used to treat schizophrenia.

Learning objective: Describe the adverse effects of olanzapine.

28. **C** Olanzapine was most likely prescribed because it has significant sedative effects. The drug, however, also has significant muscarinic-blocking activity and therefore can cause urinary retention if given to a man with prostatic hyperplasia, as in this case.

    A, B These neuroleptics have minimal antimuscarinic activity.

    D–F These drugs have more or less pronounced antimuscarinic activity but are devoid of antipsychotic properties.

Learning objective: Describe neuroleptic-induced gynecomastia.

29. **C** The history and the symptoms of the patient indicate that he was most likely suffering from gynecomastia due to a neuroleptic with D_2 antagonist activity, such as haloperidol. By blocking D_2 receptors, neuroleptics prevent the inhibitory effect of dopamine on prolactin secretion, thus causing hyperprolactinemia. High prolactin plasma levels can in turn cause amenorrhea/galactorrhea in women and gynecomastia in men.

    A Clozapine has low blocking activity on D_2 receptors and therefore does not usually cause hyperprolactinemia.

    B, D–F These drugs are not used to treat paranoid schizophrenia.

Learning objective: Describe the hematological adverse effects of clozapine.

30. **A** The low white blood cell count and the low neutrophil percentage indicate that the man was most likely suffering from drug-induced agranulocytosis. Agranulocytosis is the most fatal adverse drug reaction, accounting for 26% of all drug-related deaths. Clozapine can cause agranulocytosis in about 0.8% of patients (a rate lower than the original estimate of 1 to 2%). The onset of the disorder is variable, as it can occur a few days after starting the treatment or even several years after a daily chronic treatment. However, the first 6 months of clozapine therapy is the period of greatest risk. Discontinuation of the drug usually results in correction of neutrophil count within 30 days.

    B, D Phenothiazines can cause agranulocytosis, but the risk is only 1/10 that of clozapine.

    C, E, F Agranulocytosis due to these drugs can occur, but it is exceptionally rare.

NEUROLEPTIC DRUGS Answer key		
1. C	6. D	11. B
2. D	7. E	12. C
3. A	8. C	13. D
4. D	9. A	14. F
5. B	10. B	15. B
16. C	21. D	26. B
17. E	22. B	27. D
18. E	23. B	28. C
19. C	24. C	29. C
20. D	25. B	30. A

Answers and Explanations: III-9 Drugs for Depressive and Anxiety Disorders

Questions 1–5

1. **A**
2. **F**
3. **D**
4. **A**
5. **H**

Learning objective: Describe the leading hypothesis about the mechanism of action of antidepressant drugs.

6. **C** A leading hypothesis of depression suggests that the disease is associated with a loss of neurotrophic support in cortical areas, such as the hippocampus. The nerve growth factors, such as brain-derived neurotrophic factor (BDNF), are critical for this neurotrophic support, that is, for the regulation of neural plasticity and neurogenesis. All drugs used to treat depression share, at some level, primary effects on serotonergic and/or noradrenergic neurotransmission, as chronic treatment with these drugs increases the availability of central serotonin and/or norepinephrine. Compelling evidence suggests that sustained signaling via these neurotransmitters increases the expression of specific downstream gene products, particularly BDNF. This appears to be the ultimate mechanism of action of antidepressants.

    A Monoamine oxidase inhibitors, but not other antidepressants, inhibit monoamine metabolism.

    B Actually, downregulation, not upregulation, of central adrenoceptors was an earlier hypothesis of the mechanism of action of antidepressants.

    D According to the neurotrophic hypothesis, antidepressants should increase, not decrease, hippocampal neurogenesis.

    E Actually, some studies suggest that glutamate antagonists, not agonists, could have a role as antidepressants.

Learning objective: Describe poisoning with tricyclic antidepressants.

7. **E** The history and signs of the patient suggest that he took a toxic dose of a tricyclic antidepressant. These drugs have pronounced antimuscarinic activity (mydriasis and tachycardia) and antiadrenergic activity (low blood pressure) and prolong the QT interval on ECG by a quinidine-like action.

    A–D, F Poisoning by these drugs does not cause all the signs exhibited by the patient.

Learning objective: Describe the adverse effect of tricyclic antidepressants.

8. **C** Amitriptyline is a tricyclic antidepressant drug. All tricyclic antidepressants block α_1-adrenoceptors and therefore can cause postural hypotension, especially during the first week of treatment. Drowsiness is another common adverse effect, most likely due to central muscarinic and histaminic receptor blockade. At least partial tolerance usually develops to autonomic effects, so the symptoms tend to diminish over time.

    A, B, D–F These drugs very rarely cause postural hypotension.

Learning objective: Explain the mechanism of action of serotonin–norepinephrine reuptake inhibitors (SNRIs).

9. **C** Venlafaxine is currently a first-line agent for anxiety disorders. The drug blocks both norepinephrine and serotonin transporters. The resulting decreased reuptake of these neurotransmitters increases their availability in the synaptic cleft of central nervous system neurons. The relationship between this molecular mechanism of action and the therapeutic efficacy of the drug in anxiety disorders is still uncertain, but contemporary hypotheses implicate dysregulation of adrenergic and/or serotonergic systems in chronic anxiety.

    A Tricyclic antidepressants such as amitriptyline also block monoamine transporters, but they are not used as antianxiety agents.

    B Citalopram blocks the serotonin transporter but not the norepinephrine transporter.

    D Benzodiazepines such as lorazepam do not alter monoamine reuptake.

    E, F These drugs block only norepinephrine transporter (bupropion) or serotonin transporter (trazodone) and are not used as antianxiety agents.

Learning objective: Explain the mechanism of action of selective serotonin reuptake inhibitors (SSRIs).

10. **C** The patient's symptoms indicate that she was most likely suffering from an obsessive-compulsive disorder. Drugs that inhibit the serotonin transporter have been shown to be effective in obsessive-compulsive disorders. Classes of drugs able to act with this mechanism are SSRIs, serotonin–norepinephrine reuptake inhibitors (SNRIs), and tricyclic antidepressants. SSRIs are currently considered first-line treatment for obsessive-compulsive disorders. Tricyclic antidepressants (mainly clomipramine) are used as second-choice drugs.

    A, B, D, E See correct answer explanation.

Learning objective: Outline the appropriate therapy for depression and insomnia associated with a malignant disease.

11. **C** The patient's symptoms suggest that she was suffering from depression and anxiety, likely because of the tumor diagnosis. Pancreatic carcinoma is a type of cancer most frequently associated with depressive symptoms. Because the patient is elderly and had been suffering from an arrhythmia, tricyclic antidepressants are contraindicated. Selective serotonin reuptake inhibitors (SSRIs) such as paroxetine are best suited for depressed patients of older age with considerable attendant anxiety, as in this case. Because the patient was suffering from initial insomnia, a short-acting hypnotic such as zaleplon taken before bedtime is appropriate, as SSRIs may cause insomnia.

    A, B See correct answer explanation.

    D, E Neuroleptics are devoid of antidepressive properties.

Learning objective: Explain the mechanism of tricyclic-induced postural hypotension.

12. **D** The patient's symptoms indicate that she was most likely suffering from postural hypotension. Tricyclic antidepressants such as imipramine can cause several adverse effects due to blockade of some autonomic receptors. Blockade of α_1 adrenoceptors can result in substantial postural hypotension.

    A–C, E, F See correct answer explanation.

Learning objective: Describe the use of paroxetine in treating social anxiety disorder.

13. **E** The patient was most likely suffering from a social anxiety disorder (SAD). Several trials have provided evidence of the efficacy of pharmacotherapy with selective serotonin reuptake inhibitors (SSRIs) or serotonin–norepinephrine reuptake inhibitors (SNRIs) in SADs. Approximately one fifth of patients with SAD also suffer from an alcohol use disorder, as in this case. Paroxetine significantly reduces social anxiety and decreases the frequency of alcohol use in patients with both disorders.

    A Benzodiazepines such as diazepam should be reserved as last-line agents in patients with SAD.

    B–D, F These drugs are not effective in SAD.

Learning objective: Describe poisoning with tricyclic antidepressants.

14. **F** Tricyclic antidepressant poisoning may produce any of three major toxic syndromes:

- Anticholinergic syndrome: sedation, delirium, tachycardia, mydriasis, dry mucous membranes, hyperthermia, constipation, and urinary retention
- Cardiovascular syndrome: hypotension, sinus tachycardia with prolongation of QT intervals, torsade de pointes (rare). Bradyarrhythmias (various degrees of atrioventricular block) can occur in severe poisoning and carry a poor prognosis. They are due to the quinidine-like activity common to all tricyclic antidepressants, which can severely impair cardiac conduction.
- Convulsing syndrome: seizures may be recurrent or persistent.

Depending on the dose, patients may experience some or all of these toxic effects. The patient's coma indicates that the poisoning was severe and most likely included all three toxic syndromes.

A–E Tricyclic antidepressants tend to cause symptoms opposite to those listed.

Learning objective: Explain the mechanism of paroxetine-induced diarrhea.

15. **B** By blocking serotonin reuptake, selective serotonin reuptake inhibitors (SSRIs) such as paroxetine increase serotonin availability at serotonergic synapses in both the central and enteric nervous systems. Serotonin activation of serotonin receptors (mainly 5-HT$_{2A}$) is known to increase intestinal peristalsis, thus causing diarrhea, which occurs in up to 20% of patients taking SSRIs.

A, C–F Paroxetine does not cause these actions. Moreover, all of these actions would lead to constipation, not diarrhea.

Learning objective: Describe the therapeutic uses of serotonin-norepinephrine reuptake inhibitors (SNRIs) in neuropathic pain.

16. **D** The patient's history and symptoms suggest he was suffering from chronic phantom limb pain, a pain that is referred to a limb that no longer exists. Phantom limb pain is a type of neuropathic pain, which is caused by damage to neural structures. Unlike nociceptive pain, which is effectively alleviated by nonsteroidal antiinflammatory drugs (NSAIDs) and opioids, neuropathic pain often responds poorly to these drugs but is relieved by antidepressants, including tricyclic antidepressants and SNRIs. Phantom limb pain is sometimes very difficult to treat, but venlafaxine and duloxetine are often effective and are the drugs most frequently used. They are equivalent to tricyclics but have the substantial advantage of fewer adverse effects.

A–C, E, F These drugs are all minimally or not effective in neuropathic pain.

Learning objective: Explain the mechanism of action of amitriptyline.

17. **A** Amitriptyline is a tricyclic antidepressant drug. Drugs from this class are the most powerful inhibitors of norepinephrine and serotonin reuptake into presynaptic terminals. The resulting increased availability of those neurotransmitters in the synaptic cleft most likely mediates their antidepressant properties. Amitriptyline can cause hypersomnia in up to 88% of patients taking the drug.

B Trazodone can exert a weak blockade on serotonin reuptake but has no effect on norepinephrine reuptake.

C Bupropion can exert a weak blockade on norepinephrine reuptake but has no effect on serotonin reuptake.

D, E Citalopram and sertraline are selective serotonin reuptake inhibitors.

Learning objective: Describe the main adverse effects of selective serotonin reuptake inhibitors/serotonin–norepinephrine reuptake inhibitors (SSRIs/SNRIs).

18. **C** Most antidepressants can cause sexual dysfunction, but its incidence seems the highest with SSRIs/SNRIs (mainly paroxetine and fluoxetine) and the lowest with bupropion and mirtazapine. Sexual dysfunction seems to be primarily related to the increased activity of the central serotonergic system, as serotonin is mainly an inhibitory neurotransmitter in the central nervous system.

A, E, F Lithium, bupropion, and mirtazapine rarely cause sexual dysfunction.

B Tricyclic antidepressants such as amitriptyline frequently cause sexual dysfunction but are contraindicated in this patient because they can cause cardiac arrhythmias in patients at risk (patients with a previous episode of ventricular arrhythmia have a very high risk of recurrent arrhythmia).

D Chlorpromazine is not used for depressive disorder and may cause arrhythmias in patients at risk.

Learning objective: Describe the serotonin syndrome due to selective serotonin reuptake inhibitors/serotonin–norepinephrine reuptake inhibitor (SSRIs/SNRIs).

19. **C** The history, signs, and symptoms of the patient indicate that she was most likely suffering from serotonin syndrome. This disorder is a rare but potentially fatal interaction that can be caused by several drugs either alone or in combination, when given in high doses. These include antidepressants, opioids, psychostimulants, triptans, psychedelics, and herbs (e.g., St. John's wort, ginseng, and nutmeg). The combination of two drugs that enhance serotonin transmission (i.e., SSRIs/SNRIs with monoamine oxidase inhibitors or with

tricyclic antidepressants) can be particularly dangerous. The syndrome involves mental, autonomic, and neurologic disorders of sudden onset less than 24 hours after the beginning of treatment or of an overdose. For mild cases, discontinuation of the offending drug is the only needed treatment. For more serious cases, therapy includes benzodiazepines for agitation and somatic effects, serotonin antagonists (cyproheptadine) or atypical neuroleptics with serotonin-blocking activity (e.g., olanzapine), β-blockers for tachycardia and autonomic instability, and dantrolene for hyperthermia.

A, B, D–F These disorders do not cause the signs and symptoms reported by the patient.

Learning objective: Outline the therapeutic use of selective serotonin reuptake inhibitors (SSRIs) in major depressive disorder.

20. **B** When given in equivalent doses, all antidepressants are about equally effective in the general depressed patient population, so the choice of the drug in a specific patient is influenced mainly by the patient's medical history, the presenting symptoms, and contraindications. Selective serotonin reuptake inhibitors (SSRIs) such as fluoxetine are currently the most used drugs for depression and are especially suited for this patient because of the presence of concomitant symptoms of anxiety. Moreover, in this patient:

A Tricyclic antidepressants are contraindicated because of the exertional angina.

C, D Trazodone and mirtazapine are not indicated because they have pronounced sedative properties, and the patient is suffering from hypersomnia.

E, F Lithium and haloperidol are devoid of antidepressant activity.

Learning objective: Describe the molecular mechanism of action of mirtazapine.

21. **D** Mirtazapine can block presynaptic α_2 receptors, thus increasing the release of both norepinephrine and serotonin. In addition, it can also block serotonin (5-HT$_{2A}$ and 5-HT$_{2C}$) receptors. All of these actions probably contribute to the antidepressant effect. The drug is a second-choice agent in depressive disorders, but sometimes it is highly effective.

A–C, E, F See correct answer explanation.

Learning objective: Describe the mechanism of action of bupropion.

22. **A** Because the patient obtained partial relief from fluoxetine therapy, a reasonable next step is to add a second drug to the treatment, rather than changing the antidepressant. Bupropion has been used as augmentation therapy for many years, and its use is supported by several trials. Patients taking fluoxetine who continue to complain of fatigue and hypersomnia are good candidates for bupropion augmentation, as

in this case. Bupropion is unique among all currently available antidepressants, as it has negligible activity on serotonin neurotransmission. It most likely acts by enhancing norepinephrine and dopamine activity.

B Methylphenidate blocks the reuptake of catecholamines but is not active as an antidepressant.

C–E These drugs are sometimes used for antidepressant augmentation therapy, but they act through different mechanisms.

Learning objective: Describe the main therapeutic uses of monoamine oxidase inhibitors.

23. **A** Phenelzine is a nonselective monoamine oxidase inhibitor (MAOI). These drugs are rarely prescribed today because of frequent adverse effects and the risk of serious drug–drug and drug–food interactions. However, for the treatment of atypical depression, MAOIs are among the most effective agents available and are still prescribed for patients with this depressive subtype, usually after failure of a selective serotonin reuptake inhibitor (SSRI) therapy, as in this case.

B Entacapone acts by inhibiting an enzyme involved in neurotransmitter metabolism but is an antiparkinson, not an antidepressant, drug.

C–F These antidepressant drugs do not act by enzyme inhibition.

Learning objective: Outline the therapeutic uses of selective serotonin reuptake inhibitors (SSRIs) in obsessive-compulsive disorder.

24. **C** The patient's symptoms suggest that he is suffering from an obsessive-compulsive disorder. SSRIs are currently first-line agents for obsessive-compulsive disorders, and their effectiveness gives support to the hypothesis that these disorders are due to a dysfunction in central serotonergic transmission.

A, B, D–F These drugs have minimal or no efficacy in treating obsessive-compulsive disorders.

Learning objective: Describe the main adverse effects of selective serotonin reuptake inhibitors/serotonin–norepinephrine reuptake inhibitors (SSRIs/SNRIs).

25. **B** Abrupt discontinuation of SSRIs or SNRIs can cause a variety of symptoms that can be distressing. These include dizziness, nausea and vomiting, flulike symptoms, irritability, and anxiety. Symptoms usually emerge 1 to 3 days after the last dose. Paroxetine and sertraline are most likely to cause the discontinuation syndrome, and they should be tapered over several weeks.

A, C–F These disorders do not cause the symptoms reported by the patient.

Learning objective: Describe the main drug interactions with selective serotonin reuptake inhibitors (SSRIs).

26. **D** The patient's symptoms indicate that he was suffering from an extrapyramidal adverse effect. SSRIs are inhibitors of the cytochrome P-450 enzymes and can increase the activity of other drugs given concomitantly. Specifically, paroxetine is a potent inhibitor of the CYP2D6 isozyme, which is the main isozyme that metabolizes metoclopramide. Therefore, the dopamine-blocking actions of metoclopramide are enhanced, leading to extrapyramidal effects. Moreover, SSRIs can indirectly affect dopaminergic transmission. In fact, serotonin and dopamine appear to have an inverse relationship in certain areas of the brain, whereby stimulation of central serotonin receptors results in inhibition of dopaminergic transmission. The SSRI–metoclopramide interaction is well known and occurs rapidly, within hours of metoclopramide administration, as in this case.

    A–C, E, F The interaction of these drugs with metoclopramide is negligible.

Learning objective: Describe the use of selective serotonin reuptake inhibitors (SSRIs) in treating panic disorders.

27. **E** The patient's symptoms suggest that she was most likely suffering from a panic disorder. The disease responds to a variety of psychotropic drugs, including SSRIs, benzodiazepines, and tricyclic antidepressants. SSRIs/SNRIs are the current first-line agents for the chronic treatment of these disorders.

    A–D, F These drugs are not effective in treating panic disorders.

Learning objective: Outline the therapeutic efficacy of selective serotonin reuptake inhibitors (SSRIs) in treating bulimia nervosa.

28. **A** The patient's history and symptoms indicate that she was affected by bulimia nervosa, a chronic disorder with multiple episodes of relapse and remission that usually occurs in late adolescence. If medications are required, antidepressants are considered drugs of choice for bulimia nervosa. Selective serotonin reuptake inhibitors (SSRIs) are the preferred agents because of their tolerability and because they have been studied in the largest number of patients.

    B–F These drugs are not effective in treating bulimia nervosa.

Learning objective: Describe the main adverse effects of selective serotonin reuptake inhibitors (SSRIs)/serotonin–norepinephrine reuptake inhibitors (SNRIs).

29. **B** Most antidepressants can cause sexual dysfunction, but its incidence seems the highest with SSRIs/SNRIs. Symptoms of sexual dysfunction in males include erectile dysfunction, priapism, delayed ejaculation, decreased libido, and partial or complete anorgasmia.

    A, C–F SNRIs do not cause these symptoms.

Learning objective: Describe the adverse effect of tricyclic antidepressants.

30. **D** The symptoms of the patient indicate that he was suffering from obstructive uropathy, most likely due to prostatic hyperplasia. Drugs with antimuscarinic properties, such as amitriptyline, can precipitate complete anuria in patients with prostatic hyperplasia, as these patients already have a urethral obstruction, and the drug inhibits bladder contraction.

    A–C, E None of these drugs have antimuscarinic properties.

Learning objective: Describe the latency of effect of antidepressant medications.

31. **B** The patient most likely started a therapy with a selective serotonin reuptake inhibitor (SSRI), such as paroxetine, drugs that are currently the most commonly used antidepressants. All antidepressant medications have a similar delayed pattern of therapeutic response. Typically, patients are informed that approximately 2 to 6 weeks must elapse before they will experience any therapeutic benefit. However, researchers in the field consider this a conservative estimate, and more rigorous studies have led to the conclusion that patients can exhibit some improvement during the first 2 weeks of treatment and a maximum improvement during the fourth week. Despite a variety of explanations for this delay, there is no consensus, and the exact reason remains unknown.

    A Tricyclic antidepressants are absolutely contraindicated in patients with atrioventricular block.

    C Bupropion can cause arrhythmias and can increase blood pressure. Therefore, it should be avoided in a patient with a recent myocardial infarction.

    D Phenelzine is a nonselective and irreversible monoamine oxidase inhibitor. These drugs should be avoided in patients with cardiovascular diseases.

    E Benzodiazepines, such as diazepam, are not used as antidepressant drugs.

Learning objective: Describe the increased risk of suicide that can occur in a young person taking antidepressant drugs.

32. **E** Of these drugs, fluoxetine is thought to be the greatest risk for enhancing suicide potential in patients such as the one described here. All antidepressants have U.S. Food and Drug Administration (FDA) black box warnings, because apparently they increase the risk of suicide during the first 4 weeks of treatment in children and at-risk patients younger than

age 24, as in this case. However, the risk of suicide seems to decrease after 12 weeks of therapy. It is worth noting that, despite the FDA's decision, the issue of antidepressant-related risk of suicidality remains controversial, because this risk is strongly related to severity of depression in both youths and adults, and long-term antidepressant treatment can decrease depression severity.

A Zolpidem is a hypnotic drug, most likely given to the patient because insomnia is a frequent adverse effect of fluoxetine.

B–E These drugs are anticancer drugs used to treat Hodgkin lymphoma.

DRUGS FOR DEPRESSIVE AND ANXIETY DISORDERS Answer key					
1.	A	6.	C	11.	C
2.	F	7.	E	12.	D
3.	D	8.	C	13.	E
4.	A	9.	C	14.	F
5.	H	10.	C	15.	B
16.	D	21.	D	26.	D
17.	A	22.	A	27.	E
18.	C	23.	A	28.	A
19.	C	24.	C	29.	B
20.	B	25.	B	30.	D
				31.	B
				32.	E

Answers and Explanations: III-10 Drugs for Bipolar Disorders

Questions 1–4

1. **A**
2. **G**
3. **G**
4. **D**

Learning objective: Explain the molecular mechanisms of action of lithium.

5. **E** Lithium inhibits inositol monophosphatase, an enzyme involved in the phosphatidylinositol pathway. This leads to depletion of phosphatidylinositol 4,5-bisphosphate (PIP_2), which is the precursor of both IP_3 and DAG. Therefore, the synthesis of IP_3 and DAG is inhibited, and the activity of many receptors that are IP_3/DAG linked is depressed. This may cause an inhibition of overactive circuits in mania.

A–D, F Lithium tends to cause actions opposite to those listed.

Learning objective: Outline the use of quetiapine in bipolar disorder.

6. **D** The man was most likely affected by a bipolar disorder resistant to lithium therapy and was suffering from an acute depressive episode. Because the patient experienced five mood swings over the past year, he meets the criteria for rapid cycling, defined as occurrence of four or more mood swings or episodes of mania or depression in a year. About 70 to 80% of rapid cyclers have poor response to lithium. Quetiapine and a combination of olanzapine and fluoxetine are the drugs approved by the U.S. Food and Drug Administration for the treatment of acute episodes of depression in bipolar disorder.

A, C Typical neuroleptics, such as haloperidol and fluphenazine, could be used in the acute manic phase of bipolar disorders, but not in the depressive phase.

B, E These drugs are not effective in bipolar disorders.

F Tricyclic antidepressants are used only exceptionally in bipolar disorders. Moreover, they are contraindicated in elderly persons, as in this case.

Learning objective: Explain the mechanism of action of olanzapine.

7. **D** An acute manic attack often requires treatment with a two- or three-drug combination, usually lithium plus an anticonvulsant plus an atypical neuroleptic. All neuroleptics most likely act by blocking D_2 receptors in mesolimbic and mesocortical pathways. In addition, they block $5-HT_2$ receptors, and this action may contribute to their clinical effects. Atypical neuroleptics such as olanzapine seem to have a higher affinity for $5-HT_2$ receptors than for D_2 receptors.

A–C, E, F None of these drugs block both D_2 and $5-HT_2$ receptors.

Learning objective: Describe the adverse effects of lithium.

8. **A** Lithium likely decreases thyroid function in most patients, but few of them show symptoms of hypothyroidism. However, in this case, the symptoms are most likely due to hypothyroidism. The effect is due to inhibition of thyroid hormone synthesis. The mechanism of this effect is likely related to lithium-induced inhibition of adenylyl cyclase, which in turn inhibits thyrotropin-induced production of cyclic adenosine monophosphate (cAMP) in thyroid cells.

B Lithium is not metabolized and is excreted as such by the kidney.

C Cimetidine does not cause the pattern of adverse effects exhibited by the patient.

D Central effects of loratadine are negligible, as the drug does not cross the blood–brain barrier.

E See correct answer explanation.

Learning objective: Describe the main drug interactions with lithium.

9. **B** The patient's symptoms indicate that she was most likely suffering from adverse effects due to an excessive plasma concentration of lithium. The patient was treated with hydrochlorothiazide, and it is known that the clearance of lithium is reduced about 25% by thiazides. Lithium is 80% reabsorbed in the proximal tubule by the same mechanism as Na⁺ and competes with Na⁺ for reabsorption. Therefore, lithium retention can be increased by Na⁺ loss related to some illnesses or to diuretic use, as in this case.

    A Thiazides tend to induce hyponatremia, not hypernatremia.

    C The hepatic metabolism of lithium is zero.

    D, E See correct answer explanation.

Learning objective: Outline the therapeutic uses of lithium.

10. **E** The history and symptoms of the patient indicate that she was most likely suffering from the depressive phase of a bipolar disorder. The depression is often difficult to control and puts patients at significant risk of suicide. Lithium (alone or in combination) remains the first-line agent for maintenance therapy of bipolar disorder.

    A Antidepressant use in bipolar depression is controversial, and current guidelines suggest that they can be used (together with lithium) in the severe acute phase of bipolar depression. However, tricyclics are contraindicated in patients with suicidal ideation, as in this case.

    B, C Lorazepam and haloperidol are indicated in the acute manic phase of bipolar disorder, not in the depressive phase.

    D, F Anxiolytic and hypnotic drugs are not indicated in bipolar disorders.

Learning objective: Describe the adverse effects of lithium.

11. **C** The symptoms of the patient suggest that she was likely suffering from adverse effects of lithium. Tremor is an adverse effect of lithium that is dose-dependent and may occur in up to 60% of patients receiving high doses. When tremor is not disturbing, treatment is not necessary. Otherwise a concomitant treatment with a β-blocker can help. Polyuria, acne, and folliculitis are other adverse effects of lithium that usually subside with the discontinuation of the drug.

    A, B, D–F These drugs do not cause all the adverse effects reported by the patient.

Learning objective: Describe the duration of lithium therapy in recurrent major bipolar disorder.

12. **E** The duration of maintenance therapy with lithium in major bipolar disorder is at least 9 months. A period of successful maintenance therapy means that the individual is controlled, not cured, as most patients that stop lithium therapy eventually relapse. Furthermore, as individuals experience successive episodes, they tend to recover less completely. Therefore, in a case of serious and repeated episodes of bipolar disorder, as in this case, the person may require lithium for the rest of his or her life.

    A–D See correct answer explanation.

Learning objective: Describe the use of atypical antipsychotics for the maintenance therapy of bipolar disorder during pregnancy.

13. **C** Lithium is classified by the U.S. Food and Drug Administration (FDA) in pregnancy risk category D and therefore must be avoided during pregnancy. Some anticonvulsants (valproic acid, lamotrigine, and carbamazepine) and some atypical antipsychotics (aripiprazole, olanzapine, quetiapine, and risperidone) have become good alternative and adjunctive treatments to lithium for maintenance therapy of bipolar disorder. Among atypical antipsychotics, quetiapine has the lowest ratio of umbilical cord to maternal plasma concentration and does not seem to cause significant teratogenic risk to the fetus. Therefore, it is a rational choice for maintenance therapy in a pregnant woman with bipolar disorder.

    A, B Carbamazepine and valproic acid are effective in maintenance therapy of bipolar disorder but are contraindicated during pregnancy because of a substantial teratogenic risk (both are classified by FDA in the pregnancy risk category D).

    D–F These drugs have no proven efficacy for maintenance therapy of bipolar disorder.

Learning objective: Describe the adverse effects of lithium.

14. **B** Polyuria and polydipsia are common adverse effects of lithium due, at least in part, to inhibition of the vasopressin-induced increase of cAMP in the kidney (lithium inhibits adenylyl cyclase). Circulating levels of vasopressin are normal or elevated, but there is a lack of responsiveness of the collecting tubule (i.e., nephrogenic diabetes insipidus).

    A Lithium has no effect on renal reabsorption of sodium in this part of the nephron.

    C Lithium has no effect on plasma glucose levels.

    D Stimulation of the thirst center in the hypothalamus is the consequence, not the cause, of polyuria.

    E In nephrogenic diabetes insipidus, vasopressin secretion is normal or stimulated, not blocked.

Learning objective: Explain the molecular mechanisms of action of lithium.

15. **F** The two main proposed mechanisms of action of lithium are related to inhibition of two signal transduction pathways, that is, inositol and glycogen synthase kinase 3 signaling. The inhibition of this enzyme causes suppression of the expression of proapoptotic genes and increased expression of antiapoptotic genes. The ultimate effect is neuroprotection, which may underlie the long-term mood stabilization.

A–E All of these drugs have been used in augmentation therapy, but they do not have the above-mentioned mechanism of action.

Learning objective: Describe the adverse effects of lithium.

16. **E** Edema is a frequent adverse effect of lithium, especially during the first 5 to 7 days of therapy. Edema is likely due to increased Na^+ in the extracellular fluid, as lithium is not pumped out by Na^+/K^+-ATPase and therefore tends to accumulate inside the cells, displacing Na^+.

    A–D Lithium tends to cause adverse effects opposite to those listed.

Learning objective: Outline the therapeutic uses of lithium.

17. **E** The signs and symptoms of the patient suggest that he is suffering from an acute manic disorder. General guidelines for acute mania suggest a two- or three-drug combination that includes lithium, as it reduces both the frequency and the magnitude of mood swings. However, it has a slow onset of action, taking as long as 1 to 2 weeks to fully exert its therapeutic effects. Therefore, an adjunctive medication is used during the first days of therapy. Benzodiazepines are often given for agitation and insomnia, but second-generation neuroleptics with substantial sedative properties, such as risperidone, are preferred when there are delusions or hallucinations, as in this case.

    A–D All of these combinations have at least one drug that is not effective in treating manic disorders.

Learning objective: Describe the use of lithium in augmentation therapy for major depressive disorder.

18. **D** More than 40% of patients with major depressive disorder do not achieve remission even after two antidepressant trials. An accepted strategy used when dealing with negligible or poor antidepressant response is to add another agent to the therapy (augmentation therapy). Drugs used effectively for augmentation therapy include lithium, bupropion, buspirone, lamotrigine, and triiodothyronine.

    A, B Currently, antidepressants are not used in augmentation therapy. Moreover, amitriptyline and mirtazapine have sedating activity that could worsen the patient's sleepiness.

    C, E, F These drugs are not effective for antidepressant augmentation therapy.

Learning objective: Calculate the time to withhold lithium therapy in case of lithium overdose toxicity.

19. **D** By definition, the plasma concentration of a drug halves every half-life. Therefore, the plasma level will be 1.5 mEq/L

after one half-life and 0.75 mEq/L after two half-lives (i.e., after 40 hours).

A–C, E, F See correct answer explanation.

Learning objective: Explain the molecular mechanisms of action of lithium.

20. **D** Maintenance therapy with lithium reduces the frequency and severity of episodes of both mania and depression in patients with bipolar disorder. The drug appears to act mainly by inhibiting the inositol second messenger system, as it inhibits inositol monophosphatase, the rate-limiting enzyme in inositol recycling.

    A–C, E, F All of these drugs are effectively used in maintenance therapy of mania, but they do not have the above-mentioned mechanism of action.

Learning objective: Describe the treatment of lithium-induced diabetes insipidus.

21. **C** The patient's history and symptoms indicate that he was most likely suffering from lithium-induced nephrogenic diabetes insipidus, the most common complication of chronic lithium therapy. In the collecting tubule, lithium (Li^+) is reabsorbed through the Na^+ channels and is therefore concentrated inside the principal cells. This high concentration blocks the action of vasopressin, likely by inhibiting adenylyl cyclase, and causes nephrogenic diabetes insipidus. Amiloride is a K^+-sparing diuretic that blocks Na^+ channels in the late distal tubule and collecting duct, inhibiting the reabsorption of Li^+ through those channels. It is therefore the first-line agent for the therapy of lithium-induced diabetes insipidus.

    A, B These diuretics are dangerous in patients taking lithium because they tend to cause Na^+ depletion. Because Na^+ and Li^+ go through the same channels, Na^+ depletion promotes a clinically important degree of lithium retention

    D Spironolactone cannot affect Li^+ reabsorption because it does not block Na^+ channels in the late distal tubule and collecting duct.

    E Conivaptan is a vasopressin antagonist and therefore would increase, not decrease, the patient's polyuria.

DRUGS FOR BIPOLAR DISORDERS Answer key							
1.	A	6.	D	11.	C	16.	E
2.	G	7.	D	12.	E	17.	E
3.	G	8.	A	13.	C	18.	D
4.	D	9.	B	14.	B	19.	D
5.	E	10.	E	15.	F	20.	D
						21.	C

Answers and Explanations: III-11 Drugs for Childhood Behavioral Disorders

Questions 1–3

1. **D**
2. **A**
3. **I**

Learning objective: Identify the neural pathway underlying the therapeutic action of methylphenidate in attention deficit hyperactivity disorder.

4. **C** Attention deficit hyperactivity disorder (ADHD) is associated with alterations in regulation of motor behavior and attention. The prefrontal cortex (PFC) is important for sustaining attention over a delay, inhibiting distractions, and dividing attention. The PFC in the right hemisphere is especially important for behavioral inhibition. Lesions to the PFC produce a profile of distractibility, forgetfulness, impulsivity, poor planning, and locomotor hyperactivity. The PFC is very sensitive to its neurochemical environment, and optimal levels of norepinephrine and dopamine are needed for proper PFC control of behavior and attention. Recent electrophysiological studies in animals suggest that norepinephrine enhances "signals" through postsynaptic α_{2A} adrenoceptors in the PFC, whereas dopamine decreases "noise" through modest levels of D_1 receptor stimulation. Stimulant medications such as methylphenidate and amphetamines most likely cause some of their therapeutic effects by increasing endogenous activation of α_{2A} adrenoceptors and dopamine D_1 receptors in the PFC, optimizing PFC regulation of behavior and attention.

A, B, D, E See correct answer explanation.

Learning objective: Describe the adverse effects of methylphenidate.

5. **B** The mother's report indicated that the child was most likely affected by a tic disorder, which is fairly common in childhood. In some cases the disorder appears to be caused or worsened by prescription medications. The drugs most commonly involved are psychomotor stimulants, such as methylphenidate and amphetamines. Because the child was most likely under methylphenidate therapy, the drug probably caused his tic disorder.

A Fluphenazine can cause tics and dystonias, but the drug is not used for attention deficit hyperactivity disorder (ADHD).

C Atomoxetine is approved for ADHD, but the appearance of tics with this drug is exceedingly rare.

D, E These drugs are not used in ADHD.

Learning objective: Describe the adverse effects of atomoxetine.

6. **A** Atomoxetine is an antidepressant drug approved for the treatment of attention deficit hyperactivity disorder (ADHD). The drug selectively inhibits norepinephrine reuptake in noradrenergic terminals; this mechanism most likely underlies the increase in blood pressure, which occurs in about 10% of patients treated with the drug, especially during the first days of therapy.

B, C Norepinephrine phenylephrine can increase blood pressure but they are not used to treat ADHD.

D, E Guanfacine and clonidine are used to treat ADHD but are also used as antihypertensive agents.

Learning objective: Outline the therapy of attention deficit hyperactivity disorder (ADHD) in a patient with a concomitant depressive disorder.

7. **B** ADHD and depression frequently occur together. When this is the case, a combined therapy with two drugs can be appropriate. Methylphenidate is a commonly used drug for ADHD, and sertraline is a selective serotonin reuptake inhibitor antidepressant drug.

A, C–E None of these options have a drug that is appropriate for use as an antidepressant.

Learning objective: Explain the molecular mechanism of action of atomoxetine in attention deficit hyperactivity disorder (ADHD).

8. **B** Although the precise mechanism by which atomoxetine produces beneficial effects in ADHD is still uncertain, it is thought that the drug exerts its effects through selective inhibition of norepinephrine reuptake in noradrenergic terminals. The drug-binding sites in the brain are consistent with the known distribution of norepinephrine-containing neurons. It is hypothesized that the atomoxetine-induced increase in norepinephrine in the prefrontal cortex, a region involved in attention and memory, mediates the therapeutic effect of atomoxetine in ADHD.

A, C, E Cocaine, atomoxetine, and bupropion are nonselective inhibitors of catecholamine transporters.

D Dextroamphetamine acts by increasing catecholamine release from adrenergic terminals.

Learning objective: Outline the use of aripiprazole in Tourette syndrome.

9. **B** The patient's symptoms suggest that the boy is affected by Tourette syndrome, a chronic familial disorder characterized by motor and phonic tics. The syndrome usually appears at about the age of 5 and occurs in 1 out of 1000 males and 1 out of 10,000 females. Tics are sudden, involuntary movements or

sounds that can be suppressed voluntarily with difficulty and are often accompanied with coprolalia (foul language). Prognosis is generally good, as the syndrome usually disappears in adulthood, but some cases can persist later in life. Expert consensus recommends a trial with atypical neuroleptics before considering haloperidol, which is approved by the U.S. Food and Drug Administration, because of established efficacy and lower risk of extrapyramidal side effects. Unlike other atypical neuroleptics, aripiprazole does not cause weight gain. Because potential obesity is a problem in children, the drug can be a good choice for this age group. Other drugs approved for Tourette syndrome are clonidine and guanfacine.

A, C–F These drugs are ineffective in treating Tourette syndrome.

Learning objective: Identify the site of the central anorectic action of amphetamines.

10. **D** Amphetamines are thought to suppress appetite by increasing norepinephrine and serotonin release in the lateral hypothalamus. This increase can interfere with several peptides that increase food intake by activating the feeding center (neuropeptide Y, orexins A and B, etc.).

A–C, E, F See correct answer explanation.

Learning objective: Outline the therapeutic effects of bupropion.

11. **C** Bupropion is an antidepressant that was also found to be effective in treating attention deficit hyperactivity disorder (ADHD) and is approved as an adjunct in the management of smoking cessation. Because the patient has symptoms of both depression and ADHD and wants to quit smoking, bupropion can be an appropriate drug.

A, D Methylphenidate and guanfacine are effective in ADHD but are not antidepressants.

B, E The antidepressants paroxetine and amitriptyline are not effective in ADHD.

Learning objective: Outline the use of desmopressin in the treatment of nocturnal enuresis.

12. **A** Desmopressin acetate, a synthetic analogue of the natural human antidiuretic hormone arginine vasopressin, is approved as nasal spray and oral tablet for the treatment of nocturnal enuresis. Some studies have shown that some patients with enuresis do not have a normal circadian rhythm of vasopressin secretion and as a result produce a large amount of urine during the night. Desmopressin increases renal water reabsorption, thus reducing the volume of urine entering the bladder. It is effective in reducing the number of wet nights in 70% of children.

B Imipramine was used in the past with some success in nocturnal enuresis, even though its mechanism of action in this disorder remains unknown. However, the drug has several disadvantages (relapse is high, overdose toxicity can be lethal, etc.) and is therefore rarely prescribed today. Moreover, it is not available by nasal spray.

C Some anticholinergics were used in the past for nocturnal enuresis, but they have a vast array of adverse effects, and their efficacy is minimal.

D–F These drugs are not effective in nocturnal enuresis.

Learning objective: Explain the molecular mechanism of action of dextroamphetamine.

13. **B** The symptoms and signs of the patient suggest that he was affected by attention deficit hyperactivity disorder (ADHD). Dysregulation of central noradrenergic and dopaminergic networks has long been hypothesized as underlying the pathophysiology of ADHD. This hypothesis derives largely from pharmacological data documenting that drugs that modulate noradrenergic and dopaminergic function are effective in treating ADHD. Amphetamines increase the availability of catecholamines in the synaptic cleft mainly because they stimulate the release of catecholamines from adrenergic terminals.

A, C, E These drugs act by blocking the reuptake of catecholamines into adrenergic terminals.

D Guanfacine activates centrally acting α_2-adrenoceptors.

Learning objective: Describe the adverse effects of methylphenidate.

14. **D** Nervousness and insomnia are the most common adverse reactions to methylphenidate and may occur with all formulations. Insomnia occurs in up to 16% of adult patients but typically resolves within a few days of use, provided the dosage is appropriate and doses are not administered within 6 hours of bedtime. Insomnia is most likely related to the drug-induced increase in norepinephrine and dopamine availability, which causes a stimulation of the brainstem arousal system.

A Adrenergic drugs actually cause decreased, not increased, appetite.

B Methylphenidate-induced growth suppression has been reported in children (even if the issue is controversial) but cannot occur in an adult patient.

C Methylphenidate has the potential to lower the seizure threshold mainly in patients with a prior history of seizures. However, seizures are exceptionally rare in nonepileptic patients.

E Hallucinations and delusions can occur with methylphenidate, but their frequency is low (less than 0.1%).

Learning objective: Describe the use of atypical neuroleptics in autistic disorder.

15. **B** There is no specific treatment or cure for autism, but pharmacological treatment, behavioral therapy, and special education can improve some symptoms. Antipsychotic medications have been used widely and appear to be effective in reducing stereotypies, irritability, and self-injurious behavior. Atypical neuroleptics seem to offer some advantage over classical ones, and aripiprazole and risperidone are approved by the U.S. Food and Drug Administration for treating irritability in autistic children.

    A, C–F All of these drugs are useless or even contraindicated in autistic disorder.

Learning objective: Describe the molecular mechanism of action of methylphenidate.

16. **A** Methylphenidate exerts many of its effects through blockade of dopamine uptake by central adrenergic neurons. As a result, sympathomimetic activity in the central nervous system (CNS) is increased. The main sites of CNS activity appear to be the brainstem arousal system and the cerebral cortex.

    B–E Methylphenidate does not elicit these effects.

Learning objective: Outline the therapy of attention deficit hyperactivity disorder (ADHD) in a patient at risk of drug abuse.

17. **E** Atomoxetine is a drug approved for the treatment of ADHD. The drug is not a psychostimulant and lacks abuse potential. It is therefore suitable for patients at risk of drug abuse.

    A, C These drugs are psychostimulants with a high abuse potential.

    B, D, F These drugs are not used for treating ADHD.

Learning objective: Explain the molecular mechanism of action of guanfacine.

18. **C** Guanfacine is an oral, centrally acting α_2-adrenoceptor agonist approved for the treatment of hypertension and attention deficit hyperactivity disorder (ADHD). It has been theorized that ADHD is the result of dysfunction in frontostriatal pathways, possibly related to dysregulation of neurotransmitters such as catecholamines. Frontal networks control attention and motor intentional behavior. Animal studies have demonstrated that guanfacine improves prefrontal cortical function through postsynaptic α_2-receptor agonist effects in the prefrontal cortex.

    A, B, D These drugs are not α_2-adrenoceptor agonists.

E Epinephrine is an α_2-receptor agonist but does not cross the blood–brain barrier and is not used to treat ADHD.

Learning objective: Describe the adverse effects of guanfacine.

19. **A** Guanfacine is an α_2 selective agonist. It is approved for the therapy of attention deficit hyperactivity disorder (ADHD) and hypertension. Its mechanism of antihypertensive action is close to that of clonidine. Hypotension and palpitations are the most frequently reported cardiovascular adverse effects of the drug. These tend to diminish or subside with continued therapy or with reduced dosage.

    B Guanfacine tends to cause anorexia.

    C Dry mouth, not salivation, is a frequent adverse effect of the drug.

    D Aggressive behavior can occur very rarely in some children with risk factor for bipolar disease.

    E Sweating, not anhidrosis, is a reported adverse effect of the drug.

Learning objective: Outline the use of clonidine in both attention deficit hyperactivity disorder (ADHD) and Tourette syndrome.

20. **B** Over 90% of children with Tourette syndrome have coexisting conditions, such as ADHD (75%), mood disorders (60%), obsessive-compulsive disorder (40%), other anxiety disorders, or a combination of comorbidities.

    Clonidine is extensively used and approved by the U.S. Food and Drug Administration for the treatment of Tourette syndrome; it has been recently approved for the treatment of ADHD. The drug is an α_2-receptor agonist, and this mechanism of action likely mediates its therapeutic efficacy in both disorders.

    A, C The psychostimulants methylphenidate and dextroamphetamine are currently used in ADHD, but their use in Tourette syndrome is controversial, as they can exacerbate tics.

    D, E Haloperidol and risperidone have been used in Tourette syndrome with various success, but they are ineffective in ADHD.

DRUGS FOR CHILDHOOD BEHAVIORAL DISORDERS Answer key			
1. D	6. A	11. C	16. A
2. A	7. B	12. A	17. E
3. I	8. B	13. B	18. C
4. C	9. B	14. D	19. A
5. B	10. D	15. B	20. B

Answers and Explanations: III-12 Opioid Analgesics and Antagonists

Questions 1–5

1. **A**
2. **F**
3. **E**
4. **I**
5. **H**

Learning objective: Identify the anatomical sites of the analgesic action of opioids.

6. **D** The analgesic effect of opioids is mediated by both spinal and supraspinal actions. At the spinal level, activation of opioid receptors on posterior horn interneurons and output neurons of the substantia gelatinosa inhibits nociceptive transmission in the lateral spinothalamic tract. At the supraspinal level, activation of opioid receptors occurs in several brain areas, but the best characterized of these areas is the mesencephalic periaqueductal gray matter. Microinjections of morphine in this region block nociceptive responses in every species examined, from rodents to primates. Naloxone reverses these effects.

   A–C, E None of these brain areas are involved in the analgesic effect of opioids, but they may be the sites for other effects of opioids.

Learning objective: Identify the main site of the spinal analgesic action of morphine.

7. **B** When an opioid is given by the epidural route, it provides an exceptionally long analgesic action with limited systemic effects. In this situation, the analgesia is mainly spinal and mainly due to activation of receptors in the substantia gelatinosa, with consequent inhibition of nociceptive transmission in the lateral spinothalamic tract.

   A, C, F Activation of opioid receptors in these areas can contribute to the analgesic effect of morphine by enhancing the descending inhibitory pain pathways, but they are minimally involved when morphine is given locally by the epidural route.

   D This area is involved in the gratifying effects of opioids.

   E This area is not involved in the analgesic action of morphine.

Learning objective: Identify the main brain site of the emetic action of morphine.

8. **B** Opioids can cause nausea and vomiting mainly through stimulation of the chemoreceptor trigger zone, a group of neurons located in the area postrema on the floor of the fourth ventricle.

   A, C–F See correct answer explanation.

Learning objective: Describe the neurophysiological actions that mediate the analgesic effects of opioids.

9. **A** Opioids can affect nociceptive information in two ways:

   • Directly through inhibition of ascending transmission of information by impairment of ascending nociceptive pathways at various levels in the central nervous system

   • Indirectly through activation (likely via μ [mu] receptor-mediated inhibition of GABAergic neurons) of descending aminergic bulbospinal pathways (from the rostral ventral medulla, locus ceruleus, periaqueductal gray area, nucleus raphe magnus, etc.) that control the processing of pain transmission in the spinal cord.

   B Opioids inhibit the release of substance P, an excitatory neurotransmitter present in afferent sensory fibers.

   C Opioids can induce dissociative feelings and dysphoria, but this has nothing to do with the analgesic action.

   D, E Opioids indirectly activate these pathways (see correct answer explanation).

Learning objective: Identify the opioid that is a partial μ (mu) opioid agonist.

10. **D** Buprenorphine is a partial μ agonist and a κ (kappa) antagonist. It is much more potent than morphine (0.3 mg buprenorphine is considered equianalgesic to 10 mg morphine), and its effects are not readily antagonized by naloxone, likely because buprenorphine dissociates very slowly from opioid receptors.

    A–C, E, F These drugs are not partial opioid agonists.

Learning objective: Describe the main opioid postreceptor mechanisms.

11. **D** Opioid receptors are mainly inhibitory receptors coupled to G proteins. The primary transduction mechanisms of these receptors are activation of phospholipase C or inhibition of adenylyl cyclase. Two well-established consequences of this transduction are

    • At the presynaptic level, blockade of voltage-gated Ca^{2+} channels, which in turn reduces the release of a large number of neurotransmitters (most often glutamate but also acetylcholine, norepinephrine, serotonin, and substance P)

    • At the postsynaptic level, opening of ligand-gated K^+ channels, which in turn evokes an inhibitory postsynaptic potential

    A See correct answer explanation.

    B, E Opioids do not act on chloride or Na^+ channels.

    C, F Opioids have actions opposite to those listed.

Learning objective: Explain the molecular mechanisms of action of opioids.

12. **B** The analgesic action of morphine (as well as that of most opioids) is mainly due to direct activation of μ (mu) receptors in various areas of the central nervous system.

    A By activating μ receptors, opioids can cause the release of endogenous opioid peptides. This can contribute to the final analgesic effect but is not the main cause of this effect.

    C Activation, not blockade, of κ (kappa) receptors can contribute to the analgesic effect of opioids.

    D, E Opioids decrease the release of many neurotransmitters, including substance P and glutamate, so these listed effects are unlikely.

    F Opioids can decrease the release of norepinephrine, causing decreased activity of β adrenoceptors, but this action is not related to the analgesic action of opioids.

Learning objective: Describe the mechanism of opioid-induced miosis.

13. **C** Opioids can stimulate the Edinger–Westphal nucleus (also known as the accessory oculomotor nucleus), which is the accessory parasympathetic cranial nerve nucleus of the oculomotor nerve supplying the sphincter muscle of the iris and the ciliary muscle. Therefore, miosis is seen with virtually all opioid agonists. Tolerance to this opioid effect is negligible.

    A, B, D–F See correct answer explanation.

Learning objective: Describe the effects of an activation of μ (mu) opioid receptors on the cell membrane of a nociceptive neuron.

14. **E** Activation of postsynaptic μ opioid receptors on the cell membrane of pain transmission neurons in the spinal cord causes opening of K⁺ channels, hyperpolarizing the membrane. An inhibitory postsynaptic potential ensues; therefore, the transmission of nociceptive stimuli is impaired.

    A–D See correct answer explanation.

Learning objective: Describe the mechanism of action of pentazocine.

15. **A** Pentazocine is a partial agonist at μ (mu) receptors and a full agonist at κ (kappa) receptors. Because of this mechanism of action, it is generally less effective as an analgesic than other full opioid agonists. However, there is a large individual variability in opioid sensitivity that has been ascribed to genetic diversity of receptors. For example, some red-headed, pale skin phenotypes have a more active κ opioid system and are therefore more sensitive to the analgesic action of pentazocine. This can explain the choice in this case.

    B–E See correct answer explanation.

Learning objective: Describe the main features of the analgesic effect of opioids.

16. **F** The use of opioids to treat chronic noncancer pain is still controversial because some clinicians believe that these situations should never be treated with opioids. However, current guidelines recommend opioid therapy as a second-line option for patients who have inadequate response to other therapies, as in this case. Opioids are the only analgesic that can reduce both the sensory and the affective components of the pain experience. The affective component (i.e., suffering) is the one most effectively targeted. Methadone is often the preferred opioid for two reasons: it has excellent oral bioavailability (about 90%), and it has a long half-life (about 25 hours) that allows for a single daily dose.

    A, B Nonsteroidal antiinflammatory drugs such as indomethacin and ketorolac have no significant effect on the emotional aspect of pain.

    C–E Drugs with anxiolytic properties such as sertraline, diazepam, and venlafaxine can reduce the emotional aspect of pain, but they have negligible analgesic properties.

Learning objective: Describe the actions that mediate the therapeutic effect of morphine in pulmonary edema.

17. **D** The therapeutic effect of morphine in pulmonary edema likely involves

    - Reduced perception of shortness of breath
    - Reduced fear and apprehension (pain anticipatory anxiety is reduced).
    - Reduced preload due to peripheral venous dilation and afterload due to arteriolar vasodilation, likely due both to histamine release and decreased sympathomimetic activity secondary to decreased anxiety

    However, good evidence supporting a beneficial hemodynamic effect is lacking, and some physicians believe that the risks of morphine may outweigh the benefits.

    A–C, E Morphine causes actions opposite to those listed.

Learning objective: Describe the mechanism of the constipating action of opioids.

18. **B** Opioids increase the tone of nonvascular smooth muscle (both sphincteral and nonsphincteral) that in turn causes a contraction of the colon and a decrease of its peristaltic activity. Opioids also increase the internal anal sphincter tone and reduce the reflex relaxation response to rectal distention. All of these actions, combined with decreased normal sensory stimuli for defecation because of the central nervous system depressant action, contribute to the final constipating effect.

A, C, D Opioids cause actions opposite to those listed.

E The morphine-induced decrease of intestinal peristalsis delays passage of the fecal mass and allows increased absorption of water. Therefore, the feces become harder, not softer.

Learning objective: Describe the action of opioids on the respiratory system.

19. **D** Morphine depresses all phases of respiratory activity (respiratory rate, minute volume, and tidal exchanges) mainly because the drug reduces the responsiveness of the brainstem respiratory centers to partial pressure of arterial carbon dioxide (P_aCO_2).

A The cough reflex is depressed, not stimulated, by morphine, due, at least in part, to depression of the cough center.

B Morphine causes bronchoconstriction, not bronchodilation, which is due, at least in part, to histamine release.

C, E See correct answer explanation.

Learning objective: List the morphine effects that undergo negligible tolerance.

20. **B** Tolerance develops to most effects of morphine, including the lethal effect. Notable exceptions are the effects on the eye (which lead to miosis) and the effects on the enteric smooth muscle (which lead to constipation) for which tolerance is negligible.

A, C–F See correct answer explanation.

Learning objective: Describe the adverse effects of opioids.

21. **D** Codeine is commonly used as an antitussive when a dry, nonproductive cough is disturbing the patient. Most opioids can cause constipation when used repeatedly, as in this case.

A, B, F Most opioids can depress the cough reflex, but opioids such as buprenorphine, fentanyl, and morphine are not commonly used as antitussives.

C, E Albuterol and theophylline can be used in cases of acute bronchitis because of their bronchodilating properties, but they usually do not cause constipation.

Learning objective: Describe the adverse effects of opioids.

22. **F** An intramuscular injection of morphine can release histamine, which can cause a local reaction (weal at the injection site and pruritus).

A Most opioids can release histamine, but fentanyl and congeners (alfentanil, remifentanil, and sulfentanil) do not.

B–E These drugs do not cause histamine release.

Learning objective: Describe the adverse effects of opioids.

23. **D** Opioids can have additive central nervous system depressant actions when given to a patient treated with a sedative hypnotic drug, such as diazepam. In the most serious instances, these actions can lead to stupor, as in this case.

A–C, E, F These analgesic drugs do not have central nervous system depressant properties.

Learning objective: Describe the adverse effects of opioids.

24. **C** Pentazocine is an opioid that can cause dose-dependent dysphoria and psychotomimetic symptoms. It is sometimes sold illegally when heroin is not available. The drug is a partial agonist at μ (mu) receptors and a full agonist at κ (kappa) receptors. Dysphoria and psychotomimetic symptoms have been ascribed to activation of brain κ receptors. Chronic users of cannabis and hallucinogens are more sensitive to hallucinogenic effects of drugs, as in this case.

A, B, D, E With these drugs, the risk of hallucinogenic effects is negligible.

Learning objective: Describe the adverse effects of opioids.

25. **B** Opioid analgesics have stimulant effects on the nucleus of Edinger–Westphal, the parasympathetic portion of cranial nerve III. The increase in parasympathetic firing causes constriction of the sphincter muscle of the iris (miosis) and the ciliary muscle (cyclospasm). This impairs the accommodation of the eye for far vision.

A Opioids tend to cause euphoria in patients with pain, whereas dysphoria is more likely to occur in normally pain-free people.

C, D Opioids tend to cause constipation, not diarrhea, and hypotension, not hypertension.

E Opioids are given to treat dry cough because they depress the cough center.

Learning objective: Describe the adverse effects of opioids.

26. **C** Fentanyl is a μ (mu) receptor agonist that can be administered by transdermal patch. Because the drug is very lipid soluble, it can be absorbed slowly over about 3 days, providing a long-lasting analgesic effect. However, fever can increase the drug absorption, leading to an overdose effect, as in this case. Occasional fatalities due to this action of fentanyl are reported in the literature.

A, B Pentazocine and codeine are less likely to cause respiratory depression and are not administered by transdermal patch.

D–F Ibuprofen, ketorolac, and indomethacin are not administered by transdermal patch and have negligible risk of respiratory depression.

Learning objective: Describe the use of laxatives to manage opioid-induced constipation.

27. **C** Constipation is one of the most common side effects of opioids, affecting up to 40% of patients under chronic treatment. Therefore, all patients on chronic opioids should receive concomitant prophylaxis for constipation with laxatives (bulking laxatives, e.g., lactulose and agar; stimulant laxatives, e.g., senna and bisacodyl; or softening laxatives, e.g., docusate). It should be noted that, because the constipating effect does not undergo tolerance, concomitant therapy with laxatives should be continued indefinitely.

    A Diazepam would increase, not counteract, the sedative effect of morphine.

    B Selective serotonin reuptake inhibitors are contraindicated, or should be used with great caution, in patients taking opioids because of the risk of serotonin syndrome.

    D Opioids tend to cause bradycardia, which would be enhanced, not prevented, by β-blockers.

    E Opioids tend to cause hypotension, which would be enhanced, not prevented, by calcium channel blockers.

    F Opioids tend to decrease gastric secretion, which would be enhanced, not prevented, by omeprazole.

Learning objective: Describe the opioid postreceptor mechanisms.

28. **B** Opioid receptors are mainly inhibitory receptors coupled to G_i/G_0 proteins. The transduction mechanisms triggered by activation of these receptors include

    - Inhibition of N- and P-type Ca^{2+} channels in nerve terminals, which in turn reduces the release of a large number of neurotransmitters (mainly glutamate, but also acetylcholine, norepinephrine, serotonin, and substance P)
    - Activation of K^+ channels, which in turn leads to hyperpolarization
    - Activation of phospholipase C, which in turn increases the synthesis of IP_3/DAG
    - Activation or inhibition of adenylyl cyclase, leading to either stimulation or inhibition

    A By increasing the activity of phospholipase C, opioids increase the synthesis of IP_3/DAG.

    C Opioids have negligible effect on Na^+ channels.

    D, E Opioids have actions opposite to these.

Learning objective: Explain the rationale of the acetaminophen/codeine combination to treat pain.

29. **E** Acetaminophen and opioid analgesics provide pain relief by different mechanisms of action; thus, they have additive or synergistic effects when given concomitantly.

    A, B The two drugs do not antagonize each other's adverse effects.

    C Tolerance to the codeine analgesic effect does occur with chronic use of the combination.

    D Acetaminophen does not affect codeine biotransformation.

Learning objective: Explain the main contraindications of opioids.

30. **A** Opioids can induce smooth muscle spasm in the sphincter of Oddi, thereby increasing intrabiliary pressure. The resulting intraductal back pressure can aggravate pain symptoms. Because the duration of biliary hypertension can outlast the analgesic effect, it is better to avoid opioid analgesics in treating biliary colic.

    B Patients with hypothyroidism may have prolonged and exaggerated responses to opioids.

    C, D Opioids do not have these effects.

    E Opioids can cause nausea and vomiting, but they decrease the risk of nausea and vomiting when these symptoms are due to visceral pain.

Learning objective: Describe the main contraindications of opioids.

31. **D** Pentazocine is an opioid drug that can cause a dose-dependent increase in arterial pressure, pulmonary pressure, and heart rate. For this reason, the drug is generally contraindicated in myocardial infarction.

    A–C These opioids are indicated, not contraindicated, in myocardial infarction.

    E Methadone is not contraindicated in myocardial infarction, but it is less suitable than morphine or meperidine because of its slow onset of action.

Learning objective: Explain the main contraindications of opioids.

32. **B** Morphine and other μ (mu) opioid receptor agonists are universally used for the treatment of acute postsurgical pain. However, they have an inhibitory effect on gastrointestinal tract motility and are therefore absolutely contraindicated in treating ileus that can occur mainly after abdominal surgery, as in this case.

    A, C–E These are analgesic-antipyretic drugs that are not contraindicated for this patient.

Learning objective: Explain the main contraindications of opioids.

33. **D** The patient's vital signs suggest that head trauma had increased intracranial pressure. When this pressure is substantially elevated over a short period, there is a stimulation of the vasomotor area (which causes hypertension) and stimulation of vagal outflow (which causes bradycardia). Opioid analgesics generally are avoided in patients with head injury for the following reasons:

    - Opioids induce carbon dioxide retention, which in turn causes vasodilation of the cerebral arteries and a consequent increase in intracranial pressure, which might be already elevated because of the head injury, as in this case.
    - Head injury potentiates the respiratory depressant effects of opioids.

    A–C, E Nonsteroidal antiinflammatory drugs are not contraindicated in cases of head trauma.

Learning objective: Outline the therapeutic uses of opioids.

34. **D** The patient's signs and symptoms indicate that he was most likely receiving an opioid analgesic. Opioid analgesics such as morphine are the only analgesics that can reduce the affective aspect of pain experience ("It doesn't bother me so much"). The sedative effect of opioids can explain the patient's drowsiness during the day, and the opioid-induced increased tone of the internal sphincter of the bladder can explain the difficulty in voiding.

A Amitriptyline can have analgesic effects (mainly in neuropathic pain) but does not alter the affective aspect of pain experience.

B, F Acetaminophen and ketorolac are less effective than opioids as analgesics and do not reduce the affective aspect of pain experience.

C, E Haloperidol and diazepam can alter the affective aspect of the environment, but they are devoid of analgesic properties.

Learning objective: Outline the therapeutic uses of opioids.

35. **E** When cancer pain is severe and no longer relieved by nonsteroidal antiinflammatory drugs, an opioid analgesic is usually needed. Methadone is a strong opioid with excellent oral bioavailability and a long half-life (about 25 hours). Therefore, its administration is most convenient for the patient, and a single daily dose can provide adequate, continuous coverage.

A See correct answer explanation.

B, D Morphine and fentanyl are effective analgesics, but the administration route is more difficult and can be painful in cachectic patients with terminal cancer, as in this case.

C Tramadol is a mild analgesic and is not appropriate for strong pain.

Learning objective: Outline the therapeutic uses of opioids.

36. **D** Conscious sedation is aimed at providing alleviation of anxiety and pain, together with a diminished (but not abolished) state of consciousness. Benzodiazepines and opioids are used most often to obtain conscious sedation because this treatment has the advantage of being reversible by specific receptor antagonists (flumazenil and naloxone, respectively). The use of opioids must be very cautious in cases of head trauma because these drugs tend to increase intracranial pressure. In this case, the fact that the patient did not lose consciousness and had intact reflexes suggests that intracranial injury was unlikely and that the behavior of the patient was mainly related to pain.

A Ibuprofen and codeine are mild analgesic drugs and therefore are not useful in this setting.

B Buspirone is an anxiolytic drug with negligible hypnotic activity, and its antianxiety effect may take more than a week to become established. Therefore, it is not useful for acute treatments.

C Zolpidem is a hypnotic drug used only for treatment of insomnia.

E Diazepam could be appropriate, but acetaminophen is a mild analgesic and therefore not useful in this setting.

Learning objective: Outline the therapeutic uses of tramadol.

37. **D** The patient's history and symptoms indicate that he was most likely suffering from postherpetic neuralgia, a painful condition that develops after a case of shingles. Shingles is a very common disease (about one million cases every year in the United States), and a number of shingles cases convert to postherpetic neuralgia. Three major classes of medications are commonly used in the treatment of neuropathic pain: antidepressants, especially tricyclics; anticonvulsants, especially gabapentin and carbamazepine; and sodium channel blockers, especially mexiletine. Opioids are usually not very effective, but tramadol is a unique dual-acting opioid agent, as it is a weak agonist at μ (mu) receptors but also inhibits the neuronal reuptake of serotonin and norepinephrine. It has shown effectiveness in a number of neuropathic pain states, including postherpetic neuralgia.

A, F Antipyretics-analgesics are minimally effective against neuropathic pain.

B Some anticonvulsants are effective in neuropathic pain, but ethosuximide is ineffective.

C Benzodiazepines have no analgesic effects.

E Serotonin and norepinephrine reuptake inhibitors such as venlafaxine and duloxetine are effective in neuropathic pain, but selective serotonin reuptake inhibitors are not.

Learning objective: Outline the therapeutic uses of meperidine.

38. **D** Postanesthetic shivering is a common symptom after anesthesia, affecting 40 to 60% of patients who receive volatile anesthetics. Postanesthetic shivering can be subdivided into

- Thermoregulated shivering (with vasoconstriction), which is a normal response to hypothermia
- Nonthermoregulated shivering (without vasoconstriction). The mechanism is unknown but seems related to postoperative pain.

Because many neuronal systems appear to modulate central thermoregulation, numerous drugs can have antishivering properties, including α_2 agonists (clonidine), cholinergic agonists (physostigmine), 5-HT$_3$ antagonists (ondansetron), and opiates (meperidine, morphine, fentanyl, and tramadol). Meperidine is more effective than equianalgesic concentration of other opiates and is currently used for postanesthetic shivering. The mechanism is still uncertain but seems to be related to activation of κ (kappa) receptors and/or to activation of a subtype of α_2 receptors.

A–C, E See correct answer explanation.

Learning objective: Outline the therapeutic uses of opioid antagonists.

39. **C** The signs of the patient suggest that the mother was treated with morphine during labor. In this instance, the newborn baby can present signs of morphine overdose (pinpoint pupil, respiratory and central nervous system [CNS] depression) because the drug easily crosses the placenta. Naloxone, injected into the umbilical vein, easily counteracts the morphine-induced respiratory and central nervous system depression. Because naloxone actions are short, additional doses may be needed to maintain morphine reversal.

A Flumazenil can counteract the depressive CNS effects induced by benzodiazepines, but not the ones induced by opioids. Moreover, diazepam is not an analgesic drug and does not cause all the symptoms shown by the baby.

B, D Theophylline and caffeine can have respiratory stimulant properties, but they are functional antagonists of morphine-induced respiratory depression and therefore much less effective than naloxone, which is a pharmacological antagonist.

E, F Albuterol and ipratropium are bronchodilating agents and are therefore useless in case of depression of the respiratory center.

Learning objective: Outline the therapeutic uses of codeine/acetaminophen combination.

40. **C** The codeine/acetaminophen combination is the one most frequently used to treat mild or moderate postsurgical pain. The onset of action is rapid, and it can be titrated to effect.

A, B, D, E These combinations are not currently used to treat moderate postsurgical pain. Moreover, all these combinations include a nonsteroidal antiinflammatory drug. These agents are contraindicated in patients with present or past history of peptic ulcer, as in this case.

Learning objective: Explain the reason for the use of buprenorphine/naloxone combination in the treatment of opioid dependence.

41. **D** Naloxone is combined with buprenorphine in a sublingual preparation called suboxone. The aim of the combination was to prevent intravenous (IV) buprenorphine abuse. It is known that opioid addicts often dilute an opioid preparation and inject it IV. When given by the sublingual route, naloxone

is minimally absorbed, whereas buprenorphine absorption is good (about 70%). If the combination is given IV, naloxone should block buprenorphine's rewarding effects and even throw the addict into precipitated withdrawal. However, it is worth noting that these effects of the combination can be achieved, at best, only partially, because buprenorphine has a higher affinity for opioid receptors than naloxone and dissociates very slowly from opioid receptors.

A–C, E None of these effects will occur, as the sublingual absorption of naloxone is negligible.

Learning objective: Identify the drug whose analgesic effect is most likely due to its conversion to morphine.

42. **B** Nonsteroidal antiinflammatory drugs (NSAIDs) are particularly useful in the management of cancer-related bone pain, but when they cannot control it, the addition of an opioid is the best course of action. Because the pain is moderate, a mild opioid such as codeine can be appropriate. About 10% of the administered codeine is demethylated to morphine. Because codeine has an exceptionally low affinity for opioid receptors, its analgesic effect is most likely the result of its conversion to morphine. This conclusion is supported by pharmacokinetic data. It is known that an oral codeine dose of 120 mg is about equieffective to the standard intramuscular morphine dose of 10 mg. The oral bioavailability of codeine reported in the literature is 70 to 90%. Therefore, about 96 mg of the 120-mg dose can be absorbed, and 10% of that dose (i.e., 9.6 mg) is converted to morphine.

A, C–E None of these opioids are biotransformed to morphine.

OPIOID ANALGESICS AND ANTAGONISTS Answer key			
1. A	6. D	11. D	16. F
2. F	7. B	12. B	17. D
3. E	8. B	13. C	18. B
4. I	9. A	14. E	19. D
5. H	10. D	15. A	20. B
21. D	26. C	31. D	36. D
22. F	27. C	32. B	37. D
23. D	28. B	33. D	38. D
24. C	29. E	34. D	39. C
25. B	30. A	35. E	40. C
			41. D
			42. B

Answers and Explanations: III-13 Drugs of Abuse

Questions 1–5

1. **N**
2. **A**
3. **F**
4. **B**
5. **G**

Learning objective: Describe the adverse effects of cocaine.

6. **C** The patient's signs and symptoms indicate that he most likely took a high dose of cocaine. Formication ("Bugs are crawling under my skin"), stereotyped behavior, and paranoid delusions, together with signs of sympathetic overactivity (hypertension and tachycardia), are classic symptoms of cocaine overdose.

    A, B, D These drugs do not cause all the symptoms exhibited by the patient.

    E Phencyclidine can cause many signs and symptoms similar to those of cocaine, but the patient is usually disoriented, and nystagmus is a prominent sign. Both are absent in this patient.

Learning objective: Describe the adverse effects of cocaine.

7. **D** Behavioral stereotypy is a prominent symptom of chronic use of high doses of psychostimulants such as cocaine and amphetamines. Stereotyped behavior is characterized by repetitive and purposeless motor actions, and it has been postulated to result from an abnormal dopamine response after long-term use.

    A Even after high doses of cocaine, the person usually remains alert and oriented.

    B, C, E These symptoms usually occur when cocaine is withdrawn, but opposite symptoms occur as long as sufficient cocaine levels are present in the body.

Learning objective: Explain the mechanism of action of cannabinoids.

8. **A** The boy's signs and symptoms indicate that he was most likely using cannabis. Cannabinoid receptors have been found in the human brain, and endogenous ligands (anandamide and 2-arachidonyl glycerol) have been identified that act as neurotransmitters. These receptors are widely distributed in the cerebral cortex, hippocampus, striatum, and cerebellum and are mainly located presynaptically, thus inhibiting the release of glutamate or gamma-aminobutyric acid (GABA). The physiological role of these receptors and their endogenous ligands is not completely understood, but they most likely have important functions because of their wide location. For example, in the hippocampus, they may contribute to induction of synaptic plasticity during memory formation.

    B–E These actions would not cause all the symptoms exhibited by the patient.

Learning objective: Describe the adverse effects of marijuana.

9. **B** The two most characteristic somatic effects of cannabinoids in humans are increased pulse rate and reddening of conjunctiva, which is related to the general vasodilation induced by these drugs.

    A Cannabinoids can cause vasodilation, which in turn causes a dose-related decrease in blood pressure. Postural hypotension, not hypertension, is evident.

    C Cannabinoids produce changes in mood, but the most common psychic effects are euphoria and disinhibition, not depression.

    D In fact, cannabinoids have a weak but clinically significant analgesic action.

    E Although cannabinoids cause subjective feelings of confidence and heightened creativity, they usually lead to impairment of cognitive functions, learning, and memory.

    F Cannabinoids cause generalized vasodilation, so pale skin is unlikely.

Learning objective: Describe the adverse effects of LSD.

10. **C** The fact that the man perceived symptoms typical of LSD intoxication 2 months after taking the offending drug points out that he was most likely experiencing a flashback, a particularly troubling aftereffect of LSD and related drugs. The flashback (now called hallucinogen-persisting perception disorder) is a recurrence of part or all of a hallucinogenic drug experience, weeks or months after the drug was last taken. Some users have reported these perceptual sensations even years after the drug exposure. Precipitating conditions include stress, fatigue, anxiety states, emergence into a dark environment, and neuroleptics.

    A, B, D–F These syndromes lack the symptoms described by the patient.

Learning objective: Describe the pharmacological therapy of nicotine dependence.

11. **B** Bupropion is an atypical antidepressant structurally similar to diethylpropion, an amphetamine-like appetite suppressant. The drug inhibits reuptake of dopamine, noradrenaline, and serotonin in the central nervous system, is a noncompetitive nicotine receptor antagonist, and at high concentrations inhibits the firing of noradrenergic neurons in the locus ceruleus. It is not clear which of these effects accounts for the usefulness of bupropion during smoking cessation, but all could be important. During nicotine withdrawal, there is a reduction in central dopamine and norepinephrine levels and increased firing in the locus ceruleus. The antismoking effect of bupropion does not seem to be related to the antidepressant effect, as bupropion is equally effective as a smoking cessation therapy in smokers with and without depression. The drug can achieve long-term abstinence in about 20% of smokers. Other drugs used for smoking cessation are clonidine and varenicline.

    A, C–F See correct answer explanation.

Learning objective: Outline the pharmacological therapy of opiate withdrawal.

12. **B** The patient's symptoms indicate that he was most likely experiencing heroin withdrawal. Administration of an opioid drug acting mainly on μ (mu) receptors is the best strategy to attenuate withdrawal from opiates. Methadone was the preferred drug in the past, because it has a long duration of action and can be tapered slowly to minimize abstinence symptoms. More recently, buprenorphine has been shown to work better than other opioids for treating withdrawal from opiates and is now the drug most frequently used for this purpose.

    A, C–F See correct answer explanation.

Learning objective: Outline the use of buprenorphine in the long-term management of opiate dependence.

13. **B** Detoxification from opioids follows the general principles that are valid for all drugs of abuse. It is convenient to change the patient from an intravenous opioid such as heroin to an orally active and pharmacologically equivalent opioid, then to reduce the dose of that opioid gradually. Methadone was extensively used in the past, but more recently the introduction of buprenorphine, a partial μ (mu) opioid agonist, has represented a major change in the treatment of opiate addiction. The drug produces minimal withdrawal symptoms when stopped and has low potential for overdose, a long duration of action, and the ability to block heroin effects.

A Benzodiazepines are sometimes used to sedate a person under heroin withdrawal, but they are not suitable to achieve the goal of a drug-free patient.

C Naltrexone blocks the euphoric effect of opioids and is therefore used to prevent relapse and eventually to extinguish the habit, once the addict has become drug-free, but it can precipitate withdrawal if used in a person still physically dependent on opioids.

D–F These drugs are not used in opioid detoxification.

Learning objective: Describer the symptoms and signs of steroid abuse.

14. **E** The patient's signs and symptoms, as well as his personal history (he is a body builder), suggest that an anabolic steroid is most likely the culprit drug. Anabolic steroids are often abused by people engaging in competitive sports; by body builders, for example. The primary effects sought are increased muscle mass and strength. Among the manifestations of heavy use are increased irritability and aggression (common), changes in libido and sexual functions, and mood changes with occasional psychotic features.

    A–C Overdose of these drugs rarely causes aggressive behavior, and all can be detected by routine drug screening.

    D, F Mifepristone and danazol are not abused drugs.

Learning objective: Describe the pharmacological effects of marijuana.

15. **B** The girl's signs and symptoms indicate that she most likely smoked marijuana cigarettes. Tachycardia and reddening of the conjunctiva are the two most characteristic somatic effects of cannabinoids in humans. Other symptoms are euphoria, uncontrollable laughter, depersonalization, and sharpened vision, as in this case.

    A, C–E The behavioral signs and symptoms caused by these drugs are different from those exhibited by this girl. Moreover, a typical somatic effect of LSD and cocaine is mydriasis, whereas heroin and phencyclidine cause miosis, neither of which occurred in this girl.

Learning objective: Describe the use of naltrexone in ethanol dependence.

16. **D** Experimental studies in animals suggest that alcohol drinking is influenced by opiate receptor activity and is reduced by opiate antagonist action. Several clinical trials have shown that naltrexone decreases the rate of relapse to alcohol consumption and reduces alcohol craving. The drug has been approved by the U.S. Food and Drug Administration for this purpose.

    A, B Diazepam and clonidine are used to treat ethanol abstinence syndrome, but they do not reduce ethanol craving in alcoholics.

C Disulfiram is used to induce a conditioned aversion to alcohol, but the rationale for its use is not based on a relationship between ethanol craving and opioid activity.

E, F Methadone and buprenorphine are not used to treat ethanol dependence.

Learning objective: Describe the signs and symptoms of opiate withdrawal.

17. **A** The patient's signs and symptoms indicate that heroin was the drug from which he was experiencing withdrawal. Opioid abstinence syndrome includes

- Prodromal phase, characterized by autonomic activation (rhinorrhea, lacrimation, salivation, yawning, and sweating) that lasts 6 to 10 hours
- Acute withdrawal syndrome, characterized by a high degree of behavioral, somatic, and autonomic activation (restlessness, shaking chills, piloerection, nausea, abdominal cramps, etc.) that lasts about 7 to 10 days.
- Protracted withdrawal syndrome, characterized by subtle signs and symptoms that can persist for up to 6 months. During this period, the recidivism rate is high.

B, C Abstinence syndrome from these drugs is primarily characterized by depressive symptoms (depression, sleepiness, and fatigue).

D–F There is no evidence of a clinically significant withdrawal syndrome for these drugs in humans.

Learning objective: Describe the signs and symptoms of opiate poisoning.

18. **B** The triad of coma, miosis, and respiratory depression indicates that heroin was most likely the drug the woman had self-injected. Accidental overdosage is not uncommon in addicts, as the dose of an illicit drug is never accurate. The respiratory rate can be very low, or the patient may even be apneic, and cyanosis is often present. The pupils are symmetrical and pinpoint in size, although if hypoxia is severe, they may be dilated. Blood pressure can be near normal at first but falls progressively.

A, C–F Overdose of these drugs is not characterized by pinpoint pupils.

Learning objective: Describe the main symptoms of nicotine abstinence.

19. **A** Upon sudden cessation of smoking tobacco, individuals who smoke 20 or more cigarettes daily develop an abstinence syndrome, which is usually not severe. Its main features are

- Irritability and restlessness (the most common symptoms)
- Craving for cigarettes (usually intense and persistent)
- Insomnia

- Fatigue
- Difficulty in concentrating
- Dysphoric, anxious, or depressed mood
- Cough, dry throat, nasal drip
- Constipation, stomach pain
- Decreased heart rate, hypotension
- Increased appetite and weight gain

B–E Nicotine abstinence symptoms are opposite to those listed in these options.

Learning objective: Describe the signs and symptoms of benzodiazepine withdrawal.

20. **C** People who have been using high doses of benzodiazepines, such as alprazolam, for long periods can experience withdrawal symptoms on abrupt termination of the administration. The withdrawal syndrome may include the following symptoms:

- Following moderate dose usage: anxiety, agitation, increased sensitivity to light and sound, paresthesias, myoclonic jerks, sleep disturbances, dizziness
- Following high-dose usage: delirium, seizure

The abrupt onset of the withdrawal syndrome, as well as its severity, is a function of the half-life of the drug. Benzodiazepines with shorter elimination half-lives (alprazolam, lorazepam, temazepam, and midazolam) produce a rapidly evolving and severe withdrawal syndrome (symptoms within 12 to 24 hours after the last dose), whereas those with longer half-lives usually have a built-in tapering-off action that makes the withdrawal syndrome less severe but longer in duration.

A No withdrawal syndrome from a hallucinogenic drug such as LSD has been observed.

B, D–F Seizures are exceptionally rare in withdrawal syndromes from these drugs.

Learning objective: Explain the mechanism of action of disulfiram.

21. **B** The history and symptoms of the patient point out that the administered drug was most likely disulfiram, an agent approved by the U.S. Food and Drug Administration for the treatment of alcoholism. By inhibiting aldehyde dehydrogenase, disulfiram causes an accumulation of acetaldehyde, the substance responsible for the toxic symptoms exhibited by the patient. The rationale behind the therapy with disulfiram is based on the premise that the patient will not drink ethanol because of the unpleasant effect that occurs when ethanol is administered with disulfiram. Although effective pharmacologically, the drug has not been found effective in clinical trials because compliance with this therapy is often very low.

A, C–E See correct answer explanation.

Learning objective: Describe the adverse effects of cannabis.

22. **E** The signs of the patient (reddening of the conjunctiva with no change in pupil diameter, a fast pulse, and a diffuse tremor) suggest that the boy was smoking marijuana and was experiencing an acute panic reaction. This reaction is the most frequently reported adverse effect of cannabis, and several surveys indicate that about one half of cannabis users have reported at least one panic experience.

    A, B Amphetamine and cocaine would have caused pronounced mydriasis.

    C A panic reaction is exceptionally rare with gamma-hydroxybutyric acid.

    D Heroin would have caused pronounced miosis.

Learning objective: Describe the signs and symptoms of delirium tremens.

23. **E** Delirium tremens characterizes stage 4 of ethanol abstinence syndrome. It includes terrifying visual (or, less frequently, auditory or tactile) hallucinations, marked weakness, gross disorientation in space and time, confusion, aggression, extreme psychic agitation, coarse tremors of the hands, head, and trunk, marked ataxia, nystagmus, muscular cramps, and signs of autonomic activation (sweating, nausea and vomiting, abdominal pain, hypertension, mydriasis, tachycardia, tachypnea, and hyperthermia). The life-threatening potential of alcohol abstinence syndrome is the highest of all such syndromes. When delirium tremens occurs, the mortality ranges from 5 to 15%, despite appropriate treatment, and is about 35% in untreated cases. Death usually occurs from respiratory failure and cardiac arrhythmias.

    A Mydriasis, not miosis, is a prominent symptom.

    B Hypertension, not hypotension, is present in most cases.

    C Hyperthermia, not hypothermia, is a prominent symptom.

    D Muscular cramps, not relaxation, is a prominent symptom.

Learning objective: Describe the symptoms of ethanol withdrawal.

24. **C** Ethanol withdrawal can occur when an alcoholic person is forced to stop drinking because of some external event, such as the hospital admission in this case. The signs and symptoms of the patient (agitation, tremulousness, and hallucinations) are consistent with the first phase of alcohol withdrawal that typically occurs 8 to 48 hours after the last ethanol intake.

    A, B, D, E These events do not cause the syndrome exhibited by the patient.

Learning objective: Describe the adverse effects of cocaine.

25. **E** Smoking freebase cocaine (crack) is a common cause of diffuse alveolar hemorrhage. Other causes are Goodpasture syndrome, systemic lupus erythematosus, systemic vasculitis, and rapidly progressing glomerulonephritis. Bilateral alveolar infiltrates are typical of diffuse alveolar hemorrhage. Bronchoscopy is the most useful procedure in defining bleeding sites and determining whether they are local or diffuse.

    A–D None of these drugs cause diffuse alveolar hemorrhage.

Learning objective: Describe the illicit uses of gamma-hydroxybutyric acid (GHB).

26. **F** The girl was most likely raped after a drug was added to her drink. Such "date rape" drugs can be used to assist in the commission of a sexual assault. Drugs used to facilitate rape may have sedative, hypnotic, dissociative, or amnesiac effects and can be added to food or drink without the victim's knowledge. The three most commonly used date rape drugs are alcohol, gamma-hydroxybutyric acid (GHB), and benzodiazepines (e.g., flunitrazepam). Alcohol is most frequently implicated in substance-assisted sexual assault. Both benzodiazepines and GHB can cause anterograde amnesia, thus making the victim unable to recall the sexual assault.

    A–E These are not "date rape" drugs.

Learning objective: Describe the signs and symptoms of methanol poisoning.

27. **F** Methanol (methyl alcohol) is extensively used in cleaning products, fuel for small stoves, paint strippers, and gas line antifreeze. Poisoning sometimes occurs in homeless alcoholics who drink methanol when they are out of money and cannot purchase the daily amount of alcohol they require. Symptoms of methanol poisoning may appear as soon as 12 hours following ingestion, but they usually develop 24 hours after ingestion. These may resemble ethanol intoxication and consist of drowsiness, confusion, and ataxia, as well as weakness, headache, nausea, vomiting, and abdominal pain. Methanol toxicity in humans is primarily due to metabolism to formaldehyde and formic acid, a reaction catalyzed by the enzyme alcohol dehydrogenase. As methanol metabolism proceeds, the accumulation of these metabolites leads to a severe anion gap metabolic acidosis. Severe metabolic acidosis in conjunction with visual effects is the hallmark of methanol poisoning. Patients usually describe blurred or misty vision (e.g., being in a snowstorm), double vision, or changes in color perception. There may be constricted visual

field and, occasionally, total loss of vision. Characteristic visual dysfunctions include pupillary dilation and loss of pupillary reflex. Treatment of methanol poisoning includes suppression of its metabolism to toxic products. Because ethanol is metabolized preferentially by alcohol dehydrogenase, its administration (orally or intravenously) can retard the biotransformation of methanol to its toxic metabolites. A more specific inhibitor of alcohol dehydrogenase, fomepizole, has been approved for treatment of methanol and ethylene glycol poisoning.

A–E These syndromes do not cause the signs and symptoms exhibited by the patient.

Learning objective: List the main risks of cannabis use in people with a history of schizoaffective disorder.

28. **C** The ordinary use of cannabis produces little or no disturbances of behavior in people with stable personality. However, there are numerous clinical reports that cannabis use can precipitate a recurrence in people with a history of schizophrenia.

A A depressive episode after cannabis use is extremely rare.

B, D, E Cannabis use does not increase the risk of these disorders.

Learning objective: Identify the drug of abuse that does not result in physical or psychological dependence.

29. **C** Unlike most recreational drugs, hallucinogenic agents such as LSD induce neither physical nor psychological dependence and therefore do not lead to addiction. A likely reason for this is that these drugs primarily influence cortical and thalamic circuits and do not activate the mesolimbic dopamine reward system.

A, B, D–F All of these drugs can cause more or less pronounced physical dependence when used chronically.

Learning objective: Describe the syndrome of cocaine overdose.

30. **G** The patient's syndrome was most likely due to cocaine overdose. This syndrome is often rapidly fatal because of seizures, respiratory depression, and arrhythmias, as in this case.

A Death can occur from heroin overdose, but the syndrome is characterized by coma, shallow breathing, and miotic, not mydriatic, pupils.

B Death can occur from gamma-hydroxybutyric acid overdose, but the syndrome is characterized by coma, myoclonic

movements, bradycardia (about 30% of patients), and hypothermia, not hyperthermia.

C–F The risk of death from overdose by these drugs is negligible.

Learning objective: Explain the mechanism of action of phencyclidine.

31. **E** The vertical and horizontal nystagmus showed by the patient suggests that she smoked phencyclidine-drugged cigarettes. Nystagmus (vertical, horizontal, or rotatory) is considered a hallmark of phencyclidine intoxication, as it is present in up to 69% of cases. Phencyclidine binds with high affinity and blocks the *N*-methyl-D-aspartate (NMDA) subtype of glutamate receptors in the brain. This seems to be the main mechanism of action of the drug, but other mechanisms have been proposed, including the activation of μ (mu) opioid receptors, which may account for its analgesic properties.

A–D See correct answer explanation.

Learning objective: Describe the adverse effects of LSD.

32. **F** The symptoms and signs of the patient indicate that she had taken LSD (lysergic acid diethylamide) and was experiencing a mild adverse mental effect that in the users' jargon is a "bad trip." A more severe psychotic reaction can rarely occur with terrifying hallucinations, panic reactions, loss of emotional control, and cataleptic behavior. The users refer to this as a "freak-out."

A Cocaine can cause some of the patient's signs and symptoms (mydriasis, tachycardia, increased blood pressure, sweating, and tremor), but the type of illusion she experienced (room furniture being "alive") is an extremely rare effect of cocaine overdose.

B Opioid effects are mainly depressant in nature, and miosis, not mydriasis, is a prominent sign.

C A very large dose of cannabinoids can cause distortion of visual perception and hallucinations, but these are usually accompanied by drowsiness and lethargy, not by excitation.

D Amyl nitrite is a volatile liquid that is sometimes abused to enhance orgasm. It can only produce a transient feeling of "rush," flushing, and dizziness.

E Phencyclidine causes effects that can be similar to those of LSD, but nystagmus is a prominent effect of the drug and is absent in this patient.

Learning objective: Describe the adverse effects of phencyclidine.

33. **C** The signs and symptoms of the patient suggest that phencyclidine was most likely the self-administered drug. Phencyclidine causes effects that are different from those of psychedelic drugs such as LSD. In low doses, the drug causes emotional withdrawal, inebriation, ataxia, changes in body image, and a mind–body dissociative feeling. Horizontal nystagmus, vertical nystagmus, or both are often present and are considered hallmarks of phencyclidine intoxication. As the dose of phencyclidine increases, the patient may manifest agitation, hostile and assaultive behavior (unlike psychedelic drugs, which very rarely cause such behavior). The action of the drug on the autonomic nervous system becomes more prominent and is characterized by a confusing combination of adrenergic, cholinergic, and dopaminergic effects. A hypertensive response is typically encountered. Tachycardia, tachypnea, hyperthermia, and miosis (or, more rarely, mydriasis) may also be noted. The agitated, combative patient often has feelings of great strength. This, combined with the anesthetic effect of the drug, can result in serious injury because there is no pain sensation to stop the physical activity. With very large doses, catatonia and coma can occur with muscular rigidity that can cause rhabdomyolysis.

    A, B, D, E All of these drugs can cause some or many of the symptoms exhibited by the patient, but nystagmus is rare.

Learning objective: Describe the use of ethanol in ethylene glycol poisoning.

34. **C** Poisoning by ethylene glycol is not uncommon in young children because of its sweet taste. The chemical itself is relatively nontoxic, but it is biotransformed into hippuric, oxalic, and glycolic acids by the enzyme alcohol dehydrogenase. These metabolites are toxic and can cause severe metabolic acidosis, renal failure, and coma. Metabolism of ethylene glycol to its toxic products can be blocked by inhibiting alcohol dehydrogenase. Ethanol is metabolized preferentially by alcohol dehydrogenase; therefore, its administration (orally or intravenously) can retard the biotransformation of ethylene glycol to its toxic metabolites.

    A, B, D, E See correct answer explanation.

Learning objective: List the main risks of cannabinoid use.

35. **D** Because cannabis alters the sense of time and spatial perception, the risk of driving or work accidents is increased in people who are using cannabis.

    A There is no recorded death from parenteral injection of pure hashish oil. The therapeutic index of cannabinoids is exceedingly high.

    B A mild abstinence syndrome has been described following chronic use of very high doses. The syndrome includes increased restlessness, irritability, confusion, insomnia, sleep disturbances, nausea, cramping, and sweating. The syndrome is never lethal.

    C, E There are no data reported in the literature of an increased risk of these diseases with the use of cannabis.

Learning objective: Explain the mechanism of action of methylenedioxymethamphetamine (MDMA).

36. **B** The patient's signs and symptoms (hyperthermia, mental status changes, and muscle rigidity) suggest that he was most likely suffering from serotonin syndrome. MDMA causes the release of monoamines by reversing the action of their respective transporters. It has a preferential affinity for serotonin transporter resulting in increased synaptic levels of serotonin. The release of this neurotransmitter is so great that there is a marked intracellular depletion for 24 hours after a single dose

    A, C–F See correct answer explanation.

Learning objective: Calculate the quantity of ethanol consumed by a subject, given sufficient data.

37. **B** The quantity of a drug in a person's body can be calculated by

$$\text{Amount} = C_p \times V_d,$$

    where C_p is plasma concentration and V_d is volume of distribution. Therefore, the quantity in the patient's body on admission was about 225 g, a quantity close to the lethal dose for 50% of subjects (LD_{50}) of ethanol.

    A, C–F See correct answer explanation.

Learning objective: Describe the mechanism of action of LSD.

38. **D** LSD (lysergic acid diethylamide) is a semisynthetic ergot alkaloid. Extensive studies have shown that the drug, like most ergot derivatives, interacts with several serotonin receptor subtypes in the brain (mainly 5-HT_{1A} and 5-HT_{2A}) as a full or partial agonist. It appears to act as a full agonist at 5-HT_{1A} autoreceptors in raphe neurons, producing a marked slowing of the firing rate of serotonergic neurons. Action on 5-HT_{2A} receptors appears to disrupt thalamic gating, which in turn causes sensory overload of the brain cortex.

    A–C, E, F See correct answer explanation.

Learning objective: Describe the symptoms of amphetamine withdrawal.

39. **D** Signs and symptoms of withdrawal from an abused drug tend to be opposite to the original effects produced by that drug. Therefore, the withdrawal syndrome from psychostimulant drugs such as amphetamines and cocaine is manly depressant in nature and includes somnolence, headache, depression, and lack of motivation. Because amphetamine-like drugs cause anorexia, a ravenous appetite is also a prominent

symptom of withdrawal. The withdrawal syndrome from amphetamine-like drugs may last for several days.

A–C, E The withdrawal syndrome from these drugs is mainly excitatory in nature.

Learning objective: Describe the adverse effects of chronic ethanol use.

40. **E** Chronic use of high doses of ethanol can damage several organs, but the liver, brain, and heart are the ones most frequently involved. Dilated cardiomyopathy is due to extensive myocardial fibrosis with diffuse loss of myocytes. This results in thinning of heart walls, consequent dilation of ventricular chambers, and heart failure. Patients with advanced alcoholic cardiomyopathy and severe heart failure have a poor prognosis, particularly if they continue to drink; less than one quarter of such patients survive 3 years.

A–D, F The increased risk of these diseases due to alcoholism is low or negligible.

Learning objective: Describe the polyneuropathy that can occur after chronic administration of nitrous oxide.

41. **B** The patient was most likely suffering from polyneuropathy due to chronic administration of nitrous oxide. This gas can be found easily because it is used in the food and car industries. Common sources are cartridges used to recharge whipped cream containers. The brief euphoria produced by nitrous oxide makes it prone to abuse. The mechanism of nitrous oxide–induced neuropathy is still uncertain but seems related to a deficiency of vitamin B_{12}, because the drug inactivates the vitamin by oxidation of the cobalt atom. The deficiency is more likely in persons already at risk of vitamin B_{12} deficiency, as in this case (see the long history of alcoholism).

A Amyl nitrite is sometimes abused but does not cause polyneuropathy.

C–E These are not abused drugs.

Learning objective: Describe the pattern of central effects caused by inhalants.

42. **E** Inhalants are a group of substances whose chemical vapors can be inhaled to produce pleasant effects. Whereas other abused substances can be inhaled, the term *inhalants* is used to describe substances that are rarely, if ever, taken in any other way. A variety of products common in the home and workplace contain substances that can be inhaled. These include volatile solvents, such as glues and stain removers, and aerosols that contain propellants and solvents, such as deodorant sprays and whipped cream aerosols. Children and adolescents are particularly prone to this form of abuse because the chemicals can be easily found at home. Gases and vapors are rapidly absorbed when inhaled and tend to distribute preferentially in lipid-rich and highly perfused organs,

such as the brain and the liver. Nearly all inhalants have central nervous system (CNS) depressant effects, and evidence from animal studies suggests that their effects and mechanism of action are similar to those of alcohol and other sedative-hypnotics. They produce a temporary stimulation and reduced inhibition before the depressive CNS effects occur. Inhalant abuse is typically episodic in nature; thus, users may not be exposed to levels with sufficient frequency necessary to develop physical dependence. However, it is a very dangerous habit because inhaling highly concentrated amounts of the chemicals can cause heart failure and death within minutes after repeated inhalation (a syndrome known as "sudden sniffing death").

A–D See correct answer explanation.

Learning objective: Describe the interaction between ethanol and other central nervous system (CNS) depressants.

43. **C** The patient's history and blood exams suggest that his death was most likely due to a combination of heroin (which is converted to morphine) and alcohol. Ethanol enhances the sedative effects of most other CNS depressants, including sedative-hypnotics, opioids, several neuroleptics, and some antihistamines, as well as the effects of some psychostimulant drugs, including cocaine and amphetamine. The interaction between alcohol and sedative-hypnotics or opioids is particularly prominent, and several studies indicate that ethanol substantially decreases the minimum lethal concentration of heroin, as in this case.

A, B, D, E These drugs do not enhance the CNS depressant effects of opioids. Death due to a combination of an opioid and one of the listed drugs is exceptionally rare.

Learning objective: Differentiate between cocaine and methamphetamine effects.

44. **D** The patient's history and symptoms indicate that he was most likely suffering from a psychostimulant overdose. Cocaine and amphetamines have very similar physiological and psychological effects. Although the specific mechanisms of action are different, the final molecular action is quite similar; that is, both can increase the availability of monoamines in the synaptic cleft of brain neurons. This explains why even experienced drug users cannot distinguish the effect of the two drugs when they are injected intravenously; the orgasm-like sensation is practically the same. The patient's history, however, indicates that amphetamine was most likely the culprit drug, as the effects of amphetamine can last several hours, whereas the effects of cocaine generally last less than 1 hour.

A See correct answer explanation.

B, C, E, F These drugs do not cause the pattern of effects shown by the patient.

DRUGS of ABUSE			
	Answer key		
1. N	6. C	11. B	16. D
2. A	7. D	12. B	17. A
3. F	8. A	13. B	18. B
4. B	9. B	14. E	19. A
5. G	10. C	15. B	20. C
21. B	26. F	31. E	36. B
22. E	27. F	32. F	37. B
23. E	28. C	33. C	38. D
24. C	29. C	34. C	39. D
25. E	30. G	35. D	40. E
			41. B
			42. E
			43. C
			44. D

IV Cardiovascular and Renal Systems

Questions: IV-1 Diuretics

Directions for questions **1–5**

Match each diuretic with the appropriate description (each lettered option can be selected once, more than once, or not at all).

A. Acetazolamide
B. Amiloride
C. Conivaptan
D. Ethacrynic acid
E. Indapamide
F. Mannitol
G. Spironolactone
H. Triamterene

Difficulty level: Easy

1. This drug inhibits Na$^+$ reabsorption in the proximal tubule.

Difficulty level: Easy

2. This drug inhibits the synthesis of new Na$^+$ channels in the collecting duct.

Difficulty level: Easy

3. This drug causes an initial extracellular volume expansion in normal subjects.

Difficulty level: Easy

4. This drug increases the renal reabsorption of Ca^{2+}.

Difficulty level: Easy

5. This drug competitively blocks antidiuretic hormone receptors.

Difficulty level: Easy

6. A 56-year-old woman recently diagnosed with congestive heart failure started a therapy that included furosemide. Acetazolamide was added to counteract the potential metabolic alkalosis induced by furosemide. Which of the following molecular actions most likely mediated the therapeutic effect of acetazolamide in this patient?

A. Inhibition of carbonic acid dehydration in the tubular lumen
B. Stimulation of bicarbonate reabsorption in the proximal tubule
C. Inhibition of Na$^+$ reabsorption in the early distal tubule
D. Stimulation of H$^+$ reabsorption in the proximal tubule
E. Stimulation of carbonic acid formation inside the tubular cells

Difficulty level: Medium

7. A 27-year-old woman with a history of high altitude sickness was placed on prophylactic treatment with a diuretic drug prior to going on a hiking trip in the Rocky Mountains. Which of the following urine electrolyte profiles is most consistent with this drug treatment?

	HCO$_3^-$	Na$^+$	Ca^{2+}	K$^+$
P	++	+	0	+
Q	+	++	+	+
R	+	++	–	++
S	+	+++	+	++
T	0	+	–	–

Note: +, increased; –, decreased; 0, negligible changes.

A. Profile P
B. Profile Q
C. Profile R
D. Profile S
E. Profile T

Difficulty level: Medium

8. A 69-year-old depressed man with a 10-year history of glaucoma was admitted to the emergency department after he took several tablets of one of his medications in a suicide attempt. The patient was drowsy and complained of nausea, paresthesias, and tiredness. Physical examination revealed erythematous skin eruptions. Lab tests indicated hyperchloremic metabolic acidosis. Which of the following medications might have caused the patient's symptoms?

A. Mannitol
B. Latanoprost
C. Timolol
D. Acetazolamide
E. Pilocarpine

Difficulty level: Hard

9. A 55-year-old alcoholic man was admitted to the emergency department because of disorientation, amnesia, confusion, and bizarre behavior for the past 24 hours. His wife reported that the man was being treated for hypertension and for recently diagnosed glaucoma. Physical examination revealed a cachectic male in a confused mental state. His abdomen appeared tense with prominent veins and ascites, and a musty, pungent odor was noted in his breath. Neurologic signs included nystagmus, ataxia, and asterixis. Which of the following drugs most likely triggered the patient's syndrome?

A. Acetazolamide
B. Nifedipine
C. Losartan
D. Timolol
E. Lovastatin

Difficulty level: Easy

10. A 54-year-old woman recently diagnosed with open-angle glaucoma was prescribed topical timolol. Two weeks later, intraocular pressure was decreased but was still above the normal value. The ophthalmologist decided to add a topical drug that acts by decreasing aqueous humor production. Which of the following drugs was most likely prescribed as the second drug?

A. Pilocarpine
B. Carbachol
C. Latanoprost
D. Dorzolamide
E. Mannitol

Difficulty level: Hard

11. A 15-year-old boy awoke with weakness and 1 hour later realized that he could not move his legs. The attack lasted about 2 hours but then disappeared without residual symptoms. The boy was referred to a neurologic clinic, where the diagnosis of familial hypokalemic periodic paralysis was made. He was prescribed potassium chloride and a diuretic that is able to prevent the attacks in many cases. Which of the following drugs was most likely prescribed?

A. Mannitol
B. Hydrochlorothiazide
C. Ethacrynic acid
D. Triamterene
E. Acetazolamide

Difficulty level: Medium

12. A 67-year-old man was found to have a plasma calcium level of 12.2 mg/dL during a follow-up visit. The man had a 3-year history of Hodgkin lymphoma. He was recently diagnosed with nephrolithiasis for which he had been treated with hydrochlorothiazide for the past 3 weeks. Which of the following best explains the most likely mechanism of thiazide-induced hypercalcemia?

A. Activation of the Na^+/Ca^{2+} exchanger in the distal tubule
B. Increased Ca^{2+} reabsorption in the proximal tubule
C. Decreased secretion of parathyroid hormone
D. Decreased renal excretion of vitamin D
E. Activation of $Na^+/K^+/2Cl^-$ symporter in the thick ascending loop of Henle
F. Increased glomerular filtration of Ca^{2+}

Difficulty level: Medium

13. A 67-year-old woman was found to have a plasma level of potassium 2.8 mEq/L (normal 3.5–5.0 mEq/L) during a follow-up visit. The woman had been receiving hydrochlorothiazide for 1 month to treat her recently diagnosed essential hypertension. Which of the following actions most likely contributed to the thiazide-induced increase in renal excretion of potassium?

A. Increased Na^+ load in the lumen of the collecting tubule
B. Blockade of $Na^+/K^+/2Cl^-$ cotransporter
C. Thiazide-induced decrease in renal secretion of uric acid
D. Stimulation of Na^+/K^+ pump
E. Decreased delivery of bicarbonate to the collecting duct

Difficulty level: Hard

14. A 52-year-old alcoholic man suffering from liver cirrhosis was admitted to the emergency department because of a 2-week history of nausea, vomiting, and lower abdominal cramps. Physical examination showed a tense abdomen with prominent veins, and 3+ ascites was noted by shifting dullness and a fluid wave. A diagnosis of ascites was made, and an appropriate therapy was started. Which of the following diuretics would be contraindicated for this patient?

A. Ethacrynic acid
B. Spironolactone
C. Acetazolamide
D. Furosemide
E. Triamterene

Difficulty level: Hard

15. A 76-year-old woman from a nursing home presented to the emergency department with a change in her mental state over the past few hours. She had a medical history of coronary artery disease and hypertension. Her medications included aspirin, captopril, lovastatin, and a diuretic. On physical examination she showed decreased skin turgor, orthostatic hypotension, and disorientation to time, place, and person without focal neurologic deficits. Pertinent blood test results on admission were Na^+ 125 mEq/L, creatinine 2.7 mg/dL. Which of the following drugs most likely caused the patient's syndrome?

A. Captopril
B. Spironolactone
C. Lovastatin
D. Triamterene
E. Acetazolamide
F. Indapamide

Difficulty level: Hard

16. A 47-year-old woman suffering from metastatic breast cancer was admitted to the emergency department because of persistent thirst and polyuria. Pertinent serum values on admission were serum K^+ 2.8 mEq/L (normal 3.5–5.0 mEq/L); Ca 16.2 mg/dL (normal 8.5–10.5 mg/dL); Na^+ 155 mEq/L (normal 136–145 mEq/L). Urinalysis: specific gravity 1.001; osmolality 80 mOsm/L (range 50–1440 mOsm/L); chemistry and sediment negative. The patient was given a water deprivation test: all fluids were withheld until serum osmolality increased into the hyperosmolar range (> 310), then 5 units of vasopressin were given subcutaneously. Results are shown in the following table.

	Urine Osmolality (mOsm/L)	Serum Osmolality (mOsm/L)
Onset of test	80	292
Water deprivation	82	312
After vasopressin	84	310

Which of these drugs would be most appropriate to treat the patient's condition?

A. Desmopressin
B. Hydrochlorothiazide
C. Demeclocycline
D. Amiloride
E. Furosemide

Difficulty level: Medium

17. A 63-year-old man with a long history of heart failure was admitted to the emergency department because of severe dyspnea and edema in his legs, thighs, and lower abdominal wall. Pertinent lab results on admission included a glomerular filtration rate of 20 mL/min. A diuretic with which of the following mechanism of action would be appropriate to relieve the edema in this patient?

A. Blockade of Na^+ reabsorption in the proximal tubule
B. Blockade of Na^+ channels in the collecting tubule
C. Blockade of $Na^+/K^+/2Cl^-$ symport in the loop of Henle
D. Inhibition of aldosterone actions in the collecting tubule
E. Blockade of Na^+/Cl^- symport in the early distal tubule

Difficulty level: Medium

18. A 42-year-old obese woman was hospitalized because of hypokalemia despite daily administration of a potassium supplement. Laboratory tests on admission revealed metabolic alkalosis. The patient admitted taking furosemide tablets in an effort to lose weight. Which of the following actions most likely contributed to furosemide-induced metabolic alkalosis in this patient?

A. Increased reabsorption of uric acid
B. Increased delivery of Na^+ to the distal tubule
C. Mild inhibition of carbonic anhydrase
D. Decreased reabsorption of Ca^{2+} in the loop of Henle
E. Inhibition of renin secretion

Difficulty level: Hard

19. A 78-year-old man from a nursing home was admitted to the emergency department because of a change in his mental state over the past few hours. He had a medical history of angina and hypertension presently treated with isosorbide mononitrate, losartan, and hydrochlorothiazide. Physical examination showed a person with decreased skin turgor and disorientation to time and place without focal neurologic deficits. Blood pressure was 110/65 mm Hg on standing and 140/88 mm Hg on lying. Pertinent blood tests on admission were Na^+ 116 mEq/L (normal 136–145 mEq/L); K^+ 3.1 mEq/L (normal 3.5–5.0 mEq/L); uric acid 10.2 mg/dL (normal 3.0–8.2 mg/dL); creatinine 3.1 mg/dL (normal 0.6–1.2 mg/dL). The physician thought that the syndrome was due to diuretic therapy. Which of the following drug-induced adverse effects most likely caused the patient's signs and symptoms?

A. Kidney insufficiency
B. Hypokalemia
C. Hypovolemic hyponatremia
D. Hyperuricemia
E. Hypervolemic hyponatremia

Difficulty level: Medium

20. A 66-year-old woman suffering from systolic cardiac failure was brought to the emergency department because of a sudden onset of extreme dyspnea. She presented with cyanosis, tachypnea, hyperpnea, restlessness, anxiety, and a sense of suffocation. Cough was prominent and produced pink-tinged, frothy sputum. Pulse was thready and fast (120 bpm), blood pressure 80/45 mm Hg, and rales were audible at the lung bases. Which of the following drugs was most likely included in the immediate medical treatment of this patient?

    A. Hydrochlorothiazide
    B. Amiloride
    C. Mannitol
    D. Epinephrine
    E. Furosemide
    F. Metoprolol

Difficulty level: Hard

21. A 63-year-old woman was brought to the emergency department because she had become more lethargic and unresponsive over the past several days. Her past medical history was significant for bone metastases from breast cancer. Physical examination revealed a dehydrated, cachectic female responsive only to painful stimuli. Pertinent serum values were Na$^+$ 148 mEq/L (136–145 mEq/L); Ca 19.2 mg/dL (8.5–10.5 mg/dL). An intravenous saline infusion was started, and a diuretic was given concurrently. Which of the following diuretics was most likely administered?

    A. Acetazolamide
    B. Hydrochlorothiazide
    C. Furosemide
    D. Amiloride
    E. Spironolactone

Difficulty level: Medium

22. A 64-year-old woman suffering from stage C heart failure had her diuretic medication changed because of a serious allergic reaction to furosemide. Which of the following diuretics was most likely prescribed?

    A. Spironolactone
    B. Acetazolamide
    C. Mannitol
    D. Ethacrynic acid
    E. Triamterene
    F. Indapamide

Difficulty level: Easy

23. A 49-year-old woman was admitted to the hospital because of generalized weakness, continuous nausea, and diarrhea.

Bowel movements were frequent and watery. The patient's own report was vague, but notes in the chart from other hospitals revealed that she had a very long history of laxative abuse. Blood test results on admission showed pronounced hypokalemia (K$^+$ 2.8 mEq/L). An appropriate therapy was started that included the administration of triamterene. Which of the following actions best explains the potassium-sparing effect of this drug?

    A. Enhancement of K$^+$ reabsorption in the proximal tubule
    B. Blockade of Na$^+$ channels in the collecting duct
    C. Enhancement of K$^+$ reabsorption in the loop of Henle
    D. Blockade of aldosterone receptors in the collecting duct
    E. Blockade of Na$^+$ reabsorption in the proximal tubule

Difficulty level: Medium

24. A 60-year-old man was admitted to the hospital because of symptoms of episodic weakness, polydipsia, and polyuria over the past 2 weeks. Vital signs on admission were blood pressure 136/95 mm Hg; heart rate 80 bpm; respirations 13/min. Significant serum results on admission were K$^+$ 3.1 mEq/L (normal 3.5–5.0 mEq/L); aldosterone 45 ng/dL (normal 7–30 ng/dL). A computed tomography scan showed bilateral adrenal hyperplasia. Which of the following drugs was most likely included in the therapeutic regimen of this patient?

    A. Hydrochlorothiazide
    B. Mannitol
    C. Furosemide
    D. Fenoldopam
    E. Nitroprusside
    F. Spironolactone

Difficulty level: Medium

25. A 54-year-old alcoholic man was admitted to the emergency department with a 2-week history of nausea, vomiting, and lower abdominal cramps. Physical examination revealed an afebrile, jaundiced, and cachectic male in moderate distress. The abdomen appeared very tense with prominent veins, and 2+ ascites was noted by shifting dullness and a fluid wave. Pertinent serum values on admission were Na$^+$ 144 mEq/L (normal 136–145 mEq/L); K$^+$ 2.9 mEq/L (normal 3.5–5.0 mEq/L); bicarbonate 34 mEq/L (normal 22–28 mEq/L); albumin 2.3 g/dL (normal 3.3–4.8 mEq/L). Which of the following diuretics would be the drug of choice for this patient?

    A. Indapamide
    B. Mannitol
    C. Spironolactone
    D. Furosemide
    E. Triamterene

Difficulty level: Easy

26. A 65-year-old patient was scheduled for surgery to remove a glioma located on his left parietal lobe. Which of the following drugs would be most appropriately given before and after surgery to prevent increased intracranial pressure?

    A. Mannitol
    B. Hydrochlorothiazide
    C. Triamterene
    D. Verapamil
    E. Propranolol

Difficulty level: Easy

27. A 57-year-old Black woman, recently diagnosed with closed-angle glaucoma, was scheduled for iridotomy. Which of the following agents was most likely given intravenously before and after surgery to reduce intraocular pressure?

    A. Furosemide
    B. Triamterene
    C. Mannitol
    D. Hydrochlorothiazide
    E. Homatropine
    F. Phenylephrine

Difficulty level: Hard

28. A 52-year-old woman was admitted to the hospital with a 1-week history of muscle cramps, lethargy, and confusion. Past history of the patient was significant for depression treated with amitriptyline. Vital signs on admission were blood pressure 134/82 mm Hg (with no significant changes upon standing); heart rate 85 bpm; respirations 14/min. Physical examination was unremarkable. Pertinent lab test results on admission were serum Na^+ 118 mEq/L (normal 136–145 mEq/L); serum osmolality 220 mOsm/kg (normal 275–295 mOsm/kg); urine osmolality 950 mOsm/kg (normal 50–1400 mOsm/kg). A diagnosis was made, and an appropriate therapy was prescribed. Which of the following drugs was most likely included in the patient's treatment?

    A. Mannitol
    B. Triamterene
    C. Conivaptan
    D. Acetazolamide
    E. Hydrochlorothiazide
    F. Furosemide

Difficulty level: Medium

29. A 69-year-old man was recently diagnosed with severe cardiac failure, and the physician started treatment with propranolol, captopril, and digoxin. Diuretic therapy was also included. Which of the following pairs of diuretics would have been most appropriate for this patient?

    A. Hydrochlorothiazide and acetazolamide
    B. Furosemide and spironolactone
    C. Triamterene and acetazolamide
    D. Hydrochlorothiazide and mannitol
    E. Furosemide and mannitol

Difficulty level: Medium

30. A 63-year-old man was admitted to the emergency department because of a 12-hour history of dyspnea and bradycardia. He was taking propranolol, captopril, furosemide, and amiloride because of a previous myocardial infarction, as well as ibuprofen for osteoarthritis. Physical examination showed the patient was in respiratory distress with the following vital signs: blood pressure 150/86 mm Hg; heart rate 40 bpm; respirations 20/min. A lab analysis was ordered. Which of the following substances was most likely increased in the patient's serum?

    A. Sodium
    B. Calcium
    C. Glucose
    D. Potassium
    E. Urea nitrogen
    F. Triglycerides

Difficulty level: Easy

31. A 32-year-old woman suffering from idiopathic hypercalciuria was diagnosed with a large urinary stone in the right renal pelvis. She was scheduled for surgical removal of the calculus. Which of the following drugs would be appropriate for this patient to prevent new stone production after the operation?

    A. Acetazolamide
    B. Hydrochlorothiazide
    C. Furosemide
    D. Triamterene
    E. Spironolactone

Difficulty level: Hard

32. In a phase 1 clinical trial, the same dose of four new diuretics (P, Q, R, and S) was given intravenously to a healthy volunteer on four separate occasions. Lab studies had shown that all drugs were acidic molecules that were able to block the Na^+/Cl^- cotransporter in the early distal tubule with the same affinity. They had about the same plasma protein binding levels and were not metabolized in the body. The acid dissociation constant (pK_a) levels of the drugs were

> P = 3.5
>
> Q = 7.2
>
> R = 5.1
>
> S = 10.1

Which of the following drugs most likely produced the greatest increase in diuresis in the subject?

A. Drug P
B. Drug Q
C. Drug R
D. Drug S

Questions: IV-2 Drugs for Ischemic Heart Disease

Directions for questions **1–4**

Match each antianginal drug with the appropriate description (each lettered option can be selected once, more than once, or not at all).

A. Amyl nitrite
B. Diltiazem
C. Isosorbide mononitrate
D. Metoprolol
E. Nifedipine
F. Nicardipine
G. Nitroglycerin
H. Verapamil

Difficulty level: Easy

1. This drug is sometimes used to treat cyanide toxicity.

Difficulty level: Easy

2. This drug has no therapeutic effect on variant angina.

Difficulty level: Easy

3. This drug has a good transdermal bioavailability.

Difficulty level: Easy

4. This drug has high affinity for calcium channels of cerebral vessels.

Difficulty level: Easy

5. A 55-year-old woman recently diagnosed with variant angina started treatment with isosorbide mononitrate and diltiazem. Which of the following actions most likely mediated the therapeutic effect of nitrates in the patient's disease?

A. Increased left ventricular end-diastolic volume
B. Increased blood flow in large epicardial vessels
C. Increased heart rate
D. Decreased diastolic perfusion time
E. Increased cardiac contractility

Difficulty level: Medium

6. A 59-year-old man recently diagnosed with exertional angina started treatment with verapamil, one tablet daily. Which of the following cardiac and smooth muscle Ca^{2+} channels is most likely the main site of action of this drug?

A. Ligand-gated channels in cell membranes
B. Store-operated channels in mitochondria
C. Voltage-gated channels in the sarcoplasmic reticulum
D. Voltage-gated channels in cell membranes
E. Ligand-gated channels in the sarcoplasmic reticulum

Difficulty level: Easy

7. A 57-year-old man complained of dizziness and palpitations shortly after taking a tablet of his prescribed medication. The man was recently diagnosed with variant angina for which he had started an appropriate therapy 4 days earlier. Which of the following actions most likely caused the patient's symptoms?

A. Coronary vasodilation
B. Decreased total peripheral resistance
C. Increased venous return to the heart
D. Decreased myocardial contractility
E. Coronary steal phenomenon

Difficulty level: Medium

8. A 47-year-old man recently diagnosed with exertional angina started treatment with sublingual nitroglycerin, as needed, and oral isosorbide mononitrate. Which of the following is a potential detrimental effect of nitrates in the prophylactic treatment of exertional angina?

   A. Decreased ejection time
   B. Increased cardiac rate
   C. Increased capacitance of systemic veins
   D. Decreased arterial pressure
   E. Increased ventricular end-diastolic volume

Difficulty level: Medium

9. A 58-year-old man complained to his physician of severe chest pain when he walked rapidly despite the therapy he had carefully followed for 3 weeks. The man was recently diagnosed with exertional angina and had started treatment with transdermal nitroglycerin and atenolol. The physician decided to add a drug and prescribed diltiazem. Which of the following effects was most likely common to all the drugs the patient was taking?

   A. Decreased cardiac rate
   B. Increased cardiac contractility
   C. Decreased arterial pressure
   D. Decreased left ventricular end-diastolic volume
   E. Increased ejection time

Difficulty level: Hard

10. A 51-year-old man was admitted to the hospital in acute distress with extreme dyspnea, restlessness, and anxiety. The patient had been suffering from chronic heart failure for 3 years. Vital signs were blood pressure 115/90 mm Hg, pulse 120 bpm, respirations 22/min. A chest x-ray done immediately showed marked interstitial edema. An appropriate therapy was started that included an intravenous infusion of nitroglycerin. Which of the following actions most likely mediated the therapeutic effect of the drug in the patient's disorder?

   A. Decreased ventricular end diastolic volume
   B. Reflex increase in heart rate
   C. Reflex increase in cardiac contractility
   D. Decreased ventricular ejection time
   E. Decreased afterload
   F. Decreased platelet aggregation

Difficulty level: Hard

11. A 48-year-old man was brought to the emergency department because of severe chest pain that had been ongoing for over 3 hours. The man had been suffering from chronic stable exertional angina for 1 year and from duodenal ulcer for 3 months. His current medication included isosorbide mononitrate and verapamil for angina and famotidine for duodenal ulcer. One week earlier, the patient stopped the antianginal medications because he had not had anginal attacks during the past month. Which of the following events most likely triggered the patient's present chest pain?

   A. Chronic progression of ischemia uncovered by discontinuing therapy
   B. Famotidine-induced inhibition of verapamil metabolism
   C. Abrupt withdrawal from nitrate therapy
   D. Famotidine-induced inhibition of isosorbide mononitrate metabolism
   E. Reflex tachycardia due to nitrate therapy

Difficulty level: Medium

12. A 48-year-old woman presented to the clinic because of chest pain on exertion for the past 2 days. Physical examination showed a woman in no apparent distress. Physical signs were blood pressure 105/60 mm Hg, pulse 85 bpm, respirations 15 breaths/min. Cardiac auscultation revealed a regular rhythm with no abnormal cardiac sounds or murmurs. An electrocardiogram after exercise stress testing confirmed the diagnosis of exertional angina, and therapy with sublingual nitroglycerin and isosorbide mononitrate was started. Which of the following adverse effects would be most likely to occur in this patient?

   A. Cough and wheezing
   B. Postural hypotension
   C. Reflex bradycardia
   D. Methemoglobinemia
   E. Diarrhea
   F. Venous thrombosis

Difficulty level: Medium

13. A 46-year-old man complained to his physician of insomnia, nightmares, fatigue, diminished libido, and blanching of the fingers when exposed to cold. The man, recently diagnosed with exertional angina, had been taking an antianginal drug for 1 month. Which of the following drugs most likely caused the patient's symptoms?

   A. Propranolol
   B. Isosorbide mononitrate
   C. Nitroglycerin
   D. Nifedipine
   E. Verapamil

Difficulty level: Medium

14. A 47-year-old man complained to his physician that he experienced mild angina attacks during exertion. The patient, recently diagnosed with exertional angina, had started a therapy with a transdermal nitroglycerin preparation 2 weeks previously. He carefully applied a new patch every morning immediately after removing the old one. Anginal attacks had disappeared completely during the first week of therapy but were back thereafter. Which of the following best explains the reason for his anginal episodes?

A. Vasospastic angina complicating the exertional angina
B. Cellular tolerance to nitroglycerin
C. Increased metabolism of nitroglycerin
D. Insufficient original nitroglycerin dosage
E. Decreased absorption of nitroglycerin from the skin

Difficulty level: Hard

15. A 54-year-old man had been diagnosed recently with variant angina. The patient had been suffering from a cerebellar astrocytoma for 2 years and from a second-degree atrioventricular block for 1 year. Which of the following antianginal drugs would be appropriate for this patient?

A. Isosorbide mononitrate
B. Diltiazem
C. Verapamil
D. Nifedipine
E. Propranolol

Difficulty level: Hard

16. A 55-year-old woman complained to her physician of palpitations, flushing of the face, and vertigo. The woman, suffering from diabetes mellitus, was giving herself three daily doses of insulin. She had been recently diagnosed with exertional angina for which nitrate therapy was started with transdermal nitroglycerin and oral isosorbide mononitrate. After 3 weeks of therapy, her anginal attacks were less frequent but not completely prevented. Which of the following would be an appropriate next therapeutic step for this patient?

A. Reduce the dosage of both nitrates
B. Add propranolol
C. Add nifedipine
D. Stop isosorbide mononitrate
E. Add diltiazem

Difficulty level: Easy

17. A 77-year-old woman was brought to the emergency department with an acute myocardial infarction (MI). Six months ago, she suffered from an MI and began taking propranolol, aspirin, and lovastatin. Her current medications also included captopril and hydrochlorothiazide for hypertension. Two days

ago, she became nauseous and vomited, and she stopped taking all her medications. The abrupt withdrawal from which of the following drugs most likely triggered the recent MI?

A. Aspirin
B. Propranolol
C. Lovastatin
D. Captopril
E. Hydrochlorothiazide

Difficulty level: Medium

18. A 48-year-old man was brought to the emergency department with an acute myocardial infarction (MI). The man regularly used sildenafil in preparation for sexual intercourse because of an erectile dysfunction. He had recently been diagnosed with exertional angina, and he had been taking an appropriate prescribed therapy. Which of the following drugs most likely caused the patient's MI?

A. Propranolol
B. Nitroprusside
C. Nitroglycerin
D. Nifedipine
E. Verapamil

Difficulty level: Hard

19. A 54-year-old man complained to his physician of palpitations, facial flushing, and vertigo. The man had been suffering from gastroesophageal reflux disease for 3 years. Two week earlier, he was diagnosed with exertional angina and started the prescribed therapy. Which of the following drugs most likely caused the patient's symptoms?

A. Propranolol
B. Verapamil
C. Diltiazem
D. Nitroglycerin
E. Nifedipine

Difficulty level: Medium

20. A 50-year-old woman was admitted to the hospital with a 3-week history of early morning chest pain that caused her to awaken from sleep. The pain lasted 10 to 15 minutes and frequently radiated to her left arm. An exercise tolerance test failed to elicit precordial pain. A diagnosis of angina was made, and she was discharged from the hospital with a prescription for nifedipine. Which of the following actions most likely mediated the therapeutic effect of the drug in the patient's disease?

A. Decreased preload
B. Decreased afterload
C. Increased myocardial contractility
D. Increased heart rate
E. Decreased coronary vascular tone

Difficulty level: Hard

21. A 53-year-old man was taken to the emergency department because of dizziness and chest discomfort that apparently had been ongoing for over 5 hours. His vital signs were blood pressure 165/100 mm Hg, heart rate 50 bpm, respirations 22/min. Physical examination revealed signs of severe pulmonary congestion, and an electrocardiogram was consistent with an anterior acute myocardial infarction. An appropriate therapy was instituted that included an intravenous infusion of which of the following drugs?

   A. Epinephrine
   B. Metoprolol
   C. Nitroglycerin
   D. Verapamil
   E. Nifedipine

Difficulty level: Easy

22. A 65-year-old man suddenly collapsed in the dining room of his home. Upon arrival by ambulance at the emergency department, he regained consciousness and complained of a severe headache. Physical examination was significant for a stiff neck and mild mental confusion. A computed tomography scan revealed blood in the subarachnoid space. Which of the following drugs would be appropriate to prevent delayed cerebral ischemia in this patient?

   A. Verapamil
   B. Isosorbide mononitrate
   C. Propranolol
   D. Dobutamine
   E. Nicardipine
   F. Clonidine

Difficulty level: Easy

23. A 53-year-old man diagnosed with exertional angina was prescribed inhaled nitroglycerin and oral isosorbide mononitrate. Which of the following molecular actions most likely mediated the therapeutic efficacy of these drugs in the patient's disease?

   A. Conversion of nitrite ions into nitrous oxide (N_2O)
   B. Increased intracellular Ca^{2+} concentration
   C. Dephosphorylation of the myosin light chain
   D. Decreased synthesis of guanylyl cyclase
   E. Phosphorylation of myosin light chain kinase

Difficulty level: Hard

24. A 59-year-old man was recently diagnosed with exertional angina. The patient, who was a heavy smoker, had been suffering from chronic obstructive pulmonary disease for 15 years and from gastroesophageal reflux disease for 3 years. Which of the following drugs would be appropriate to prevent anginal attacks in this patient?

   A. Propranolol
   B. Verapamil
   C. Diltiazem
   D. Isosorbide mononitrate
   E. Nifedipine

Difficulty level: Medium

25. A 47-year-old man recently diagnosed with exertional angina started treatment with transdermal nitroglycerin and oral propranolol. Which of the following was most likely a purpose for the combination therapy in this case?

   A. To enhance nitrate-induced coronary vasodilation
   B. To prevent nitrate-induced tachycardia
   C. To prevent nitrate-induced decrease in arterial pressure
   D. To enhance propranolol-induced decrease in cardiac rate
   E. To enhance propranolol-induced decrease in cardiac contractility

Difficulty level: Easy

26. A 50-year-old man was discharged from the hospital after recovery from an acute myocardial infarction. His postdischarge medications included propranolol. How long should the patient continue to take this drug?

   A. Three months
   B. Six months
   C. One year
   D. Two years
   E. Indefinitely

Difficulty level: Medium

27. A 46-year-old man complained to his family physician of throbbing headaches and severe constipation. The man, recently diagnosed with exertional angina, had started an antianginal treatment 2 weeks ago. Which of the following pairs of drugs was he most likely taking?

   A. Verapamil and isosorbide mononitrate
   B. Nitroglycerin and isosorbide mononitrate
   C. Nitroglycerin and propranolol
   D. Propranolol and isosorbide mononitrate
   E. Propranolol and verapamil

Difficulty level: Easy

28. A 24-year-old man complained to his family physician of episodes of precordial pain precipitated by exertion and relieved by rest. The man had been recently diagnosed with hypertrophic cardiomyopathy. Which of the following pairs of drugs would be appropriate for this patient?

    A. Isosorbide mononitrate and nifedipine
    B. Nitroglycerin and captopril
    C. Nitroglycerin and verapamil
    D. Verapamil and metoprolol
    E. Nifedipine and captopril
    F. Isosorbide mononitrate and metoprolol

Difficulty level: Easy

29. A 48-year-old man presented to the hospital with a 5-day history of burning pain in his right hand and arm. The pain occurred mainly when he was using his hands at work and was accompanied by the middle fingers of his right hand turning cold and somewhat blue. The man was a construction worker and frequently used vibrating machinery. Several white splotches appeared when the hand was placed in cold water, and tingling was felt in the hand. Which of the following drugs would be appropriate to treat the patient's disorder?

    A. Nitroprusside
    B. Albuterol
    C. Nifedipine
    D. Clonidine
    E. Labetalol
    F. Fenoldopam

Difficulty level: Medium

30. A 43-year old man was admitted to the hospital with a myocardial infarction (MI) and was started on a therapy that included atenolol. Which of the following actions most likely contribute to mortality reduction obtained by β-blockers in MI?

    A. Increased myocardial oxygen supply
    B. Decreased atrioventricular conduction
    C. Decreased myocardial remodeling
    D. Increased systemic vascular resistance
    E. Increased left ventricular end-diastolic pressure

Questions: IV-3 Drugs for Cardiac Failure

Directions for questions **1–5**

Match each drug used in cardiac failure with the appropriate description (each lettered option can be selected once, more than once, or not at all).

    A. Captopril
    B. Digoxin
    C. Dobutamine
    D. Furosemide
    E. Losartan
    F. Milrinone
    G. Nesiritide
    H. Propranolol
    I. Spironolactone

Difficulty level: Easy

1. This drug can cause peripheral vasodilation by blocking phosphodiesterase type 3.

Difficulty level: Easy

2. This drug can increase the synthesis of cyclic adenosine monophosphate (cAMP) in the heart.

Difficulty level: Easy

3. The chronic use of this aldosterone antagonist can reduce mortality in patients with severe heart failure.

Difficulty level: Easy

4. This drug can cause peripheral vasodilation by increasing the synthesis of cyclic guanosine monophosphate (cGMP).

Difficulty level: Easy

5. This drug can increase central parasympathetic firing.

Difficulty level: Easy

6. A 68-year-old man recently diagnosed with stage C heart failure started a treatment with metoprolol, losartan, furosemide, and digoxin. Which of the following molecular actions most likely mediated the positive inotropic action of digoxin?

    A. Closing of calcium channels in cardiac cell membranes
    B. Increased release of Ca^{2+} from the sarcoplasmic reticulum during systole
    C. Activation of Na^+/K^+ ATPase
    D. Activation of the Ca^{2+}/Na^+ exchanger in cardiac cell membranes
    E. Opening of K^+ channels in cardiac cell membranes

Difficulty level: Medium

7. A 57-year-old man suffering from persistent atrial fibrillation started a treatment with digoxin, one tablet daily. Which of the following types of receptors most likely mediated the therapeutic effect of the drug in this patient?

A. Beta-2 adrenergic

B. M_2 cholinergic

C. D_1 dopaminergic

D. Serotoninergic

E. Nm cholinergic

Difficulty level: Easy

8. A 57-year-old woman suffering from persistent atrial flutter started a treatment with digoxin. Which of the following cardiac actions most likely occurred during the therapy?

A. Increased end-systolic volume

B. Decreased abnormal cardiac automaticity

C. Decreased diastolic time

D. Increased atrial refractoriness

E. Decreased heart rate

Difficulty level: Easy

9. A 61-year-old man recently diagnosed with stage C heart failure was admitted to the hospital for evaluation. It was found that he had an ejection fraction of 30% at rest. A treatment that included digoxin was started. Which of the following cardiovascular parameters did digoxin most likely increase in this patient?

A. Stroke volume

B. Total peripheral resistance

C. Oxygen consumption of the heart

D. End-diastolic volume

E. Heart rate

Difficulty level: Medium

10. A 42-year-old man was admitted to the emergency department in acute distress with breathlessness, markedly distended neck veins, and atrial fibrillation. His blood pressure was 100/90 mm Hg, pulse 120 bpm. An echocardiogram revealed an ejection fraction of 35%. Treatment was started with furosemide, captopril, and digoxin. In this patient, digoxin most likely decreased which of the following cardiovascular parameters?

A. Stroke volume

B. End-systolic volume

C. End-diastolic volume

D. Systolic pressure

E. Pulse pressure

Difficulty level: Medium

11. A 68-year-old woman recently diagnosed with stage C heart failure started a treatment with digoxin. Knowing that digoxin has a clearance of about 7 L/h and an oral bioavailability of about 70%, which of the following doses (in milligrams) was most likely given to achieve a mean steady-state plasma concentration of 1 μg/L?

A. 1.4

B. 0.125

C. 0.24

D. 2.0

E. 0.5

F. 2.4

Difficulty level: Easy

12. A 63-year-old man complained to his physician of nausea, vomiting, and a visual sensation of green-yellow halos around bright objects. The man, recently diagnosed with cardiac failure and atrial fibrillation, had started an appropriate treatment 2 weeks earlier. Which of the following drugs most likely caused the patient's symptoms?

A. Verapamil

B. Propranolol

C. Digoxin

D. Lidocaine

E. Furosemide

F. Captopril

Difficulty level: Hard

13. A 63-year-old woman was found to have a third-degree atrioventricular block. The woman, who had been suffering from stage C heart failure, had been receiving captopril, furosemide, and digoxin for 2 months, and the disease was well controlled. The physician believed that the block was due to digoxin therapy. Which of the following would be an appropriate therapeutic adjustment for this patient?

A. Discontinue digoxin and start milrinone

B. Add physostigmine and decrease the digoxin dose

C. Add atropine and decrease the digoxin dose

D. Discontinue digoxin and start metoprolol

E. Add dobutamine and decrease the digoxin dose

F. Discontinue digoxin and start losartan

Difficulty level: Medium

14. A 54-year-old woman presented to the clinic complaining of palpitations. One month earlier, the woman was diagnosed with stage C heart failure and started treatment with metoprolol, digoxin, and captopril. Her medications also included estrogen and a calcium supplement for postmenopausal osteoporosis. The patient's vital signs were blood pressure 145/90, pulse 130 bpm. An electrocardiogram showed ventricular tachycardia. Significant plasma levels on admission were K^+ 5.8 mEq/L, Ca^{2+} 12.2 mEq/L, creatinine 3.5 mg/dL. Which of the following events most likely triggered the patient's arrhythmia?

A. Metoprolol-induced decrease in cardiac contractility
B. Increased serum K^+ level
C. Captopril-induced vasodilation
D. Increased serum Ca^{2+} level
E. Estrogen-induced hypertension

Difficulty level: Medium

15. A 61-year-old alcoholic man was admitted to the hospital with a 2-day history of epigastric pain associated with nausea and vomiting. The man had been suffering from systolic heart failure for 1 year, and his disease was well controlled with captopril, furosemide, and digoxin. Pertinent serum data on admission were K^+ 2.8 mEq/L, creatinine 3.2 mg/dL. An electrocardiogram showed a heart rate of 65 bpm with occasional premature ventricular contractions and runs of bigeminy. Which of the following would be an appropriate therapeutic adjustment for this patient?

A. Add potassium supplementation and reduce the digoxin dose
B. Add atropine and reduce the digoxin dose
C. Increase the furosemide dose and reduce the digoxin dose
D. Discontinue digoxin and start losartan
E. Discontinue digoxin and start milrinone

Difficulty level: Medium

16. A 72-year-old man was admitted to the hospital because of anuria. The man had a long history of severe systolic cardiac failure and chronic obstructive pulmonary disease. Shortly after admission, the patient started vomiting, then became agitated, verbally abusive, and disoriented in space and time. He was telling the nurse that he heard loud voices cursing him. An electrocardiogram showed atrial tachycardia with atrioventricular block. Which of the following drugs most likely caused the patient's symptoms?

A. Captopril
B. Digoxin
C. Ipratropium
D. Metoprolol
E. Ethacrynic acid
F. Albuterol

Difficulty level: Medium

17. A 65-year-old woman presented to the hospital with a chief complaint of palpitations. The woman was suffering from stage C heart failure and had been receiving digoxin, furosemide, and losartan for 6 months. Laboratory data on admission included potassium 3.9 mEq/L (normal 3.5–5.0 mEq/L), calcium 9.2 mg/dL (normal 8.5–10.5 mg/dL), magnesium 2.5 mEq/L (normal 1.5–2.0 mEq/L), total thyroxine (T_4) 42 ng/mL (normal 50–110 ng/mL), thyroid-stimulating hormone (TSH) 15 mIU/mL (normal 0.5–5.5 mIU/mL). An electrocardiogram showed junctional tachycardia, which, according to her physician, was most likely due to digoxin treatment. Which of the following pathologic conditions most likely increased the risk of digoxin toxicity in this patient?

A. Hypermagnesemia
B. Hyperaldosteronism
C. Hyperparathyroidism
D. Concomitant furosemide treatment
E. Hypothyroidism

Difficulty level: Easy

18. A 65-year-old man was brought to the emergency department in acute distress. He was agitated, incoherent, disoriented in time and space, and seemed to be hallucinating. The patient had been suffering from severe chronic cardiac failure for 2 years, and his wife reported that she had found an empty bottle of digoxin tablets near her husband's bed. Vital signs were blood pressure 100/50 mm Hg, heart rate 45 bpm. An emergency treatment was instituted, and a drug was given intravenously. Which of the following drugs was most likely administered?

A. Lidocaine
B. Atropine
C. Phenytoin
D. Potassium chloride
E. Digoxin antibodies
F. Amiodarone

Difficulty level: Medium

19. A 73-year-old man complained to his physician of increasing fatigue and shortness of breath that was often worse at night, forcing him to "sit bolt upright." He also noticed that his feet were getting swollen. Past history was unremarkable. Vital signs were blood pressure 150/90, respirations 17/min. On examination, mild pitting edema was seen on the legs. An electrocardiogram disclosed a second-degree atrioventricular block. His physician diagnosed initial cardiac failure and prescribed an appropriate therapy. Which of the following drugs would be contraindicated for this patient?

A. Captopril

B. Hydrochlorothiazide

C. Digoxin

D. Losartan

E. Furosemide

F. Spironolactone

Difficulty level: Hard

20. A 62-year-old woman was admitted to the hospital complaining of nausea, mental confusion, dizziness, and palpitations. The woman, suffering from hypertension and recurrent atrial fibrillation, had been receiving hydrochlorothiazide, captopril, and digoxin for several months. One week ago, she started erythromycin and ibuprofen for an acute upper respiratory tract infection. Which of the following events most likely caused the patient's symptoms?

A. Hydrochlorotiazide-induced hypokalemia

B. Erythromycin-induced increase in digoxin oral bioavailability

C. Hydrochlorotiazide-induced hypocalcemia

D. Captopril-induced decrease in digoxin clearance

E. Ibuprofen-induced decrease in digoxin clearance

Difficulty level: Medium

21. A 62-year-old man was seen at a clinic because of nausea, vomiting, diarrhea, dizziness, and confusion for 8 hours. The man, suffering from systolic heart failure, had been receiving captopril, digoxin, and furosemide for 8 months. A few days earlier, his physician added amiodarone to the therapy because of the appearance of multifocal premature ventricular beats. Which of the following would be the most plausible explanation of the patient's symptoms?

A. Captopril-induced hyperkalemia

B. Amiodarone-induced increase in digoxin plasma levels

C. Amiodarone-induced decrease in atrioventricular conduction

D. Furosemide-induced increase in diuresis

E. Furosemide-induced hyperuricemia

Difficulty level: Easy

22. A 52-year-old man complained to his physician of diarrhea, palpitations, and blurred vision. Five days earlier, the man was diagnosed with stage C systolic heart failure and started a treatment with captopril, atenolol, and a standard dose of digoxin. Past history was significant for hereditary nephrogenic diabetes insipidus, presently controlled by hydrochlorothiazide (100 mg daily). Which of the following conditions could have facilitated the appearance of the patient's symptoms?

A. Advanced age

B. Thiazide treatment

C. Hypernatremia due to water depletion

D. Decreased clearance of digoxin

E. Worsening of the heart failure

Difficulty level: Easy

23. A 61-year-old man recently diagnosed with stage C heart failure started a treatment that included digoxin. Which of the following cardiovascular parameters was most likely increased after few days of therapy?

A. Cardiac reserve

B. Coronary vasoconstriction

C. Oxygen consumption

D. End-diastolic volume

E. Heart rate

Difficulty level: Easy

24. A 66-year-old man with a long history of heart failure was admitted to the hospital because of a heart failure exacerbation. His current medications included furosemide, captopril, and carvedilol. On admission, the patient showed the following hemodynamic profile: blood pressure 100/60 mm Hg, pulse 118/min, cardiac output 2.6 L/min. Physical examination confirmed the diagnosis of acute heart failure, and an intravenous infusion of milrinone was started. Which of the following molecular events most likely mediated the positive inotropic action of the drug?

A. cAMP-mediated increase in cardiac intracellular Ca^{2+} levels

B. cGMP-mediated dephosphorylation of the myosin light chain

C. Opening of K^+ channels in cardiac cell membranes

D. Increased binding of Ca^{2+} to calmodulin

E. Activation of the $1Ca^{2+}/3Na^+$ antiport

Difficulty level: Medium

25. A 61-year-old man presented to the hospital with shortness of breath, decreased exercise capacity, and distended neck veins. The man had a history of severe hypertension currently treated with hydrochlorothiazide and captopril. Despite the treatment, his blood pressure was still 170/110. After physical examination and laboratory tests, a diagnosis of diastolic cardiac failure was made. Which of the following would be a useful drug to add to the patient's therapeutic regimen?

   A. Metoprolol
   B. Digoxin
   C. Dobutamine
   D. Milrinone
   E. Phenylephrine
   F. Mannitol

Difficulty level: Hard

26. A 22-year-old previously healthy woman was brought to the emergency room because she had collapsed while jogging. She denied orthopnea, paroxysmal nocturnal dyspnea, chest pain, or edema. Her younger brother was known to have had two episodes of syncope after exertion. An electrocardiogram indicated left ventricular hypertrophy, and an echocardiogram showed a normal ejection fraction and asymmetric septal hypertrophy. Which of the following drugs would be most appropriate for this patient?

   A. Prazosin
   B. Atenolol
   C. Digoxin
   D. Nitroglycerin
   E. Furosemide

Difficulty level: Hard

27. A 60-year-old man was admitted to the cardiac unit because of progressive, debilitating symptoms of cardiac failure that had confined him to bed for the past month. The man had a 2-year history of chronic cardiac failure that was symptomatic despite treatment with maximal doses of furosemide, enalapril, metoprolol, and digoxin. Physical examination showed significant jugular venous distention, warm and wet skin, bilateral rales, and hepatomegaly. The hemodynamic profile was blood pressure 100/66 mm Hg, heart rate 105 bpm, central venous pressure 23 mm Hg, cardiac output 3.9. L/min. Furosemide and dopamine were given intravenously, but 15 minutes later, the central venous pressure was still 20 mm Hg. Another drug was given intravenously. Which of the following drugs would be most appropriate for the patient at this time?

   A. Digoxin
   B. Norepinephrine
   C. Lidocaine
   D. Nesiritide
   E. Verapamil
   F. Losartan

Difficulty level: Medium

28. A 67-year-old man was admitted to the coronary unit with an acute inferior myocardial infarction. Despite the initial therapy, his condition deteriorated, and 2 hours after admission, he had the following hemodynamic profile: blood pressure 94/50, cardiac output 2.9 L/min, cardiac index 1.5 L/min/m^2 (normal 2.6–4.2 L/min/m^2). An intravenous infusion of dobutamine was started. Which of the following actions most likely mediated the positive inotropic action of dobutamine?

   A. Inhibition of phosphodiesterase
   B. Protein kinase–mediated increase in cytoplasmic Ca^{2+} availability
   C. Inhibition of the Ca^{2+}/Na$^+$ exchanger in cardiac cell membrane
   D. Activation of phospholipase A$_2$
   E. Inhibition of Na$^+$/K$^+$ ATPase in cardiac cell membranes

Difficulty level: Easy

29. A 68-year-old man was diagnosed with systolic heart failure with normal ejection fraction and normal sinus rhythm at rest. A treatment with captopril was started. Which of the following actions most likely mediated the therapeutic effect of captopril in this patient?

   A. Increased cardiac contractility
   B. Reduction of angiotensin-mediated vasoconstriction in the kidney
   C. Reduction of preload and afterload
   D. Stimulation of epinephrine release from adrenergic nerves
   E. Stimulation of bradykinin metabolism

Difficulty level: Medium

30. A 52-year-old woman was discharged from the hospital after recovery from an acute MI. Her postdischarge medications included captopril. Which of the following actions most likely contributes to mortality reduction obtained by the use of angiotensin-converting enzyme (ACE) inhibitors in MI?

   A. Decreased cardiac contractility
   B. Increased preload
   C. Coronary vasodilation
   D. Decreased ventricular automaticity
   E. Reduction of myocardial remodeling

Difficulty level: Medium

31. A 58-year-old man presented to a clinic with the chief complaint of increasing shortness of breath and a 10-lb weight gain over the past 2 weeks. Physical examination revealed a dyspneic and cyanotic male with the following vital signs: blood pressure 135/100 mm Hg, pulse 125 bpm, respirations 22/min. His liver was enlarged, and pitting edema was seen on the legs. A Doppler echocardiogram showed an ejection fraction of 35%. An appropriate drug therapy was started that included metoprolol. Which of the following actions most likely contribute to the therapeutic effect of metoprolol in this patient?

A. Increased renin secretion
B. Decreased preload
C. Prevention of chronic sympathetic overactivity
D. Increased myocardial remodeling
E. Downregulation of cardiac β receptors

Difficulty level: Medium

32. A 58-year-old African-American man diagnosed with stage B systolic heart failure started a treatment that included a hydralazine/isosorbide dinitrate combination. Which of the following actions most likely mediated the therapeutic effect of the drug in the patient's disease?

A. Increased cardiac contractility
B. Reduction of angiotensin II secretion
C. Reduction of preload and afterload
D. Inhibition of sympathetic activity
E. Decreased heart rate

Difficulty level: Easy

33. A 64-year-old woman complained to her physician of fatigue, increasing shortness of breath, and ankle edema. The patient's vital signs were blood pressure 145/85 mm Hg, pulse 78 bpm, respirations 18/min. After further exams, a diagnosis of stage C systolic heart failure was made. An appropriate multidrug therapy was prescribed that included furosemide. Which of the following is a primary reason for the use of loop diuretics in chronic systolic heart failure?

A. They inhibit angiotensin II synthesis.
B. They increase venous return to the heart.
C. They inhibit renal prostaglandin biosynthesis.
D. They act even when the glomerular filtration rate is very low.
E. They increase the contractility of the failing heart.

Difficulty level: Medium

34. A 53-year-old man with stage C heart failure continued to experience symptoms of peripheral edema and dyspnea on exertion despite treatment with maximal doses of captopril, metoprolol, furosemide, and digoxin. His cardiologist decided to add a drug to the patient's therapy. Which of the following drugs would be appropriate for the patient at this time?

A. Losartan
B. Triamterene
C. Spironolactone
D. Indapamide
E. Milrinone
F. Nesiritide

Difficulty level: Medium

35. A 63-year-old woman recently diagnosed with systolic heart failure started a treatment with furosemide and captopril. Plasma levels of which of the following pairs of compounds were most likely increased after the administration of captopril?

A. Vasopressin and sodium
B. Norepinephrine and angiotensin II
C. Bradykinin and angiotensin I
D. Atrial natriuretic peptide and serotonin
E. Angiotensin III and prostaglandins

Difficulty level: Easy

36. A 65-year-old woman complained to her physician of dyspnea of exertion despite ongoing therapy and of a frequent dry, nonproductive cough. The patient had been diagnosed with stage C systolic heart failure for which she had been taking captopril and furosemide for the past month. The physician told the patient that the cough was most likely due to captopril and substituted another drug that he believed to be more effective, as it is able to antagonize the actions of non-angiotensin-converting enzyme (ACE)–generated angiotensin II. Which of the following drugs was most likely prescribed?

A. Enalapril
B. Fenoldopam
C. Diltiazem
D. Spironolactone
E. Losartan
F. Nitroprusside

Difficulty level: Medium

37. A 59-year-old woman recently diagnosed with stage C heart failure started a therapy that included spironolactone. Which of the following molecular actions most likely mediated the therapeutic effect of spironolactone in the patient's disease?

A. Inhibition of potassium excretion in the collecting duct
B. Blockade of the Na^+/H^+ antiporter in the proximal tubule
C. Decreased Na^+ conductance in aldosterone-controlled Na^+ channels
D. Inhibition of renin secretion by the macula densa
E. Blockade of the Na^+/Cl^- symporter in the early distal tubule

Difficulty level: Easy

38. A 57-year-old woman recently diagnosed with systolic heart failure started a treatment with captopril and carvedilol. Which of the following laboratory results was most likely to occur in this patient?

A. Hypercalcemia
B. Hyperkalemia
C. Hypervolemia
D. Hypernatremia
E. Hyperglycemia

Difficulty level: Hard

39. A 61-year-old man recently diagnosed with stage C systolic heart failure started a therapy with captopril and carvedilol. Which of the following sets of effects on diuresis, arteriolar tone and myocardial oxygen consumption most likely occurred after 1 week of therapy?

	Diuresis	Arteriolar Tone	Myocardial Oxygen Consumption
A	Increased	Decreased	Decreased
B	Increased	Unchanged	Increased
C	Decreased	Decreased	Unchanged
D	Unchanged	Decreased	Unchanged
E	Decreased	Increased	Decreased

Difficulty level: Easy

40. A 54-year-old man complained to his physician of an abnormal increase in the size of his breasts. The man had been suffering from systolic heart failure for 3 years. Two months earlier, the cardiologist had added a drug to the patient's therapeutic regimen. Which of the following drugs most likely caused the patient's symptom?

A. Furosemide
B. Losartan
C. Carvedilol
D. Spironolactone
E. Indapamide

Questions: IV-4 Antihypertensive Drugs

Directions for questions **1–5**

Match each antihypertensive drug with its appropriate mechanism of action (each lettered option can be selected once, more than once, or not at all).

A. Aliskiren
B. Clonidine
C. Diazoxide
D. Enalapril
E. Fenoldopam
F. Furosemide
G. Hydralazine
H. Hydrochlorothiazide
I. Labetalol
J. Losartan

K. Methyldopa
L. Nifedipine
M. Nitroprusside
N. Prazosin
O. Propranolol
P. Spironolactone
Q. Verapamil

Difficulty level: Easy

1. Nitric oxide is the active metabolite.

Difficulty level: Easy

2. Activation of dopamine D_1 receptors

Difficulty level: Easy

3. Blockade of angiotensin AT$_1$ receptors

Difficulty level: Easy

4. Potassium channel opening in smooth muscle cells

Difficulty level: Easy

5. Competitive inhibition of renin

Difficulty level: Medium

6. A 63-year-old man recently diagnosed with stage 1 essential hypertension started a treatment with hydrochlorothiazide. After several weeks of treatment, the antihypertensive action of the drug was most likely associated with which of the following effects?

   A. Remarkable postural hypotension
   B. Decreased cardiac output
   C. Decreased peripheral vascular resistance
   D. Increased interstitial fluid volume
   E. Decreased renal blood flow

Difficulty level: Medium

7. A 52-year-old man complained to his physician of acute pain at the base of his right big toe. The man, who had been working as a painter for 15 years, was recently diagnosed with essential hypertension and started an antihypertensive therapy 1 month ago. A lab test showed a plasma uric acid level of 17 mg/dL. Which of the following drugs is most likely to have caused the signs and symptoms of this patient?

   A. Captopril
   B. Hydrochlorothiazide
   C. Methyldopa
   D. Furosemide
   E. Prazosin
   F. Minoxidil

Difficulty level: Medium

8. During a routine physical, a 65-year-old woman was found to have a blood pressure of 165/90 mm Hg. Past medical history was significant for a second-degree heart block and for osteoporosis. One year ago, she had suffered from a severe episode of angioedema. Which of the following antihypertensive drugs would be most appropriate for this patient?

   A. Captopril
   B. Propranolol
   C. Verapamil
   D. Hydrochlorothiazide
   E. Minoxidil

Difficulty level: Hard

9. A 52-year-old woman suffering from hypertension still had a blood pressure of 156/92 mm Hg after 3 months of therapy with hydrochlorothiazide and losartan. Her physician decided to add a third drug that acts by decreasing central sympathetic outflow. Which of the following adverse effects was most likely to occur after a few days of therapy with the new drug?

   A. Severe postural hypotension
   B. Megaloblastic anemia
   C. Palpitations
   D. Pronounced sedation
   E. Sialorrhea

Difficulty level: Medium

10. A 65-year-old man was admitted to the emergency department because of restlessness, apprehension, tremor, sweating, and tachycardia. Vital signs on admission were blood pressure 190/100 mm Hg, pulse 110 bpm, respirations 18/min. History revealed that the patient had been taking a thiazide diuretic and losartan for 3 months for stage 2 hypertension. However, his blood pressure was still not well controlled, and recently his physician had added a third drug to the therapeutic regimen. Because the patient was experiencing daytime somnolence and dry mouth, he decided to discontinue the newly prescribed medication the day before admission. Which of the following drugs was most likely the new drug that the patient decided to stop taking?

   A. Captopril
   B. Minoxidil
   C. Nifedipine
   D. Hydralazine
   E. Clonidine
   F. Fenoldopam

Difficulty level: Easy

11. A 35-year-old woman in her 29th week of gestation was found to have a positive direct Coombs test during a routine prenatal visit. Two months after she became pregnant, she was diagnosed with stage 1 hypertension and started an antihypertensive therapy. Which of the following drugs was she most likely taking?

   A. Captopril
   B. Propranolol
   C. Nifedipine
   D. Methyldopa
   E. Prazosin
   F. Losartan

Difficulty level: Easy

12. A 47-year-old man with a history of hypertension had been taking hydrochlorothiazide for 1 month, but his blood pressure was not controlled despite adherence to medication and nonpharmacologic measures. The patient was also trying to quit smoking without success. The physician decided to add a second drug to the therapeutic regimen that could help the patient as an adjunct to a smoking cessation program. Which of the following drugs was most likely prescribed?

   A. Minoxidil
   B. Propranolol
   C. Nifedipine
   D. Clonidine
   E. Hydralazine

Difficulty level: Easy

13. A 60-year-old man reported to his physician that for the past 2 days he felt very dizzy and faint when he stood up rapidly. The man had a history of essential hypertension that was poorly controlled with losartan and hydrochlorothiazide. One week earlier, he was diagnosed with prostatic hyperplasia, and the physician added a new drug to the therapy. Which of the following drugs most likely caused this adverse effect?

   A. Propranolol
   B. Minoxidil
   C. Hydralazine
   D. Prazosin
   E. Methyldopa
   F. Fenoldopam

Difficulty level: Easy

14. A 61-year-old man suffering from hypertension had been taking hydrochlorothiazide and propranolol for 2 months, but the therapy failed to completely control his blood pressure. The man was recently diagnosed with benign prostatic hyperplasia and experienced frequent nocturia. His physician decided to add a third drug that could also help with the patient's difficulty in urinating. A drug from which of the following drug classes was most likely prescribed?

   A. Alpha-1 blockers
   B. Ca^{2+} channel blockers
   C. Angiotensin-converting enzyme (ACE) inhibitors
   D. Dopamine D_1 blockers
   E. Alpha-2 agonists
   F. Beta-blockers

Difficulty level: Medium

15. A 50-year-old woman came to her physician complaining of dizziness and vertigo for the past 3 days. The woman was recently diagnosed with hypertension and diastolic dysfunction and had started a hypertensive therapy 1 week earlier. Physical examination showed supine blood pressure of 166/94 mm Hg and standing blood pressure of 140/83 mm Hg. Which of the following antihypertensive drugs was the patient most likely taking?

   A. Propranolol
   B. Clonidine
   C. Captopril
   D. Hydrochlorothiazide
   E. Labetalol

Difficulty level: Hard

16. A 38-year-old man was diagnosed with hypertension (156/95 mm Hg) during a routine physical exam. Subsequent exams indicated he was affected by hypertrophic cardiomyopathy. Which of the following antihypertensive drugs would be most appropriate for this patient?

   A. Minoxidil
   B. Hydralazine
   C. Clonidine
   D. Prazosin
   E. Propranolol
   F. Captopril

Difficulty level: Hard

17. A 64-year-old man with a long history of hypertension was admitted to the emergency department because of the sudden onset of severe, sharp, diffuse chest pain that radiated to his back. Physical examination revealed a pulse of 110 bpm and blood pressure of 230/120 mm Hg. A computed tomography scan showed a dissection of the arch of the aorta. An emergency intravenous treatment was started. Which of the following pairs of drugs were most likely administered?

   A. Labetalol and prazosin
   B. Diazoxide and hydralazine
   C. Clonidine and captopril
   D. Nitroprusside and esmolol
   E. Minoxidil and nifedipine

Difficulty level: Medium

18. A 56-year-old woman recently diagnosed with hypertension and atrial fibrillation started a treatment with atenolol. Which of the following sets of physiologic changes was most likely after the administration of the drug?

	Cardiac Output	Venous Tone	Postural Hypotension
A	Decreased	Unchanged	Negligible
B	Increased	Unchanged	Negligible
C	Decreased	Decreased	Marked
D	Unchanged	Decreased	Marked
E	Decreased	Increased	Slight

Difficulty level: Medium

19. A 56-year-old man complained to his physician that for the past 2 days he had experienced palpitations, sweating, and flushing. History revealed that the man had been diagnosed with hypertension 3 months earlier. He had started a therapy with hydrochlorothiazide and captopril, but his blood pressure was still 170/100 mm Hg. One week ago, his physician decided to add a third antihypertensive agent to the treatment. Which of the following drugs was most likely added to the patient's therapy resulting in his present complaint?

A. Hydralazine
B. Propranolol
C. Verapamil
D. Clonidine
E. Nitroprusside

Difficulty level: Easy

20. A 61-year-old man who had been suffering from stage 2 hypertension for many years had recently added minoxidil to his antihypertensive therapy. Which of the following actions best explains the antihypertensive effect of this drug?

A. Decreased cardiac output
B. Decreased central adrenergic tone
C. Decreased extracellular fluid volume
D. Decreased synthesis of angiotensin II
E. Decreased total peripheral resistance

Difficulty level: Easy

21. A 45-year-old woman was admitted to the hospital with a 2-day history of nausea, blurred vision, confusion, and intractable headache. Physical examination revealed an alert but disoriented female with a blood pressure of 240/130 mm Hg and a pulse of 95 bpm. A preliminary diagnosis of hypertensive encephalopathy was made, and an intravenous infusion of diazoxide was started. Which of the following molecular actions most likely mediated the therapeutic effect of this drug?

A. Increased synthesis of cyclic guanosine monophosphate (cGMP)
B. Activation of dopamine D_1 receptors
C. Opening of K^+ channels
D. Increased synthesis of cyclic adenosine monophosphate (cAMP)
E. Increased synthesis of inositol triphosphate/diacylglycerol (IP_3/DAG)
F. Blockade of Ca^{2+} channels

Difficulty level: Medium

22. A 47-year-old Black man presented to his physician complaining of a pounding morning headache. The patient had been suffering from chronic obstructive pulmonary disease for 3 years and had his right kidney removed after a car accident 5 years ago. His blood pressure was 170/115 mm Hg, and physical examination revealed a systolic-diastolic bruit on the epigastrium. The diagnosis of renovascular hypertension due to arteriosclerotic stenosis of the renal artery was confirmed later by arteriography. Which of the following would be a suitable drug treatment for this patient?

A. Hydrochlorothiazide and captopril
B. Furosemide and captopril
C. Furosemide and propranolol
D. Propranolol and nifedipine
E. Hydrochlorothiazide and nifedipine

Difficulty level: Hard

23. A 45-year-old African-American woman with known hypertension has been receiving hydrochlorothiazide and propranolol for several months. Now she has been diagnosed with variant angina, and her physician wants to revise her therapy. Which of the following would be the most appropriate therapeutic change to make at this time?

A. Substitute nifedipine for the propranolol,
B. Add nitroglycerin to the therapeutic regimen,
C. Substitute captopril for the propranolol,
D. Substitute nifedipine for the hydrochlorothiazide,
E. Add captopril to the therapeutic regimen,

Difficulty level: Hard

24. A 63-year-old hypertensive woman had been receiving an antihypertensive drug for 15 days. The following serum values were obtained from the patient before and after drug therapy:

Plasma Levels	Before	After
Aldosterone	High	Low
Potassium (mEq/L)	3.5	4.3
Renin	Normal	High
Angiotensin II	High	Low

Which of the following drugs was most likely administered?

A. Hydrochlorothiazide
B. Propranolol
C. Captopril
D. Hydralazine
E. Spironolactone

Difficulty level: Easy

25. A 33-year-old woman with known hypertension is now 2 weeks' pregnant. Which of the following antihypertensive drug classes is absolutely contraindicated in this woman?

A. Potassium channel openers
B. Angiotensin-converting enzyme (ACE) inhibitors
C. Ca^{2+} channel blockers
D. Alpha-1 blockers
E. Central sympatholytics

Difficulty level: Easy

26. A 67-year-old man complained to his physician of a dry, disturbing cough. In addition, he noted that food seemed to have lost its flavor. The man was recently diagnosed with stage 2 essential hypertension and had started a multidrug treatment 1 week earlier. Which of the following drugs most likely caused the patient's signs and symptoms?

A. Nifedipine
B. Clonidine
C. Propranolol
D. Minoxidil
E. Captopril

Difficulty level: Medium

27. A 59-year-old Black man presented to the clinic complaining of pruritic swelling of the eyelids, nose, lips, hands, feet, and genitalia. The man had recently been discharged from the hospital after an acute myocardial infarction. He had been prescribed an appropriate multidrug treatment. He noted that the swelling appeared a few hours after starting the therapy. Which of the following drugs most likely caused the patient's presenting symptoms?

A. Clopidogrel
B. Isosorbide mononitrate
C. Atenolol
D. Captopril
E. Lovastatin

Difficulty level: Medium

28. A 57-year-old man was admitted to the emergency department because he had not urinated for the past 12 hours. He had recently been diagnosed with moderate hypertension and had started taking two antihypertensive drugs 10 days ago. After a Foley catheter was inserted, only 30 mL of urine was obtained. A Doppler ultrasonography revealed bilateral renal artery stenosis. Which of the following pairs of drugs was the patient most likely taking?

A. Nifedipine and furosemide
B. Hydralazine and propranolol
C. Captopril and hydrochlorothiazide
D. Prazosin and methyldopa
E. Clonidine and verapamil

Difficulty level: Hard

29. A 60-year-old woman was found to have a blood pressure of 155/95 mm Hg during a routine doctor's visit. The patient had been suffering from type 1 diabetes for 12 years and from gouty arthritis for 5 years. Urinalysis showed microhematuria. Further blood pressure checks supported the diagnosis of stage 1 essential hypertension. Which of the following would be the most appropriate antihypertensive drug for this patient?

A. Hydrochlorothiazide
B. Propranolol
C. Captopril
D. Clonidine
E. Nitroprusside
F. Aliskiren

Difficulty level: Hard

30. A 52-year-old man was recently diagnosed with stage 1 hypertension and stage 1 systolic heart failure. Which of the following would be an appropriate antihypertensive treatment for this patient?

A. Hydrochlorothiazide and verapamil
B. Hydrochlorothiazide and minoxidil
C. Furosemide and hydralazine
D. Hydrochlorothiazide and captopril
E. Furosemide and methyldopa

Difficulty level: Easy

31. A 65-year-old Black woman recently diagnosed with stage 1 essential hypertension started a treatment with a thiazide diuretic. Which of the following molecular mechanisms is most likely to mediate the long-term antihypertensive effect of the thiazide drug in this patient?

A. Increased nitric oxide release from vascular endothelium

B. Decreased potassium in the extracellular fluid

C. Decreased sodium in smooth muscle cells

D. Increased calcium in the extracellular fluid

E. Increased cyclic guanosine monophosphate (cGMP) in smooth muscle cells

Difficulty level: Easy

32. A 55-year-old African-American woman was found to have a blood pressure of 165/100 mm Hg during a routine visit. Further analyses showed similar blood pressure values on multiple readings, a normal electrocardiogram, normal lab values, and no evidence of left ventricular hypertrophy or retinopathy. Which of the following antihypertensive drugs would be most appropriate for this patient?

A. Captopril

B. Furosemide

C. Nitroprusside

D. Fenoldopam

E. Hydrochlorothiazide

F. Atenolol

Difficulty level: Medium

33. A 66-year-old man recently diagnosed with stage 2 essential hypertension started a treatment with hydrochlorothiazide and losartan. Which of the following statements best explains the rationale for the association of these two drugs?

A. Thiazides enhance the antihypertensive effect of losartan.

B. Losartan counteracts thiazide-induced hypercalcemia.

C. Thiazides inhibit the appearance of tolerance to losartan.

D. Persons over age 65 rarely respond to a therapy with losartan alone.

E. Losartan inhibits thiazide-induced hypovolemia.

Difficulty level: Medium

34. A 70-year-old man with a recent history of stage 2 hypertension came to the clinic for a checkup. He smoked one pack of cigarettes daily and consumed three to five ethanol-containing drinks weekly. His present medications included captopril and verapamil. The patient's vital signs were blood pressure 166/96 mm Hg, heart rate 68 bpm. Pertinent lab values on admission were serum creatinine 1.6 mg/dL, potassium 5.1 mEq/L. Which of the following would be the most appropriate change in the patient's antihypertensive regimen?

A. Add furosemide.

B. Change captopril to losartan.

C. Add hydrochlorothiazide.

D. Change verapamil to nifedipine.

E. Add minoxidil.

Difficulty level: Easy

35. A 38-year old woman in week 16 of gestation was diagnosed with stage 1 chronic hypertension and started a treatment with methyldopa. Which of the following molecular actions most likely mediated the antihypertensive effect of this drug?

A. Opening K^+ channels in vascular smooth muscle cells

B. Blockade of β_1 adrenoceptors in juxtaglomerular cells

C. Activation of α_2 adrenoceptors in the vasomotor center

D. Activation of dopamine D_1 receptors in renal vessels

E. Blockade of α_1 receptors in vascular smooth muscle cells

Difficulty level: Easy

36. A 55-year-old woman with a long history of poorly controlled essential hypertension had recently added atenolol to her therapeutic regimen. Which of the following was most likely a primary mechanism that mediated the antihypertensive effect of atenolol in this patient?

A. Dilation of large veins

B. Inhibition of epinephrine release from the adrenal medulla

C. Blockade of β_2 receptors of the vascular wall

D. Decreased sympathetic outflow from vasomotor area

E. Decreased cardiac output

F. Decreased total blood volume

Difficulty level: Easy

37. A 46-year-old man underwent surgery to remove a glioma of the left brain lobe. An intravenous infusion of a drug was started to induce controlled hypotension to minimize blood loss during surgery. Which of the following drugs would be most appropriate for this purpose?

A. Labetalol

B. Hydralazine

C. Nifedipine

D. Nitroprusside

E. Enalaprilat

F. Diazoxide

Difficulty level: Medium

38. A 48-year-old woman was admitted to the emergency department with a 1-day history of nausea, blurred vision, confusion, and intractable headache. Her history showed that she was a heavy smoker and had been suffering from toxic tobacco amblyopia for 2 years. Physical examination revealed an alert but disoriented woman with a blood pressure of 220/140 mm Hg and a pulse of 90 bpm. An electrocardiogram showed a second-degree atrioventricular block. A preliminary diagnosis of hypertensive encephalopathy was made, and an intravenous infusion of a drug was started. Which of the following drugs would be most appropriate for this patient?

    A. Verapamil
    B. Diazoxide
    C. Labetalol
    D. Clonidine
    E. Captopril
    F. Nitroprusside

Difficulty level: Medium

39. A 55-year-old man at a routine checkup was found to have a blood pressure of 175/105 mm Hg. He had a long history of hypertension and had previously experienced adverse effects with verapamil (severe constipation) and captopril (annoying cough). He was presently taking hydrochlorothiazide, clonidine, and propranolol. His physician decided to add a fourth drug to the patient's regimen. Which of the following drugs would be appropriate at this time?

    A. Nifedipine
    B. Diazoxide
    C. Methyldopa
    D. Enalaprilat
    E. Minoxidil
    F. Fenoldopam

Difficulty level: Medium

40. A 31-year-old woman complained to her physician of pounding headache and occasional palpitations. The woman was recently married, and the couple wanted to have children. She had been suffering from moderate asthma for 5 years, presently treated with inhaled albuterol. She was found to have a high blood pressure (160/92 mm Hg), and subsequent exams confirmed the diagnosis of essential hypertension and atrial tachycardia. Which of the following drugs would be an appropriate antihypertensive therapy for this patient?

    A. Furosemide
    B. Captopril
    C. Prazosin
    D. Propranolol
    E. Diltiazem
    F. Fenoldopam

Questions: IV-5 Antiarrhythmic Drugs

Directions for questions **1–6**

Match each antiarrhythmic drug with the appropriate description (each lettered option can be selected once, more than once, or not at all).

    A. Adenosine
    B. Amiodarone
    C. Diltiazem
    D. Esmolol
    E. Flecainide
    F. Ibutilide
    G. Lidocaine
    H. Magnesium sulfate
    I. Metoprolol
    J. Mexiletine
    K. Phenytoin
    L. Procainamide
    M. Quinidine
    N. Sotalol

Difficulty level: Easy

1. This drug is an anticonvulsant frequently used to treat generalized tonic-clonic seizures.

Difficulty level: Easy

2. This drug acts on acetylcholine-sensitive K^+ channels.

Difficulty level: Easy

3. This drug is the most effective antiarrhythmic agent for both supraventricular and ventricular arrhythmias.

Difficulty level: Easy

4. This drug blocks inactivated (but not activated) Na^+ channels.

Difficulty level: Easy

5. This drug blocks both β receptors and K^+ channels.

Difficulty level: Easy

6. This drug may be used for treating malaria.

Difficulty level: Medium

7. A 51-year-old woman at a routine office visit was found to have a heart rate of 110 bpm. The woman had a history of atrial flutter for which she had been receiving quinidine for the past 2 weeks following a successful electrical cardioversion. The physician thought that her tachycardia was caused by quinidine. Which of the following actions best explains the mechanism of this adverse effect of quinidine?

A. Blockade of muscarinic receptors
B. Activation of α_1 receptors
C. Stimulation of arterial baroreceptors
D. Activation of calcium channels
E. Activation of potassium channels

Difficulty level: Hard

8. A Purkinje fiber was isolated from an animal heart and placed in a recording chamber. Action potentials were recorded before and after a low dose of quinidine was added to the perfusate. Which of the following electrophysiological responses would quinidine most likely produce in this preparation?

A. Decreased action potential duration
B. Increased slope of phase 3
C. Decreased slope of phase 0
D. Decreased effective refractory period
E. Increased slope of phase 4

Difficulty level: Easy

9. A 63-year-old man was admitted to the hospital because of fever, chills, and profuse epistaxis. The man, suffering from a reentrant supraventricular arrhythmia, had started a new antiarrhythmic drug the day before. Lab results on admission disclosed a platelet count of 50,000/mm³. Which of the following drugs most likely caused the patient's disorder?

A. Lidocaine
B. Verapamil
C. Quinidine
D. Adenosine
E. Sotalol
F. Diltiazem

Difficulty: Hard

10. A 24-year-old man presented to the emergency department with a chief complaint of palpitations for the past 3 hours. He had experienced no prior symptoms and had no significant past medical history. Vital signs were blood pressure 100/60 mm Hg, pulse 190 bpm, respirations 14/min. An electrocardiogram showed a picture compatible with Wolff–Parkinson–White syndrome. An appropriate therapy was instituted that included intravenous administration of a drug. Which of the following drugs was most likely given?

A. Digoxin
B. Verapamil
C. Propranolol
D. Procainamide
E. Nifedipine

Difficulty level: Easy

11. A 47-year-old woman suffering from sustained ventricular tachycardia had been receiving mexiletine for 1 month. In this patient's abnormal pacemaker cells, the drug most likely decreased which of the following electrophysiological parameters of the heart?

A. Refractoriness
B. Slope of phase 4
C. Action potential duration
D. Length of phase 2
E. Diastolic interval

Difficulty level: Easy

12. A 47-year-old man developed increasing ectopic beats followed by sustained tachycardia after being admitted to the coronary unit following a myocardial infarction. An electrocardiogram showed a frequency of 175 bpm, wide QRS complexes, and atrioventricular dissociation. He was given an intravenous infusion of an antiarrhythmic drug that restored the normal sinus rhythm, but 1 hour later the patient showed increased agitation, loss of coordination, confusion, slurred speech, nystagmus, trembling, and muscle twitching. Which of the following drugs was most likely administered?

A. Lidocaine
B. Phenytoin
C. Sotalol
D. Mexiletine
E. Verapamil
F. Digoxin

Difficulty level: Easy

13. A 65-year-old woman admitted to the emergency department with a myocardial infarction developed sustained ventricular tachycardia. Neither amiodarone nor lidocaine was effective, and the cardiologist decided to try another drug that acts mainly by blocking activated Na⁺ channels and K⁺ channels. Which of the following drugs was most likely administered?

A. Mexiletine
B. Adenosine
C. Sotalol
D. Verapamil
E. Procainamide

Difficulty level: Medium

14. A 54-year-old woman complained to her physician of palpitations, insomnia, diarrhea, and increased sweating for the past 3 weeks. Physical examination revealed a patient in moderate distress with mild hand tremors and exophthalmos. Vital signs were blood pressure 146/62 mm Hg, pulse 122 bpm, respirations 18/min. An electrocardiogram showed atrial tachycardia. Which of the following drugs would be most appropriate to treat the patient's arrhythmia?

A. Quinidine
B. Amiodarone
C. Verapamil
D. Propranolol
E. Digoxin

Difficulty level: Hard

15. A 34-year-old man was admitted to the emergency department with severe dyspnea and chest pain. Family history revealed that his father died suddenly from a heart attack that was apparently related to a gene defect. Auscultation of the heart showed an ejection-type murmur, and chest x-ray disclosed massive cardiomegaly. The electrocardiogram showed atrial fibrillation. An appropriate therapy was prescribed. Which of the following drugs was most likely given?

A. Procainamide
B. Quinidine
C. Flecainide
D. Atenolol
E. Nitroglycerin

Difficulty level: Easy

16. A 78-year-old man was admitted to the hospital because of dyspnea, a nonproductive cough, and fever. The man had been receiving an antiarrhythmic drug for 2 months to treat refractory supraventricular tachycardia. A chest x-ray showed diffuse bilateral infiltrates. Bacterial, fungal, and viral cultures were negative. Which of the following drugs most likely caused the patient's pulmonary disorder?

A. Flecainide
B. Mexiletine
C. Amiodarone
D. Sotalol
E. Procainamide

Difficulty level: Easy

17. A 44-year-old man complained to his physician of joint pains in his elbows and knees and of an unusual masklike rash over his face. The man, who was suffering from Wolff–

Parkinson–White syndrome, had been receiving an antiarrhythmic drug for 1 month. Discontinuation of the drug caused the symptoms to abate. Which of the following drugs did the patient most likely take?

A. Quinidine
B. Lidocaine
C. Amiodarone
D. Adenosine
E. Procainamide
F. Ibutilide

Difficulty level: Hard

18. A 56-year-old woman was admitted to the intensive care unit because she had been experiencing chest palpitations for the past 3 hours. Vital signs on admission were blood pressure 96/70 mm Hg, heart rate 210 bpm, respiration 15 breaths/min. An electrocardiogram indicated atrial fibrillation with wide QRS. A diagnosis was made, and amiodarone was given intravenously (IV). Fifteen minutes later, the heart rate was still 180 bpm. Another appropriate drug was administered IV. Which of the following was most likely the second drug administered?

A. Lidocaine
B. Mexiletine
C. Phenytoin
D. Nifedipine
E. Nitroglycerin
F. Procainamide

Difficulty level: Hard

19. A 53-year-old woman with a history of major depression was brought to the clinic by her husband because she was experiencing ongoing lethargy. Her medications included amitriptyline, and the husband said that he found an empty bottle of the medication in her room. Physical examination showed a lethargic, oriented patient with blood pressure 113/64, pulse 135 bpm, respirations 22/min. An electrocardiogram showed a ventricular arrhythmia with widened QRS complexes. An appropriate therapy was instituted, and an antiarrhythmic drug was prescribed. Which of the following antiarrhythmic drugs would be absolutely contraindicated for this patient?

A. Mexiletine
B. Lidocaine
C. Quinidine
D. Phenytoin
E. Propranolol

Difficulty level: Medium

20. A 54-year-old woman was admitted to the hospital because of an episode of dizziness and near-syncope. Her medical history was significant for urinary tract infection, presently treated with ciprofloxacin. A few days earlier, she was diagnosed with atrial fibrillation and started a treatment with sotalol. An electrocardiogram strip recorded by a Holter monitor during another episode of near-syncope clarified the diagnosis. From which of the following disorders did the patient most likely suffer?

A. Premature ventricular contractions
B. Atrial fibrillation
C. Second-degree atrioventricular block
D. Polymorphic ventricular tachycardia
E. Atrial tachycardia
F. Ventricular fibrillation

Difficulty level: Medium

21. A 55-year-old woman who had been suffering from atrial flutter for 3 months was admitted to the hospital for cardioversion. She received an intravenous infusion of a drug for 10 minutes, and a few minutes later the heart reverted to a normal sinus rhythm. Which of the following drugs was most likely administered?

A. Mexiletine
B. Lidocaine
C. Adenosine
D. Amiodarone
E. Ibutilide
F. Phenytoin

Difficulty level: Hard

22. A 50-year-old woman was brought to the emergency department by her brother, who stated she consumed a full bottle of one of her medications in a suicide attempt. The woman had a long history of depression, chronic obstructive pulmonary disease (treated by ipratropium), and recurrent supraventricular tachycardia. The patient was confused and drowsy. Vital signs were blood pressure 85/45 mm Hg, pulse 45 bpm, respirations 23/min. Which of the following drugs most likely caused the patient's signs and symptoms?

A. Ipratropium
B. Adenosine
C. Propranolol
D. Lidocaine
E. Verapamil

Difficulty level: Hard

23. A 59-year-old woman presented with an abrupt onset of palpitations accompanied by a vague complaint of "feeling ill." Subsequent Holter monitoring revealed atrial fibrillation with a ventricular response up to 152 bpm. The patient's past history included primary hyperparathyroidism and intermittent claudication for 3 years, apparently due to peripheral occlusive arteriosclerosis. Which of the following drugs would be appropriate for the chronic control of the patient's arrhythmia?

A. Digoxin
B. Propranolol
C. Verapamil
D. Lidocaine
E. Phenytoin
F. Adenosine

Difficulty level: Easy

24. A 44-year-old man presented to the emergency department complaining of fatigue and palpitations of 3-hour duration. Vital signs were heart rate 160 bpm, blood pressure 100/60 mm Hg, respirations 15/min. Physical examination was unremarkable. An electrocardiogram confirmed the diagnosis of narrow complex supraventricular tachycardia. An intravenous injection of adenosine was given, and 10 minutes later the heart rate went back to normal. Which of the following molecular actions most likely mediated the therapeutic efficacy of the drug in the patient's disease?

A. Blockade of Na^+ channels
B. Opening of Ca^{2+} channels
C. Activation of M_2 receptors
D. Blockade of β_1 receptors
E. Opening of K^+ channels

Difficulty level: Medium

25. 45-year-old man was admitted to the coronary unit because of a myocardial infarction in the posterior wall. Two hours after admission, his heart rate started decreasing (40 bpm), and an electrocardiogram indicated sinus bradycardia. Which of the following drugs would be most appropriate for this patient?

A. Isoproterenol
B. Epinephrine
C. Dobutamine
D. Dopamine
E. Atropine

Difficulty level: Easy

26. A 46-year-old woman complained to her physician of sleepiness, fatigue, cold intolerance, weight gain, and constipation. The woman, who had been suffering from ventricular tachycardia, had been receiving an antiarrhythmic drug for 2 months. A blood test revealed a high level of thyrotropin. Which of the following drugs most likely caused the patient's signs and symptoms?

   A. Mexiletine
   B. Sotalol
   C. Flecainide
   D. Lidocaine
   E. Procainamide
   F. Amiodarone

Difficulty level: Easy

27. A 56-year-old alcoholic man presented to the emergency department with a chief complaint of chest palpitations for the past 3 hours. Vital signs were blood pressure 170/90, pulse 170 beats/min. An electrocardiogram confirmed atrial fibrillation, and the physician was considering prescribing one of the following drugs: atenolol, verapamil, or digoxin. Which of the following actions best explains the therapeutic effectiveness of all of these drugs in treating atrial fibrillation?

   A. Decreased atrioventricular conduction
   B. Increased intra-atrial conduction
   C. Increased ventricular refractoriness
   D. Increased myocardial contractility
   E. Decreased cardiac preload

Difficulty level: Medium

28. A 52-year-old man with a long history of chronic obstructive pulmonary disease was recently diagnosed with atrial fibrillation. Which of the following drugs would be appropriate for the chronic control of the patient's arrhythmia?

   A. Amiodarone
   B. Verapamil
   C. Nifedipine
   D. Lidocaine
   E. Mexiletine
   F. Sotalol

Difficulty level: Hard

29. A 63-year-old man who had been suffering from hypertension and mild cardiac failure for 3 years was recently diagnosed with sustained atrial fibrillation. The arrhythmia was refractory to therapy with verapamil and was only partially controlled by sotalol. Which of the following drugs would be appropriate to prescribe to the patient at this time?

   A. Diltiazem
   B. Mexiletine
   C. Amiodarone
   D. Lidocaine
   E. Propranolol

Difficulty level: Medium

30. A 33-year-old woman presented to the emergency department complaining of fatigue and palpitations for the past 3 hours. Physical examination revealed a female in no apparent distress with the following vital signs: blood pressure 100/60 mm Hg, heart rate 172 bpm, respirations 12/min. An electrocardiogram showed a regular rhythm with heart rate 168 bpm. A Valsalva maneuver and a carotid sinus massage were attempted with no success. An intravenous injection of a drug was given. Which of the following drugs would be appropriate for this patient?

   A. Lidocaine
   B. Mexiletine
   C. Adenosine
   D. Phenytoin
   E. Verapamil
   F. Diltiazem

Difficulty level: Medium

31. A 24-year-old man complained to his physician of frequent bursts of palpitations for the past week. Further exams led to the diagnosis of idiopathic left ventricular tachycardia. Which of the following drugs would be appropriate for the chronic control of the patient's arrhythmia?

   A. Lidocaine
   B. Digoxin
   C. Quinidine
   D. Flecainide
   E. Adenosine

Difficulty level: Hard

32. A 57-year-old man admitted to the coronary unit after coronary bypass surgery developed increasing ectopic beats followed by sustained tachycardia. An electrocardiogram showed a frequency of 170 bpm, wide QRS complexes, and atrioventricular dissociation. An intravenous (IV) loading dose of an appropriate drug was given, then an IV infusion of the same drug was started. Which of the following drugs was most likely administered?

   A. Phenytoin
   B. Verapamil
   C. Quinidine
   D. Mexiletine
   E. Lidocaine

Difficulty level: Easy

33. A 62-year-old man suffering from atrial flutter was electrically cardioverted and discharged from the hospital with a postdischarge therapy for rhythm control. The prescribed drug primarily blocks activated Na$^+$ channels and has negligible effects on action potential duration. Which of the following drugs was most likely given?

   A. Amiodarone
   B. Flecainide
   C. Lidocaine
   D. Adenosine
   E. Diltiazem

Difficulty level: Hard

34. A 35-year-old man with a long history of heroin abuse was admitted to the emergency department because of nausea and vomiting, blurred vision, dizziness, ringing in the ears, and headache. The man said he had intravenously (IV) self-injected a dose of heroin bought from a new vendor. One hour after the admission, he was found unresponsive by the nursing staff. An electrocardiogram showed torsade de pointes. Cardiopulmonary life support was initiated, and a drug was given IV. Which of the following drugs would be appropriate for the patient at this time?

   A. Ibutilide
   B. Amiodarone
   C. Procainamide
   D. Sotalol
   E. Magnesium sulfate
   F. Verapamil
   G. Lidocaine

Difficulty level: Easy

35. A 58-year-old-woman admitted to the coronary unit with a myocardial infarction developed ventricular tachycardia and was given an intravenous injection of amiodarone. The therapeutic effect of the drug was most likely mediated by an increase in which of the following electrophysiological parameters?

   A. Slope of phase 4
   B. Slope of phase 0
   C. Action potential duration
   D. Length of phase 2
   E. Maximum diastolic potential

Difficulty level: Medium

36. A 53-year-old woman is in her cardiologist's office for a routine visit. The woman has been suffering from paroxysmal atrial fibrillation for 4 months. Her current medications are digoxin and warfarin. Now the cardiologist would like to attempt to restore and maintain sinus rhythm with oral amiodarone. Which of the following would be an appropriate adjustment of the ongoing therapy of this patient?

   A. Decrease the warfarin dose only.
   B. Decrease the digoxin dose only.
   C. Decrease both warfarin and digoxin doses.
   D. Increase the digoxin dose before starting amiodarone.
   E. Discontinue warfarin as soon as sinus rhythm is restored.

Difficulty level: Hard

37. A 67-year-old woman complained to her physician of frequent palpitations for the past 2 weeks. The woman had been suffering from severe asthma for 5 years and from exertional angina for 2 years. An electrocardiogram showed absence of P waves and an "irregularly irregular" ventricular rate. Which of the following antiarrhythmic drugs would be appropriate for this patient?

   A. Sotalol
   B. Flecainide
   C. Mexiletine
   D. Lidocaine
   E. Labetalol
   F. Adenosine
   G. Diltiazem

Difficulty level: Easy

38. A 55-year-old man, admitted to the coronary unit with a myocardial infarction developed ventricular fibrillation and was successfully cardioverted. To prevent further fibrillatory episodes, he was given an intravenous antiarrhythmic drug that is effective in both supraventricular and ventricular arrhythmias and has a half-life of about 1 month. Which of the following drugs was most likely administered?

   A. Mexiletine
   B. Sotalol
   C. Quinidine
   D. Amiodarone
   E. Procainamide
   F. Lidocaine

Difficulty level: Easy

39. A Purkinje fiber was isolated from an animal heart and placed in a recording chamber. Action potentials were recorded before and after a low dose of ibutilide was added to the perfusate. Which of the following was the most likely electrophysiological action of the drug on this preparation?

   A. Decreased action potential duration
   B. Decreased slope of phase 0
   C. Increased action potential duration
   D. Decreased effective refractory period
   E. Increased slope of phase 4

Questions: IV-6 Antihyperlipidemic Drugs

Directions for questions **1–4**

Match each antihyperlipidemic drug with the appropriate description (each lettered option can be selected once, more than once, or not at all).

A. Cholestyramine
B. Ezetimibe
C. Gemfibrozil
D. Niacin
E. Lovastatin

Difficulty level: Easy

1. This drug can sometimes cause hypertriglyceridemia.

Difficulty level: Easy

2. Facial flushing is the most common adverse effect of this drug.

Difficulty level: Easy

3. High doses of this drug can cause metabolic acidosis.

Difficulty level: Easy

4. This drug activates a nuclear transcription receptor.

Difficulty level: Easy

5. A 21-year-old woman recently diagnosed with familial combined hyperlipidemia started a treatment with lovastatin. Which of the following molecular actions most likely mediated the therapeutic efficacy of the drug in the patient's disease?

A. Downregulation of hepatic low-density lipoprotein (LDL) receptors
B. Increased synthesis of lipoprotein lipase
C. Decreased synthesis of mevalonic acid
D. Decreased storage of LDL in hepatic endosomes
E. Increased plasma levels of hepatic aminotransferases
F. Increased plasma levels of creatine phosphokinase

Difficulty level: Easy

6. A 28-year-old woman recently diagnosed with familial combined hyperlipidemia started a treatment with a low-fat diet and cholestyramine. This therapy most likely caused the greatest reduction in plasma levels of which of the following compounds?

A. Very-low-density lipoprotein (VLDL)
B. High-density lipoprotein (HDL)
C. Low-density lipoprotein (LDL)
D. Chylomicrons
E. Triglycerides

Difficulty level: Medium

7. A 54-year-old obese man had plasma low-density lipoprotein (LDL) cholesterol of 270 mg/dL despite 4 months of therapy with lovastatin. The physician decided to add cholestyramine to the patient's regimen. Recently, the patient had been found to have stage 1 hypertension for which he was currently taking propranolol and hydrochlorothiazide. Which of the following changes in the pharmacokinetics of these two drugs was most likely to occur when the patient began to take cholestyramine?

A. Clearance of propranolol increased.
B. Clearance of hydrochlorothiazide decreased.
C. Oral bioavailability of propranolol increased.
D. Oral bioavailability of hydrochlorothiazide decreased.
E. Volume of distribution of propranolol increased.
F. Volume of distribution of hydrochlorothiazide decreased.

Difficulty level: Hard

8. A 52-year-old man was found to have total cholesterol of 380 mg/dL and triglycerides of 230 mg/dL despite 3 months of a diet low in saturated fat. The man had been suffering from hemophilia since birth and from external hemorrhoids for 2 years. An antihyperlipidemic therapy was prescribed. Which of the following drugs would be contraindicated in this patient?

A. Lovastatin
B. Cholestyramine
C. Ezetimibe
D. Niacin
E. Gemfibrozil

Difficulty level: Medium

9. A 24-year-old woman suffering from familial hypertriglyceridemia was screened with a blood lipid profile during a routine visit. Relevant laboratory test results were uric acid 15 mg/dL (normal 4.0–8.5 mg/dL), total cholesterol 170 mg/dL (normal < 200 mg/dL), triglycerides 1230 mg/dL (normal < 200 mg/dL). A lipid-lowering drug was prescribed. Which of the following was most likely the mechanism of action of that drug?

A. Increase of lipid synthesis by adipose tissue
B. Downregulation of low-density lipoprotein (LDL) receptors in the liver
C. Inhibition HMG-CoA (3-hydroxy-3-methylglutaryl–coenzyme A) reductase activity in the liver
D. Stimulation of lipoprotein lipase synthesis
E. Decreased absorption of exogenous cholesterol

Difficulty level: Easy

10. A 55-year-old obese woman was found to have a total cholesterol level of 360 mg/dL (normal < 200 mg/dL), despite many months of lovastatin treatment. The physician decided to add ezetimibe to the therapeutic regimen. Which of the following cells represents the main site of action of the added drug?

    A. Adipocytes
    B. Capillary endothelial cells
    C. Platelets
    D. Hepatocytes
    E. Intestinal epithelial cells

Difficulty level: Easy

11. A 57-year-old man was found to have low-density lipoprotein (LDL) cholesterol of 360 mg/dL (normal < 130 mg/dL) despite 5 months of treatment with lovastatin. The physician decided to add ezetimibe to the therapeutic regimen. Which of the following statements best explains the rationale of adding ezetimibe to lovastatin therapy?

    A. The combination decreases the risk of lovastatin-induced myopathy.
    B. The combination results in synergistic cholesterol-lowering effects.
    C. Ezetimibe slows down the metabolism of lovastatin.
    D. Ezetimibe increases the intestinal absorption of lovastatin.
    E. The combination strongly increases high-density lipoprotein (HDL) plasma levels.

Difficulty level: Easy

12. A 46-year-old man suffering from familial hypercholesterolemia was found to have total cholesterol of 430 mg/dL despite many months of treatment with lovastatin. Triglyceride levels were normal. His physician decided to add niacin to the therapeutic regimen. Which of the following molecular actions most likely mediated the therapeutic efficacy of niacin in the patient's disease?

    A. Inhibition of very-low-density lipoprotein (VLDL) production by the hepatocyte
    B. Inhibition of high-density lipoprotein (HDL) synthesis by the liver
    C. Increase of circulating fibrinogen
    D. Stimulation of lipolysis in adipose tissue
    E. Decreased absorption of exogenous cholesterol

Difficulty level: Easy

13. A 49-year-old man was brought by ambulance to the emergency department with the admitting diagnosis of myocardial infarction. Emergency therapy was started, which included alteplase, aspirin, heparin, and metoprolol. The next day lovastatin and ezetimibe were added to the therapeutic regimen. Which of the drugs received by the patient acts primarily in the cytoplasmic compartment of liver cells?

    A. Alteplase
    B. Aspirin
    C. Lovastatin
    D. Heparin
    E. Ezetimibe
    F. Metoprolol

Difficulty level: Medium

14. A 52-year-old obese man suffering from gout and hypertension was found to have low-density lipoprotein (LDL) cholesterol of 360 mg/dL (normal < 130 mg/dL) and a serum uric acid of 15.5 mg/dL (normal 4.0–8.5 mg/dL). Other laboratory values were within normal limits. A lipid-lowering therapy was prescribed. Which of the following antihyperlipidemic drugs would be relatively contraindicated in this patient?

    A. Cholestyramine
    B. Niacin
    C. Ezetimibe
    D. Lovastatin
    E. Gemfibrozil

Difficulty level: Medium

15. A 56-year-old woman suffering from familial hypercholesterolemia was found to have total cholesterol of 470 mg/dL (normal < 200 mg/dL) despite many months of treatment with lovastatin. Triglyceride levels were normal. The physician decided to add niacin to the therapeutic regimen. Which of the following drugs should be given during the first days of therapy to avoid niacin-induced flushes?

    A. Warfarin
    B. Atropine
    C. Aspirin
    D. Prazosin
    E. Gemfibrozil

Difficulty level: Hard

16. A 40-year-old obese man suffering from type I diabetes mellitus and hyperlipidemia was admitted to the hospital because of vomiting and circulatory collapse. The patient had started an antihyperlipidemic therapy 1 month ago. Pertinent plasma data on admission were pH 7.32, HCO_3^- 12 mEq/L (normal 22–26 mEq/L), partial pressure of arterial carbon dioxide (P_aCO_2) 16 mm Hg (normal 25–45 mm Hg), Cl^- 125 mEq/L (normal 90–105 mEq/L). Which of the following drugs could have contributed to the syndrome the patient was suffering from?

A. Lovastatin
B. Insulin
C. Niacin
D. Gemfibrozil
E. Cholestyramine

Difficulty level: Easy

17. A 57-year-old woman was found to have triglyceride levels of 630 mg/dL (normal < 200 mg/dL). Therapy with gemfibrozil was prescribed. Which of the following cellular structures most likely represents the site of action of this drug?

A. Smooth endoplasmic reticulum
B. Nucleus
C. Cell membrane
D. Cytoplasm
E. Rough endoplasmic reticulum
F. Mitochondria

Difficulty level: Medium

18. A 45-year-old man complained to his physician of muscle aches, soreness, and weakness. The patient had been suffering from duodenal ulcer for 2 years, from familial hypercholesterolemia for 5 years, and from open-angle glaucoma for 1 year. Current therapy included famotidine and sucralfate for ulcer, lovastatin for hyperlipidemia, and timolol and latanoprost for glaucoma. A urinalysis showed myoglobinuria. Which of the following drugs most likely caused this finding?

A. Latanoprost
B. Famotidine
C. Timolol
D. Sucralfate
E. Lovastatin

Difficulty level: Medium

19. A 49-year-old man at a routine checkup was found to have the following lipid profile: low-density lipoprotein (LDL) cholesterol 180 mg/dL (normal < 200 mg/dL), high-density lipoprotein (HDL) cholesterol 14 mg/dL (normal > 35 mg/dL), triglycerides 150 mg/dL (normal < 200 mg/dL). The man

weighed 295 lb (134 kg) and was a heavy cigarette smoker. Which of the following antihyperlipidemic drugs would be most appropriate for this patient?

A. Gemfibrozil
B. Lovastatin
C. Cholestyramine
D. Niacin
E. Ezetimibe

Difficulty level: Easy

20. A 26-year-old obese woman who was found to have a low-density lipoprotein (LDL) cholesterol level of 270 mg/mL (normal <130 mg/mL) despite 4 months of diet, started a lipid-lowering therapy with cholestyramine. Which of the following is the primary site of action of this drug?

A. Liver
B. Small intestine
C. Colon
D. Plasma
E. Adipose tissue
F. Gall bladder

Difficulty level: Medium

21. A new antihyperlipidemic drug was tested on patients with high cholesterol levels during a phase 3 clinical trial. Which of the following populations would be best suited to show the potential protective effect of the drug against coronary artery disease?

A. Women ages 40 to 50
B. Men ages 50 to 60
C. Obese children
D. Women over age 75
E. Men over age 75

Difficulty level: Medium

22. A 53-year-old woman was brought to the hospital because of sudden unilateral blindness and inability to move the extremities of the contralateral body side. All symptoms disappeared a half hour later. An angiogram revealed a 55% stenosis of the right carotid artery. An appropriate therapy was prescribed. Which of the following drugs given chronically would be most likely to contribute to a decreased risk of further stroke in this patient?

A. Isosorbide mononitrate
B. Furosemide
C. Lovastatin
D. Esmolol
E. Alteplase
F. Gemfibrozil

Difficulty level: Medium

23. A 35-year-old man with familial combined hyperlipidemia was found to have a total cholesterol level of 380 mg/mL (normal < 200 mg/mL) and a triglyceride level of 720 mg/mL (normal < 150 mg/mL). His family doctor decided to start therapy with lovastatin and gemfibrozil. The physician was aware that with this therapy the patient was at increased risk of myopathy. To prevent this disorder, which of the following enzymes should be measured every 2 weeks?

   A. HMG-CoA (3-hydroxy-3-methylglutaryl–coenzyme A) reductase
   B. Aminotransferase
   C. Alkaline phosphatase
   D. Cyclooxygenase
   E. Creatine kinase

Difficulty level: Easy

24. A 57-year-old obese woman had low-density lipoprotein (LDL) cholesterol of 350 mg/dL (normal < 130 mg/dL) despite 3 months of therapy with lovastatin. The physician decided to add to the patient's regimen a drug that acts by increasing the elimination of bile acids. Which of the following drugs was most likely prescribed?

   A. Cholestyramine
   B. Gemfibrozil
   C. Atorvastatin
   D. Niacin
   E. Ezetimibe

Difficulty level: Medium

25. A 53-year-old man continued to have a low-density lipoprotein (LDL) cholesterol level of 270 mg/dL (normal < 130 mg/dL) after a 6-month trial of diet therapy. His triglyceride levels were in the normal range. The patient had been suffering from type II diabetes mellitus for 2 years and peptic ulcer for 4 months. Current therapy included glyburide and metformin for diabetes and omeprazole for peptic ulcer. Which of the following drugs would be most appropriate to treat this patient's hyperlipidemia?

   A. Niacin
   B. Cholestyramine
   C. Lovastatin
   D. Nicotinamide
   E. Gemfibrozil

Difficulty level: Medium

26. During a routine follow-up visit, a 52-year-old man was found to have the following lab results: alanine aminotransferase 120 U/L (normal 8–20 U/L), aspartate aminotransferase 108 U/L (normal 8–20 U/L). The man had been discharged from the hospital after an acute myocardial infarction 2

months earlier and was on an appropriate postdischarge therapy. Which of the following drugs most likely caused the lab results?

   A. Atenolol
   B. Lovastatin
   C. Warfarin
   D. Clopidogrel
   E. Captopril

Difficulty level: Hard

27. A 51-year-old man suffering from hyperlipidemia was screened with a lipoprotein profile during a follow-up medical evaluation. He was found to have a low-density lipoprotein (LDL) cholesterol level of 440 mg/dL (normal <130 mg/dL) despite many months of lovastatin therapy. Triglyceride levels were 120 mg/dL. The patient had been suffering from type I diabetes for 15 years. Because a substantial reduction of LDL cholesterol was needed, a combination of two antihyperlipidemic drugs was considered. Which of the following would be the most appropriate drug combination for this patient?

   A. Lovastatin and cholestyramine
   B. Lovastatin and niacin
   C. Cholestyramine and niacin
   D. Gemfibrozil and ezetimibe
   E. Gemfibrozil and cholestyramine

Difficulty level: Hard

28. Each of the following patients (1 to 5) was found to have an abnormal lipid profile and was placed on a lipid-lowering diet for 4 months. None had any history of ischemic heart disease. The results of the patients' fasting lipid profile after 4 months of diet are given in the following table.

	Triglycerides (mg/dL)	LDL (mg/dL)	HDL (mg/dL)
1	300	120	20
2	190	130	25
3	300	210	20
4	230	180	65
5	180	120	45
Normal values	< 200	< 130	> 35

Abbreviations: HDL, high-density lipoprotein; LDL, low-density lipoprotein.

For which one of the following patients would it be most important to recommend an antihyperlipidemic drug at this time?

   A. Patient 1
   B. Patient 2
   C. Patient 3
   D. Patient 4
   E. Patient 5

Difficulty level: Medium

29. A 63-year-old obese man presented to the hospital with the admitting diagnosis of acute renal failure. He reported that 2 days earlier, he realized his urine was clear and red. One month earlier, the man was found to have plasma cholesterol of 310 mg/dL (normal < 200 mg/dL) and triglycerides of 950 mg/dL (normal < 150 mg/dL). He started an appropriate lipid-lowering therapy at that time. Which of the following pharmacotherapies most likely caused the patient's renal failure?

    A. Cholestyramine alone
    B. Cholestyramine and niacin
    C. Lovastatin and gemfibrozil
    D. Lovastatin alone
    E. Niacin alone

Difficulty level: Medium

30. A 54-year-old man suffering from familial hypercholesterolemia started treatment with lovastatin and cholestyramine. Which of the following actions most likely mediated the therapeutic effect of both drugs in the patient's disease?

    A. Decreased intestinal reabsorption of bile acids
    B. Decreased conversion of cholesterol to bile acids
    C. Decreased synthesis of cholesterol by the liver
    D. Upregulation of hepatic low-density lipoprotein (LDL) receptors
    E. Decreased synthesis of triglycerides by the liver

Questions: IV-7 Drugs Affecting Hemostasis

Directions for questions **1–4**

Match each drug affecting hemostasis with the appropriate description (each lettered option can be selected once, more than once, or not at all).

    A. Abciximab
    B. Alteplase
    C. Aminocaproic acid
    D. Aspirin
    E. Clopidogrel
    F. Desmopressin
    G. Enoxaparin
    H. Factor VIII
    I. Heparin
    J. Protamine sulfate
    K. Vitamin K
    L. Warfarin

Difficulty level: Easy

1. This drug binds noncompetitively to glycoprotein IIb/IIIa receptor complex.

Difficulty level: Easy

2. This drug increases the activity of factor VIII.

Difficulty level: Easy

3. This drug blocks the conversion of plasminogen to plasmin.

Difficulty level: Easy

4. This drug catalyzes the conversion of plasminogen into active plasmin.

Difficulty level: Easy

5. A 54-year-old woman suffering from asthma was brought to the emergency department because of a sudden onset of left-side paralysis. Imaging studies confirmed the diagnosis of thromboembolic stroke, and the patient started a treatment that included a drug that acts by blocking platelet adenosine diphosphate (ADP) receptors. Which of the following drugs has this mechanism of action?

    A. Warfarin
    B. Aminocaproic acid
    C. Alteplase
    D. Clopidogrel
    E. Heparin
    F. Aspirin

Difficulty level: Easy

6. A 34-year-old man admitted to the emergency department with a presumptive diagnosis of pulmonary thromboembolism started a treatment that included a drug that acts by accelerating the binding between antithrombin III and clotting factor proteases. Which of the following drugs has this mechanism of action?

    A. Warfarin
    B. Aminocaproic acid
    C. Alteplase
    D. Clopidogrel
    E. Heparin
    F. Aspirin

Difficulty level: Medium

7. A 30-year-old woman presented to her family physician complaining of black, tarry stools. The woman had had a prosthetic valve replacement 4 months earlier for severe aortic stenosis secondary to rheumatic disease and had been receiving daily oral anticoagulant therapy since then. Physical examination revealed subconjunctival hemorrhage and bruises on her arms and legs. Which of the following drugs most likely caused the patient's signs and symptoms?

A. Streptokinase
B. Aspirin
C. Heparin
D. Warfarin
E. Aminocaproic acid
F. Bivalirudin

Difficulty level: Hard

8. A 42-year-old woman suffering from systemic lupus erythematosus presented to the clinic with substernal, nonradiating pain that awakened her from sleep. Physical examination showed a patient in moderate distress, complaining of chest pain that was worsened by thoracic motion. Vital signs included temperature 103°F (39.4°C), pulse 90 bpm, blood pressure 150/90 mm Hg, respirations 18/min. Auscultation revealed a precordial systolic and diastolic friction rub. Which of the following drug classes would be absolutely contraindicated for this patient?

A. Nonsteroidal antiinflammatory drugs
B. Fibrinolytic drugs
C. Glucocorticoids
D. Opioids
E. Antibiotics

Difficulty level: Medium

9. A 55-year-old man complained to his physician of red blood in his stools and pink urine. Two weeks earlier, the man had started a treatment with warfarin for recurrent deep vein thrombosis. On physical examination, the patient appeared pale and diaphoretic. Vital signs were blood pressure 85/55 mm Hg, heart rate 105 bpm, respirations 20/min. An appropriate therapy was started. Which of the following drugs was most likely administered intravenously to the patient?

A. Vitamin K
B. Aminocaproic acid
C. Protamine sulfate
D. Alteplase
E. Fresh frozen plasma

Difficulty level: Medium

10. A 32-year-old man suffering from hemophilia A was at his dentist's office for a tooth extraction. In preparation for minor surgery, the patient received a subcutaneous injection of desmopressin, a drug that was effective for him in the past. Which of the following statements best explains why desmopressin was an appropriate therapy for the patient?

A. It increases the plasma levels of factor VIII.
B. It increases the intestinal absorption of vitamin K.
C. It has a pronounced antifibrinolytic activity.
D. It inhibits the activity of antithrombin III.
E. It inhibits the activity of proteins C and S.

Difficulty level: Easy

11. A 72-year-old man recently diagnosed with atrial fibrillation started a treatment that included dabigatran. The inhibition of which of the following molecular actions most likely mediated the therapeutic effect of the drug in this patient?

A. Prothrombin synthesis
B. Thromboxane A_2 activity
C. Thrombin activity
D. Plasminogen synthesis
E. Antithrombin III activity

Difficulty level: Medium

12. A 62-year-old woman complained to her physician of nose bleeds and red eyes. The woman had been receiving warfarin for 1 month because of deep venous thrombosis. Four days earlier, she had started treatment with erythromycin for acute pharyngitis. Which of the following drug-induced changes was most likely responsible for the patient's symptoms?

A. Erythromycin-induced inhibition of clotting factors synthesis
B. Erythromycin-induced inhibition of warfarin metabolism
C. Warfarin-induced thrombosis of the nasal mucosal microvasculature
D. Erythromycin-induced decrease of intestinal absorption of vitamin K
E. Warfarin-induced decreased of vitamin K production by intestinal flora

Difficulty level: Medium

13. A 56-year-old man admitted to the hospital with a myocardial infarction underwent a percutaneous coronary angioplasty for the revascularization of his left coronary. Which of the following drugs was most likely given intravenously during the procedure?

A. Warfarin
B. Clopidogrel
C. Protamine
D. Aminocaproic acid
E. Recombinant factor VIIa
F. Abciximab

Difficulty level: Medium

14. A 64-year-old man was admitted to the emergency department with the presumptive diagnosis of pulmonary embolism. He was started on an appropriate emergency therapy. Three days later, his fingers became discolored, and laboratory tests showed the following: white blood cell count (WBC) $10.2 \times 10^3/mm^3$ (normal $4.3–10.8 \times 10^3/mm^3$), red blood cell count (RBC) $4.8 \times 10^6/mm^3$ (normal $3.5–5.0 \times 10^6/mm^3$), platelets $75 \times 10^3/mm^3$ (normal $140–440 \times 10^3/mm^3$). Which of the following drugs most likely caused the patient's signs and symptoms?

   A. Vitamin K
   B. Aspirin
   C. Heparin
   D. Warfarin
   E. Alteplase
   F. Aminocaproic acid

Difficulty level: Easy

15. A 63-year-old man told his physician that in the morning he discovered his urine was cloudy and red. The man was suffering from persistent atrial fibrillation and had been stabilized on warfarin therapy for 1 month. Three days earlier, he had started taking an over-the-counter preparation containing cimetidine for heartburn. Which of the following statements best explains the cause of the patient's symptoms?

   A. Decreased renal clearance of warfarin
   B. Decreased intestinal absorption of vitamin K
   C. Inhibition of hepatic metabolism of warfarin
   D. Anticoagulant effect of cimetidine
   E. Warfarin displacement from plasma protein–binding sites

Difficulty level: Medium

16. A 71-year-old woman who underwent hip replacement was discharged from the hospital with an appropriate postdischarge therapy that included daily subcutaneous injection of regular heparin. Which of the following lab exams should be performed frequently during the heparin treatment?

   A. Red blood cell count (RBC)
   B. Platelet count
   C. Plasma K^+ level
   D. Plasma Na^+ level
   E. Bleeding time
   F. Fibrinolysis time

Difficulty level: Medium

17. A 50-year-old man was brought to the emergency department by ambulance for management of severe, unrelenting chest pain for the past hour. The man had been suffering from exertional angina for 5 years. Physical examination revealed a middle-aged man in obvious distress with the following vital signs: blood pressure 165/100 mm Hg, heart rate 110 bpm, respirations 22/min. An electrocardiogram showed ST-segment depression in multiple leads. Which of the following pairs of drugs should be included in the immediate treatment of this patient?

   A. Clopidogrel and aminocaproic acid
   B. Alteplase and warfarin
   C. Heparin and aspirin
   D. Abciximab and warfarin
   E. Aminocaproic acid and abciximab
   F. Aspirin and desmopressin

Difficulty level: Easy

18. A 67-year-old woman presented to the clinic because of progressive swelling and soreness of the left calf. After physical examination and lab exams, a diagnosis of deep venous thrombosis was made, and a treatment with enoxaparin was started. Which of the following is the main advantage of this drug over the standard unfractionated heparin?

   A. Complete absence of bleeding complications
   B. Good oral bioavailability
   C. Lower incidence of drug-induced thrombocytopenia
   D. Pronounced antiplatelet activity
   E. Inhibitions of a larger number of coagulation factors

Difficulty level: Hard

19. A 65-year-old man developed sudden dyspnea and chest pain 2 days after surgery to remove a gastric carcinoma. Physical examination revealed an anxious man in severe respiratory distress with the following vital signs: temperature 99.5°F (37.5°C), pulse 120 bpm, blood pressure 90/50 mm Hg, respirations 28 breaths/min. A computed tomography scan showed complete obstruction of a branch of the left pulmonary artery. Which of the following drugs should be included in the acute parenteral treatment of this patient?

   A. Nitroglycerin
   B. Aspirin
   C. Alteplase
   D. Warfarin
   E. Heparin
   F. Clopidogrel

Difficulty level: Medium

20. A 48-year-old woman who had been suffering from breast cancer for 2 years was admitted to the hospital with a diagnosis of deep venous thrombosis. An intravenous (IV) loading dose of heparin was administered, followed by an IV infusion. After 6 hours of heparin therapy, the patient's activated partial thromboplastin time (aPTT) had not increased relative to her heparin pretreatment levels. Which of the following statements best explains this finding?

A. The patient had high plasma levels of heparin-binding proteins.

B. The patient's therapy included a vitamin K supplement.

C. Heparin has a very short half-life (2 to 4 minutes).

D. Heparin effects are delayed at least 12 hours after administration.

E. The patient had high plasma levels of antithrombin III.

Difficulty level: Medium

21. A 63-year-old man suddenly collapsed at home and was brought unconscious to the emergency department. Physical examination showed a comatose patient with flaccid paralysis on both left extremities. Vital signs were blood pressure 132/70 mm Hg, pulse 90 bpm, respirations 8 breaths/min. A diffusion magnetic resonance imaging (MRI) scan disclosed complete occlusion of the right internal carotid artery. Emergency therapy was ordered. Which of the following drugs was most likely included in the emergency treatment of this patient?

A. Aminocaproic acid

B. Desmopressin

C. Alteplase

D. Dabigatran

E. Bivalirudin

F. Warfarin

Difficulty level: Medium

22. A 69-year-old obese man presented to the clinic because of left calf swelling and pain of 1-day duration. He stated that a few days before the onset of symptoms, he had arrived home after a 14-hour flight from India. Duplex scanning was performed and revealed clot formation in the patient's left calf. The patient did not exhibit signs of pulmonary embolism. Which of the following pairs of drugs were most likely prescribed to the patient?

A. Heparin and abciximab

B. Warfarin and abciximab

C. Heparin and warfarin

D. Alteplase and warfarin

E. Alteplase and heparin

F. Alteplase and abciximab

Difficulty level: Medium

23. A 50-year-old woman admitted to the coronary unit because of a myocardial infarction received an appropriate multidrug therapy. The next day she complained of an abrupt headache, followed shortly by vomiting and loss of consciousness. A computed tomography scan of the brain confirmed the diagnosis of stroke due to cerebral hemorrhage. Which of the following drugs most likely contributed to the appearance of the patient's stoke?

A. Aspirin

B. Propranolol

C. Nitroglycerin

D. Alteplase

E. Warfarin

Difficulty level: Medium

24. A 55-year-old woman recently diagnosed with atrial flutter started a treatment that included warfarin. The time of onset of the anticoagulant effect of this drug mainly depends on the half-life of which of the following endogenous compounds?

A. Already-formed factor VII

B. Circulating antithrombin

C. Already formed factor II

D. Vitamin K

E. Circulating fibrinogen

Difficulty level: Medium

25. A 68-year-old man with no past medical history was admitted to the emergency department because of severe substernal crushing chest pain with radiation to the left arm for the past 2 hours. An electrocardiogram confirmed the diagnosis of acute anterior myocardial infarction. Which of the following pairs of drugs were most likely immediately given intravenously to the patient?

A. Alteplase and heparin

B. Alteplase and warfarin

C. Dobutamine and milrinone

D. Dobutamine and aspirin

E. Clopidogrel and heparin

F. Aspirin and warfarin

Difficulty level: Hard

26. A 64-year-old woman was diagnosed with hypothyroidism and started on levothyroxine replacement therapy. For the previous 8 months, she had been receiving warfarin therapy for the treatment of recurrent deep venous thrombosis. Her warfarin dose was adjusted to maintain her international normalized ratio (INR) between 2 and 3. When she started thyroxine replacement therapy, her physician reduced the dosage of warfarin by 50% and advised her that her INR would need to be monitored on a weekly basis until a new appropriate dose of warfarin was determined. Which of the following statements best explains why the warfarin dose was reduced?

   A. Warfarin decreases the renal clearance of levothyroxine.
   B. Warfarin decreases the hepatic clearance of levothyroxine.
   C. Levothyroxine decreases the hepatic clearance of warfarin.
   D. Levothyroxine increases the catabolism of clotting factors.
   E. Levothyroxine increases the intestinal absorption of warfarin.

Difficulty level: Easy

27. A 67-year-old man recently diagnosed with atrial fibrillation started a treatment that included warfarin. Which of the following molecular actions most likely mediated the efficacy of the drug in the patient's disease?

   A. Potentiation of the activity of antithrombin III in the blood
   B. Blockade of the reduction of vitamin K epoxide
   C. Stimulation of the metabolism of factors II, VII, IX, and X in the liver
   D. Activation of endogenous anticoagulant proteins in the liver
   E. Blockade of the synthesis of vitamin K in the liver

Difficulty level: Medium

28. A 65-year-old man with congestive heart failure presented to the clinic complaining of several days of fatigue and fast heart rate. On physical examination, his pulse was irregular, and his heart rate was 130 bpm. After doing an electrocardiogram, a diagnosis of atrial fibrillation was made, and cardioversion was planned for this patient in 6 weeks. Which of the following drugs did the patient most likely receive during the 6 weeks before cardioversion?

   A. Heparin
   B. Streptokinase
   C. High-dose aspirin
   D. Warfarin
   E. Abciximab

Difficulty level: Easy

29. A 57-year-old man was admitted to the emergency department because of unrelenting chest pain for the past 3 hours. After physical examination and lab tests, a diagnosis of unstable angina was made, and the patient received an emergency therapy that included abciximab. Which of the following steps of thrombus formation was most likely inhibited by this drug?

   A. Binding of fibrinogen to platelet surface
   B. Activation of factor X
   C. Synthesis of thromboxane A_2
   D. Synthesis of factor II
   E. Binding of adenosine diphosphate (ADP) to its platelet receptor
   F. Activation of factor IX

Difficulty level: Easy

30. A 65-year-old man leaving the hospital after a myocardial infarction received an appropriate postdischarge therapy that included aspirin, one low-dose tablet daily. Which of the following actions most likely mediated the therapeutic effect of the drug in the patient's disease?

   A. Competitive inhibition of cyclooxygenase
   B. Competitive inhibition of lipoxygenase
   C. Irreversible blockade of adenosine diphosphate (ADP) receptors
   D. Activation of the glycoprotein IIb/IIIa receptor complex
   E. Irreversible acetylation of cyclooxygenase
   F. Blockade of the synthesis of prostaglandin I_2 (PGI_2, prostacyclin)

Answers and Explanations: IV-1 Diuretics

Questions 1–5

1. **A**
2. **G**
3. **F**
4. **E**
5. **C**

Learning objective: Explain the molecular mechanism of diuretic action of carbonic anhydrase inhibitors.

6. **A** Acetazolamide is a carbonic anhydrase inhibitor. Carbonic anhydrase is an enzyme located in the brush border and cytoplasm of renal proximal convoluted tubule epithelial cells. In the proximal tubule, a large amount of H^+ is secreted into the lumen via the Na^+/H^+ exchanger. Most of this H^+ combines with bicarbonate ion in the tubular fluid to form carbonic acid, which is rapidly dehydrated to CO_2 and water (this reaction is catalyzed by carbonic anhydrase). The CO_2 diffuses into the proximal tubular cells, where the opposite reaction takes place to form H^+ and HCO_3^- (this reaction is also catalyzed by carbonic anhydrase). The HCO_3^- exits the cell on the basolateral side and is reabsorbed as bicarbonate. Hydrogen ion is secreted into the lumen via the Na^+/H^+ exchanger. By blocking carbonic anhydrase, acetazolamide blocks the reabsorption of bicarbonate and Na^+, resulting in increased diuresis.

    B Acetazolamide causes an inhibition, rather than a stimulation, of bicarbonate reabsorption.

    C This is the mechanism of action of thiazide diuretics.

    D Hydrogen is not reabsorbed by the kidney. By inhibiting carbonic anhydrase, acetazolamide inhibits the formation of carbonic acid inside the tubular cells, which in turn inhibits the secretion of hydrogen into the lumen.

    E Acetazolamide causes inhibition, not stimulation, of carbonic acid formation inside the tubular cells.

Learning objectives: Outline the use of carbonic anhydrase inhibitors in the prophylaxis of altitude sickness; describe the urine profile of a patient treated with carbonic anhydrase inhibitors.

7. **A** Acetazolamide, a carbonic anhydrase inhibitor, is the only diuretic used to prevent mountain sickness in people who are at risk for this disorder and have to go to a high altitude. The mechanism of this action is not clear, but it may be related to the induction of metabolic acidosis. Carbonic anhydrase inhibitors produce urine that is very rich in bicarbonate. Urinary sodium is only slightly increased (the efficacy of the diuretic is low). Urinary K^+ excretion is also increased (all diuretics except potassium-sparing diuretics increase urinary K^+ excretion).

    B This urine profile would be caused by osmotic diuretics.

    C This urine profile would be caused by thiazide diuretics.

    D This urine profile would be caused by loop diuretics.

    E This urine profile would be caused by K^+-sparing diuretics.

Learning objective: Describe the main adverse effects of carbonic anhydrase inhibitors.

8. **D** The symptoms of the patient are classic for acetazolamide overdose. The drug is used to treat glaucoma, because it decreases the production of aqueous humor, a fluid rich in bicarbonate. High doses of carbonic anhydrase inhibitors such as acetazolamide can cause metabolic acidosis as they profoundly increase the urinary excretion of bicarbonate. Because the plasma loss of bicarbonate is counterbalanced by an increase of extracellular Cl^-, most incidents of metabolic acidosis are hyperchloremic.

    A–C, E All of these drugs are used for glaucoma, but they do not cause hyperchloremic metabolic acidosis.

Learning objectives: Outline comorbidity contraindications for the use of carbonic anhydrase inhibitors; describe the main adverse effects of carbonic anhydrase inhibitors.

9. **A** The history, symptoms, and signs of the patient suggest that he was suffering from portal-systemic encephalopathy, a syndrome that can occur when extensive portal-systemic collaterals have developed as a result of portal hypertension. Liver cirrhosis is one of the most common causes of portal-systemic encephalopathy, and this was most likely the cause in this case. Carbonic anhydrase inhibitors cause urine alkalinization, which in turn reduces urinary excretion of ammonia. The resulting hyperammonemia is an important cause of portal-systemic encephalopathy, as NH_4^+ causes brain toxicity. Most likely, the ophthalmologist overlooked the possibility that the patient had liver cirrhosis and prescribed acetazolamide for glaucoma.

    B–E These drugs do not trigger liver encephalopathy in patients at risk for liver cirrhosis.

Learning objective: Describe the main therapeutic uses of carbonic anhydrase inhibitors.

10. **D** Dorzolamide is a carbonic anhydrase inhibitor. The rationale for the use of carbonic anhydrase inhibitors in open-angle glaucoma is based on the fact that aqueous humor is rich in bicarbonate. By inhibiting bicarbonate synthesis, the production of aqueous humor is decreased.

    A–C, E All of these drugs are used to treat glaucoma, but they act by increasing the outflow of aqueous humor, not by decreasing its production.

Learning objective: Describe the therapeutic uses of carbonic anhydrase inhibitors.

11. **E** Familial hypokalemic periodic paralysis is a rare autosomal condition characterized by episodes of flaccid paralysis with loss of deep tendon reflex. Potassium flows from the bloodstream into muscle cells during attacks. Acetazolamide may help to prevent the attacks; the mechanism of action is still uncertain, but it could be related to the production of metabolic acidosis, which decreases the activity of Na^+/K^+ ATPase, thus lowering the entry of potassium into muscle cells.

    A–C These diuretics can cause hypokalemia and are therefore contraindicated in this disease.

    D Potassium-sparing diuretics are sometimes used in hypokalemic periodic paralysis, but they are not needed in this case, as a potassium supplementation was prescribed.

Learning objective: Explain the mechanism of thiazide-induced hypercalcemia.

12. **A** In the kidney, the distal convolute tubule reabsorbs about 8% of the filtered Ca^{2+} load. This reabsorption occurs through epithelial Ca^{2+} channels. In the steady state, however, the cell must extrude all the entered Ca^{2+}; this occurs through a plasma membrane Ca^{2+}-ATPase (the Ca^{2+} pump) and also through the Na^+/Ca^{2+} exchanger located on the basolateral surface of cells of the distal tubule. Thiazides inhibit the Na^+/Cl^- symporter in the early distal convoluted tubule, thus decreasing the intracellular concentration of Na. This likely enhances the activity of the Na^+/Ca^{2+} exchanger, which in turn creates a greater driving force for reabsorption of Ca^{2+} through the epithelial Ca^{2+} channels. The final effect is an increased reabsorption of Ca^{2+} that can cause hypercalcemia or, more often, can unmask hypercalcemia due to other causes, as in this case (malignancy is a common cause of hypercalcemia).

    B–F Thiazides do not cause these effects.

Learning objective: Explain the mechanism of thiazide-induced increase in renal excretion of potassium.

13. **A** Potassium secretion by the distal tubule is a passive process that depends on the electrochemical gradient between the distal tubular cells and the tubular lumen. The higher the Na^+ load in the distal tubule, the higher the Na+ reabsorption. This creates a lumen-negative potential that favors K^+ excretion.

    B Thiazides do not inhibit the $Na^+/K^+/2Cl^-$ cotransporter.

C Thiazides can decrease the secretion of uric acid, but this has nothing to do with the thiazide-induced increase in K^+ excretion.

D Thiazides do not stimulate the Na^+/K^+ pump.

E Thiazides are weak carbonic anhydrase inhibitors and therefore tend to increase, not decrease, the delivery of bicarbonate to the collecting duct.

Learning objective: Explain the main contraindications to carbonic anhydrase inhibitors.

14. **C** Drugs that can cause alkaline urine are usually contraindicated in serious hepatic disease for the following reason: ammonia (NH_3) is secreted by the proximal tubule by a countertransport mechanism in exchange for Na^+, which is reabsorbed. If the urine is acidic, it accepts a proton and exists almost entirely as NH_4^+, which is trapped there. If the urine is alkaline, fewer protons are available, and ammonia can return to the systemic circulation. In patients with serious hepatic disease, ammonia cannot be converted into urea and can cause hyperammonemia, which in turn can trigger a hepatic coma.

    B Spironolactone is the preferred diuretic in ascites due to hepatic cirrhosis

    A, D, E All of these diuretics can be used in ascites due to hepatic cirrhosis.

Learning objectives: Outline the signs of hyponatremia; identify the diuretics that can cause hyponatremia.

15. **F** Indapamide is a sulfonamide compound categorized as a "thiazide-like" diuretic. The patient's signs and symptoms suggest the diagnosis of dilutional hyponatremia, which is a rare but sometimes fatal adverse effect of thiazide and thiazide-like diuretics. These drugs affect the diluting ability of the kidney while increasing Na^+ excretion. Once volume depletion occurs, the release of antidiuretic hormone (ADH) causes water retention and worsens the hyponatremia. In contrast, loop diuretics (not included in the question) also affect the concentrating ability of the kidney, thus limiting ADH-mediated water retention. The effect of thiazides may last 1 to 2 weeks after cessation of the therapy. Elderly patients are especially prone to thiazide-induced hyponatremia, particularly if a preexisting renal insufficiency exists, as in this case (see the high creatinine level).

    A–E The risk of dilutional hyponatremia with these drugs is negligible.

Learning objective: Describe the therapeutic use of thiazides in diabetes insipidus.

16. **B** Polyuria with low urine osmolality suggests the diagnosis of diabetes insipidus. To determine the cause of this syndrome, vasopressin is used. Because nephrogenic diabetes insipidus is vasopressin-resistant, urine osmolality would not change significantly after vasopressin, as in this case. A common cause of nephrogenic diabetes insipidus is hypercalcemia, which is common in bone metastases of various tumors. Thiazide diuretics can reduce polyuria and polydipsia in diabetes insipidus. The mechanism of this paradoxical effect is likely related to the extracellular volume reduction, which in turn causes an activation of the renin–angiotensin system. Angiotensin enhances the reabsorption of Na^+ and water in the proximal tubule by stimulating the Na^+/H^+ exchanger. This in turn causes a decreased delivery of fluid to the distal tubule. Thus, there is a decrease in the maximum volume of dilute urine that can be produced.

    A Desmopressin is effective in neurogenic diabetes insipidus, but it is ineffective in nephrogenic diabetes insipidus. Neurogenic diabetes insipidus is unlikely in this case, because it is vasopressin-sensitive; therefore, urine osmolality would have been increased significantly after vasopressin.

    C Demeclocycline is appropriate for the treatment of syndrome of inappropriate antidiuretic hormone secretion (SIADH). This syndrome leads to hyponatremia (not hypernatremia, as in diabetes insipidus) and low serum osmolality.

    D Amiloride is used effectively in case of lithium-induced nephrogenic diabetes insipidus because the drug blocks lithium transport into the cells of the collecting tubule. However, it is not effective in other forms of diabetes insipidus.

    E Furosemide is not effective in nephrogenic diabetes insipidus. It can be used in case of chronic renal failure, but this diagnosis is unlikely in this case because urine osmolality is lower than serum osmolality (in chronic renal failure, urine osmolality is usually fixed close to that of serum).

Learning objective: Explain the molecular mechanism of action of loop diuretics.

17. **C** When the glomerular filtration rate (GFR) is less than 30 mL/min (as can occur in severe heart failure), the only diuretics that are still active are loop diuretics. This is likely related, at least in part, to the fact that by inhibiting Na^+ and Cl^- transport into the macula densa, the macula densa is no longer able to sense salt concentration in the tubular fluid and therefore increases renin secretion, leading to an increase in angiotensin II. Because angiotensin II preferentially constricts the efferent arteriole, GFR is enhanced.

    A, B, D, E See correct answer explanation.

Learning objective: Explain the molecular mechanism of furosemide-induced metabolic alkalosis.

18. **B** There are three main causes of alkalosis induced by loop diuretics. The most important is increased delivery of Na^+ to the distal tubule. The consequent increased reabsorption of Na^+ creates a lumen-negative potential that favors both H^+ and K^+ excretion. The second cause is the stimulation of aldosterone release due to volume contraction and increased renin secretion. The third cause occurs only when hypokalemia is severe. In this case, K^+ tends to leave the cell, and H^+ enters to maintain electroneutrality, with the final result of extracellular alkalosis and intracellular acidosis.

    A, C, D All of these are actions of loop diuretics, but they do not lead to metabolic alkalosis.

    E Loop diuretics actually increase renin secretion.

Learning objective: Explain the mechanism of thiazide-induced extracellular volume depletion.

19. **C** The patient's signs and symptoms suggest the diagnosis of hypovolemic hyponatremia, which is a rare but sometimes fatal adverse effect of thiazide diuretics. These drugs affect the diluting ability of the kidney while increasing Na^+ excretion. Once volume depletion occurs, the release of antidiuretic hormone causes water retention and worsens hyponatremia. This effect of thiazides may last 1 to 2 weeks after cessation of the therapy. Elderly patients are especially prone to thiazide-induced hyponatremia, particularly if preexisting renal insufficiency exists, as in this case (see the high creatinine level).

    A, B, D These disorders do not cause the signs and symptoms shown by the patient.

    E The patient is hyponatremic, but the postural hypotension and the diuretic therapy indicate that hyponatremia is hypovolemic, not hypervolemic.

Learning objective: Describe the main therapeutic uses of loop diuretics.

20. **E** The patient exhibits the classic symptoms of pulmonary edema. Furosemide is the diuretic of first choice for this condition because it is able to quickly reduce preload (and therefore the left ventricular filling pressure) through the following actions:

    • Rapid increase in venous capacitance, likely mediated by prostaglandin release (the initial beneficial effect may result more from this action than from diuresis)
    • Brisk and abundant natriuresis

    A, B Hydrochlorothiazide and amiloride are less effective than loop diuretics and do not have acute vasodilating properties.

    C, D, F Mannitol, epinephrine, and metoprolol are contraindicated in pulmonary edema.

Learning objective: Describe the main therapeutic uses of loop diuretics.

21. **C** Lab values of this patient indicate very high Ca^{2+} levels, and her symptoms and history are in accordance with the diagnosis of profound hypercalcemia. Malignancy and hyperparathyroidism are the most common causes of hypercalcemia. The first-line emergency treatment for this disorder is hydration and volume expansion, as such patients are volume depleted due to the accompany polyuria, nausea, and vomiting.

    Furosemide is administered because it can increase urinary Ca^{2+} excretion. Ca^{2+} and Mg^{2+} are reabsorbed in the thick ascending limb of the loop of Henle, because the action of the $Na^+/K^+/2Cl^-$ cotransporter in that portion of the nephron leads to excess K^+ accumulation within the tubular cells. This results in back-diffusion of K^+ into the tubular lumen and development of a lumen-positive electrical potential. This potential provides the driving force for reabsorption of Ca^{2+} and Mg^{2+} via the paracellular pathway. By blocking the $Na^+/K^+/2Cl^-$ cotransporter, furosemide decreases the reabsorption of these ions.

    A Acetazolamide has no significant effect on urinary Ca^{2+} excretion.

    B, D, E These diuretics actually decrease urinary Ca^{2+} excretion.

Learning objective: Determine the choice of a loop diuretic in a patient with a serious allergic reaction to sulfa drugs.

22. **D** The only loop diuretic that is not a sulfonamide is ethacrynic acid. Therefore, ethacrynic acid represents a suitable alternative to the use of furosemide when furosemide is contraindicated because of serious adverse effects, as in this case.

    A Spironolactone is used in heart failure as an adjunct drug, but it cannot substitute for a loop diuretic in a patient with stage C heart failure.

    B, E Acetazolamide and triamterene are not used in heart failure because they are much less effective than loop diuretics.

    C Mannitol is absolutely contraindicated in patients with heart failure.

    F All thiazides and thiazide-like drugs are sulfonamides and are therefore relatively contraindicated in a patient who experienced a serious allergic reaction to a sulfonamide drug even though the risk of an allergic reaction after administration of a thiazide diuretic in a patient with sulfonamide hypersensitivity appears to be very low. Moreover, the patient had stage C heart failure, and loop diuretics are usually necessary to restore and maintain euvolemia.

Learning objective: Explain the molecular mechanism of action of potassium-sparing diuretics.

23. **B** Potassium-sparing diuretics are administered in cases of hypokalemia, which may occur in laxative abusers, as in this case. Epithelial cells in the late distal tubule and collecting duct have luminal membrane Na^+ channels that provide a conductive pathway for the entry of Na^+ into the cells down an electrochemical gradient created by the basolateral Na^+/K^+ pump. This entry creates a lumen-negative potential that supplies a driving force for the secretion of K^+ into the lumen through K^+ channels located in the luminal membrane. Triamterene and amiloride block Na^+ channels in the late distal tubule and collecting duct. Because K^+ secretion is coupled with Na^+ entry in these segments, the blockade of Na^+ channels causes a K^+-sparing effect.

    A, C–E See correct answer explanation.

Learning objective: Describe the therapeutic uses of spironolactone.

24. **F** The signs of the patient and lab results indicated that he was most likely suffering from primary hyperaldosteronism due to adrenal hyperplasia, which is more common in elderly men. Unlike adrenal adenoma, surgery is not recommended for bilateral adrenal hyperplasia; the hyperaldosteronism usually can be controlled by spironolactone, an aldosterone receptor antagonist. However, about 50% of such patients need additional antihypertensive treatment.

    A–C These diuretics are contraindicated, as they can worsen the hypokalemia and the metabolic alkalosis.

    D, E Patients with primary hyperaldosteronism usually need antihypertensive treatment, but fenoldopam and nitroprusside are used only in hypertensive emergencies.

Learning objective: Describe the therapeutic uses of spironolactone.

25. **C** The history and symptoms of the patient suggest that he has been suffering from liver cirrhosis. Moreover, the low K^+ and high bicarbonate levels suggest that high levels of aldosterone are present. Secondary hyperaldosteronism is common in advanced liver cirrhosis for the following reasons:

    • Ascites-induced hypovolemia activates the renin–angiotensin–aldosterone system.
    • Liver metabolism of aldosterone is reduced because of liver impairment.
    • Hypoalbuminemia is a known consequence of liver cirrhosis. Because aldosterone is highly bound to albumin, cirrhotic patients have a higher free, active concentration of aldosterone.

    Spironolactone is an aldosterone receptor antagonist and therefore is a rational diuretic choice.

A, B, D All of these diuretics would cause hypokalemia, which would worsen the disease. A thiazide or furosemide can be added to spironolactone if diuresis remains insufficient after 4 or more days of increasingly large doses of spironolactone.

E Triamterene is a potassium-sparing diuretic, like spironolactone, but is not an aldosterone antagonist.

Learning objective: Describe the therapeutic uses of osmotic diuretics.

26. **A** Osmotic diuretics are often given to patients with a brain tumor before and after neurosurgery to reduce cerebrospinal fluid volume and therefore intracranial pressure. These drugs cannot cross the blood–brain barrier, and they enhance the diffusion of water back into the plasma by elevating plasma osmolality.

    B, C Other diuretics are useless in decreasing intracranial pressure.

    D, E Increased intracranial pressure often causes hypertension and bradycardia. Drugs that decrease the heart rate are therefore contraindicated.

Learning objective: Describe the therapeutic uses of osmotic diuretics.

27. **C** Hyperosmotic agents such as mannitol can lower intraocular pressure by creating an osmotic gradient between the ocular fluid and plasma. They are used to decrease intraocular pressure before and after iridotomy and, together with other drugs that lower intraocular pressure, in acute attacks of glaucoma.

    A, B, D Furosemide, triamterene, and hydrochlorothiazide do not reduce intraocular pressure.

    E, F Homatropine and phenylephrine are actually contraindicated in glaucoma, as they can increase intraocular pressure.

Learning objective: Describe the therapeutic uses of antidiuretic hormone antagonists.

28. **C** The signs and lab values of this patient suggest the diagnosis of syndrome of inappropriate antidiuretic hormone secretion (SIADH), which is usually characterized by hypervolemic (or sometimes normovolemic) hyponatremia, low serum osmolality, and urine osmolality higher than serum osmolality. The syndrome is associated with myriad disorders, including chronic treatment with tricyclic antidepressants, as in this case. The majority of patients with SIADH do not require therapy because plasma Na^+ usually stabilizes in the range of 125 to 130 mEq/L; these patients are asymptomatic. However, when plasma Na^+ is more than 120 mEq/L, and symptoms supervene, as in this case, therapy should be initiated. Because the syndrome is due to excessive ADH secretion, the use of an ADH antagonist, conivaptan, is a rational choice. Patients with very high urine osmolality (like this patient) benefit most from ADH antagonists.

    A, B, D–F These drug are useless or even dangerous in SIADH.

Learning objective: Describe the therapeutic uses of loop and potassium-sparing diuretics.

29. **B** The majority of patients with cardiac failure will require the chronic administration of a loop diuretic to maintain euvolemia. However, these drugs cause hypokalemia, which increases the risk of adverse effects with cardiac glycosides. In fact, a decrease in serum K^+ concentration increases the binding of cardiac glycosides to Na^+/K^+ ATPase. The concurrent administration of potassium-sparing diuretics such as spironolactone will prevent furosemide-induced hypokalemia.

    A This combination would prevent the thiazide-induced metabolic alkalosis (as acetazolamide tends to cause acidosis) but does not prevent hypokalemia.

    C Potassium-sparing diuretics have low diuretic efficacy and therefore are not suitable for treating a patient with cardiac failure.

    D, E Mannitol is absolutely contraindicated in heart failure because the resulting extracellular volume expansion can cause a dangerous circulatory overload.

Learning objective: Identify the drugs that can cause hyperkalemia.

30. **D** The history and the signs of the patient (extreme bradycardia) suggest that he was most likely suffering from hyperkalemia due to several causes. He received amiloride, a potassium-sparing diuretic, and captopril, which indirectly decreases aldosterone formation, thus hindering the body's ability to counteract the hyperkalemia (normally, a small increase in K^+ concentration will increase aldosterone secretion several fold). The patient was also treated with propranolol and ibuprofen. Beta-blockers can cause hyperkalemia by suppressing renin release and by decreasing K^+ uptake by skeletal muscle, and nonsteroidal antiinflammatory drugs can cause hyperkalemia by reducing renal K^+ excretion. The patient was also taking furosemide, but the hypokalemic action of the furosemide most likely was not enough to counteract all the hyperkalemic actions mentioned above.

    A–C, E, F See correct answer explanation.

Learning objective: Describe the use of thiazides to prevent kidney stone production.

31. **B** Thiazide diuretics decrease urinary Ca^{2+} excretion and therefore are often used in cases of kidney stones and idiopathic hypercalciuria.

    A Carbonic anhydrase inhibitors such as acetazolamide have negligible effects on the urinary excretion of Ca^{2+}.

    C Loop diuretics such as furosemide increase urinary Ca^{2+} excretion.

    D, E Potassium-sparing diuretics such as triamterene and spironolactone decrease Ca^{2+} excretion, but their action is weak, and they are not used for idiopathic hypercalciuria.

Learning objective: Explain the relationship between the pharmacokinetics of diuretics and their concentration at the site of action.

32. **A** In order to act, all diuretics must reach a certain concentration in the tubular lumen, as the tubular cells in different parts of the nephron are the molecular targets of these agents. The diuretics under study are given at the same dose and have the same plasma protein binding, which indicates that the same amount was filtered by the glomerulus. The reabsorption of the drug by the proximal tubule will be related to the lipid solubility in the urine. An acidic drug is mainly water soluble when its acid dissociation constant (pK_a) is less than the pH of the medium. Because the pH range of the urine is from 4.0 to 8.5, drug P will be the one with the lowest lipid solubility and be the least reabsorbed by the proximal tubule. This means that its concentration in the late distal tubule will be the highest. The four diuretics have equal affinity for the Na^+/Cl^- transporter, so their diuretic effect will be proportional to their concentration at the site of action.

    B–D See correct answer explanation.

DIURETICS Answer key					
1.	A	6.	A	11.	E
2.	G	7.	A	12.	A
3.	F	8.	D	13.	A
4.	E	9.	A	14.	C
5.	C	10.	D	15.	F
16.	B	21.	C	26.	A
17.	C	22.	D	27.	C
18.	B	23.	B	28.	C
19.	C	24.	F	29.	B
20.	E	25.	C	30.	D
				31.	B
				32.	A

Answers and Explanations: IV-2 Drugs for Ischemic Heart Disease

Questions 1–4

1. **A**
2. **D**
3. **G**
4. **F**

Learning objective: Outline the actions leading to the therapeutic effect of nitrates in variant angina.

5. **B** Nitrates dilate large epicardial vessels, thus increasing epicardial blood flow. This action is the most important for the therapeutic effect of these drugs in variant angina, which is characterized by coronary spasm.

    A By causing venous dilation, nitrates can cause a decrease, not an increase, of left ventricular end-diastolic volume.

    C, E Nitrates can cause reflex tachycardia and reflex increase in cardiac contractility, but these are detrimental, not therapeutic, effects in patients with angina.

    D Nitrates can decrease diastolic perfusion time (as a consequence of reflex tachycardia), but this is a detrimental effect in patients with angina.

Learning objective: Identify the site of action of verapamil.

6. **D** Calcium channel blockers with heart activity, such as verapamil and diltiazem, act on voltage-gated channels in cardiac and smooth muscle cell membranes. The blockade of channels in cardiac muscle leads to a reduction in cardiac contractility and rate, whereas the blockade in vascular smooth muscle causes vasodilation, which in turn reduces the afterload of the heart. Both actions are useful for the therapeutic effect of these drugs in exertional angina.

    A These channels are not blocked by calcium channel blockers.

    B Calcium is exchanged between cytosol and mitochondria, which are storage sites for calcium, through specific mitochondrial store-operated calcium channels, but these channels are not blocked by calcium channel blockers.

    C, E Calcium channels in the sarcoplasmic reticulum are opened by depolarization and blocked by ryanodine. Calcium channel blockers affect these channels only at very high concentration.

Learning objective: Describe the peripheral vascular actions of antianginal drugs.

7. **B** The prescribed drug was most likely nifedipine, a drug of choice in variant angina. The symptoms were most likely due to a decrease in total peripheral resistance that in turn can induce dizziness (due to decreased cerebral blood flow) and palpitations (due to reflex tachycardia). These are two common adverse effects of nifedipine.

A Coronary vasodilation is a nifedipine effect but does not cause the symptoms reported by the patient.

C A decrease in total peripheral resistance causes a decrease, not an increase, of venous return to the heart.

D A decrease in cardiac contractility cannot explain the palpitations reported by the patient.

E Coronary steal is a phenomenon where an alteration of circulation patterns leads to a reduction in the blood directed to the coronary circulation. It is caused when there is narrowing of the coronary arteries (as in exertional angina), and an arteriolar vasodilator is used. This happens because the coronary arteries downstream of the narrowing are maximally dilated to compensate for the decreased upstream blood supply. Thus, dilating the resistance vessels upstream of the narrowing causes blood to be shunted (stolen) away from the coronary vessels supplying the ischemic zones, creating more ischemia. The coronary steal phenomenon cannot occur in variant angina, where there is no anatomical narrowing but only an arterial spasm, and cannot explain the symptoms reported by the patient.

Learning objective: Describe the main potential detrimental effects of nitrates in exertional angina.

8. **B** By causing peripheral vasodilation, high doses of nitrates can induce reflex tachycardia, which in turn increases oxygen consumption. This detrimental effect can be prevented by the concomitant use of a β-blocker.

A, C, D These are all useful effects of nitrates in exertional angina.

E Nitrates tend to decrease, not increase, ventricular end-diastolic volume.

Learning objective: Describe the cardiovascular effects of antianginal drugs.

9. **C** Arterial pressure (AP) is equal to stroke volume (SV) by heart rate (HR) by peripheral vascular resistance (PVR):

$$AP = SV \times HR \times PVR.$$

Nitrates mainly decrease SV (by dilating the large veins), calcium channel blockers mainly decrease HR and PVR, and β-blockers mainly decrease HR and SV (by decreasing heart contractility). Therefore, all can lower the blood pressure.

A Cardiac-active calcium channel blockers and β-blockers decrease cardiac rate. On the contrary, nitrates and dihydropyridines have no direct effect on heart rate but can cause reflex tachycardia because of drug-induced vasodilation.

B Cardiac-active calcium channel blockers and β-blockers decrease cardiac contractility. Nitrates and dihydropyridines have no direct effect on heart contractility, but they can cause reflex increase in contractility because of drug-induced vasodilation.

D Left ventricular end-diastolic volume is decreased by nitrates (because of the predominant venous vasodilation), but calcium channel blockers with heart activity and β-blockers tend to increase it because of the increased duration of diastole.

E Ejection time is increased by calcium channel blockers with heart activity and β-blockers due to the decrease in cardiac contractility, but it can be decreased by nitrates and dihydropyridines due to reflex increase in cardiac contractility.

Learning objective: Outline the actions leading to the therapeutic effect of nitrates in pulmonary edema.

10. **A** The signs and symptoms of the patient indicate that he is suffering from pulmonary edema. By increasing cyclic guanosine monophosphate production, nitrates cause relaxation of both resistance and capacitance vessels, but relaxation of the latter (especially large veins) is more pronounced, with standard therapeutic doses, probably because the enzyme that converts nitrates to nitric oxide is more abundant in veins than in arteries. This venodilation reduces preload to the heart by pooling blood in the periphery, thus reducing ventricular end-diastolic volume. In this way, pulmonary congestion is reduced, and pulmonary edema is relieved.

B–D The nitrate-induced peripheral vasodilation tends to cause reflex tachycardia and reflex increase in cardiac contractility when high doses are given, but this would adversely affect pulmonary edema by increasing the pulmonary pressure. A decreased ventricular ejection time is usually the consequence of tachycardia, so it would adversely affect pulmonary edema.

E By causing arteriolar vasodilation, nitrates also decrease afterload, but this action is less pronounced than the venous vasodilation. Thus, the decreased afterload is not the main reason for the therapeutic efficacy of nitrates in pulmonary edema.

F Nitrates decrease platelet aggregation, but this is not the reason that they are effective in treating pulmonary edema.

Learning objective: Discuss the risk of abrupt withdrawal from nitrate therapy.

11. **C** Long-term nitrate therapy should be discontinued gradually, as there is clinical evidence that severe myocardial ischemia may occur in persons withdrawing suddenly from long-term organic nitrate exposure.

   A Unlike unstable angina, stable exertional angina very rarely progresses to myocardial infarction. Moreover, the fact that the patient had no attacks during the past month indicates that the therapy was appropriate.

   B, D Unlike cimetidine, famotidine has no inhibitory effects on drug metabolism.

   E A too-high dose of nitrates may cause reflex tachycardia by reducing the blood pressure, but this is unlikely in this patient because he was receiving verapamil, which actually decreases the heart rate.

Learning objective: Describe nitrate-induced postural hypotension.

12. **B** Nitrates can cause postural hypotension because venodilation decreases preload. In fact, insufficient left ventricular end-diastolic volume (due to decreased venous return, hypovolemia, etc.) is the most common cause of postural hypotension. Postural hypotension is even more likely in this patient because her blood pressure is low.

   A Nitrates tend to cause bronchodilation, so cough and wheezing are unlikely.

   C Nitrates tend to cause reflex tachycardia, not bradycardia.

   D Nitrates very rarely cause methemoglobinemia when given at therapeutic doses. To get this effect, the doses given must be huge. However, therapeutic doses of nitrites can cause methemoglobinemia.

   E Nitrates tend to cause relaxation of the gut smooth muscle, so diarrhea is unlikely.

   F Nitrates decrease platelet aggregation, so venous thrombosis is unlikely.

Learning objective: Describe the main adverse effects of β-blockers.

13. **A** All the symptoms reported by the patient are classic adverse effects of β-blockers. These drugs block β_2-mediated vasodilation and cause a reflex vasoconstriction because of the decreased cardiac output. These actions can account for the blanching of the fingers when exposed to cold. Fatigue is likely due to decreased cardiac output. The other effects are centrally mediated, but the mechanisms are still uncertain.

   B–E The other listed drugs do not cause all the effects reported by the patient.

Learning objective: Discuss the problem of tolerance development to nitrates.

14. **B** Tolerance to nitrates does occur. Because it appears rapidly (24 hours) and disappears rapidly (6 to 10 hours), brief periods of no therapy (overnight) can be sufficient to permit recovery, but this patient was continuously receiving the drug.

   A Vasospastic angina complicating exertional angina is an unlikely possibility.

   C Nitroglycerin does not induce the cytochrome P-450 system.

   D Anginal attacks disappeared completely during the first week of therapy, so the dosage was most likely appropriate.

   E Transdermal bioavailability of nitroglycerin is 50 to 90% and does not change over time.

Learning objective: Choose the appropriate antianginal therapy for a patient with concomitant diseases.

15. **D** Calcium channel blockers are considered drugs of first choice in variant angina. Moreover, in the present case:

   A A brain tumor is likely to increase the intracranial pressure, so nitrates are contraindicated.

   B, C The atrioventricular (AV) block also contraindicates drugs that tend to decrease atrioventricular conduction, such as verapamil and diltiazem.

   E Beta-blockers such as propranolol are not effective in variant angina, and they may be dangerous by causing coronary vasoconstriction. Moreover, they are contraindicated in this case because of the AV block.

Learning objective: Explain the main approaches to combination therapy for angina.

16. **E** The patient's current symptoms are most likely due to nitrate therapy. The addition of a cardiac-active calcium channel blocker such as diltiazem can attenuate the nitrate-induced reflex tachycardia and reflex increase in cardiac contractility. Moreover, in this patient:

   A, D Because anginal attacks are not completely prevented, it is useless to reduce nitrate dosage, which would decrease adverse effects but also decrease therapeutic effects.

   B Beta-blockers such as propranolol are relatively contraindicated in patients receiving insulin treatment, because they can mask some symptoms of hypoglycemia and inhibit gluconeogenesis, thus impairing the body's capacity to recover from hypoglycemia.

   C Nifedipine could increase palpitations because it can cause reflex tachycardia.

Learning objective: Discuss the risk of abrupt withdrawal from β-blocker therapy.

17. **B** Abrupt discontinuation of β-blockers such as propranolol can precipitate myocardial infarction and can increase the risk of sudden death in cardiac patients. The underlying mechanism is unclear, but it is well established that there is enhanced sensitivity to β-adrenoceptor agonists in patients who have undergone long-term treatment with β-blockers, likely due to upregulation of β receptors. Abrupt withdrawal from the β-blocker allows an increased number of receptors to be exposed to norepinephrine. This supersensitivity can be attenuated by tapering the dose of the β-blocker for several weeks before discontinuation.

A, C–E All of the other listed drugs do not cause abrupt withdrawal symptoms.

Learning objective: Describe the interaction between nitrates and sildenafil.

18. **C** Erection requires relaxation of the nonvascular smooth muscle of the corpora cavernosa. Sildenafil is used in erectile dysfunction because it inhibits isoform 5 of phosphodiesterase, which is found in high concentration in smooth muscle cells of the corpora cavernosa. This increases the concentration of cyclic guanosine monophosphate (cGMP), which in turn stimulates the dephosphorylation of the myosin light chain. Because of this mechanism of action, sildenafil potentiates the action of nitrates (which also cause an increase in cGMP), and severe hypotension and a few myocardial infarctions have been reported in men using both drugs.

B Nitroprusside can cause an increase in cGMP, and its actions are potentiated by sildenafil, but the drug is not used to treat angina.

A, D, E None of these drugs have actions potentiated by sildenafil.

Learning objective: Describe the main adverse effects of nitrates.

19. **D** The dose of nitroglycerin given to this patient was likely too high, as the symptoms the patient is referring to are classic for nitrate toxicity.

A–C Beta-blockers such as propranolol, verapamil, and diltiazem tend to decrease heart rate, so palpitations are unlikely.

E Nifedipine can cause all the adverse effects reported by the patient. However, all calcium channel blockers are contraindicated in gastroesophageal reflux disease because they tend to relax the lower esophageal sphincter.

Learning objective: Outline the actions leading to the therapeutic effect of nifedipine in variant angina.

20. **E** The signs and symptoms of the patient indicate that she was most likely suffering from variant angina. Nifedipine is a dihydropyridine calcium channel blocker that causes vasodilation by blocking L-type calcium channels in smooth muscle membranes. The antianginal effect of both calcium channel blockers and nitrates in variant angina is mainly due to coronary vasodilation, which in turn increases oxygen supply to the heart. Today, calcium channel blockers are considered the drug of choice to prevent attacks of variant angina that are characterized by coronary spasms. Dihydropyridines, verapamil and diltiazem, are considered equally efficacious in this disease.

A Because dihydropyridines are mainly arteriolar vasodilators, they minimally affect preload.

B Dihydropyridines decrease afterload, but this is not the main mechanism of antianginal action in variant angina. In fact, by decreasing either preload or afterload, the oxygen demand of the heart is decreased, which is good in case of exertional angina. By contrast, an increase in oxygen supply is needed in variant angina, and this can be accomplished only by coronary vasodilation.

C, D In therapeutic doses, dihydropyridines have no direct effect on the heart. Large doses can cause a reflex increase in cardiac contractility and rate, but these are not useful actions in a patient with angina.

Learning objective: Describe the use of nitroglycerin in myocardial infarction.

21. **C** Recent studies have reinvestigated the use of nitrate therapy in myocardial infarction (MI) in the setting of concomitant thrombolytic therapy and aspirin administration. The pooled effects from several studies have shown a small but statistically significant decrease in mortality in patients receiving nitrates. Therefore, intravenous nitroglycerin is currently recommended for routine use during the first 24 to 48 hours in most patients with MI, particularly if they have signs of acute heart failure (impending pulmonary edema) and are hypertensive, as in this case.

A Epinephrine is contraindicated in MI because it increases cardiac work and oxygen demand.

B Intravenous β-blockers such as metoprolol given within the first few hours after onset of MI improve prognosis by reducing infarct size and incidence of ventricular fibrillation. In this case, however, they are contraindicated because of bradycardia and the impending pulmonary edema (these patients are dependent on sympathetic activation to increase the heart rate and to maintain blood pressure to vital organs).

D Verapamil and diltiazem have been shown to reduce the rate of reinfarction and death in patients with preserved left ventricular function, but they are contraindicated in this case because of bradycardia and signs of cardiac failure.

E Dihydropyridines such as nefedipine have been uniformly unsuccessful in reducing either mortality or reinfarction in patients with MI.

Learning objective: Choose the appropriate drug therapy for a patient with subarachnoid hemorrhage.

22. **E** Subarachnoid hemorrhage should always be considered in patients who present with headache and syncope. The diagnostic test of choice for this disease is computed tomography scan, which has a sensitivity greater than 90%. Delayed ischemic deficit due to vasospasm is the most common cause of morbidity and mortality following subarachnoid hemorrhage. Nicardipine is a calcium channel blocker with some affinity for cerebral blood vessels and is used by intravenous infusion to prevent cerebral vasospasm associated with subarachnoid hemorrhage or stroke.

    A All of the other calcium channel blockers, including verapamil, lack selectivity for cerebral blood vessels and therefore are not indicated in subarachnoid hemorrhage.

    B–D, F All of these drugs are useless or dangerous in subarachnoid hemorrhage.

Learning objective: Explain the molecular mechanism of the antianginal action of nitrates.

23. **C** Nitrates release free nitrite ions, which in turn are converted to nitric oxide. Nitric oxide causes the activation of guanylyl-cyclase, thereby causing an increase in cyclic guanosine monophosphate. This second messenger causes dephosphorylation of the myosin light chain. Myosin is no longer able to interact with actin, and vascular smooth muscle relaxes.

    A Nitrite ions are converted to nitric oxide, not to N_2O.

    B Intracellular Ca^{2+} concentration is actually reduced by nitrates.

    C The synthesis of guanylyl cyclase is actually increased, not decreased, by nitrates.

    E Phosphorylation of myosin light chain kinase would increase, not decrease, smooth muscle contraction.

Learning objective: Choose the appropriate antianginal therapy for a patient with concomitant diseases.

24. **D** A long-acting nitrate, a β-blocker, or a calcium channel blocker can all be used for exertional angina prophylaxis. However, in this patient

    A Propranolol is contraindicated because of the chronic obstructive pulmonary disease.

    B, C, E Calcium channel blockers relax the lower esophageal sphincter and therefore should be avoided in the presence of gastroesophageal reflux disease.

Learning objective: Explain the main reasons for combination therapy of angina.

25. **B** Because the three classes of antianginal drugs use different mechanisms of actions, a combination of two of these agents may increase the effectiveness and reduce the incidence of adverse effects. Sometimes β-blockers are administered with nitrates in the therapy of exertional angina because

- Beta-blockers can offset the nitrate-induced increase in cardiac contractility and rate.
- Nitrates can prevent the β-blocker-induced increase in end-diastolic volume and ejection time.

    A Beta-blockers cause vasoconstriction of coronary vessels, mainly as a consequence of the reduced heart rate.

    C Beta-blockers do not prevent the nitrate-induced decrease in arterial pressure. Moreover, this is a useful effect of nitrates, and it would be irrational to prevent it.

    D, E Nitrates counteract, not enhance, the effect of propranolol on cardiac rate and contractility.

Learning objective: Describe the use of β-blockers in the postdischarge therapy of myocardial infarction.

26. **E** Beta-blocker therapy after a myocardial infarction should be continued indefinitely (unless there are contraindications or adverse effects supervene) because of proven long-term morbidity and mortality benefits.

    A–D See correct answer explanation.

Learning objective: Describe the adverse effects of calcium channel blockers and nitrates.

27. **A** Calcium channel blockers sometimes are added to nitrates to attenuate the nitrate-induced tachycardia. Throbbing headache is a typical adverse effect of nitrates, and severe constipation is a typical adverse effect of verapamil.

    B–D Nitrates and β-blockers do not cause severe constipation.

    E Beta-blockers and verapamil do not cause throbbing headache (in fact, both are used in the therapy of headache).

Learning objective: Choose the appropriate antianginal therapy for a patient with hypertrophic cardiomyopathy.

28. **D** Calcium channel blockers acting on the heart and β-blockers (alone or in combination) are the treatment of choice in angina associated with hypertrophic cardiomyopathy. In this disease, there is a marked hypertrophy and thickening of the upper interventricular septum below the aortic valve. During systole, the septum thickens, and the anterior leaflet of the mitral valve is sucked toward the septum, producing outflow tract obstruction. The major consequence of hypertrophy is that the stiff, noncompliant ventricle resists diastolic filling. Beta-blockers and calcium channel blockers decrease myocardial contractility. This action increases ventricular compliance and decreases outflow obstruction. Beta-blockers and calcium channel blockers acting on the heart also slow the heart rate, which allows a more complete diastolic filling.

    A–C Nitrates, as well as other drugs that reduce preload (diuretics, angiotensin-converting enzyme [ACE] inhibitors, etc.), are contraindicated in this disease because they decrease the already deficient ventricular end-diastolic volume.

E Dihydropyridines are devoid of cardiac activity and therefore are not useful in hypertrophic cardiomyopathy. ACE inhibitors are relatively contraindicated in this disease because they can reduce preload.

Learning objective: Describe the use of calcium channels blockers in Raynaud phenomenon.

29. **C** The signs and symptoms of the patient suggest the diagnosis of Raynaud phenomenon, a vasospasm of part of the hand in response to cold, emotional stress, or vibration (which is likely a causal factor in this case). The disorder can be primary or secondary to several pathological conditions (mostly connective tissue disorders). Nifedipine has become the arteriolar vasodilator of choice in patients with Raynaud phenomenon not controlled by conservative measures.

A, B, D–F These drugs are not used for the therapy of Raynaud phenomenon.

Learning objective: Explain why β-blockers can decrease mortality in myocardial infarction.

30. **C** Several studies have shown that β-blockers decrease infarct-associated mortality (by about 25% when given in the first 2 days and by about 13% when given later). They reduce myocardial remodeling (an increase in myocardial mass that is enhanced by catecholamines and angiotensin II). They also decrease myocardial oxygen demand (by decreasing heart contractility and rate) and the risk of ventricular fibrillation (by decreasing heart conduction and automaticity), and they limit the infarct size, thus decreasing the risk of myocardial rupture.

A By decreasing heart contractility and rate, β-blockers decrease, not increase, myocardial oxygen supply.

B Beta-blockers decrease atrioventricular conduction, but this is not a major factor contributing to reduced mortality.

D Beta-blockers can increase systemic vascular resistance (by blocking β_2 receptors in the vascular smooth muscle), but this would increase mortality.

E Beta-blockers can increase left ventricular end-diastolic pressure (if given in too high doses, due to the increased diastolic time), but this would increase mortality.

DRUGS FOR ISCHEMIC HEART DISEASE Answer key		
1. A	6. D	11. C
2. D	7. B	12. B
3. G	8. B	13. A
4. F	9. C	14. B
5. B	10. A	15. D
16. E	21. C	26. E
17. B	22. E	27. A
18. C	23. C	28. D
19. D	24. D	29. C
20. E	25. B	30. C

Answers and Explanations: IV-3 Drugs for Cardiac Failure

Questions 1–5

1. **F**
2. **C**
3. **I**
4. **G**
5. **B**

Learning objective: Explain the molecular mechanism of action of digoxin.

6. **B** At the molecular level, all cardiac glycosides inhibit Na^+/K^+ ATPase, the membrane-bound transporter called the sodium pump. The increased amount of sodium inside the cell inhibits the Ca^{2+}/Na^+ exchanger, an antiporter that uses the electrochemical potential for Na^+ to drive Ca^{2+} extrusion. The consequence of this inhibition is that less Ca^{2+} is removed from the cell. The increased intracellular calcium is stored in the sarcoplasmic reticulum during diastole, so a greater amount of Ca^{2+} is released from the sarcoplasmic reticulum during systole.

A Digitalis glycosides at high concentration can open, not close, cardiac calcium channels.

C, D See correct answer explanation.

E Digitalis glycosides have no direct effect on potassium channels.

Learning objective: Identify the main receptors involved in the therapeutic effect of digoxin in atrial fibrillation.

7. **B** Digoxin is still used in persistent atrial fibrillation (although it is no longer a first-line therapy) because it can decrease the atrioventricular conduction, thus decreasing the high ventricular rate. This is accomplished by a stimulation of vagal activity due to

• Stimulation of vagal nuclei in the brainstem
• Sensitization of carotid sinus baroreceptors
• Facilitation of muscarinic transmission at the cardiac muscle cells.

The receptors involved in vagal activity on the heart are mainly muscarinic.

A, C–E See correct answer explanation.

Learning objective: Describe the cardiac actions of digoxin.

8. **E** Digoxin decreases heart rate both in the normal and the failing heart (unless toxic effects of the drug supervene) due to decreased atrioventricular (AV) conduction, which is a consequence of a direct action and of a parasympathomimetic action on the AV node.

A By increasing contractility, digoxin decreases, not increases, the end-systolic volume.

B Digoxin dose-dependently increases abnormal cardiac automaticity, as indicated by the many varieties of arrhythmia caused by the drug.

C By causing bradycardia, digoxin increases, not decreases, the diastolic time.

D Atrial refractoriness is decreased, not increased, by digoxin, due to both a direct action and a parasympathomimetic action of the drug.

Learning objective: Describe the hemodynamic actions of digoxin in the failing heart.

9. **A** The increase in stroke volume is a direct consequence of the positive inotropic action of digitalis glycosides.

B Digoxin can cause peripheral vasoconstriction in the normal subject, but in patients with cardiac failure, digoxin causes peripheral vasodilation because the increased cardiac output offsets the reactive vasoconstriction.

C Digoxin actually decreases oxygen consumption in the failing heart because

- Increased contractility reduces the left ventricular end-diastolic volume and the associated stretch of the cardiac fibers (oxygen consumption of the heart is directly proportional to the stretch of the cardiac fibers).
- Increased cardiac output offsets the tachycardia induced by the sympathetic activation.

D, E See explanation C.

Learning objective: Describe the hemodynamic actions of cardiac glycosides in the failing heart.

10. **B** An inotropic drug increases the force of heart contraction; therefore, a higher fraction of the end-diastolic volume is ejected during systole. Consequently, the end-systolic volume (i.e., the volume of blood remaining in the ventricle at the end of the systole) is decreased.

A All inotropic drugs increase, not decrease, the stroke volume.

C The end-diastolic volume is the sum of the end-systolic volume plus the stroke volume. Because the stroke volume is increased and the end-systolic volume is decreased by inotropic drugs, the end-diastolic volume is not significantly changed.

D Digoxin increases, not decreases, the systolic blood pressure in patients in cardiac failure because of the increase in cardiac output.

E Pulse pressure may be sharply decreased in patients with cardiac failure because of the decrease in stroke volume, the main determinant of pulse pressure. Moreover, diastolic pressure is normal or increased because of sympathetic activation. By increasing cardiac contractility, digoxin increases the stroke volume and offsets the reactive, sympathetically mediated vasoconstriction. Therefore, the pulse pressure is increased, not decreased.

Learning objective: Calculate the maintenance dose of digoxin, given sufficient data.

11. **C** A maintenance dose of a drug is given by

$$D = (C_{ss} \times CL)/F,$$

where D is dose, C_{ss} is concentration at steady state, CL is clearance, and F is oral bioavailability.

Therefore:

Dose = $(1\ \mu g/L \times 7L/h)/0.7 = 10\ \mu g/h = 0.24$ mg daily

A, B, D–F See correct answer explanation.

Learning objective: Describe the main adverse effects of digoxin.

12. **C** The most solid indication for digoxin is still the combination of chronic cardiac failure with atrial fibrillation. Because of its direct atrioventricular (AV) blocking effects and vagomimetic properties, digoxin reduces the number of impulses conducted through the AV node and therefore controls the ventricular response rate in patients with atrial fibrillation. Most likely, digoxin was included in the patient's management, and the symptoms of the patient are classic symptoms of digitalis toxicity.

A, B Verapamil and propranolol can control the ventricular response rate in patients with atrial fibrillation by decreasing AV conduction. However, they do not cause the patient's symptoms.

D, E Lidocaine and furosemide do not decrease AV conduction and are of no value in atrial fibrillation.

Learning objective: Outline the therapy for digoxin-induced atrioventricular block.

13. **C** Digoxin-induced atrioventricular (AV) block is most likely due, at least in part, to the parasympathomimetic action of digoxin. Therefore, treatment with atropine and a reduction of the digoxin dose is a rational therapeutic approach.

A Milrinone is used only for short-term intravenous treatment of patients with end-stage heart failure.

B Because physostigmine is a cholinergic drug, it would worsen the AV block.

D To discontinue digoxin would be irrational because the ongoing therapy was effective. Moreover, metoprolol is contraindicated in the presence of AV block.

E Beta-adrenergic agonists are used only for short-term intravenous treatment of patients with acute cardiac failure. Additionally, even if a β-adrenergic agonist can increase the ventricular rate in patients with AV block due to increased vagal activity, it would be acting as a physiological antagonist of the acetylcholine-mediated effect. In this case, atropine is a much better choice, as a pharmacological antagonist is superior to a physiological antagonist in most cases.

F See answer explanation D.

Learning objective: Describe the factors that enhance the risk of digoxin toxicity.

14. **D** Ventricular tachycardia is a serious adverse effect of digoxin. The patient's reduced renal function (see the creatinine serum level) most likely decreased the renal excretion of digoxin, thus increasing the risk of adverse effects. Digoxin toxicity is enhanced by many factors, including hypercalcemia, which accelerates the overloading of intracellular calcium stores. Increased intracellular calcium appears to be responsible for an increased abnormal automaticity.

A–C, E See correct answer explanation.

Learning objective: Describe the therapy of digoxin toxicity.

15. **A** The patient's symptoms (nausea and vomiting), as well as the arrhythmia shown by the electrocardiogram, are classic signs of digoxin toxicity. Furosemide treatment most likely caused hypokalemia, which is a well-recognized predisposing factor to digoxin toxicity. In fact, in patients with serum K^+ of 3 mEq/L, the dose of digoxin needed to produce toxicity is about one half of that needed in patients with serum K^+ of 5 mEq/L. Moreover, the patient had reduced renal function (see the creatinine serum level), which most likely decreased the renal excretion of digoxin. Potassium supplementation is the rational therapy for hypokalemia. The dose of digoxin must also be reduced because of the renal insufficiency.

B This strategy would be used when digoxin toxicity is due to excessive parasympathomimetic activity of the drug, which is usually suggested by the presence of severe bradycardia or by an atrioventricular block.

C This option is irrational; a reduced digoxin dose would, of course, reduce toxicity, but an increased furosemide dose would worsen the hypokalemia.

D Digoxin was effective for 1 year, which indicates that the heart failure was serious enough to require an inotropic drug. Therefore, it would be irrational to withdraw an inotropic medication.

E Milrinone is an effective inotropic drug, but because of its toxicity, it is used only when other drugs are not able to improve the symptoms of the disease. When a drug is effective but causes adverse effects, as in this case, the first thing to do is to adjust the dosage.

Learning objective: Describe digoxin-induced arrhythmias.

16. **B** A patient with severe systolic dysfunction was most likely receiving cardiac therapy that included digoxin. The patient probably developed acute renal failure (as indicated by the sudden anuria) that substantially increased the toxicity of digoxin. In fact, the patient's symptoms are typical of so-called digitalis delirium.

A, C–E These drugs do not cross the blood–brain barrier, so central effects are unlikely.

F Albuterol crosses the blood–brain barrier and may cause feelings of apprehension and anxiety but not the symptoms exhibited by the patient.

Learning objective: Describe the factors that enhance the risk of digoxin toxicity.

17. **E** The patient is suffering from hypothyroidism, as indicated by the low thyroxine (T_4) and high thyroid-stimulating hormone (TSH) levels. Hypothyroidism increases the risk of digoxin toxicity because elimination of digoxin is decreased, and the heart is more sensitive to digoxin.

A Hypomagnesemia, not hypermagnesemia, can increase digoxin toxicity.

B Hyperaldosteronism is unlikely, as potassium levels are normal.

C Hyperparathyroidism is unlikely, as calcium levels are normal.

D Concomitant furosemide treatment can increase digoxin toxicity mainly by causing hypokalemia, but this is unlikely in this case, as the patient has been receiving furosemide and digoxin for several months without adverse effects, and potassium levels are normal.

Learning objective: Describe the treatment for digoxin poisoning.

18. **E** The patient's history and symptoms indicated that the patient attempted suicide by ingesting several digoxin tablets. The best way to treat digoxin poisoning is to administer digoxin antibodies (digoxin immune Fab) that bind digoxin with very high affinity, thus removing the drug from its tissue-binding sites. This approach is extremely effective in reversing digoxin intoxication.

A–D, F All of these drugs may be used in digoxin toxicity to treat specific digoxin-induced cardiac symptoms (e.g., lidocaine in case of ventricular tachycardia and atropine in case of atrioventricular block). However, when poisoning is severe and many body functions are seriously affected (see the psychic symptoms of the patient), digoxin antibodies must be administered first.

Learning objective: Describe the main contraindication of digoxin.

19. **C** Digoxin is relatively contraindicated in patients with significant atrioventricular (AV) block because the drug decreases AV conduction via both parasympathomimetic actions and a direct depressive effect on the AV node. Moreover, digoxin is not indicated for mild cardiac failure. Because the patient is hypertensive, all the other listed drugs are appropriate for initial heart failure or for hypertension.

    A, B, D–F See correct answer explanation.

Learning objective: Describe a digoxin–drug interaction of clinical importance.

20. **B** Broad-spectrum antibiotics such as erythromycin can increase the oral bioavailability of digoxin because they kill bacteria present in normal intestinal flora (mainly *Eubacterium lentum*) that are able to metabolize digoxin. This is a major and clinically important drug interaction with digoxin.

    A Although hypokalemia can increase digoxin toxicity, it is unlikely in this case because the patient has been receiving hydrochlorothiazide and digoxin for several months without adverse effects.

    C Hydrochlorothiazide can cause hypercalcemia, not hypocalcemia.

    D Captopril rarely decreases digoxin renal excretion, but it is unlikely in this case for the reasons explained above.

    E Although ibuprofen rarely decreases digoxin renal excretion, the effect is transient and clinically unimportant.

Learning objective: Describe a digoxin–drug interaction of clinical importance.

21. **B** The patient's symptoms suggest digoxin overdose. Some antiarrhythmic drugs (e.g., quinidine, amiodarone, and verapamil) can substantially increase the plasma concentration of digoxin, leading to adverse effects. In fact, the plasma levels of digoxin can be doubled by concomitant treatment with amiodarone. The mechanism of the interaction is unknown and probably multifactorial.

    A Captopril-induced hyperkalemia is usually mild. A mild hyperkalemia actually counteracts most adverse effects of digoxin.

    C Amiodarone can decrease atrioventricular conduction, but this cannot explain the patient's symptoms.

    D, E These effects of furosemide do not increase digoxin toxicity.

Learning objective: Identify a digoxin–drug interaction of clinical importance.

22. **B** The patient's symptoms are classic signs of digitalis toxicity. The fairly high dose of thiazide most likely caused hypokalemia and hypercalcemia, which are two well-recognized predisposing factors to digitalis toxicity. Twice as much digoxin is required to produce toxicity in patients with serum K+ of 5 mEq/L as in those with a serum K+ of 3 mEq/L.

    A Advanced age can increase the risk of digitalis toxicity, but this patient is not old (an old person is defined as 65 years of age or more).

    C Hypernatremia is not a predisposing factor for digitalis toxicity.

    D, E There is no evidence to support these options.

Learning objective: Describe the hemodynamic actions of digoxin in the failing heart.

23. **A** By definition, cardiac reserve is the capacity of the heart to function well beyond its basal level. In cardiac failure, the heart is unable to increase its force of contraction when the demand for work is increased. Therefore, cardiac output might be adequate under resting conditions, but be insufficient when the body is exercising. This would explain why dyspnea of exertion is one of the most common symptoms of cardiac failure. By increasing heart contractility, digoxin can increase the stroke volume under exercise; that is, it increases cardiac reserve.

    B An increase in cardiac contractility would cause coronary vasodilation, not vasoconstriction.

    C Oxygen consumption is decreased, not increased, in a failing heart under digoxin treatment because the increased contractility diminishes the stretch of cardiac fibers, which is the major determinant of oxygen consumption.

    D, E These cardiovascular parameters are decreased, not increased, by digoxin.

Learning objective: Explain the molecular mechanism of the positive inotropic action of milrinone.

24. **A** A patient with acute decompensated heart failure usually needs positive inotropic agents. Because the patient was using β-blockers, phosphodiesterase inhibitors are preferred over dobutamine. Phosphodiesterase inhibitors inhibit the cyclic adenosine monophosphate (cAMP) phosphodiesterase 3 isozyme with a resulting increase in cAMP levels. The cascade of events that follows this increase is equal to that triggered by other inotropic drugs (β₁ agonists, glucagon, etc.), which also increase (although by a different mechanism) cAMP levels. It involves opening of voltage-gated Ca^{2+} channels, which in turn increases intracellular Ca^{2+} levels.

    B Phosphodiesterase inhibitors do not inhibit the cyclic guanosine monophosphate (cGMP) phosphodiesterase isozyme. Also, the dephosphorylation of the myosin light chain would lead to relaxation, not contraction, of muscle cells.

    C The increased cAMP level does not trigger the opening of K+ channels. Additionally, this opening would cause hyperpolarization of the cell membrane, which would adversely affect myocyte contractility.

Learning objective: Explain the use of β-blockers in diastolic cardiac failure.

25. **A** Beta-blockers are drugs of choice in diastolic heart failure because

- They slow the heart rate, thus allowing more time for complete ventricular filling.
- They increase heart relaxation, thus counteracting the stiffness of the ventricular wall.
- They reduce myocardial oxygen demand.

B–D Inotropic drugs are usually contraindicated in diastolic heart failure because they do not relieve the high end-diastolic pressure and may induce arrhythmias.

E Phenylephrine is a pure α agonist and would further increase the blood pressure.

F Mannitol is an osmotic diuretic, which can be dangerous in patients with heart failure.

Learning objective: Explain the use of β-blockers in hypertrophic obstructive cardiomyopathy.

26. **B** The history and exam results indicate that the patient was most likely suffering from hypertrophic obstructive cardiomyopathy, a disorder usually inherited in an autosomal dominant pattern. In this disease, the asymmetric hypertrophy of the ventricular septum leads to left ventricular outflow obstruction. Syncope usually occurs after exercise, probably because the increased epinephrine causes an increased contractile function that worsens the obstruction and a decreased diastolic time that reduces diastolic ventricular filling.

Other classic symptoms of the disease are angina (a limited coronary blood flow reserve is present in hypertrophied states) and diastolic heart failure (due to the reduced compliance of the hypertrophied left ventricle). Beta-blockers and calcium channel blockers that act on the heart (verapamil and diltiazem) are drugs of choice in this disease, because they decrease cardiac contractility and increase diastolic ventricular filling.

A, C–E All of the other listed drugs are contraindicated in hypertrophic obstructive cardiomyopathy because either they decrease venous return (prazosin, nitrates, or diuretics) or increase contractile function (inotropic agents).

Learning objective: Outline the use of nesiritide in stage D heart failure.

27. **D** The patient was most likely suffering from stage D cardiac failure despite maximal doses of the standard recommended therapy. On admission, the patient was in acute heart failure, as indicated by the high central venous pressure and poor cardiac output. Because the central venous pressure is very high, a venous vasodilator such as nitroglycerin or nesiritide is indicated to reduce preload. Nesiritide (recombinant atrial natriuretic peptide) has the advantage of having both natriuretic and vasodilatory properties and can add to the diuretic effect of furosemide in refractory patients.

A The patient has been receiving maximal doses of digoxin without effect, and the long half-life of the drug suggests that a steady-state plasma level of digoxin has already been attained in the patient. To add digoxin would most likely be without therapeutic effect and would substantially increase the risk of toxicity.

B, C, E, F These drugs are without effect and could be dangerous in a patient in acute cardiac failure.

Learning objective: Explain the molecular mechanism of the positive inotropic action of dobutamine.

28. **B** Dobutamine activates mainly β_1 adrenoceptors. The subsequent activation of cyclic adenosine monophosphate (cAMP)–dependent protein kinase A increases the opening of membrane voltage-gated calcium channels (causing an increased speed and strength of myocyte contraction), as well as the opening of sarcoplasmic calcium channels (causing an increased reuptake of Ca^{2+} by the sarcoplasmic reticulum). Therefore, both the speed of contraction and the speed of relaxation of myocytes are increased.

A This is the mechanism of action of milrinone.

C, E These molecular actions are triggered by digoxin, not dobutamine.

D The increase of this enzyme is triggered by activation of α receptors, not β receptors.

Learning objective: Explain the reasons for the beneficial effect of angiotensin-converting enzyme (ACE) inhibitors in heart failure.

29. **C** Captopril is an ACE inhibitor, and most effects of the drug are the consequence of decreased plasma angiotensin levels. This decrease in turn reduces peripheral resistance, both directly and through a reduction in sympathetic activity (thus decreasing afterload), and reduces aldosterone secretion (thus decreasing preload). These effects relieve the workload of the heart and result in improved systolic contractile function.

B Although this action is beneficial, this is not at all the main reason why captopril is useful in heart failure.

A, D By inhibiting angiotensin II formation, captopril actually would inhibit all angiotensin-mediated effects, including increased cardiac contractility and epinephrine release from adrenergic nerves.

E By inhibiting ACE, captopril inhibits, not stimulates, bradykinin metabolism.

Learning objective: Explain angiotensin-converting enzyme inhibitor (ACE)–induced mortality reduction in myocardial infarction.

30. **E** ACE inhibitors block the vasoconstricting activity of angiotensin II, thus reducing both preload and afterload, which in turn reduces the workload of the heart. In addition, they reduce the growth effects of angiotensin II on cardiac myocytes and attenuate the cardiac fibrosis induced by angiotensin II. These actions lead to reduction of myocardial remodeling. The initial remodeling phase after a myocardial infarction (repair of the necrotic area and myocardial scarring) may be considered beneficial, but over time remodeling causes an increase of ventricular mass and volume that adversely affects cardiac function. By reducing cardiac remodeling, ACE inhibitors improve ejection fraction and decrease mortality.

    A ACE inhibitors do not appreciably affect cardiac contractility.

    B By blocking aldosterone formation, ACE inhibitors decrease, not increase, preload.

    C By decreasing the workload of the heart, ACE inhibitors actually can indirectly cause coronary vasoconstriction.

    D ACE inhibitors have negligible effects on ventricular automaticity.

Learning objective: Explain the role of β-blockers in the therapy of systolic heart failure.

31. **C** The patient's symptoms indicate that he was suffering from stage C heart failure. His decreased ejection fraction points out that his heart failure was systolic. The left ventricular ejection fraction is the best way to differentiate between systolic and diastolic heart failure. Today, β-blockers are first-line agents for both systolic and diastolic heart failure, but the clinical use is different:

    - For systolic heart failure, guidelines suggest early use, low dose, gradual titration, and selected agents. There is fairly strong evidence that the benefits of β-blockers in systolic heart failure are not a class effect. Metoprolol, bisoprolol, and carvedilol are the β-blockers shown to reduce mortality in large heart failure trials.
    - For diastolic heart failure, higher doses are used, there is less need to titrate, and a wider range of drugs is acceptable.

    Beneficial effects of β-blockers in systolic heart failure include

    - Prevention of chronic overactivity of the sympathetic nervous system, which leads to decreased heart rate and reduced myocardial remodeling through inhibition of the mitogenic activity of catecholamines
    - Inhibition of renin secretion by blocking β_1 receptors in juxtaglomerular cells
    - Upregulation of β_1 receptors (in heart failure, β_1 receptors are downregulated due to the chronic activation of the sympathetic nervous system)

    A, B, D, E Beta-blockers elicit actions opposite to those listed.

Learning objective: Explain the mechanism of the therapeutic effect of the hydralazine/isosorbide dinitrate combination in Black patients with heart failure.

32. **C** It has been shown that the hydralazine/isosorbide dinitrate combination can be effective primarily in Black patients with systolic heart failure. Because of this, the U.S. Food and Drug Administration has approved the combination product for the treatment of heart failure as an adjunct to standard heart failure therapy in Black patients. The mechanism of the therapeutic effect of the combination is most likely related to the nitrate-mediated reduction of preload and the hydralazine-mediated reduction of afterload.

    A Both hydralazine and nitrates can cause reflex increase in cardiac contractility, but this action is not the main reason that the combination is useful in heart failure.

    B By causing the reflex activation of the sympathetic system, both drugs can increase, not decrease, the angiotensin II formation.

    D Both drugs can activate, not inhibit, the sympathetic system.

    E By causing the reflex activation of the sympathetic system, both drugs can increase, not decrease, the heart rate.

Learning objective: Describe the role of loop diuretics in the therapy of chronic systolic heart failure.

33. **D** Diuretics are indicated in systolic heart failure because they decrease preload. Therefore, they are used primarily in patients with pulmonary congestion and peripheral edema, as in this case.

    In most patients in heart failure, loop diuretics are preferred for two main reasons:

    - They are the most effective diuretics presently available.
    - They are the only diuretics that retain their activity even when the glomerular filtration rate is very low. Most diuretics lose their effectiveness when creatinine clearance is less than 30 mL/min. Loop diuretics retain their effectiveness until creatinine clearance is less than 5 mL/min.

    In systolic heart failure, the glomerular filtration rate is often quite low because of the decreased cardiac output; this explains why all diuretics, except loop diuretics, are minimally effective in stage C heart failure.

A Loop diuretics stimulate, not inhibit, angiotensin II synthesis by decreasing macula densa sensitivity.

B Loop diuretics decrease, not increase, venous return to the heart by increasing venous capacitance vessels (which seems mainly related to the increased synthesis of prostaglandins).

C Loop diuretics stimulate, not inhibit, prostaglandin biosynthesis.

E By decreasing preload, loop diuretics increase the stroke volume, but this is not because they increase heart contractility. By definition, contractility is the change in the peak isometric force of the cardiac fiber at any given initial fiber length. Diuretics increase contraction, not contractility, of the heart by decreasing preload, that is, by decreasing the cardiac fiber length.

Learning objective: Describe the use of spironolactone in heart failure.

34. **C** It has been shown that spironolactone significantly reduces (about 30%) mortality and hospitalization for heart failure due to left ventricular systolic dysfunction. The protective effect of the drug is most likely related to its antagonistic activity at aldosterone receptors rather than to its diuretic effect, because spironolactone is a mild diuretic and because other direct-acting potassium-sparing diuretics, such as triamterene and amiloride, are completely devoid of protective effects in systolic heart failure. Current guidelines recommend initiating aldosterone antagonists in patients with severe heart failure, as in this case.

A Losartan is an angiotensin receptor antagonist. Even if the actions of angiotensin-converting enzyme (ACE) inhibitors and angiotensin antagonists are not exactly the same, it is unlikely that losartan can be effective in a patient not responding to captopril.

B See correct answer explanation.

D Indapamide is a thiazide diuretic. It is minimally effective in severe heart failure. Moreover, the patient already received furosemide without evident improvement.

E, F Milrinone and nesiritide are used only for acute heart failure when other drugs are not effective.

Learning objective: Describe the pharmacological actions of angiotensin-converting enzyme (ACE) inhibitors.

35. **C** Captopril is an ACE inhibitor. ACE catalyzes the synthesis of angiotensin II from angiotensin I and promotes the degradation of bradykinin. By blocking the enzyme, ACE inhibitors will increase the plasma levels of angiotensin I and bradykinin. Both actions contribute to the vasodilating activity of these drugs (even if the first is by far the most important), as angiotensin II is a powerful vasoconstricting agent, and bradykinin is a vasodilator. The resultant decrease in afterload is a primary mechanism of the therapeutic effect of ACE inhibitors in systolic heart failure.

A It is known that angiotensin II promotes the secretion of vasopressin from the posterior pituitary. By inhibiting angiotensin II formation, vasopressin plasma levels are, if anything, decreased, not increased. By blocking aldosterone synthesis, plasma sodium levels are expected to decrease, not increase.

B Angiotensin II stimulates norepinephrine release from sympathetic nerve terminals. By inhibiting angiotensin II formation, ACE inhibitors decrease, not increase, plasma levels of norepinephrine.

D ACE inhibitors have negligible effects on these endogenous compounds.

E Prostaglandin plasma levels can be increased by ACE inhibitors, but angiotensin III levels would be decreased.

Learning objective: Describe the main advantages of angiotensin antagonists over angiotensin-converting enzyme (ACE) inhibitors.

36. **E** The prescribed drug was most likely losartan, an angiotensin II receptor blocker. Angiotensin II is synthesized from renin and catalyzed by ACE. However, some tissues contain nonrenin angiotensinogen-processing enzymes that catalyze the synthesis of angiotensin II without the need for ACE. ACE inhibitors reduce the biosynthesis of angiotensin II produced by the action of ACE, but they do not inhibit alternative non-ACE angiotensin II–generating pathways. Because angiotensin II antagonists block type 1 angiotensin II receptors, the actions of angiotensin II are blocked regardless of the biochemical pathways leading to angiotensin synthesis. Whether the pharmacological differences between angiotensin blockers and ACE inhibitors result in significant differences in therapeutic outcome is still an open question. It is common to substitute an ACE inhibitor with an angiotensin blocker when the first is not effective and can cause adverse effects, as in this case.

A–D, F See correct answer explanation.

Learning objective: Explain the most likely molecular mechanism of the therapeutic effect of spironolactone in systolic heart failure.

37. **C** Spironolactone is a competitive aldosterone receptor antagonist that significantly reduces morbidity and mortality in advanced systolic heart failure. This reduction is achieved in the absence of demonstrable diuretic effect, lending support to the hypothesis that the therapeutic effect of the drug is related to its blocking activity at aldosterone receptors. The major action of aldosterone is to stimulate the kidney to reabsorb Na^+ and water. However, aldosterone has similar actions on salt and water transport in the colon, salivary glands, and sweat glands. Moreover, aldosterone receptors are present in several other tissues, including myocardium, and it is likely that the drug increases Na^+ conductance across most cell membranes. Morphologic studies indicate that chronic excess of aldosterone (plus salt loading), as occurs in heart failure, can induce a pathologic remodeling, causing fibrosis in the heart, kidney, and other organs in animals and humans. The mechanism of this effect is still uncertain, but it could be related to the increased Na^+ conductance in aldosterone-controlled Na^+ channels in several tissues, including the myocardium. By blocking aldosterone receptors, spironolactone can decrease aldosterone-controlled Na^+ conductance.

    A Spironolactone can have a potassium-sparing effect by inhibiting potassium excretion in the collecting duct, but this is not the reason for its efficacy in chronic heart failure.

    B This would be the mechanism of action of carbonic anhydrase inhibitors.

    D Spironolactone has no direct effect on renin secretion by the macula densa.

    E This would be the mechanism of action of thiazide diuretics.

Learning objective: Describe the main adverse effects of angiotensin-converting enzyme (ACE) inhibitors.

38. **B** ACE inhibitors decrease aldosterone synthesis. Lower aldosterone levels tend to decrease K^+ excretion. Carvedilol is a nonselective β-blocker and a selective α_1-blocker. Blockade of β_2 receptors in the skeletal muscle tends to decrease K^+ uptake. Hyperkalemia is uncommon if one of the two drugs is given singly, but the risk of hyperkalemia is substantially increased when they are given concomitantly.

    A ACE inhibitors and β-blockers have a negligible effect on calcium plasma levels.

    C, D Blockade of aldosterone production is expected to decrease, not increase, extracellular fluid volume and sodium plasma levels.

    E ACE inhibitors have a negligible effect on glucose metabolism. Beta-blockers can decrease, not increase, the glucose level by blocking β_2–mediated gluconeogenesis and glycogenolysis in the liver.

Learning objective: Describe the effects of angiotensin-converting enzyme (ACE) inhibitors and β-blockers in a patient with stage C systolic heart failure.

39. **A** A patient suffering from stage C systolic heart failure most likely shows decreased diuresis (because of the decreased cardiac output), increased arteriolar tone (because of angiotensin II actions and sympathetic overactivity), and increased myocardial oxygen consumption (because the high preload increased the stretch of the cardiac fibers, which is a major determinant of oxygen consumption).

    By decreasing preload and afterload, ACE inhibitors increase cardiac output ,which in turn can

    • Improve kidney blood flow, leading to an increased diuresis
    • Offset the sympathetic overactivity, leading to decreased arteriolar tone
    • Decrease the diastolic stretch of cardiac fibers, leading to a decrease in myocardial oxygen consumption

    Carvedilol is an α-/β-blocker that can

    • Decrease arteriolar tone
    • Decrease heart rate, leading to a decrease in myocardial oxygen consumption

    B–E See correct answer explanation.

Learning objective: Describe the main adverse effects of spironolactone.

40. **D** The patient was suffering from gynecomastia, a well-described adverse effect of spironolactone that is related to dose and duration of treatment. High doses have been associated with up to a 50% prevalence of this adverse effect. Owing to its affinity for other steroid receptors, spironolactone can induce gynecomastia most likely by displacing androgens from androgen receptors. Generally, discontinuation of treatment results in resolution of gynecomastia.

    A–C, E The risk of gynecomastia with these drugs is negligible.

DRUGS FOR CARDIAC FAILURE Answer key			
1. F	6. B	11. C	16. B
2. C	7. B	12. C	17. E
3. I	8. E	13. C	18. E
4. G	9. A	14. D	19. C
5. B	10. B	15. A	20. B
21. B	26. B	31. C	36. E
22. B	27. D	32. C	37. C
23. A	28. B	33. D	38. B
24. A	29. C	34. C	39. A
25. A	30. E	35. C	40. D

Answers and Explanations: IV-4 Antihypertensive Drugs

Questions 1–5

1. **M**
2. **E**
3. **J**
4. **C**
5. **A**

Learning objective: Describe the main action leading to the antihypertensive effect of thiazides.

6. **C** The initial hypotensive effects of diuretics are associated with a reduction in plasma volume and cardiac output. Peripheral vascular resistance is usually unaffected (or sometimes increased). After 4 to 8 weeks of continuous therapy, blood volume and cardiac output return to normal, and peripheral vascular resistance decreases. Mechanisms underlying this decrease are probably related to a depletion of body Na^+ stores.

   A Diuretics cause negligible postural hypotension, because the baroreceptor reflex is not affected.

   B See correct answer explanation.

   D Thiazides tend to decrease, not increase, interstitial fluid volume.

   E Blood flow in any organ is related to perfusion pressure and vessel resistance. Perfusion pressure in turn is mainly related to cardiac output. After several weeks of treatment with diuretics, cardiac output is normal; therefore, renal blood flow is either normal or increased, not decreased.

Learning objective: Describe the main adverse effects of thiazides.

7. **B** The patient's symptoms and the lab results indicate that he was most likely suffering from gouty arthritis. Chronic treatment with thiazides may cause hyperuricemia and precipitate attacks of gout in at-risk patients. Hyperuricemia is likely due to both a hypovolemia-induced increase in uric acid reabsorption and competition with urates for the organic acid transport system in the proximal tubule.

   Being a painter, the patient was already at risk for gout because a strong association exists between the risk of gout and lead exposure through diet or occupation (painters, plumbers, etc.).

   A, C, E, F These drugs do not cause hyperuricemia.

   D Furosemide can cause hyperuricemia, but the drug is rarely used as an antihypertensive.

Learning objective: Identify the most appropriate antihypertensive drug in a patient with concomitant diseases.

8. **D** The patient has stage 2 essential hypertension; therefore, an antihypertensive medication is recommended in addition to lifestyle modification. The patient is a good candidate for a thiazide diuretic for several reasons. First, these drugs are usually the most appropriate initial therapy for uncomplicated hypertension because they decrease morbidity and mortality. Second, the woman is suffering from osteoporosis, and thiazides can cause retention of calcium, a potentially beneficial effect. Moreover, in this patient:

   A Angiotensin-converting enzyme (ACE) inhibitors are contraindicated because of the past episode of angioedema.

   B, C Beta-blockers and verapamil are contraindicated because of the heart block.

   E Minoxidil is never a drug of first choice for antihypertensive therapy.

Learning objective: Describe the main adverse effects of central sympathoplegic antihypertensive drugs.

9. **D** Sedation is a frequent, and sometimes pronounced, adverse effect of central sympathoplegic antihypertensive drugs (methyldopa and clonidine), probably due to decreased adrenergic transmission in the central nervous system.

   A Postural hypotension is an uncommon and usually minor adverse effect of methyldopa and clonidine, because basal central adrenergic tone is reduced, but the baroreceptor reflex is still operative.

   B Hemolytic, not megaloblastic, anemia occasionally occurs with methyldopa.

   C Methyldopa and clonidine tend to decrease the heart rate, so palpitations are unlikely.

   E Methyldopa and clonidine frequently cause xerostomia, not sialorrhea. The mechanism of the effect is still uncertain.

Learning objective: Describe the symptoms of clonidine withdrawal.

10. **E** The patient's symptoms are most likely due to sudden clonidine withdrawal. Rebound hypertension can occur (to levels above those present prior to treatment), but the syndrome can appear in the absence of an overshoot in blood pressure. The signs and symptoms of the syndrome are associated with increased sympathetic discharge (plasma levels of catecholamines are increased). The exact mechanism underlying the clonidine withdrawal syndrome is not known, but the rebound hypertension seems to be due to an up-regulation of α_1 receptors.

    A–D, F Withdrawal of none of the other listed drugs precipitates the described syndrome.

Learning objective: Identify the antihypertensive drug that can most likely cause a positive Coombs reaction.

11. **D** Methyldopa is the most commonly used drug for chronic treatment of hypertension during pregnancy, primarily because there has been the most experience with this drug during pregnancy. Positive Coombs reaction occurs in up to 30% of patients treated for more than 6 months, but hemolytic anemia occurs in only 1 to 5% of cases. This is a type II allergic drug reaction. Apparently, the drug is able to alter the red blood cell surface chemically, thereby uncovering an antigen that induces and then reacts with an antibody, thus causing cell lysis.

    A–C, E, F None of these drugs produce a positive Coombs test or hemolytic anemia.

Learning objective: Describe the therapeutic uses of clonidine.

12. **D** Clonidine is the only antihypertensive that is also used in smoking cessation programs because it reduces anxiety, irritability, and craving during tobacco withdrawal (it doubles the number of patients who remain abstinent for 6 months or more). The mechanism of this action is uncertain, but it seems to be related to the drug-induced decrease in central sympathetic outflow, which may mitigate many of the signs of sympathetic overactivity that are present during tobacco withdrawal.

    A–C, E These drugs do not affect tobacco withdrawal.

Learning objective: Describe the main adverse effects of prazosin.

13. **D** The drug taken by the patient was most likely prazosin, an antihypertensive agent sometimes given to patients with resistant hypertension and concomitant prostatic hyperplasia, because it can also facilitate urination by relaxing the bladder internal sphincter. Prazosin can cause marked postural hypotension and syncope with the first dose (the so-called first-dose phenomenon). This is probably due to the blockade of α_1 receptors both in the arterioles (which impairs the reflex vasoconstriction) and in the veins (which decreases venous return). The orthostatic effect declines over time. The mechanism responsible for the development of such tolerance is not clear. Other antihypertensive drugs that can cause syncope are labetalol, angiotensin-converting enzyme (ACE) inhibitors, losartan, and nitroprusside.

    A Beta-blockers do not cause postural hypotension and syncope because they do not significantly affect the baroreceptor reflex or venous return.

    B, C Unlike drugs that dilate capacitance vessels, arteriolar vasodilators do not cause significant postural hypotension, so the risk of fainting with these drugs is negligible.

E Centrally acting antiadrenergic agents usually do not cause significant postural hypotension because they decrease the basal adrenergic tone, but the sympathetic nervous system can still be activated by proper stimuli.

F Fenoldopam is used only for hypertensive emergencies.

Learning objective: Describe the therapeutic uses of α_1-blockers.

14. **A** Alpha-1 blockers (e.g., prazosin and terazosin) are used as antihypertensive drugs primarily in men with prostatic hyperplasia because they relax the internal sphincter of the bladder and the prostate capsule.

    B–F None of these drugs have relaxant properties on the internal sphincter of the bladder and prostate capsule.

Learning objective: Identify the antihypertensive drug that is most likely to cause postural hypotension.

15. **E** By blocking α_1 receptors, labetalol affects the baroreceptor reflex that is responsible for rapid, moment-to-moment adjustment in blood pressure, such as in transition from a reclining to an upright posture. The increased sympathetic outflow cannot induce normal vasoconstriction because α_1 receptors are blocked, so postural hypotension results.

    A In general, β-blockers such as propranolol cause negligible postural hypotension because the baroreceptor reflex is not affected.

    B Clonidine acts centrally to reduce sympathetic outflow. However, the baroreceptor reflex is only marginally affected, and postural hypotension is slight.

    C Angiotensin-converting enzyme (ACE) inhibitors such as captopril rarely cause postural hypotension. The reason is uncertain but could be due to downward resetting of baroreceptors.

    D In general, thiazide diuretics such as hydrochlorothiazide cause negligible postural hypotension because the baroreceptor reflex is not affected.

Learning objective: Choose the appropriate antihypertensive drug for a patient suffering from hypertrophic cardiomyopathy.

16. **E** Beta-blockers such as propranolol are first-line agents in hypertrophic cardiomyopathy because they increase the duration of diastole and decrease left ventricular contractility and myocardial wall stress during systole. In this case, they should also reduce the high blood pressure and are therefore the most appropriate drugs for this patient.

    A–D These drugs will not improve and may even exacerbate the hypertrophic cardiomyopathy and therefore are not suited for this patient.

    F The use of angiotensin-converting enzyme (ACE) inhibitors in hypertrophic cardiomyopathy is controversial. Some clinicians think they have no role in the disease, whereas others believe they are beneficial by limiting hypertrophy.

Learning objective: Describe the use of antihypertensive drugs in aortic dissection.

17. **D** Aortic dissection is a highly lethal disorder. Because mortality is highest in the early hours after dissection begins, drug therapy to lower the arterial pressure should be started as soon as possible. Nitroprusside is given as a constant intravenous drip with the objective of reducing the blood pressure to the lowest level compatible with adequate cerebral, coronary, and renal perfusion. Because nitroprusside used alone can cause reflex tachycardia, a β-blocker such as esmolol is usually used concomitantly. Both drugs have very short half-lives that allow blood pressure response titration from minute to minute. Surgical repair on an emergency basis usually follows the medical therapy.

    A Labetalol is used for acute aortic dissection, but the addition of prazosin is irrational, as labetalol itself is also an α₁-blocker.

    B Diazoxide is used in case of hypertensive emergency, but the addition of hydralazine is irrational, as the drug can cause reflex tachycardia.

    C, E None of these drugs are suitable for hypertensive emergencies because their onset of action is too slow.

Learning objective: Describe the hemodynamic effects of atenolol.

18. **A** Atenolol is a selective β₁-blocker. Cardiac output is decreased because of the decrease in cardiac contractility and rate; venous tone is unchanged because there are no β₁ receptors on the vessels; and postural hypotension is negligible because the drug does not cause hypovolemia, and the baroreceptor reflex is unaffected.

    B–E See correct answer explanation.

Learning objective: Describe the main adverse effects of hydralazine.

19. **A** Hydralazine is an arteriolar vasodilator that causes reflex tachycardia, which explains the subjective feeling of palpitations. Skin vasodilation causes sweating and flushing.

    B–D All of these drugs tend to cause bradycardia, so palpitations are unlikely.

    E Nitroprusside can cause tachycardia and flushing. However, it is used only in hypertensive emergencies, as its half-life is very short.

Learning objective: Describe the actions leading to the therapeutic effect of minoxidil.

20. **E** Minoxidil acts by opening potassium channels in smooth muscle cell membranes, which leads to membrane stabilization, thus making contraction less likely. Vasodilation is limited to the arterioles (the effect on capacitance vessels is negligible) and causes the reduction of total peripheral resistance.

A, B Minoxidil causes a reflex activation of the sympathetic nervous system, which results in effects opposite to those listed.

C Minoxidil can sometimes increase, not decrease, the extracellular fluid volume, leading to edema.

D By decreasing blood pressure, minoxidil can activate, not inhibit, the renin angiotensin system.

Learning objective: Explain the molecular mechanism of action of diazoxide.

21. **C** Diazoxide is an arteriolar vasodilator sometimes used for hypertensive emergencies (but not for nonemergency treatment of hypertension). It opens potassium channels in smooth muscle cell membranes, thus stabilizing the membrane potential at the resting level. In this way, it counteracts smooth muscle contraction.

    A, B, D–F See correct answer explanation.

Learning objective: Describe the antihypertensive uses of calcium channel blockers.

22. **E** The patient is suffering from stage 2 hypertension, so a combination therapy is advisable. A diuretic (hydrochlorothiazide) and a Ca^{2+} channel blocker (nifedipine) would be a rational choice because Blacks often have low-renin hypertension and may respond best to diuretics and Ca^{2+} channel blockers. Moreover, in this patient

    A, B Captopril is contraindicated because of the renal artery stenosis in a solitary kidney.

    C, D Propranolol is contraindicated because of chronic obstructive pulmonary disease.

Learning objective: Explain the antihypertensive use of nifedipine in a patient with concomitant disease.

23. **A** Beta-blockers are useless in variant angina and can even be dangerous by causing coronary vasoconstriction. Nifedipine is a drug of choice in variant angina, as it causes a generalized vasodilation that includes the coronary arteries. Because the drug is also effective in hypertension, the substitution of propranolol with nifedipine is a rational therapeutic choice.

    B Nitroglycerin is effective in variant angina (but less effective than calcium channel blockers). In this case, however, propranolol must be withdrawn, so the simple addition of another drug is not a wise choice.

    C Captopril is a good therapy for hypertension but cannot cure the variant angina.

    D, E See explanation B.

Learning objective: Describe the pharmacological effects of angiotensin-converting enzyme (ACE) inhibitors.

24. **C** Captopril is an ACE inhibitor that reduces the synthesis of angiotensin II. This in turn will reduce the plasma level of aldosterone, whereas renin will increase (short-loop negative feedback), as will potassium.

    A, B, D These drugs do not cause this pattern of effects.

    E Spironolactone causes hyperkalemia but does not change the plasma levels of aldosterone, renin, and angiotensin II.

Learning objective: List the main contraindications for angiotensin-converting enzyme (ACE) inhibitors.

25. **B** ACE inhibitors are known to cause various malformations, growth retardation, and even fetal death, primarily when given during the second and third trimester of pregnancy. They are category D (positive evidence of human risk) in the classification by the U.S. Food and Drug Administration.

    A, C–E None of the other listed drug classes are absolutely contraindicated in pregnancy.

Learning objective: Describe the main adverse effects of angiotensin-converting enzyme (ACE) inhibitors.

26. **E** A dry, disturbing cough is a typical adverse effect of ACE inhibitors that occurs in up to 20% of patients and is most likely due to the increased plasma levels of bradykinin. The loss of taste (dysgeusia) reported by the patient is another typical effect of ACE inhibitors (the reason is unknown).

    A–D None of the other listed antihypertensive drugs cause these adverse effects.

Learning objective: Describe the main adverse effects of angiotensin-converting enzyme (ACE) inhibitors.

27. **D** The signs and symptoms of the patient strongly suggest the diagnosis of angioedema. ACE inhibitors are known to cause angioedema in 0.1 to 0.3% of patients. This effect is not dose-related and nearly always develops within the first week of therapy. Airway obstruction may lead to death. The mechanism underlying the disorder seems to be related to accumulation of bradykinin produced by these drugs. Angioedema is very rare in patients taking type 1 angiotensin II receptor antagonists.

    A–C, E None of the other listed drugs cause angioneurotic edema.

Learning objective: Describe the main adverse effects of angiotensin-converting enzyme (ACE) inhibitors.

28. **C** ACE inhibitors are known to slow the progression of renal impairment in hypertensive diabetics and in hypertensive patients with chronic renal failure. On the other hand, they can produce acute renal failure in patients with bilateral renal artery stenosis (or stenosis of the renal artery of a solitary kidney), severe aortic stenosis, and even severe intrarenal microvascular disease. In fact, in these diseases, angiotensin II is the main determinant of a sufficient glomerular filtration rate (GFR). Factors that predispose a patient to acute renal failure from ACE inhibition include concomitant use of diuretics (sodium-volume depletion caused by diuretics makes patients more sensitive to ACE inhibitors) and of nonsteroidal antiinflammatory drugs, which prevent the vasodilating action of renal prostaglandins.

    A, B, D, E See correct answer explanation.

Learning objective: Choose the appropriate antihypertensive drug for a patient with concomitant diseases.

29. **C** Angiotensin-converting enzyme (ACE) inhibitors appear to be ideal agents to treat hypertension in diabetics because they do not have biochemical adverse effects on glucose regulation, like other agents may. In addition, they are drugs of choice in chronic diabetic glomerulopathy because they slow down the progression of the disease. The patient shows signs of renal impairment (microhematuria), so captopril represents a rational choice. Moreover, in this patient

    A Thiazide diuretics are contraindicated because of gouty arthritis.

    B Beta-blockers are relatively contraindicated in insulin-dependent diabetics because they can mask signs and symptoms of hypoglycemia.

    D, F Clonidine and aliskiren are not first-choice drugs in antihypertensive therapy.

    E Nitroprusside is used in hypertensive emergency only.

Learning objective: Choose the appropriate therapy for a patient suffering from hypertension and heart failure.

30. **D** Diuretics and angiotensin-converting enzyme (ACE) inhibitors are the drugs of first choice in all stages of cardiac failure. The same drugs are also first-choice agents for hypertension. Therefore, the combination of hydrochlorothiazide and captopril is a rational choice for this patient.

    A, B Verapamil and minoxidil are not useful (and can be dangerous) in heart failure.

    C, E Many patients with cardiac failure will require the chronic administration of a loop diuretic to maintain euvolemia, but hydralazine and methyldopa are not drugs of choice to treat stage 1 cardiac failure.

Learning objective: Explain the molecular mechanism of antihypertensive action of thiazides.

31. **C** Thiazide diuretics are drugs of choice for mild hypertension, and they are especially effective in the elderly and Black populations. They can lower systolic blood pressure (BP) by 15 to 20 mm Hg and diastolic BP by 8 to 15 mm Hg. The main and long-term BP lowering effect results from a decrease in peripheral vascular resistance. The mechanism of this decrease is still uncertain, but it is probably related to a depletion of body Na^+ stores, which leads to a fall in smooth muscle intracellular Na^+ concentration. This in turn decreases intracellular Ca^{2+} concentration by activating the $1Ca^{2+}/3Na^+$ exchanger. Because less calcium is available, relaxation occurs.

A Blood volume depletion can initially contribute to the antihypertensive effect of thiazides, but this is not the main long-term mechanism, because after 6 to 8 weeks of continuous therapy, intravascular volume and cardiac output return to normal, but the antihypertensive effect persists.

B, D Hypokalemia and hypercalcemia are adverse effects of thiazides. If they are severe, they can cause several signs and symptoms, including hypotension, but these are not mechanisms of the antihypertensive effect of thiazides.

E An increase in the cyclic guanosine monophosphate (cGMP) level can cause vasodilation, but thiazides do not affect this second messenger.

Learning objective: Describe the antihypertensive use of thiazides.

32. **E** The patient was most likely suffering from essential hypertension. African-Americans tend to have higher and more severe hypertension than other populations, likely because of differences in electrolyte homeostasis, glomerular filtration rate, and sodium excretion. These differences likely contribute to the higher antihypertensive effectiveness of thiazide diuretics in African-Americans.

A, F Captopril is an angiotensin-converting enzyme (ACE) inhibitor, and atenolol is a β-blocker. It appears that ACE inhibitors, angiotensin antagonists, and β-blockers are less effective in Blacks than thiazide diuretics or calcium channel blockers.

B Loop diuretics such as furosemide are by far less effective than thiazide diuretics for the long-term management of hypertension.

C, D These drugs are used only in cases of hypertensive emergencies.

Learning objective: Explain the reasons for the association of thiazides and angiotensin II antagonists.

33. **A** It has been shown that thiazides can enhance the action of most antihypertensive drugs given concomitantly. Because

of this, the association of hydrochlorothiazide and losartan is today one of the most common antihypertensive medication regimens. The combination therapy with losartan and hydrochlorothiazide can achieve a greater reduction in blood pressure than the combined effects of either of these drugs alone and is therefore a true synergistic effect.

B–E See correct answer explanation.

Learning objective: Explain the reasons for a change in antihypertensive therapy.

34. **C** The patient's blood pressure is still high despite the therapy. Moreover, serum potassium is close to the upper limit of the normal range. In this situation, a third antihypertensive drug should be added. Hydrochlorothiazide is the best choice because it is a first-choice antihypertensive drug, it enhances the action of angiotensin-converting enzyme (ACE) inhibitors, and it can lower plasma potassium levels.

A Loop diuretics are less effective than thiazide diuretics as antihypertensives, and they are not indicated unless there is a concomitant disorder, such as severe chronic kidney disease (glomerular filtration rate less than 30 mL/min), left ventricular dysfunction, or severe edema.

B, D Indications for changing a drug in antihypertensive therapy are mainly related to drug-induced adverse effects (when a drug is not effective, another drug is added without changing the first drug). There is no evidence of adverse effects due to the drugs the patient was taking.

E Minoxidil has several adverse effects and is reserved for very difficult-to-control hypertension.

Learning objective: Describe the molecular mechanism of the antihypertensive action of methyldopa.

35. **C** Hypertension is the most common medical problem encountered during pregnancy, complicating 2 to 3% of pregnancies, and is a major cause of perinatal morbidity and mortality. Methyldopa is the drug most commonly used to treat chronic hypertension in pregnancy in the United States. The antihypertensive effect of methyldopa is most likely mediated by an action on the central nervous system. The drug is taken up by the adrenergic neurons, where it is transformed into methylnorepinephrine, an α_2 receptor agonist. Methylnorepinephrine activates α_2 receptors located in the nucleus of the tractus solitarius and in the rostral ventrolateral medulla. This activation decreases the firing from the reticulospinal tract, leading to a decreased central adrenergic tone.

A This is the mechanism of action of minoxidil.
B This is the mechanism of action β–blockers.
D This is the mechanism of action of fenoldopam.
E This is the mechanism of action of prazosin.

Learning objective: Explain the mechanism of antihypertensive action of β-blockers.

36. **E** Several mechanisms of the antihypertensive action of β-blockers have been postulated, but the two main mechanisms are most likely the following:

- Reduction of cardiac output due to the decrease in cardiac contractility and rate
- Inhibition of the renin–angiotensin system due to inhibition of renin secretion

A Beta-blockers have negligible effect on large veins, but blockade of β_2 receptors should constrict, not dilate, the vessels.

B Beta-blockers have negligible effect on the release of epinephrine from the adrenal medulla.

C Blockade of β_2 receptors should increase, not decrease, blood pressure. In fact, this action of β-blockers is weak under resting conditions and is overridden by the effect on cardiac output.

D This is a postulated mechanism of antihypertensive action of β-blockers but is by no means the main one. In fact, even β-blockers that do not cross the blood–brain barrier, such as atenolol, do have antihypertensive effect.

F Beta-blockers have negligible effect on blood volume.

Learning objective: Describe the therapeutic uses of nitroprusside.

37. **D** Nitroprusside is the drug most frequently used to induce controlled hypotension during surgery. The drug has high efficacy and can induce a decrease of blood pressure to the desired level. Moreover, the drug has a very short half-life (about 2 minutes), so blood pressure will quickly return to preoperative values when the drug is discontinued.

A–C, E, F All these drugs have half-lives of hours, so they are not suited for a controlled hypotension during surgery.

Learning objective: Describe the therapeutic use of diazoxide in a patient with concomitant diseases.

38. **B** Hypertensive encephalopathy is a medical emergency, and the patient's blood pressure should be lowered at once with parenteral medications that have a rapid onset of action. Diazoxide is used for hypertensive emergencies only. It is usually given by slow intravenous infusion, and its maximum effect occurs within 2 to 3 minutes.

A, C Verapamil and labetalol can be used to treat hypertensive emergencies but are contraindicated in this case because of the atrioventricular block.

D, E Clonidine and captopril are given by oral route only and are not suited to treat hypertensive emergencies.

F Nitroprusside is a first-line drug for hypertensive crisis but is contraindicated in this patient because of toxic tobacco amblyopia. This rare condition is likely associated with defective or absent rhodanese, the mitochondrial enzyme that detoxifies cyanide by converting it to thiocyanate.

Learning objective: Explain the choice of a fourth antihypertensive drug in a patient under antihypertensive therapy.

39. **E** Minoxidil is a very effective antihypertensive drug but is usually considered a third- or fourth-line agent because of its toxicity. Because the current treatment is not effective for this patient, the rationale is to add a fourth drug with a different mechanism of action. Minoxidil, an arteriolar vasodilator that acts by opening potassium channels in smooth muscle cell membranes, is more effective than other arteriolar vasodilators (nifedipine, hydralazine, etc.) in refractory hypertension. Minoxidil-induced arteriolar vasodilation results in reflex activation of the sympathetic nervous system, which in turn causes tachycardia, increased cardiac output, and fluid retention (due to increased plasma renin activity). Therefore, concomitant β-blocker and diuretic therapy is almost always required with minoxidil treatment, as in this case.

A Nifedipine would be contraindicated in this patient because he has experienced constipation with another calcium channel blocker.

B, F These drugs are used only in case of hypertensive emergencies.

C The mechanism of antihypertensive action of methyldopa is very close to that of clonidine, so its addition would not be rational.

D Enalaprilat would be contraindicated in this patient because he has experienced cough with another angiotensin-converting enzyme (ACE) inhibitor.

Learning objective: Choose the right antihypertensive drug in a patient with concomitant disease.

40. **E** The patient was suffering from hypertension and atrial tachycardia. Diltiazem has both antihypertensive and antiarrhythmic actions and is therefore an appropriate drug. Moreover, in this patient

A, C Furosemide and prazosin are not first-choice drugs for hypertension.

B Captopril is contraindicated in women who want to get pregnant.

D Propranolol is contraindicated because of asthma.

F Fenoldopam is used in hypertensive emergencies only.

ANTIHYPERTENSIVE DRUGS Answer key							
1.	M	6.	C	11.	D	16.	E
2.	E	7.	B	12.	D	17.	D
3.	J	8.	D	13.	D	18.	A
4.	C	9.	D	14.	A	19.	A
5.	A	10.	E	15.	E	20.	E
21.	C	26.	E	31.	C	36.	E
22.	E	27.	D	32.	E	37.	D
23.	A	28.	C	33.	A	38.	B
24.	C	29.	C	34.	C	39.	E
25.	B	30.	D	35.	C	40.	E

Answers and Explanations: IV-5 Antiarrhythmic Drugs

Questions 1–6

1. **K**
2. **A**
3. **B**
4. **B**
5. **N**
6. **M**

Learning objective: Describe the mechanism of quinidine-induced paradoxical tachycardia.

7. **A** Quinidine is still sometimes used to maintain the normal sinus rhythm after cardioversion, but it can cause paradoxical tachycardia, due to its antimuscarinic action on the heart, which increases atrioventricular conduction.

    B Quinidine blocks, not activates, α_1 receptors, thus causing peripheral vasodilation.

    C By causing vasodilation, quinidine actually decreases the stimulation of arterial baroreceptors.

    D, E Quinidine can block, not activate, both calcium and potassium channels.

Learning objective: Describe the electrophysiological actions of quinidine.

8. **C** Blockade of activated sodium channels is the distinctive feature of class Ia antiarrhythmic drugs. The slope of phase 0 of the cardiac action potential in normal atrial, Purkinje, and ventricular cells is dependent on sodium current. The higher the number of sodium channels that are in the open state, the higher the sodium current and the steeper the slope of phase 0. By blocking activated sodium channels (the number of channels that are blocked is dose-dependent), the sodium current will be less intense, and the slope of phase 0 decreases.

    A, B, D By blocking potassium channels, quinidine slows down repolarization. Therefore, action potential duration is increased, the slope of phase 3 is decreased, and the effective refractory period is increased.

    E The slope of phase 4 is related to automaticity (the steeper the slope, the higher the automaticity). Most antiarrhythmic drugs decrease the slope of phase 4, unless toxic doses are given.

Learning objective: Describe the main adverse effects of quinidine.

9. **C** Quinidine is rarely used today as an antiarrhythmic drug because of its numerous adverse effects, but it is still occasionally prescribed when other antiarrhythmic drugs are either not tolerated or ineffective. More than 100 drugs have been implicated in causing thrombocytopenia, but quinidine and heparin are the two drugs that have the strongest association with this disorder. Quinidine-induced thrombocytopenia appears to be immunologically mediated and usually develops within 12 to 24 hours after ingestion of the drug by a sensitized individual.

    A, B, D–F The risk of drug-induced thrombocytopenia with these drugs is quite low.

Learning objective: Describe the therapeutic uses of procainamide.

10. **D** Wolff–Parkinson–White (WPW) is a preexcitation syndrome in which there is an accessory bypass tract (known as a Kent bundle) connecting the atrium to the ventricle. An impulse can travel down this pathway and excite the ventricle before the expected regular impulse through the atrioventricular (AV) node; hence the term *preexcitation*. WPW syndrome can occur in children and adults without overt cardiac disease. The true incidence is unknown but varies in different reports from 0.1 to 3.0 per 1000 electrocardiograms. About 20 to 30% of all supraventricular tachycardias are associated with WPW syndrome. A direct current cardioversion represents the treatment of choice for WPW syndrome (for long-term ablation of the accessory pathway). Medical therapy must be used cautiously because it may unexpectedly increase the ventricular rate. Of the drugs approved by the U.S. Food and Drug Administration, procainamide, which prolongs the refractory period of the accessory pathways, in addition to blocking sodium channels and depressing phase 0, is considered by many the drug of choice.

    A–C Digoxin, calcium channel blockers, and β-blockers may be dangerous because they can block the AV node and may redirect impulses down the bypass tract.

    E Nifedipine has no direct action on the heart, and the reflex tachycardia it induces may worsen the arrhythmia.

Learning objective: Describe the electrophysiological actions of mexiletine.

11. **B** The typical action of most antiarrhythmic drugs is the decreased slope of phase 4 in pacemaker cells, which means a decrease in automaticity.

    A, C Mexiletine is a class Ib drug. These agents can decrease action potential duration (and thus refractoriness) in normal cardiac cells, but they increase action potential duration in abnormal cells.

    D Phase 2 is due to movement of calcium across cardiac cell membrane. Class Ib drugs do not affect calcium movement.

    E Because antiarrhythmic drugs tend to decrease cardiac rate, the interval between two action potentials (i.e., the diastolic interval) is increased, not decreased.

Learning objective: Describe the main adverse effects of lidocaine.

12. **A** Lidocaine is a drug of choice for ventricular arrhythmias associated with myocardial infarction, and the patient's tachycardia was most likely ventricular in nature, as atrioventricular dissociation was noted. The patient's signs and symptoms are typical central nervous system effects of a high dose of lidocaine.

    B, C High doses of phenytoin or sotalol do not cause the pattern of signs and symptoms exhibited by the patient.

    D Mexiletine is a lidocaine-like drug that is only used orally to prevent recurrence of ventricular tachycardia.

    E, F Verapamil and digoxin are not used and may even be contraindicated in ventricular tachycardia.

Learning objective: Describe the molecular mechanism of action of procainamide.

13. **E** Procainamide is a class Ia antiarrhythmic drugs. All drugs of this class block activated sodium and potassium channels. Amiodarone and lidocaine are drugs of choice for treatment of ventricular arrhythmias in the peri-infarction period. Procainamide is an alternative agent when the above-mentioned drugs are either not tolerated or ineffective. The drug blocks activated Na^+ channels, and recovery from blockade is about 1.8 seconds (the fastest of class Ia drugs), so it exerts greater effect in depolarized and/or rapidly driven cardiac myocytes.

    A–D See correct answer explanation.

Learning objective: Describe the uses of propranolol in hyperthyroidism.

14. **D** The patient presents with classic symptoms of hyperthyroidism. When a tachyarrhythmia is associated with hyperthyroidism, β-blockers remain the drugs of choice, as many symptoms of this disease are associated with sympathetic activation.

    A–C, E All of the other listed drugs can be used to treat supraventricular arrhythmias, but in this case, a β-blocker is preferred (see correct answer explanation).

Learning objective: Describe the use of β-blockers for atrial fibrillation associated with congenital hypertrophic cardiomyopathy.

15. **D** The patient's history, symptoms, and signs indicate that he was most likely affected by congenital hypertrophic cardiomyopathy, a disorder usually inherited in an autosomal dominant pattern. Classic symptoms of the disease are angina (a limited coronary blood flow reserve is present in hypertrophied states) and diastolic heart failure (due to the reduced compliance of the hypertrophied left ventricle). Beta-blockers without partial agonist activity (and calcium channel blockers that act on the heart, e.g., verapamil and diltiazem) are drugs of choice in this disease because they decrease cardiac contractility and increase diastolic ventricular filling (by causing bradycardia). Beta-blockers are also indicated in atrial fibrillation, as they can control the ventricular rate ("rate control"), even if they cannot reinstate normal sinus rhythm ("rhythm control"). In this case, they are useful for both conditions.

    A–C All of the listed drugs can be used, albeit rarely, in atrial fibrillation, but in this case, β-blockers are definitely preferred (see correct answer explanation).

    E Nitrates are contraindicated in hypertrophic cardiomyopathy because they reduce preload, which is already low because of the reduced volume and compliance of the left ventricle.

Learning objective: Describe the main adverse effects of amiodarone.

16. **C** The patient's signs and symptoms indicate a pulmonary disorder. Microbial infection is unlikely, and diffuse bilateral lung infiltrates are consistent with pulmonary fibrosis. Amiodarone-induced pulmonary fibrosis is the most serious adverse effect of the drug. Its incidence is variable (1 to 7% of the population), and mortality is also quite variable (0.1 to 10.0% of those affected). Amiodarone toxicity is cumulative and is more common in elderly patients, as in this case.

    A, B, D, E All of the other listed drugs may be used for prophylaxis of sustained ventricular tachycardia, but they do not cause pulmonary fibrosis.

Learning objective: Describe the lupoid syndrome caused by procainamide.

17. **E** The patient's signs and symptoms are consistent with drug-induced lupus (also called lupoid syndrome), an autoimmune disorder that is similar to idiopathic systemic lupus erythematosus. The agents most commonly reported to cause the disorder are procainamide (about one third of the patients taking the drug over a 1-year period) and hydralazine. Other drugs that can cause drug-induced lupus are chlorpromazine, isoniazid, methyldopa, quinidine, sulfonamides, and penicillamine. Onset of the drug-induced lupus syndrome can occur as soon as 1 month after therapy begins, as in this case. Unlike idiopathic lupus, drug-induced lupus typically improves rapidly after the discontinuation of the drug.

    A Quinidine can cause lupus but is not used to treat Wolff–Parkinson–White syndrome.

    B–D, F The risk of drug-induced lupus with these drugs is quite low.

Learning objective: Choose the appropriate antiarrhythmic drug for a patient with atrioventricular nodal tachycardia resistant to amiodarone.

18. **F** The patient was diagnosed with a reentrant supraventricular tachycardia. The two common types of reentrant tachycardias are

- Atrioventricular nodal reentrant tachycardia (AVNRT), which is due to a functional division of the atrioventricular (AV) node into two pathways with different conduction characteristics. One is a fast conducting pathway, and the other is a slower conducting pathway. Because the electrical signal travels through the AV node, the QRS complex of this tachycardia is narrow. The tachycardia is usually responsive to vagal maneuvers or adenosine acutely, or to calcium channel blockers, β-blockers, or (historically) digoxin chronically.
- Atrioventricular reciprocating tachycardia (AVRT) is due to an extra, abnormal electrical connection in the heart (often called an accessory pathway) that joins one of the atria with one of the ventricles. Because the electrical signal travels through both the AV node and the accessory pathway, the QRS complex of this tachycardia is usually wide. In this form of tachycardia, adenosine, calcium channel blockers, β-blockers, and digoxin are usually contraindicated because they decrease the conduction through the AV node, facilitating the conduction through the accessory pathway.

The electrocardiogram of the patient indicates that she was most likely suffering from an AVRT. Drugs that primarily decrease conduction across the accessory pathway include some class I drugs (procainamide, propafenone, and flecainide) and class III drugs (amiodarone and sotalol), and they are used until the accessory pathway can be removed by ablation.

It is common to change drug class when the first drug was not effective, as in this case.

A–C Lidocaine, mexiletine, and phenytoin are minimally effective in supraventricular arrhythmias.

D, E Nifedipine and nitroglycerin are actually contraindicated in AVRT (see correct answer explanation).

Learning objective: Identify the main contraindications of quinidine.

19. **C** Class Ia and Ic antiarrhythmic drugs are absolutely contraindicated in case of poisoning with tricyclic antidepressants as they share cardiotoxic and anticholinergic side effects with these drugs. Moreover, antiarrhythmic drugs that increase action potential duration are generally contraindicated in patients with widened QRS complexes.

A, B Mexiletine and lidocaine are indicated, not contraindicated, for treatment of ventricular arrhythmias.

D Phenytoin is indicated in arrhythmias due to digitalis toxicity and is not contraindicated in ventricular arrhythmias, although its efficacy remains controversial.

E Beta-blockers such as propranolol might be effective in treating tricyclic-induced arrhythmias, but they are not drugs of choice because they can cause bradycardia and worsen tricyclic-induced hypotension.

Learning objective: Describe the main adverse effects of sotalol.

20. **D** The electrocardiographic hallmark of polymorphic ventricular tachycardia is a long Q-T interval. Prolongation of Q-T interval indicates prolongation of action potential duration, which is related to a decreased outward potassium current during phase 3 of the action potential. Long Q-T interval is present prior to the onset of tachycardia and is due to hereditary or acquired potassium channel defects. Hereditary Q-T syndromes are due to rare mutations of the genes encoding potassium channels. However, the importance of the disorder in everyday practice is related to its provocation by diseases or drugs that prolong Q-T interval. Diseases include hypothyroidism, subarachnoid hemorrhage, myocarditis, hypokalemia, and hypomagnesemia. Drugs include class Ia and III antiarrhythmic drugs, tricyclic antidepressants, neuroleptics, some antihistamines, macrolide antibiotics, and quinolones. All of these drugs are able to increase action potential duration by blocking or modifying potassium channels. High doses of these drugs can trigger polymorphic ventricular tachycardia in patients at risk. Sotalol is the only β-blocker that can block potassium channels (a property not related to β-receptor blockade), and it can cause polymorphic ventricular tachycardia. Moreover, the patient was taking a quinolone and so was already at risk of developing the disorder.

A–C, E, F See correct answer explanation.

Learning objective: Describe the use of ibutilide in pharmacological cardioversion.

21. **E** Ibutilide, a class III antiarrhythmic drug with potassium channel–blocking and sodium channel–enhancing effects, was the first drug approved by the U.S. Food and Drug Administration for the termination of atrial flutter or fibrillation. The conversion rate with this drug is lower than the conversion rate with direct current but is generally attempted first, as electrical cardioversion requires general anesthesia. Other drugs that have been used for pharmacological cardioversion are quinidine, procainamide, and flecainide, but they are usually less effective than ibutilide with more frequent adverse effects.

A–D None of these drugs are used for pharmacological cardioversion.

Learning objective: Describe the main adverse effects of verapamil.

22. **E** With increasing prescription usage, poisoning with calcium channel blockers has increased dramatically. Clinical manifestations of verapamil overdosage include decreased consciousness, hypotension, and various bradyarrhythmias (bradycardia, atrioventricular block, asystole).

    A Ipratropium is given only by the inhalation route. Moreover, systemic absorption of the drug is minimal.

    B Adenosine is used for the acute treatment of paroxysmal ventricular tachycardia but is not a drug for chronic treatment. Moreover, it is given by the intravenous route, so poisoning by this drug is unlikely in this case.

    C Propranolol is used to treat supraventricular arrhythmias but is contraindicated in this case because of chronic obstructive pulmonary disease.

    D Mexiletine is not used to treat supraventricular arrhythmias.

Learning objective: Choose the appropriate antiarrhythmic drug for a patient with concomitant diseases.

23. **C** The first treatment goal in atrial fibrillation is to slow the ventricular rate, thus allowing the ventricles to contract and empty more effectively. Digoxin, β-blockers, and calcium channel blockers all can be used effectively because they can cause an incomplete atrioventricular block, thus allowing fewer atrial impulses to pass into the ventricle. However, in this patient

    A Digoxin is contraindicated because of hyperparathyroidism, because hypercalcemia strongly increases digitalis sensitivity. Primary hyperparathyroidism is the most common cause of hypercalcemia; its incidence is higher in postmenopausal women.

    B Nonselective β-blockers are contraindicated because of peripheral occlusive arteriosclerosis.

    D, E Class Ib antiarrhythmic drugs are not effective in supraventricular arrhythmias.

    F Adenosine is only used for the acute treatment of supraventricular arrhythmias.

Learning objective: Explain the molecular mechanism of action of adenosine.

24. **E** Adenosine activates specific A_1 adenosine receptors in the heart, which in turn open acetylcholine-sensitive K^+ channels, that is, channels normally driven by parasympathetic activity. This leads to hyperpolarization of the sinoatrial and atrioventricular (AV) nodes. Adenosine is considered the agent of choice for the acute conversion of paroxysmal supraventricular tachycardia. Vagotonic maneuvers (carotid sinus massage, Valsalva maneuver, etc.), particularly if used early, may terminate the arrhythmia. If these maneuvers are ineffective, adenosine is used. Blocking conduction through the AV node for one beat interrupts the reentrant cycle. On the other hand, adenosine is contraindicated in wide complex supraventricular tachycardias because it can increase conduction through the accessory pathway.

    A–D See correct answer explanation.

Learning objective: Choose the appropriate drug for a patient with sinus bradycardia.

25. **E** Sinus bradycardia complicating a myocardial infarction is most likely due to increased vagal activity. In this case, atropine is the drug of choice.

    A–D All of the other listed drugs can increase the heart rate, but they are physiological antagonists of acetylcholine. A pharmacological antagonist is better than a physiological antagonist in most cases.

Learning objective: Describe the main adverse effects of amiodarone.

26. **F** The patient's signs and symptoms are consistent with hypothyroidism. Amiodarone can cause either hyperthyroidism or hypothyroidism, although hypothyroidism is more common. These complications are a consequence of the high iodine content in amiodarone. When amiodarone is metabolized in the liver, iodine molecules are released and can exert pharmacological effects.

    A–C, E All of these drugs may be used for sustained ventricular tachycardia prophylaxis, but they do not cause thyroid disorders.

    D Lidocaine is not used for sustained ventricular tachycardia prophylaxis.

Learning objective: Identify the electrophysiological property common to β-blockers, Ca^{2+} channel blockers, and digoxin.

27. **A** The first treatment goal in atrial fibrillation is to slow the ventricular rate, thus allowing the ventricles to contract and empty more effectively. Digoxin, β-blockers, and calcium channel blockers can all be used effectively because they can cause an incomplete atrioventricular block, thus allowing fewer atrial impulses to pass into the ventricle.

    B–E See correct answer explanation.

Learning objective: Choose the appropriate antiarrhythmic drug for a patient with a concomitant disease.

28. **B** The first treatment goal in atrial fibrillation is to slow the ventricular rate, thus allowing the ventricles to contract and empty more effectively. Calcium channel blockers such as verapamil with cardiac activity can decrease cardiac rate by causing an incomplete atrioventricular block, so that fewer atrial impulses can pass into the ventricle.

A Amiodarone is used to maintain rhythm control in atrial fibrillation but is contraindicated in this case because of the chronic obstructive pulmonary disease.

C Nifedipine is useless in this case because it has no anti-arrhythmic activity.

D, E Class Ib antiarrhythmic drugs such as lidocaine and mexiletine are not effective in supraventricular arrhythmias.

F Beta-blockers such as sotalol can be used effectively in atrial fibrillation but are contraindicated in this case because of the chronic obstructive pulmonary disease.

Learning objective: Outline the use of amiodarone in a patient with concomitant disease.

29. **C** Amiodarone is considered a second-choice drug in any instance of atrial fibrillation, but it may be a first-choice drug in patients with concomitant hypertension and left ventricular dysfunction. It is therefore an appropriate drug to be tried in this case, Moreover, in this patient

A Verapamil was not effective, so it seems unwise to try another drug (diltiazem) with the same mechanism of action.

B, D Mexiletine and lidocaine are not effective in supra-ventricular arrhythmias.

E Because sotalol was only partially effective, it is not appropriate to try another β-blocker.

Learning objective: Describe the use of adenosine for the acute treatment of supraventricular arrhythmias.

30. **C** The electrocardiogram record and the therapeutic maneuvers strongly suggest that the patient is suffering from paroxysmal supraventricular tachycardia. Adenosine is the drug of choice for the acute conversion of paroxysmal supraventricular tachycardia. The drug activates A_1 adenosine receptors, which in turn open acetylcholine-sensitive K^+ channels. This leads to hyperpolarization of sinoatrial (SA) and atrioventricular (AV) nodes, thus decreasing SA node rhythm and AV conduction.

A, B, D Class Ib drugs have no effect on most supraventricular arrhythmias.

E, F Class IV drugs with cardiac activity may be attempted to slow conduction in the AV node, but adenosine is tried first in most cases.

Learning objective: Describe the use of flecainide to treat certain forms of ventricular tachycardia

31. **D** Idiopathic left ventricular tachycardia is a ventricular arrhythmia that usually presents in patients between 15 and 40 years of age with structurally normal hearts. The arrhythmia responds well to class Ic antiarrhythmic drugs and to verapamil for acute termination, as well as for long-term control.

A, E These drugs are given intravenously and have a short half-life. They cannot be used for the chronic control of ventricular tachycardia.

B, C These drugs are useless in idiopathic ventricular tachycardia.

Learning objective: Describe the use of lidocaine in the acute treatment of ventricular arrhythmias.

32. **E** Making the distinction between supraventricular tachycardia and ventricular tachycardia (VT) is important because this distinction influences subsequent management. The hallmark of VT is atrioventricular dissociation, as in this case. The impulse arises from the ventricle without relationship to the atria, unless retrograde atrial conduction occurs. Sustained VT is a medical emergency because it can develop into ventricular fibrillation if untreated. Lidocaine and amiodarone are first-line agents in this setting. Procainamide is a backup drug for VT.

A Phenytoin is mainly effective in VT resulting from digitalis excess. Its efficacy in VT due to other causes is questionable.

B, C Calcium channel blockers such as verapamil and quinidine are usually not effective in VT.

D Mexiletine is a lidocaine-like drug that is used to prevent recurrence of VT. However, it is given orally and is not a drug for an emergency treatment.

Learning objective: Describe the use of flecainide for the chronic control of supraventricular arrhythmias.

33. **B** Drugs used to maintain sinus rhythm after cardioversion include class Ia, Ic, and III antiarrhythmics, but in a patient with no structural heart disease, flecainide is usually preferred.

A Amiodarone could be used in the present case but it blocks the inactivated Na^+ channels only and strongly increases the action potential duration.

C−E These drugs are not used for rhythm control of atrial flutter and fibrillation after cardioversion.

Learning objective: Describe the antiarrhythmic use of magnesium sulfate.

34. **E** The patient's history and symptoms suggest that he was most likely suffering from an adverse effect of quinidine, a drug currently used to cut heroin and cocaine. The electrocardiogram indicated that the patient's arrhythmia was torsades de pointes (TdP). TdP occurs in conjunction with a long Q-T interval that was present prior to the onset of tachycardia. A vast array of drugs can cause TdP, especially when given at high doses. An exception is quinidine, because it can cause the disorder even at therapeutic plasma concentrations. Magnesium is considered a first-line agent to restore and maintain normal sinus rhythm in TdP. A loading dose is usually given intravenously (IV) followed by IV infusion. The exact mechanism of action of magnesium is unknown.

A–D All of these drugs are in fact contraindicated, as they can trigger TdP in patients at risk.

F, G Verapamil and lidocaine are not effective in TdP.

Learning objective: Describe the electrophysiological actions of amiodarone.

35. **C** The increase in action potential duration is the hallmark of class III drugs. This increase primarily results from blockade of potassium channels.

A The slope of phase 4 is actually decreased by most antiarrhythmic drugs.

B Slope of phase 0 is unaffected by amiodarone because it blocks the inactivated potassium channel only.

D The length of phase 2 depends on calcium channels. Amiodarone has little effect on calcium channels unless high doses are given.

E A condition that increases (i.e., makes less negative) the maximum diastolic potential would increase the automaticity of pacemaker cells; amiodarone does the reverse.

Learning objective: Describe the main drug–drug interactions with of amiodarone.

36. **C** Amiodarone is a potent inhibitor of the cytochrome P-450 enzyme system. Two of the most significant interactions associated with amiodarone are with warfarin and digoxin. The time course of these interactions is prolonged due to the long half-life of amiodarone. Usually dosages of warfarin are reduced by 30 to 50% after amiodarone is instituted. Amiodarone can increase digoxin serum levels, with most studies reporting an approximate doubling of these levels. The exact mechanism of this interaction is unknown and is probably multifactorial.

A, B, D See correct answer explanation.

E Warfarin should be continued for at least 3 weeks after return to sinus rhythm.

Learning objective: Choose the appropriate antiarrhythmic drug for a patient with concomitant diseases.

37. **G** The electrocardiogram is diagnostic for atrial fibrillation (absence of P waves and the "irregularly irregular" ventricular rate).The aim of therapy of atrial fibrillation is to reduce the high ventricular rate to avoid the risks related to tachycardia. This can be achieved by

- Giving drugs that depress conduction and increase refractoriness in the atrioventricular node, so that fewer impulses can reach the ventricle (called "rate control")
- Restoring the normal sinus rhythm (called "rhythm control")

Usually the control of ventricular rate is instituted first, as this control may cause a dramatic diminution of the patient's symptoms. Appropriate drugs are digoxin, β-blockers, and calcium channel blockers. The choice among these agents depends on the concomitant disease.

Restoration of the sinus rhythm can be attempted with

- Electrical cardioversion, which is accomplished with a single strong electric shock that throws the entire heart into refractoriness for a few seconds; a normal sinus rhythm usually follows.
- Pharmacological cardioversion, which can be accomplished with many antiarrhythmic drugs, including flecainide, β-blockers, sotalol, and amiodarone

Today ibutilide seems the therapy of choice.

Both electrical and pharmacological cardioversion can be complicated by systemic embolism. Therefore, therapeutic anticoagulation should be given for at least 3 weeks prior to cardioversion and continued for 4 weeks after cardioversion.

It is important to note that restoration to normal sinus rhythm can be achieved easily (in over 90% of patients after cardioversion) but is difficult to maintain (sinus rhythm remains for 12 months in only 30 to 50%), and using rhythm control rather than rate control in patients with atrial fibrillation does not improve outcomes and increases the risk of torsades de pointes. This explains why many patients can simply be managed with rate control, as in this case. The choice of a calcium channel blocker for this patient is appropriate because

A, E Beta-blockers are contraindicated because the patient is suffering from severe asthma.

B Flecainide can be used for rate control in patients with atrial fibrillation, but it can provoke or exacerbate potentially lethal arrhythmias primarily when the patient has coronary artery disease, as in this case.

C, D Mexiletine and lidocaine are usually not effective in supraventricular arrhythmias.

F Adenosine has a very short half-life and is used to offset attacks of paroxysmal supraventricular tachycardia.

Learning objective: Identify the antiarrhythmic drug with a half-life of about 1 month.

38. **D** Amiodarone is the treatment of choice when antiarrhythmic therapy is chosen to prevent recurrence of ventricular tachycardia or when the tachycardia is accompanied by hemodynamic instability, as in this case. Amiodarone's half-life is extremely long (14 to 53 days) because the drug is very lipid soluble and therefore has a huge volume of distribution (about 4500 L). This very long half-life has two consequences:

    • Adverse effects persist long (4 to 6 weeks) after the discontinuation of the drug.

    • Loading doses are used to accelerate the onset of drug effect.

    A–C, E, F The half-life of these drugs does not exceed 24 hours.

Learning objective: Describe the electrophysiological actions of ibutilide.

39. **C** Blockade of activated K⁺ channels is the distinctive feature of class III antiarrhythmic drugs. The slope of phase 3 of the cardiac action potential is mainly dependent on K⁺ current. The higher the number of K⁺ channels that are in the open state, the higher the K⁺ current and the faster the repolarization phase. By blocking K⁺ channels, the K⁺ current will be less intense, and the repolarization phase will be prolonged, increasing the action potential duration.

A By blocking K^+ channels, ibutilide slows down repolarization; therefore, action potential duration is increased, not decreased.

B Ibutilide has little effect on Na^+ channels (if anything, it seems to activate some Na^+ channels); therefore, the slope of phase 0, which depends on the activation of those channels, is not decreased.

D The effective refractory period depends on the action potential duration; it is therefore increased, not decreased.

E The slope of phase 4 is related to automaticity (the steeper the slope, the higher the automaticity). Most antiarrhythmic drugs decrease the slope of phase 4, unless toxic doses are given.

ANTIARRHYTHMIC DRUGS Answer key			
1. K	6. M	11. B	16. C
2. A	7. A	12. A	17. E
3. B	8. C	13. E	18. F
4. B	9. C	14. D	19. C
5. N	10. D	15. D	20. D
21. E	26. F	31. D	36. C
22. E	27. A	32. E	37. G
23. C	28. B	33. B	38. D
24. E	29. C	34. E	39. C
25. E	30. C	35. C	

Answers and Explanations: IV-6 Antihyperlipidemic Drugs

Questions 1–4

1. **A**
2. **D**
3. **A**
4. **C**

Learning objective: Describe the mechanism of action of HMG-CoA (3-hydroxy-3-methylglutaryl–coenzyme A) reductase inhibitors.

5. **C** HMG-CoA reductase inhibitors inhibit 3-hydroxy-3-methylglutaryl–CoA reductase, which is the enzyme that catalyzes the synthesis of mevalonic acid from 3-hydroxy-3-methylglutaryl–CoA. The formation of mevalonic acid is the rate-limiting step in cholesterol biosynthesis.

A The statin-induced inhibition of cholesterol synthesis in the liver results in an upregulation, not downregulation, of hepatic high-affinity low-density lipoprotein (LDL) receptors, which in turn causes an increased removal of LDL from the blood.

B Statins have no effect on lipoprotein lipase.

D The LDLs removed from the blood fuse together in the liver, forming larger vesicles called endosomes. Because removal of cholesterol from blood is increased by statins, storage of LDL in hepatic endosomes will also be increased, not decreased.

E, F Statins can increase the plasma levels of hepatic aminotransferase and creatine phosphokinase, but this is a sign of potential toxicity, not of therapeutic efficacy of these drugs.

Learning objective: Describe the antihyperlipidemic effects of cholestyramine.

6. **C** Type II hyperlipoproteinemia is characterized by an elevation of low-density lipoprotein (LDL), which may be primary or secondary. Statins are currently used in this disease, but the physician avoided them in this case because the patient is a woman of reproductive age. Bile acid–binding resins increase the intestinal elimination of bile acids. This increased elimination causes an upregulation of hepatic LDL receptors, which in turn reduces the plasma level of LDL.

A, B, D, E These compounds are not consistently affected by bile acid–binding resins.

Learning objective: Describe the main drug interactions with cholestyramine.

7. **D** Cholestyramine is an anion exchange resin that binds bile acids in the intestinal lumen, thus preventing their reabsorption. In fact, the excretion of bile acid is increased up to 10-fold when the resin is given. This in turn causes an enhanced conversion of cholesterol to bile acids in the liver, an increased uptake of low-density lipoprotein (LDL) and intermediate-density lipoprotein from plasma, and an upregulation of high-affinity LDL receptors on cell membranes. Resins can bind many drugs (including β-blockers and thiazides), reducing their intestinal absorption.

    A, B, E, F Cholestyramine does not affect the distribution or the elimination of drugs given concomitantly.

    C Intestinal absorption of propranolol is actually decreased; therefore, the oral bioavailability is decreased, not increased.

Learning objective: Describe the main contraindications of cholestyramine.

8. **B** Cholestyramine can cause severe constipation and is therefore contraindicated in patients with hemorrhoids. In addition, the drug is contraindicated in patients with any coagulation defect because it decreases the intestinal absorption of vitamin K.

    A, C–E See correct answer explanation.

Learning objective: Explain the mechanism of action of gemfibrozil.

9. **D** The prescribed drug was most likely a fibrate. In fact, fibrates are the drugs of first choice when there is a big, isolated increase in triglyceride level. Moreover, in this patient, niacin is contraindicated because of hyperuricemia, resins can cause an increase in triglyceride level, and statins should be avoided in a woman of reproductive age. The mechanism of action of fibrates is still uncertain but most likely involves a gene-mediated increase in lipoprotein lipase synthesis.

    A Fibrates cause lipolysis, not an increase of lipid synthesis.

    B The antihyperlipidemic agents tend to cause an upregulation, not a downregulation, of low-density lipoprotein (LDL) receptors.

    C Statins, not fibrates, inhibit HMG-CoA (3-hydroxy-3-methylglutaryl–coenzyme A) reductase activity in the liver.

    E Fibrates have no effect on absorption of exogenous cholesterol.

Learning objective: Explain the mechanism of action of ezetimibe.

10. **E** Ezetimibe inhibits the absorption of cholesterol by the small intestine, apparently by blocking a specific sterol transporter, Niemann–Pick C1–like 1 (NPC1L1), located in the epithelial cells of intestinal mucosa.

    A–D See correct answer explanation.

Learning objective: Describe the main drug interactions with ezetimibe.

11. **B** Ezetimibe lowers the serum cholesterol concentration by selectively inhibiting the absorption of cholesterol from the small intestine. It has a modest cholesterol-lowering effect when used alone, but the combination with HMG (3-hydroxy-3-methylglutaryl) reductase inhibitors can reduce low-density lipoprotein (LDL) cholesterol levels up to 70%.

    A The risk of statin-induced myopathy is not affected by the concomitant administration of ezetimibe (the risk is, instead, increased by the concomitant administration of fibrates or niacin).

    C, D Ezetimibe does not affect the pharmacokinetics of lovastatin.

    E Ezetimibe does not appreciably increase the high-density lipoprotein (HDL)–raising effect of lovastatin.

Learning objective: Explain the mechanism of action of niacin.

12. **A** Niacin inhibits very-low-density lipoprotein (VLDL) production by hepatocytes, which in turn decreases production of low-density lipoprotein (LDL). The mechanism of this action is still uncertain but seems to involve

    • A decreased synthesis of triglycerides by the liver
    • An inhibition of lipolysis in adipose tissue, which in turn causes a decreased delivery of free fatty acids to the liver
    • A stimulation of lipoprotein lipase activity, which enhances hydrolysis of VLDL and delivery of triglycerides to adipose tissue

    B Niacin actually increases the synthesis of high-density lipoprotein (HDL) by the liver. It also can cause hyperuricemia in about 20% of patients by an unknown mechanism.

    C Niacin causes a substantial reduction of fibrinogen levels, which can be of value in case of atherosclerosis or thrombosis.

    D Niacin actually inhibits lipolysis of triglycerides by hormone-sensitive lipase in adipose tissue.

    E Niacin has negligible effects on exogenous cholesterol absorption.

Learning objective: Describe the site of action of HMG-CoA (3-hydroxy-3-methylglutaryl–coenzyme A) reductase inhibitors.

13. **C** HMG-CoA reductase is located in the liver endoplasmic reticulum, so all HMG-CoA reductase inhibitors such as lovastatin act in the cytoplasmic compartment of liver cells, where the endoplasmic reticulum is located

    A, D Alteplase and heparin act on plasma enzymes.

    B Aspirin inhibits thromboxane synthesis in platelets.

    E Ezetimibe acts on intestinal cell brush border membranes.

    F Metoprolol acts on receptors located in cell membranes.

Learning objective: Describe the main contraindications of niacin.

14. **B** Niacin is relatively contraindicated in patients suffering from gout and hyperuricemia because it tends to increase uric acid levels.

A Cholestyramine could be appropriate in this patient because he has an isolated increase of low-density lipoprotein (LDL).

C, D Statins are effective in all disorders involving elevated levels of LDL.

E Fibrates are useless (reduction of LDL is usually negligible) but not contraindicated in this patient.

Learning objective: Describe the clinically relevant drug interactions with niacin.

15. **C** The cutaneous vasodilation and uncomfortable flushes are adverse effects that most people experience after each dose of niacin. They seem to be primarily prostaglandin-mediated, and therefore an aspirin (or another nonsteroidal antiinflammatory drug) can alleviate the flushing in many patients. Because these effects undergo rapid tolerance, aspirin is needed only during the first days of therapy.

A There is no rationale for the use of warfarin. In fact, niacin can cause a substantial reduction of circulating fibrinogen levels, which actually reduces the risk of thrombosis.

B There is no rationale for the use of atropine. Moreover, the drug would worsen the cholestyramine-induced constipation.

D Prazosin would increase the niacin-induced vasodilation.

E Gemfibrozil is used only in case of hypertriglyceridemia. In this patient, triglyceride levels are normal.

Learning objective: Describe the adverse effects of cholestyramine.

16. **E** The signs and symptoms of the patient indicate that he is suffering from metabolic acidosis most likely due to cholestyramine overdose. A very high dose of cholestyramine can cause metabolic acidosis mainly in patients at risk, as in this patient, who is prone to metabolic acidosis because of diabetes.

Cholestyramine is an anion exchange resin that binds negatively charged bile acids. Chloride is released from binding sites in exchange for bile acids, so chloride anions can be absorbed. When an anion other than bicarbonate is increased in plasma, HCO_3^- must decrease in order to maintain electroneutrality. A reduced plasma bicarbonate concentration is defined as acidosis. Because in this case the acidosis is due to an increase in chloride anion, it is called hyperchloremic.

B Insulin protects diabetic patients from ketoacidosis, so in this case one can suspect that an insufficient insulin dosage and an inappropriate diet were unlikely contributing factors.

A, C, D These drugs do not cause or trigger metabolic acidosis.

Learning objective: Describe the site of action of gemfibrozil.

17. **B** Fibrates bind to and activate a nuclear receptor (the peroxisome proliferator-activated receptor alpha) in hepatocytes, skeletal muscle, and the heart. Activation of this receptor in turn activates transcription of genes that modulate protein expression. The main consequence is the increased expression of lipoprotein lipase.

A, C–F See correct answer explanation.

Learning objective: Describe the adverse effects of HMG-CoA (3-hydroxy-3-methylglutaryl–coenzyme A) reductase inhibitors.

18. **E** The patient was most likely affected by myopathy, a rare but serious adverse effect of statins. The disorder occurs in less than 0.1% of patients when statins are given alone, but it can occur more often when they are given together with niacin or fibrates (up to 5% when given with gemfibrozil). Myopathy can cause rhabdomyolysis with myoglobinuria, as in this case.

A–D These drugs do not cause myopathy.

Learning objective: Describe the antihyperlipidemic effects of niacin.

19. **D** Low high-density lipoprotein (HDL) level is a predictor of increased coronary artery disease (CAD), independent of all other risk factors. Therefore, it is important to raise HDL, even if the other lipid fractions are normal, especially if the patient has other risk factors for CAD, as in this case. The main factors that are correlated with low HDL are cigarette smoking, obesity, androgenic or related steroids, hypertriglyceridemia, and genetic factors. Some lipid-lowering drugs can raise HDL even if other lipid parameters are in the normal range, as in this case. Niacin (by an unknown mechanism) has the greatest ability to raise HDL, up to 30%, and is therefore the drug of choice in disorders associated with extremely low serum levels of HDL (these patients tend to have premature atherosclerosis, and the low HDL level may be the only identified risk factor).

A Gemfibrozil can raise HDL up to 10%.

B Statins can raise HDL up to 10%

C, E Resins and ezetimibe have little effect on HDL.

Learning objective: Describe the main site of action of cholestyramine.

20. **B** Cholestyramine is an acid-binding resin. These drugs act by binding bile acids and similar steroids in the small intestine, thus preventing reabsorption of bile acids secreted by the liver. In this way, they increase the need of cholesterol by the liver, which in turn induces an upregulation of liver low-density lipoprotein (LDL) receptors.

A, C–E See correct answer explanation.

Learning objective: Identify the patient population that can benefit most from antihyperlipidemic drugs.

21. **B** It is well known that there is a direct relationship between the total and low-density lipoprotein (LDL) cholesterol in blood and the risk of coronary heart disease (CHD). It is also well known that the risk of CHD increases with age and that women have a very low risk of CHD during premenopausal years, but that after menopause, the rate of developing CHD parallels that of men. Therefore, men tend to develop CHD in their 50s and 60s, whereas women tend develop it in their 60s and 70s. This explains why the antihyperlipidemic drugs are mostly beneficial for middle-aged men and least beneficial for women during premenopausal years.

    A, C–E See correct answer explanation.

Learning objective: Outline the therapeutic uses of HMG-CoA (3-hydroxy-3-methylglutaryl–coenzyme A) reductase inhibitors.

22. **C** The signs and symptoms of the patient indicate that she was most likely suffering from a transient ischemic attack, a brief episode of neurologic disturbance caused by a reduced blood supply to an area of the brain. Aspirin is the drug most frequently used to decrease the risk of stroke in these patients, but it has been consistently shown that statins can also reduce this risk.

    E Fibrinolytic drugs are first-line agents for the acute therapy of stroke but not for the chronic prophylactic treatment.

    A, B, D, F See correct answer explanation.

Learning objective: Describe the adverse effects of HMG-CoA (3-hydroxy-3-methylglutaryl–coenzyme A) reductase inhibitors.

23. **E** Creatine kinase is an enzyme found in high concentration in heart and skeletal muscle. Because this enzyme exists in relatively few organs, its serum concentration is used as a specific index of injury of myocardium or skeletal muscle. In fact, creatine kinase levels can prove helpful in recognizing muscular dystrophy before clinical signs appear.

    A This enzyme mediates the first step in cholesterol biosynthesis.

    B Aminotransferase (alanine and aspartate aminotransferase) levels are measured primarily to diagnose liver disease.

    C Alkaline phosphatase is an enzyme originating mainly in the bone and liver, with some activity in the kidney and intestine. The enzyme is measured primarily as an index of bone or liver disease.

    D This enzyme mediates the synthesis of eicosanoids.

Learning objective: Explain the mechanism of action of cholestyramine.

24. **A** Cholestyramine is a bile acid–binding resin. Drugs of this class are highly positively charged (cholestyramine is a quaternary amine) and bind negatively charged bile acids in exchange with Cl⁻. Because of their large size, resins are not absorbed, and the bound bile acids are excreted in the stool. In this way, enterohepatic circulation of bile acids is prevented (normally, more than 95% of bile acids are reabsorbed; their excretion is increased up to 10-fold when the resins are given).

    B–E None of these drugs affect bile acid elimination.

Learning objective: Choose the appropriate antihyperlipidemic drug for a patient with concomitant disease.

25. **C** Currently, statins represent the most effective and best tolerated agents for treating dyslipidemia. They are effective in all types of dyslipidemia, and when given as a single agent, they may decrease low-density lipoprotein (LDL) cholesterol up to 60% and total cholesterol up to 45%. Therefore, they are the drugs of first choice for treatment of elevated LDL cholesterol. Higher doses can also reduce triglyceride levels up to 35%. Moreover, in this patient

    A Niacin should be avoided because of diabetes and peptic ulcer.

    B Cholestyramine is relatively contraindicated because it could impair the absorption of the other currently used drugs.

    D Unlike niacin, nicotinamide is devoid of antihyperlipidemic properties.

    E Fibrates such as gemfibrozil are the drugs of choice for treating type III hyperlipidemia (familial dysbetalipoproteinemia), as well as high triglyceride levels. They do not significantly decrease LDL.

Learning objective: Describe the adverse effects of HMG-CoA (3-hydroxy-3-methylglutaryl–coenzyme A) reductase inhibitors.

26. **B** Statins are often prescribed after a myocardial infarction to prevent reinfarction. Statins cause an increase in liver enzymes in about 2% of patients. Abnormal enzyme values usually resolve with cessation of treatment, but the drug should be discontinued when the aminotransferase activity is persistently elevated to more than 3 times the normal limits because of the risk of hepatotoxicity.

    A, C–E These drugs do not cause an increase in liver enzymes.

Learning objective: Outline the therapeutic uses of antihyperlipidemic drug combinations.

27. **A** The five major classes of antihyperlipidemic drugs can be given in combination when

   - Low-density lipoprotein (LDL) and very-low-density lipoprotein (VLDL) are both elevated.
   - LDL or VLDL is not normalized with a single agent.
   - Pronounced high-density lipoprotein (HDL) deficiency coexists with other hyperlipidemias.

Statins work with resins in a highly synergistic manner, decreasing total cholesterol by up to 65%. Moreover, in this patient

B, C Niacin should be avoided because it can cause hyperglycemia in diabetics by increasing insulin resistance.

D, E Fibrates cause only a modest reduction in total cholesterol, and the combinations with other antihyperlipidemic drugs are used only in patients with combined hyperlipidemia.

Learning objective: Outline the therapeutic uses of antihyperlipidemic drugs.

28. **C** All of the patients except patient 5 should start a lipid-lowering drug therapy, as they still have an abnormal lipid profile after 4 months of diet. Patient 3, however, is the one who needs the drug therapy the most, because he has three risk factors: high triglycerides, high low-density lipoprotein (LDL), and low high-density lipoprotein (HDL) levels.

A Patient 1 has high triglycerides, normal LDL cholesterol levels, and low HDL cholesterol levels (two risk factors).

B Patient 2 has normal triglycerides and normal LDL cholesterol levels but low HDL cholesterol levels (one risk factor).

D Patient 4 has marginally high triglycerides and high LDL cholesterol levels but very high HDL cholesterol levels (an HDL > 60 mg/dL represents a negative risk factor).

Learning objective: Outline the therapeutic uses of antihyperlipidemic drug combinations.

29. **C** The patient's acute renal failure was most likely due to rhabdomyolysis, which is a consequence of myopathy, a rare but serious adverse effect of statins. The excessive release of myoglobin from the damaged muscle can explain the red and clear urine and the acute renal failure, most likely due to precipitation of myoglobin into renal tubules with secondary tubular obstruction. The incidence of myopathy is low (< 0.1%) when a statin is given alone but is much increased (up to 5%) in patients who concomitantly receive fibrates. In this case, the patient most likely received a combined therapy

with lovastatin and gemfibrozil, as both cholesterol and triglycerides were elevated.

A, B Cholestyramine does not increase the risk of rhabdomyolysis when taken with other antihyperlipidemic drugs.

D As stated above, statins alone have a low risk of myopathy.

E Niacin alone does not cause myopathy.

Learning objective: Describe the mechanism of action of antihyperlipidemic drugs.

30. **D** The increased bile acid excretion caused by anion exchange resins leads to an upregulation of hepatic low-density lipoprotein (LDL) receptors, which in turn increases the extraction of cholesterol from plasma. In the same way, the inhibition of cholesterol synthesis by statins causes an upregulation of hepatic LDL receptors.

A The intestinal reabsorption of bile acids is decreased by cholestyramine, but statins can cause a compensatory increase in cholesterol absorption.

B The conversion of cholesterol to bile acids is actually increased by cholestyramine.

C The synthesis of endogenous cholesterol by the liver is decreased by statins, but cholestyramine can cause a compensatory increase of cholesterol synthesis.

E Statins decrease triglyceride production, but the resin-induced increase in bile acid production can be accompanied by an increase in hepatic triglyceride synthesis.

ANTIHYPERLIPIDEMIC DRUGS Answer key		
1. A	6. C	11. B
2. D	7. D	12. A
3. A	8. B	13. C
4. C	9. D	14. B
5. C	10. E	15. C
16. E	21. B	26. B
17. B	22. C	27. A
18. E	23. E	28. C
19. D	24. A	29. C
20. B	25. C	30. D

Answers and Explanations: IV-7 Drugs Affecting Hemostasis

Questions 1–4

1. **A**
2. **F**
3. **C**
4. **B**

Learning objective: Explain the mechanism of actions of clopidogrel.

5. **D** Clopidogrel is an antiplatelet drug that causes an irreversible inhibition of adenosine diphosphate (ADP) receptors, thereby inhibiting ADP-mediated platelet aggregation. The drug is used to prevent recurrence of ischemic stroke mainly in people who are at risk of aspirin hypersensitivity, such as the asthmatic patient in this case.

A–C, E, F None of these drugs block platelet ADP receptors.

Learning objective: Explain the molecular mechanism of action of heparin.

6. **E** The activity of antithrombin III inhibits clotting factor proteases by forming equimolar stable complexes with them. Heparin strongly accelerates this reaction, which is the basis of its anticoagulant activity.

    A–D These drugs do not affect the binding between antithrombin III and clotting factor proteases.

Learning objective: Describe the main adverse effects of warfarin.

7. **D** The primary approach to prevent valvular thrombosis and systemic thromboembolism associated with mechanical prosthetic valve replacement is long-term anticoagulation with warfarin. Most likely, the dose of warfarin was too high, so bleeding occurred, as pointed out by the signs and symptoms of the patient.

    A Fibrinolytic drugs such as streptokinase are not indicated for long-term prevention of thrombosis.

    B Aspirin is sometimes used together with warfarin in treating patients with prosthetic valves, mainly when evidence of thromboembolism exists despite adequate anticoagulation. However, it is not effective for prevention when given alone.

    C, F The question specifies oral anticoagulant therapy. Heparin and bivalirudin must be given parenterally and therefore are not suited for long-term anticoagulation.

    E Aminocaproic acid is an antiplasmin drug and therefore would be contraindicated in this setting.

Learning objective: Describe the main contraindications for fibrinolytic drugs.

8. **B** The patient's signs and symptoms suggest that she was most likely suffering from acute pericarditis. In the current era of thrombolytic therapy for acute coronary occlusion, the distinction between myocardial infarction (MI) and acute pericarditis is crucial. If pericarditis is misdiagnosed as MI, thrombolytic drugs may cause pericardial hemorrhage and cardiac tamponade. Usually pericardial pain can be distinguished from ischemic coronary pain because the latter is not aggravated by chest motion. When present, a precordial friction rub is diagnostic, as in this case. Pericarditis may be caused by inflammation, trauma, or neoplasm. Sometimes it accompanies systemic diseases, as in this case. Most often, however, the etiology of acute pericarditis cannot be identified and is referred to as idiopathic.

    A, C Antiinflammatory drugs are used to relieve inflammation and pain of acute pericarditis.

    D If pain does not subside with antiinflammatory drugs, opioids can be used.

    E Antibiotics are employed when pericarditis is due to bacterial infection (most commonly tuberculosis).

Learning objective: Choose the appropriate therapy for a patient suffering from severe warfarin overdose.

9. **E** The symptoms of the patient strongly suggest a hemorrhagic complication of warfarin therapy. The standard treatment of warfarin overdose would be vitamin K, but the patient is diaphoretic and hypotensive, suggesting that bleeding is life-threatening. In this case, the action of vitamin K is too slow to be useful (onset is delayed for 6 hours and is complete by 24 hours). Fresh frozen plasma (which contains prothrombin and factors VII, IX, and X) or activated clotting factors should be administered in case of severe acute bleeding due to anticoagulant therapy.

    A See correct answer explanation.

    B–D These drug are either useless or dangerous in bleeding disorders.

Learning objective: Explain the mechanism of coagulant action of desmopressin.

10. **A** Vasopressin and desmopressin increase plasma levels of factor VIII and von Willebrand factor, presumably by V_2 receptor-mediated release from storage sites in vascular endothelium. Because of this, desmopressin is sometimes used after minor trauma or before elective dental surgery in patients with mild hemophilia A who have demonstrated responsiveness.

    B–E Desmopressin does not have these effects.

Learning objective: Explain the mechanism of action of dabigatran.

11. **C** Dabigatran is a new oral anticoagulant that acts by binding reversibly to thrombin, thus blocking thrombin activity. Unlike warfarin, this direct thrombin inhibitor has a rapid onset of action, does not interact with P-450-interacting drugs, and gives a predictable anticoagulant response, making routine anticoagulant monitoring unnecessary.

    A, B, D, E See correct answer explanation.

Learning objective: Describe the clinically important drug interactions of warfarin.

12. **B** Macrolide antibiotics can inhibit warfarin metabolism, resulting in increased plasma levels of the drug. This interaction is well established, and prolongation of prothrombin time may occur even with small doses of erythromycin.

    A Erythromycin does not inhibit the synthesis of clotting factors.

    C Warfarin can cause local thrombosis that seems related to the inhibition of anticoagulant protein C, but this adverse effect is rare and usually occurs during the first day of warfarin therapy when the anticoagulant effect is not yet operative.

D Erythromycin has no effect on the intestinal absorption of vitamin k.

E Warfarin does not affect production of vitamin K by intestinal flora.

Learning objective: Describe the therapeutic uses of abciximab.

13. **F** Various anticoagulation regimens are always performed before, during, and after angioplasty to reduce the incidence of thrombosis. Heparin (not listed) and abciximab are the two drugs given intravenously for this purpose.

A, B Warfarin and clopidogrel are not given intravenously. They are usually started some time before the intervention and continued for months after it.

C–E The use of protamine, aminocaproic acid, and recombinant factor VIIa during coronary angioplasty would be irrational.

Learning objective: Describe the main adverse effects of heparin.

14. **C** The lab results indicate that the patient was most likely suffering heparin-induced thrombocytopenia (HIT). The disorder can be asymptomatic (type I) or associated with peripheral vascular occlusion, which can cause stroke, myocardial infarction, tissue gangrene, or even death (type II). In fact, the mortality rate of type II HIT can be as high as 40%. HIT occurs in about 1 to 5% of patients receiving unfractionated heparin. The pathogenesis of HIT is still uncertain, but it appears that heparin-dependent immunoglobulin G (IgG) antibodies activate platelets that aggregate intravascularly. Consequently, platelet-fibrin thrombi may form, leading to vascular occlusion.

A, B, D, E The risk of thrombocytopenia with all of the other listed drugs is either low (aspirin) or negligible.

Learning objective: Describe the clinically important drug interactions of warfarin.

15. **C** Cimetidine is a potent inhibitor of the cytochrome P-450 system and can thereby increase the plasma level of several drugs, including warfarin. Blood in urine is often the first sign of bleeding from anticoagulant therapy.

A Warfarin is almost completely metabolized by the liver, so its renal clearance is negligible.

B, D, E Cimetidine has no effect on the intestinal absorption of vitamin K, on blood coagulation, or on binding of warfarin to plasma proteins.

Learning objective: List the exams that should be done frequently during heparin treatment.

16. **B** Because heparin-induced thrombocytopenia (HIT) is a serious adverse effect of heparin, a platelet count should be performed weekly during heparin treatment. Any thrombocytopenia appearing during treatment should be considered suspicious for HIT.

A, C, D These exams are not needed during heparin treatment.

E Bleeding time is normal in the presence of coagulation disorders other than thrombocytopenia or von Willebrand disease. It can be increased in case of HIT, but the platelet count is a much more reliable test.

F This test evaluates fibrinolytic activity. Heparin does not alter fibrinolysis.

Learning objective: Describe the therapeutic uses of aspirin and heparin in unstable angina.

17. **C** The patient was most likely suffering from unstable angina (see the symptoms and the electrocardiogram). Unstable angina is a medical emergency to be treated in a cardiac care unit. The immediate challenge is relief of pain and control of all ischemic episodes. Pain relief is usually accomplished with intravenous infusion of nitroglycerin, which has the advantage of fast onset of action and rapid reversibility. Opioids should be used to control pain only when it is not adequately relieved by anti-ischemic medication. To reduce intracoronary clotting, oral aspirin and intravenous heparin should be instituted immediately (these drugs have been shown to reduce the incidence of subsequent myocardial infarction).

A, D, E, F Each of these combinations has at least one drug that is useless (warfarin and desmopressin) or contraindicated (aminocaproic acid).

B Alteplase is a fibrinolytic drug. These drugs can be used to break down thrombi but not to prevent thrombus formation. Therefore, they are not useful (and may be harmful) in unstable angina. Warfarin is not used for emergency anticoagulation because of its delayed onset of action.

Learning objective: Describe the main advantages of low-molecular-weight heparins (LMWHs) over standard heparin.

18. **C** High-molecular-weight heparin (HMWH) causes transient thrombocytopenia in up to 15% of patients and severe thrombocytopenia (which is antibody-mediated) in up to 5% of patients. Enoxaparin is low-molecular-weight heparin (LMWH). LMWH-induced thrombocytopenia is seen in less than 1% of patients.

A LMWHs cause a lower incidence of bleeding complications, which could be related to the fact that these agents preferentially inhibit factor Xa more potently than they inhibit thrombin (thrombin inhibition requires a larger heparin molecule). Nevertheless, bleeding complications do occur even with LMWH.

B The oral bioavailability of both HMW and LMW heparins is zero.

D, E LMWHs do not have antiplatelet activity, and they actually inhibit fewer coagulation factors than standard heparin.

Learning objective: Describe the therapeutic uses of heparin.

19. **E** The sudden dyspnea, hypotension, and pleuritic chest pain, particularly in a high-risk setting (gastric cancer), would suggest the diagnosis of massive pulmonary embolism, which is confirmed by the computed tomography scan. Heparin is a drug of choice to prevent further thrombus formation and embolization.

    A Nitroglycerin is used only if chest pain is due to coronary disease; moreover, it is contraindicated in this case because of hypotension.

    B, F Aspirin and clopidogrel have been tried to prevent (not to treat) thromboembolism, but results are inconclusive or frankly negative. Moreover, they are not given parenterally.

    C The systemic hypotension and extreme hypoxemia warrant consideration of thrombolytic therapy. However, recent surgery (as in this case) is a major contraindication for fibrinolytic drugs.

    D Warfarin is not used for the acute treatment of pulmonary embolism because of its slow onset of action.

Learning objective: Explain the main reasons for heparin resistance.

20. **A** The lack of action of heparin in this case was most likely due to heparin resistance. Heparin can bind to different plasma proteins, including platelet factor 4, fibrinogen, and factor VIII. As many heparin-binding proteins are acute-phase reactants, the phenomenon of heparin resistance is often encountered in acutely ill patients or in patients with malignancy, as in this case.

    B Vitamin K does not affect the anticoagulant action of heparin.

    C The half-life of heparin is dose-dependent and is 30 to 150 minutes at therapeutic doses.

    D Heparin is effective immediately after intravenous injection or delayed 20 to 60 minutes after subcutaneous injection.

    E Heparin resistance can occur with very low, not high, levels of antithrombin III. This deficiency is a rare hereditary disorder that generally comes to light when the patient suffers recurrent venous thrombosis.

Learning objective: Describe the therapeutic uses of alteplase in ischemic stroke.

21. **C** The signs and symptoms of the patient suggest that he is most likely suffering from an ischemic stroke due to the occlusion of a cerebral artery. The guidelines of the American Stroke Association indicate that alteplase, administered within 3 hours of onset, can reduce the ultimate disability caused by the ischemic stroke.

    A, B These drugs can increase blood coagulability (desmopressin) or inhibit fibrinolysis (aminocaproic acid) and are therefore contraindicated in ischemic stroke.

    D, E, F No studies have clearly demonstrated that emergency treatment with anticoagulants is useful in mitigating the neurologic effects of a stroke. However, the use of a full dose of unfractionated heparin remains controversial despite years of debate and lack of evidence supporting its use.

Learning objective: Choose the appropriate drugs for a patient with deep venous thrombosis.

22. **C** The standard therapy for uncomplicated deep venous thrombosis (DVT) is an intravenous injection of unfractionated heparin followed by a short course (4 or 5 days) of subcutaneous heparin. Warfarin is started the first or second day of heparin therapy and continued for months.

    A, B Abciximab is not used for thrombosis prophylaxis.

    D–F The use of alteplase in an uncomplicated DVT is not recommended because of the potential adverse effects of fibrinolytic drugs (i.e., the induction of a lytic state). Although some studies have suggested that fibrinolytic therapy is more effective than anticoagulant therapy in DVT, fibrinolytic therapy is usually considered only when thrombosis is massive and/or complicated by hypotension or shock.

Learning objective: Describe the most serious adverse effect of alteplase.

23. **D** The standard therapy of myocardial infarction (MI) includes an intravenous thrombolytic drug (alteplase, reteplase, etc.), which is most effective in the first few hours after onset. Bleeding (most common in cerebral vessels) is the most frequent adverse effect of these drugs.

    A Aspirin, if not contraindicated, is given at presentation and daily indefinitely thereafter. Its antiplatelet effect reduces short- and long-term mortality. Bleeding, however, is not as common as with thrombolytic drugs.

    B Beta-blockers, if not contraindicated, are given within the first few hours after onset because they reduce recurrence rate and mortality. Bleeding is not an adverse effect of this drug class.

    C Nitroglycerin is recommended for the first 24 to 48 hours in patients with MI and heart failure or hypertension. Bleeding is not an adverse effect of nitrates.

    E Warfarin is not currently used in MI.

Learning objective: Explain why the onset of anticoagulant effect of warfarin is delayed.

24. **C** Warfarin has no effect on the activity of already formed clotting factors II, VII, IX, and X in the circulation. Because warfarin inhibits the synthesis of new clotting factors but not the metabolism of the already formed clotting factors, its effect depends on the time taken for the degradation of these factors, or their half-lives. Additionally, because thrombin (i.e., factor II) has the longest half-life (about 60 hours), its half-life is the main determinant of the onset of action of warfarin.

    A, B, D, E These options are unlikely.

Learning objective: Describe the therapeutic uses of anticoagulant and fibrinolytic drugs in myocardial infarction.

25. **A** All patients with myocardial infarction (MI) who seek medical care within the first 12 hours after symptom onset should be considered for urgent reperfusion of the infarct-related artery, but the earlier therapy is begun, the greater the benefit. The definitive therapies for reperfusion are fibrinolysis or percutaneous coronary intervention (PCI). The fibrinolytic drugs most often used are tissue plasminogen activators (e.g., alteplase), as it has been shown that they are "fibrin-specific"; that is, they preferentially activate plasminogen bound to fibrin. Tissue plasminogen activators clearly open coronary arteries more rapidly than nonspecific activators. Heparin should be administered to all patients with acute MI, unless a contraindication exists. Heparin given with alteplase improves the rapidity with which patency is induced and is essential for maintaining the patency, thus avoiding reocclusion, which is a problem with fibrinolytic therapy.

    B Warfarin is not an emergency anticoagulant because its onset of action is slow.

    C Inotropic drugs are administered only when cardiogenic shock is present.

    E Clopidogrel can be administered as an adjunctive therapy, but it is not given intravenously.

    D, F See correct answer explanation.

Learning objective: Describe the clinically important drug interactions of warfarin.

26. **D** Thyroid hormones increase the catabolism of many endogenous compounds, including clotting factors. This action results in a decreased coagulability of blood, so the effects of anticoagulants are enhanced. In this case, the woman's initial warfarin dose was appropriate to provide a safe level of anticoagulation therapy for her hypothyroid state, but when her thyroid level was raised to normal, the warfarin dose needed to be adjusted to adapt to the increased catabolic rate of clotting factors that would occur in the presence of higher thyroxine levels. Monitoring must be carried out to reestablish the appropriate new, lower dose of warfarin.

    A, B Warfarin has no effect on the pharmacokinetics of thyroid hormones.

    C, E Thyroid hormones have negligible effects on the absorption or metabolism of warfarin.

Learning objective: Explain the molecular mechanism of action of warfarin.

27. **B** Vitamin K is an essential cofactor for converting precursor proteins into the active coagulation factors in the liver. Vitamin K quinone is the active form. Oxidation of this quinone to vitamin K epoxide is coupled with activation of coagulation factors II, VII, IX, and X, as well as the anticoagulant factors proteins C and S. Epoxide is then reconverted to quinone, and warfarin blocks this reductive conversion.

    A This is actually the mechanism of action of heparin.

    C Warfarin does not affect clotting factor metabolism.

    D Warfarin actually blocks the activation of anticoagulant factors proteins C and S.

    E Vitamin K is not synthesized in the liver but is stored there initially, after intestinal absorption.

Learning objective: Choose the appropriate anticoagulant for a patient with atrial fibrillation.

28. **D** Chronic anticoagulant therapy is always given before cardioversion in order to prevent thromboembolism. In fact, one of the most feared consequences of atrial fibrillation is the development of atrial thrombi, with subsequent embolization. This is most likely to occur once the normal sinus rhythm is restored, due to the more effective contraction of the atria.

    A Heparin is not appropriate for long-term therapies, as it must be given parenterally.

    B Streptokinase is a thrombolytic drug and therefore not used to prevent thrombus formation.

    C Although aspirin is sometimes used as an alternative to warfarin in this setting, studies to determine its efficacy have yielded inconsistent results. Moreover, the antiplatelet dose should be a low dose, not a high dose.

    E Abciximab is a monoclonal antibody that binds noncompetitively to glycoprotein IIb/IIIa receptor complex, which regulates the final step in platelet aggregation. Its therapeutic uses are limited to percutaneous coronary intervention and unstable angina.

Learning objective: Explain the molecular mechanism of action of abciximab.

29. **A** Abciximab is a humanized monoclonal antibody directed against the IIb/IIIa receptor complex. This complex functions as a receptor mainly for fibrinogen but also for von Willebrand factor and can be activated (directly or indirectly) by most of the other mentioned molecules, including adenosine diphosphate (ADP), thrombin, collagen, and thromboxane A_2. The binding of fibrinogen to the IIb/IIIa receptor results in cross-linking between platelets and is the final common pathway in platelet aggregation. By blocking the platelet glycoprotein IIb/IIIa receptor complex, these drugs prevent platelet aggregation induced by any aggregating substance.

   B, F These steps are inhibited by heparin.

   C This step is inhibited by aspirin.

   D This step is inhibited by warfarin.

   E This step is inhibited by clopidogrel.

Learning objective: Explain the mechanism of antithrombotic action of aspirin.

30. **E** Aspirin inhibits the synthesis of thromboxane A_2 (TXA_2) through the irreversible acetylation of cyclooxygenase I. TXA_2 is a potent platelet aggregator and is released from platelets during aggregation. Because platelets do not synthesize new proteins, the action of aspirin on platelet cyclooxygenase is permanent, lasting for the life of the platelet (4 to 10 days). Complete inactivation of the enzyme is achieved with doses of 160 to 300 mg per day. Higher doses do not improve efficacy and are potentially less effective for the following reason: cyclooxygenase blockade reduces both the platelet-mediated production of TXA_2, which promotes aggregation, and the endothelial cell–mediated production of prostaglandin I_2, or prostacyclin (PGI_2), which inhibits aggregation. However, endothelial cells produce new cyclooxygenase in a matter of hours, whereas platelets cannot manufacture the enzyme. With low doses, then, only prolonged inhibition of TXA_2 synthesis occurs. If the dose of aspirin is increased, prostacyclin synthesis can be inhibited for a longer time, thus counteracting the effects of TXA_2 synthesis inhibition.

   A F See correct answer explanation.

   B Aspirin does not inhibit the lipoxygenase pathway.

   C This is the mechanism of action of clopidogrel.

   D This would cause, not inhibit, platelet aggregation.

DRUGS AFFECTING HEMOSTASIS Answer key					
1.	A	6.	E	11.	C
2.	F	7.	D	12.	B
3.	C	8.	B	13.	F
4.	B	9.	E	14.	C
5.	D	10.	A	15.	C
16.	B	21.	C	26.	D
17.	C	22.	C	27.	B
18.	C	23.	D	28.	D
19.	E	24.	C	29.	A
20.	A	25.	A	30.	E

V Endocrine System

Questions: V-1 Drugs for Hypothalamic and Pituitary Disorders

Directions for questions **1–6**

Match each endocrine drug with the appropriate description (each lettered option can be selected once, more than once, or not at all).

- **A.** Cabergoline
- **B.** Chorionic gonadotropin
- **C.** Cosyntropin
- **D.** Desmopressin
- **E.** Degarelix
- **F.** Follitropin alfa
- **G.** Leuprolide
- **H.** Octreotide
- **I.** Oxytocin
- **J.** Pegvisomant
- **K.** Somatropin

Difficulty level: Easy

1. An adrenocorticotropic hormone (ACTH) analogue

Difficulty level: Easy

2. A recombinant follicle-stimulating hormone (FSH) analogue

Difficulty level: Easy

3. A somatropin receptor antagonist

Difficulty level: Easy

4. A somatostatin analogue

Difficulty level: Easy

5. A gonadotropin-releasing hormone (GnRH) analogue

Difficulty level: Easy

6. A drug with luteinizing hormone (LH) activity

Difficulty level: Easy

7. A 27-year-old primipara woman was admitted to the obstetrical unit for labor induction because of a postdate pregnancy. An intravenous infusion of oxytocin was started. Activation of which of the following signaling pathways most likely mediates the therapeutic efficacy of this drug?

- **A.** Cyclic adenosine monophosphate (cAMP) synthesis
- **B.** Phosphoinositide hydrolysis
- **C.** Cyclic guanosine monophosphate (cGMP) synthesis
- **D.** Tyrosine residue phosphorylation
- **E.** Gene transcription

Difficulty level: Easy

8. A 37-year-old man recently diagnosed with acromegaly started a treatment with octreotide. Which of the following cells most likely represent the main site of action of the drug in this patient?

- **A.** Supraoptic neurons
- **B.** Pituitary somatotrophs
- **C.** Pituitary thyrotrophs
- **D.** Paraventricular neurons
- **E.** Ventromedial neurons

Difficulty level: Medium

9. A 33-year-old woman who had been unable to conceive a baby for 3 years started a controlled ovarian hyperstimulation treatment for in vitro fertilization. Which of the following drugs was most likely administered daily to suppress the luteinizing hormone surge that could prematurely trigger ovulation?

- **A.** Testosterone
- **B.** Octreotide
- **C.** Leuprolide
- **D.** Cosyntropin
- **E.** Somatropin

Difficulty level: Easy

10. A 34-year-old woman complained to her gynecologist of severe pelvic pain during both menstrual and nonmenstrual days. The woman, diagnosed with endometriosis 1 year earlier, had good pain relief after surgical ablation of endometriotic lesions, but her symptoms had returned. Her gynecologist prescribed a cycle of therapy with leuprolide. Which of the following adverse effects would be expected to occur during the therapy?

- **A.** Galactorrhea
- **B.** Vaginal infections
- **C.** Menorrhagia
- **D.** Hot flushes
- **E.** Venous thrombosis

11. A 54-year-old woman complained to her physician of an uncomfortable flushing for the past few days. Further exams led to the diagnosis of carcinoid syndrome due to primary carcinoid tumor of the lung, and the patient was scheduled for surgery. Which of the following drugs would be appropriate to control the patient's symptoms and to prevent a surgery-induced carcinoid crisis?

   A. Somatropin
   B. Leuprolide
   C. Desmopressin
   D. Octreotide
   E. Prolactin

12. A 64-year-old woman was found to have high serum levels of insulin-like growth factor 1 (IGF-1) during a regular clinic visit. Her medical history was significant for atrial fibrillation presently controlled with a pacemaker and for a pituitary adenoma diagnosed 8 months ago. Because radiation therapy was contraindicated, the patient had been receiving octreotide since then. Which of the following drugs would be appropriate to add to the patient's therapy at this time?

   A. Cosyntropin
   B. Mecasermin
   C. Leuprolide
   D. Cabergoline
   E. Degarelix

13. A 52-year-old woman presented to the hospital with a 3-week history of fatigue, cold intolerance, and constipation. Physical examination showed a patient with coarse, dry, scaly skin, eyelid drop, a puffy face, and a large tongue. Pertinent serum values on admission were free thyroxine (FT_4) 0.2 ng/dL (normal 0.4–2 ng/dL), thyroid-stimulating hormone (TSH) 0.3 μIU/mL (normal 0.5–4.7). An intravenous injection of thyrotropin-releasing hormone (TRH) was given to better clarify the diagnosis. Serum TSH levels measured soon after the injection showed a significant increase in TSH. Which of the following was most likely the cause of the patient's syndrome?

   A. Hashimoto thyroiditis
   B. Hypothalamic dysfunction
   C. Papillary thyroid carcinoma
   D. Graves disease
   E. Pituitary dysfunction

14. A 45-year-old woman was seen at the clinic because of episodic weakness, paresthesias, and constipation for the past week. Vital signs were blood pressure 100/55 mm Hg, pulse 95 bpm, respirations 16/min. Physical examination revealed increased pigmentation, especially on skinfolds and extensor surfaces. Bluish black discoloration of the areolae and mucous membranes was also noted. Significant serum levels on admission were Na$^+$ 122 mEq/L (normal 136–145 mEq/L), K$^+$ 6.2 mEq/L (normal 3.5–5.5 mEq/L), fasting glucose 58 mg/dL (normal 70–110 mg/dL), blood urea nitrogen (BUN) 34 mg/dL (normal 7–18 mg/dL). The serum level of a hormone was measured before and after the intravenous injection of a test drug to confirm the diagnosis. Which of the following test drugs was most likely administered?

   A. Somatropin
   B. Mecasermin
   C. Adrenocorticotropic hormone (ACTH)
   D. Octreotide
   E. Leuprolide
   F. Somatostatin

15. A 50-year-old man was admitted to the hospital because of two episodes of hematochezia and hematemesis of dark red blood over a 7-hour period. Past history of the patient was significant for alcoholism for 12 years. Physical examination showed a somnolent but easily arousable man with subicteric skin. The abdomen was mildly distended with a 10-cm liver span. Small fluid waves were present. An esophagoscopy was ordered, and a drug was given by continuous infusion after an intravenous loading dose. Which of the following drugs was most likely administered?

   A. Adrenaline
   B. Albuterol
   C. Nifedipine
   D. Prazosin
   E. Vasopressin

16. A 37-year-old woman recently diagnosed with pituitary adenoma underwent ablative radiation therapy, but the treatment failed to control the patient's symptoms. Lab tests still showed a high level of insulin-like growth factor 1. A pharmacotherapy with octreotide was prescribed. Which of the following actions most likely mediated the therapeutic effect of the drug in the patient's disorder?

   A. Stimulation of growth hormone metabolism
   B. Inhibition of growth hormone release
   C. Inhibition of insulin release
   D. Blockade of growth hormone receptors
   E. Blockade of thyroid-stimulating hormone (TSH) receptors

Difficulty level: Easy

17. A 41-year-old man was found to have growth hormone deficiency after irradiation of the hypophysis to treat a parasellar tumor. Therapy with somatropin was started. Which of the following adverse effects is most likely to occur in this patient?

- **A.** Arthralgias
- **B.** Hypoglycemia
- **C.** Weigh loss
- **D.** Osteoporosis
- **E.** Dehydration

Difficulty level: Medium

18. A 26-year-old man wishing to start a family was diagnosed with infertility due to oligospermia. He started a treatment that included intramuscular injection of human chorionic gonadotropin three times weekly. Which of the following molecular actions is the intended target for this therapy?

- **A.** Stimulation of Leydig cell testosterone production
- **B.** Activation of testosterone receptors in the hypothalamus
- **C.** Inhibition of growth hormone–releasing hormone (GnRH) secretion from the hypothalamus
- **D.** Stimulation of secretion of prostatic fluid
- **E.** Stimulation of mitotic activity of Sertoli cells

Difficulty level: Easy

19. A 62-year-old man diagnosed with metastasized prostate cancer started a treatment that included a depot preparation of goserelin. Which of the following actions most likely mediated the therapeutic effect of the drug in the patient's disease?

- **A.** Inhibition of aromatase enzyme
- **B.** Inhibition of follicle-stimulating hormone (FSH) and luteinizing hormone (LH) release
- **C.** Blockade of prostate testosterone receptors
- **D.** Inhibition of topoisomerase I
- **E.** Blockade of gonadotropin receptors

Difficulty level: Medium

20. A 56-year-old man recently diagnosed with carcinoid tumor of the lung started a treatment that included octreotide The patient was most likely at increased risk of which of the following adverse effects as a result of this therapy?

- **A.** Gallstones
- **B.** Drowsiness
- **C.** Hypoglycemia
- **D.** Heat intolerance
- **E.** Flushing

Difficulty level: Easy

21. A 6-year-old girl presented to her pediatrician with pubic hair, breast development, and regular menstruation. After clinical and laboratory evaluations, a diagnosis of true precocious puberty was made. Which of the following drugs would be appropriate for this girl?

- **A.** Somatropin
- **B.** Estradiol
- **C.** Testosterone
- **D.** Bromocriptine
- **E.** Menotropins
- **F.** Leuprolide

Difficulty level: Easy

22. A 71-year-old man suffering from symptomatic advanced prostate cancer started a treatment with a drug that functions as competitive antagonist at gonadotropin-releasing hormone (GnRH) receptors. Which of the following drugs did the patient most likely take?

- **A.** Degarelix
- **B.** Leuprolide
- **C.** Cabergoline
- **D.** Pegvisomant
- **E.** Mecasermin

Difficulty level: Medium

23. An 8-year-old healthy girl was referred to a pediatric endocrinologist for short stature. Physical examination and karyotype analysis led to the diagnosis of Turner syndrome. Which of the following drugs would be most appropriate to treat the patient's disease?

- **A.** Oxandrolone
- **B.** Somatropin
- **C.** Somatostatin
- **D.** Testosterone
- **E.** Octreotide
- **F.** Cabergoline

Difficulty level: Medium

24. An 8-year-old boy was referred to a pediatric endocrinologist because of growth retardation. Lab tests showed increased serum growth hormone levels but very low serum levels of insulin-like growth factor 1 (IGF-1). Further exams led to the diagnosis of Laron dwarfism. Which of the following drugs would be most appropriate for this boy?

- **A.** Somatropin
- **B.** Octreotide
- **C.** Mecasermin
- **D.** Oxandrolone
- **E.** Cabergoline

Difficulty level: Medium

25. A 70-year-old man, recently diagnosed with a small-cell carcinoma, was admitted to the hospital for surgical resection of the lung. On admission, the patient appeared lethargic and confused. Pertinent lab results on admission were

Serum:

Na+ 120 mEq/L (normal 136–145 mEq/L)

K^+ 4.8 mEq/L (normal 4.5–5.0 mEq/L)

Osmolality 250 mOsm/L (normal 275–300 mOsm/L)

Urine:

Na^+ 50 mEq/L (normal 40–220 mEq/L)

Osmolality 400 mOsm/L (normal 50–1200 mOsm/L)

A drug from which of the following classes would be useful in correcting the patient's electrolyte imbalance?

A. Loop diuretics
B. Thiazide diuretics
C. Antidiuretic hormone (ADH) agonists
D. Glucocorticoids
E. ADH antagonists

Difficulty level: Medium

26. A 34-year-old man presented to the hospital with a history of joint pain, headache, excessive sweating, and deepening of the voice. Physical examination revealed hypertension, enlargement of the hands, a doughy appearance of the skin, and a barrel chest. A computed tomography scan disclosed a pituitary adenoma, and the patient underwent radiotherapy. Which of the following drugs would be appropriate for this patient while waiting for radiotherapy to work?

A. Leuprolide
B. Cosyntropin
C. Somatropin
D. Octreotide
E. Degarelix

Difficulty level: Easy

27. A 36-year-old man was found to have high serum levels of insulin-like growth factor 1 (IGF-1) during a regular clinic visit. Ten months earlier, the man was diagnosed with acromegaly and underwent radiation therapy, but the treatment was only partially effective, and the man had been receiving octreotide since then. Addition of which of the following drugs would be appropriate for the patient at this time?

A. Pegvisomant
B. Degarelix
C. Leuprolide
D. Cosyntropin
E. Methimazole

Difficulty level: Medium

28. A 36-year-old woman complained to her physician of amenorrhea for the past 2 months and of a white discharge from her breasts during the past month. A computed tomography scan showed a pituitary adenoma. A drug with which of the following mechanism of action would be most appropriate for this patient?

A. Stimulation of dopamine synthesis
B. Stimulation of growth hormone (GH) metabolism
C. Blockade of GH receptors
D. Blockade of D_2 receptors
E. Inhibition of GH release
F. Activation of D_2 receptors

Difficulty level: Medium

29. A 35-year-old woman presented to her gynecologist with concern that she and her husband had not conceived despite unprotected intercourse for the past 15 months. Further exams led to the diagnosis of unexplained infertility, and the woman started a "step-up" protocol of ovulation induction that included initial daily injections of follitropin alfa. The drug can activate specific receptors located in granulosa cells of the ovary to produce which of the following enzymes?

A. Transglycosylase
B. Topoisomerase II
C. Dehydrogenase
D. Desmolase
E. Aromatase

Difficulty level: Hard

30. A 34-year-old man was admitted to the hospital because of prolonged, massive watery diarrhea for the past 2 days. Physical and lab exams indicated a pancreatic tumor, and radioimmunoassay confirmed the diagnosis of vipoma. The patient was given intravenous fluids for hydration and was scheduled for surgery. Which of the following drugs would be appropriate to control the patient's diarrhea?

A. Somatotropin
B. Hydrochlorothiazide
C. Adrenocorticotropic hormone (ACTH)
D. Octreotide
E. Cabergoline
F. Leuprolide

Difficulty level: Medium

31. A 35-year-old woman presented to the clinic complaining of continuous thirst and polyuria. She reported that she often awoke at night because of thirst and the need to urinate. History showed that 6 months previously, she had sustained

a basal skull fracture during a car accident from which she recovered completely. Lab tests showed a urine osmolality of 20 mOsm/kg (normal 50–1200 mOsm/kg) and undetectable serum antidiuretic hormone (ADH) levels. Which of the following drugs would be most appropriate for this patient?

A. Hydrochlorothiazide
B. Amiloride
C. Desmopressin
D. Carbamazepine
E. Chlorpropamide

Difficulty level: Medium

32. A 7-year-old boy recently diagnosed with idiopathic hypopituitarism started a treatment with somatropin, a recombinant growth hormone with a molecular weight of about 22,000 D. Which of the following was most likely the main site of distribution of this drug?

A. Fat tissue
B. Plasma
C. Extracellular fluids
D. Cell cytosol
E. Total body water

Difficulty level: Medium

33. A 55-year-old woman was admitted to the emergency department with the diagnosis of septic shock. Despite fluid therapy and norepinephrine, she was still hypotensive (80/50 mm Hg) and tachycardic (120 bpm), and the cardiologist decided to start an intravenous infusion of another drug. A few minutes later, her blood pressure was 106/75 mm Hg, and her pulse was 88 bpm. Which of the following was most likely the drug given to the patient?

A. Epinephrine
B. Desmopressin
C. Phenylephrine
D. Dobutamine
E. Vasopressin

Questions: V-2 Drugs for Thyroid Disorders

Directions for questions 1–3

Match each drug used in thyroid diseases with the appropriate description (each lettered option can be selected only once, more than once, or not at all):

A. Levothyroxine
B. Liothyronine
C. Methimazole
D. Potassium iodide
E. Propylthiouracil
F. Radioactive iodine

Difficulty level: Easy

1. This drug is a target for thyroid deiodinase.

Difficulty level: Easy

2. This drug causes thyroid cell necrosis.

Difficulty level: Easy

3. This drug acts mainly by inhibiting hormone release from the thyroid gland.

Difficulty level: Medium

4. A 64-year-old woman was admitted to the emergency department with the admitting diagnosis of myxedema coma. An emergency treatment was started that included an intravenous injection of triiodothyronine (T_3) every 6 hours for 2 days. Which of the following were most likely the patient's serum levels of free thyroxine (FT_4) and thyroid-stimulating hormone (TSH, thyrotropin) after 2 days of therapy?

A. FT_4 low, TSH high
B. FT_4 high, TSH low
C. FT_4 high, TSH high
D. FT_4 low, TSH low

Difficulty level: Easy

5. A 2-year-old boy was brought to the emergency department because of fever, irritability, increased lethargy, and multiple episodes of diarrhea. The mother reported that she found her levothyroxine bottle empty a few hours earlier. Vital signs of the boy were blood pressure 130/80 mm Hg, heart rate 180 bpm, respirations 26/min. Laboratory test results on admission showed a total triiodothyronine level of 472 ng/dL (normal: 40–130 ng/dL). An appropriate emergency therapy was planned. Which of the following drugs should be administered first to control hormone-related effects that could be rapidly lethal in this patient?

A. Betamethasone
B. Propranolol
C. Potassium iodide
D. Propylthiouracil
E. Radioactive iodine

Difficulty level: Medium

6. A 50-year-old woman who underwent thyroid ablation with radioactive iodine had been taking levothyroxine as replacement therapy. Which of the following best represents the percentage of drug bound to plasma proteins in this patient?

A. 10.5%
B. 30.57%
C. 50.72%
D. 75.0%
E. 99.96 %

Difficulty level: Medium

7. A few days after a normal delivery, a newborn baby boy became lethargic, had respiratory difficulties and a hoarse cry, and sucked poorly. Physical examination revealed large fontanelles, macroglossia, a distended abdomen, cyanotic skin, hypotonia, slow reflexes, and rectal temperature of 95°F (35°C). Which of the following drugs would be appropriate for this baby?

A. Methimazole
B. Somatrem
C. Levothyroxine
D. Theophylline
E. Potassium iodide
F. Prednisone

Difficulty level: Hard

8. A 51-year-old woman suffering from chronic asthma was admitted to the hospital with nausea and vomiting, extreme restlessness, insomnia, tremor, mental confusion, and fever (103.1°F, 39.5°C). After her sister died a few days ago, she experienced increased hunger, dyspnea on exertion, palpitations, and diarrhea. Laboratory data on admission included a free thyroxine (FT_4) level of 11 ng/dL (normal 0.9–2.0 ng/dL) and undetectable thyroid-stimulating hormone (TSH, thyrotropin) levels. Which of the following drugs should be included in the emergency treatment of the patient?

A. Diltiazem
B. Radioactive iodine
C. Triiodothyronine
D. Danazol
E. Propranolol
F. Aspirin

Difficulty level: Medium

9. A 30-year-old woman who was 1 month pregnant complained to her physician of swelling of the eyelids and increasing lid aperture. Subsequent blood tests gave the following results: free thyroxine (FT_4) 3.3 ng/dL (normal 0.9–2.0 ng/dL), thyroid-stimulating hormone (TSH, thyrotropin) < 0.01 mU/L (normal 0.5–5.0 mU/L). Treatment with which of the following drugs

would be appropriate for this patient during the first trimester of pregnancy?

A. Radioactive iodine
B. Octreotide
C. Potassium iodide
D. Methyldopa
E. Propylthiouracil
F. Esmolol

Difficulty level: Easy

10. A 53-year-old woman suffering from thyrotoxicosis underwent thyroid ablation with radioactive iodine. Three weeks later, she started a therapy with levothyroxine. Which of the following best describes the molecular mechanism of action of this drug?

A. Agonist at thyroid-stimulating hormone (TSH) receptors
B. Antagonist at TSH receptors
C. Agonist at thyroid hormone (TH) receptors
D. Antagonist at TH receptors
E. Agonist at thyrotropin-releasing hormone (TRH) receptors
F. Antagonist at TRH receptors

Difficulty level: Easy

11. A 50-year-old woman who underwent thyroid ablation with radioactive iodine started treatment with levothyroxine. Which of the following cell elements represent the main site of therapeutic action of the drug?

A. Cell membrane
B. Mitochondria
C. Smooth endoplasmic reticulum
D. Cell nucleus
E. Golgi apparatus
F. Lysosomes

Difficulty level: Easy

12. A 53-year-old woman recently diagnosed with hyperthyroidism started an appropriate treatment. One month later, the following laboratory values were obtained:

Red blood cell count (RBC): 4.6×10^6/mm^3 (normal 4.0–5.5×10^6/mm^3)

White blood cell count (WBC): 0.6×10^3/mm^3 (normal 3.2–9.8×10^6/mm^3)

Platelets 180×10^3/mm^3 (normal 140–400×10^6/mm^3)

Which of the following drugs most likely caused these results?

A. Radioactive iodine
B. Potassium iodide
C. Methimazole
D. Propranolol
E. Levothyroxine

Difficulty level: Medium

13. A 33-year-old woman was admitted to the hospital because of anorexia, malaise, jaundice, and right upper quadrant abdominal pain for the past 2 days. The woman, who was 2 months' pregnant, was diagnosed with hyperthyroidism 1 month ago and started an appropriate therapy. Pertinent lab results on admission included alanine aminotransferase of 410 U/L (normal 20–40 U/L). Which of the following drugs most likely caused the patient's disorder?

A. Methimazole
B. Radioactive iodine
C. Propylthiouracil
D. Propranolol
E. Potassium iodide

Difficulty level: Easy

14. A 40-year-old man complained to his physician of increased appetite, palpitations, and diarrhea. Laboratory results confirmed the diagnosis of mild hyperthyroidism, and a treatment with methimazole was started. Which of the following actions most likely contributed to the therapeutic efficacy of the drug in this patient?

A. Proteolysis of thyroglobulin
B. Stimulation of thyroid peroxidase
C. Blockade of iodine uptake by the thyroid gland
D. Accumulation of iodine into thyroglobulin
E. Inhibition of iodination of tyrosine residues

Difficulty level: Hard

15. A 59-year-old woman complained to her physician of insomnia. The woman had undergone radioiodine treatment for thyroid ablation 6 months earlier and started replacement therapy with levothyroxine. Further questioning revealed that she had recently increased her daily drug dose because she felt fatigued and sad. A lab test showed thyroid-stimulating hormone (TSH) 0.1 mU/L (normal 0.5–5.0 mU/L) and free thyroxine (FT$_4$) 2.4 ng/dL (normal 0.8–2.7 ng/dL). Which of the following signs and symptoms most likely occurred in this patient after the inappropriate increase of the drug dose?

A. Decreased heart rate
B. Fluid retention
C. Decreased diastolic pressure
D. Decreased body temperature
E. Anorexia
F. Constipation

Difficulty level: Hard

16. A 67-year-old woman complained to her physician that for the past few days she had experienced restlessness and frequent runs of tachycardia. The woman had undergone thyroid ablation 7 months earlier and started replacement therapy with levothyroxine. Further exams led to the diagnosis of hyperthyroidism, most probably due to excessive self-dosage of the drug. Which of the following disorders most likely caused the patient's tachycardia?

A. Hypertrophic cardiomyopathy
B. Atrial fibrillation
C. Mitral regurgitation
D. Mitral stenosis
E. Constrictive pericarditis

Difficulty level: Easy

17. A 44-year-old woman recently diagnosed with Graves disease started a therapy with methimazole. Inhibition of which of the following enzymes most likely mediated the therapeutic effect of the drug in the patient's disease?

A. Thyroid protease
B. Topoisomerase I
C. Thyroid monodeiodinase
D. Thyroid peroxidase
E. Thyroid aldolase

Difficulty level: Medium

18. A 60-year-old alcoholic woman was brought to the emergency department after a car accident. Medical history of the patient was significant for hepatic cirrhosis and hypothyroidism. Although she had been advised repeatedly to take her thyroxine regularly, she continued to take it sporadically. Physical examination showed a distressed patient complaining of severe pain in both legs. An intramuscular injection of morphine sulphate was given to allay pain. Soon after the injection, the patient showed disorientation, lethargy, and shallow breathing, followed by unconsciousness. Her temperature was 93°F (30°C). Which of the following drugs should be included in the emergency therapy of this patient?

A. Intravenous (IV) potassium iodide
B. Oral methimazole
C. Oral levothyroxine
D. IV triiodothyronine
E. Oral propylthiouracil

Difficulty level: Easy

19. A 45-year-old woman complained to her physician of cold intolerance and menstrual irregularities over the past 3 weeks. The woman, recently diagnosed with Graves disease, had started a treatment with methimazole 2 months earlier. The physician told the patient that her symptoms were most likely due to an excessive dose of methimazole. Which of the following effects could also occur as a result of an excessive dose of that drug?

A. Palpitations
B. Sweating
C. Insomnia
D. Tremor
E. Constipation

Difficulty level: Easy

20. A 46-year-old man was taking levothyroxine as replacement therapy following radioactive iodine-induced thyroid ablation. Which of the following molecular actions most likely mediated the majority of therapeutic effects of the drug in this patient?

A. Alteration of transcription of specific genes
B. Decreased Na$^+$/K$^+$ ATPase activity
C. Inhibition of RNA activity
D. Inhibition of mitochondrial oxidative phosphorylation
E. Increased plasma catecholamine levels

Difficulty level: Easy

21. A 29-year-old woman complained to her physician of fatigue, constipation, and menstrual irregularities for the past 2 months. Physical examination showed delayed deep tendon reflexes, mild bradycardia, and a nontender, nodular thyroid goiter. A blood analysis showed thyroid peroxidase antibodies of 120 IU/L (normal < 0.8 IU/L). Which of the following drugs would be most appropriate for this patient?

A. Methimazole
B. Potassium iodide
C. Levothyroxine
D. Ethinyl estradiol
E. Radioactive iodine

Difficulty level: Hard

22. A 50-year-old woman suffering from hyperthyroidism was admitted to the emergency department with the admitting diagnosis of thyroid storm. Further exams confirmed the diagnosis, and an emergency therapy was started that included propranolol and hydrocortisone. Which of the following pairs of drugs should also be added to the emergency treatment of this patient?

A. Diltiazem and methimazole
B. Aspirin and atenolol
C. Radioactive iodine and dexamethasone
D. Esmolol and verapamil
E. Propylthiouracil and potassium iodide

Difficulty level: Easy

23. A 48-year-old man complained to his physician of a feeling of fullness in his neck. Physical examination showed diffuse enlargement of the thyroid gland without any apparent masses. Further exams led to the diagnosis of nontoxic goiter, most likely endemic because the man lived in an iodine-deficient country. Iodide supplementation was prescribed to provide sufficient iodide ions to the thyroid. These ions cross thyroid cell membranes by active transport. Which of the following is the primary transporter carrying iodide ions through the apical membrane of thyroid follicular cells?

A. Na$^+$/iodine symporter
B. Sulfate exchanger
C. Cl$^-$/iodide exchanger
D. Na$^+$/K$^+$ exchanger
E. Na$^+$/Cl$^-$ symporter

Difficulty level: Medium

24. A 64-year-old man complained to his physician of constipation, cold intolerance, and abnormal sensations in his hands and feet. A blood test showed the following results:

Free triiodothyronine (FT$_3$) 0.02 ng/dL (normal 0.23–0.42 ng/dl)

Free thyroxine (FT$_4$) 0.2 ng/dL (normal 0.8–2.7 ng/dL)

Thyroid-stimulating hormone (TSH) 0.1 mU/L (normal 0.5–5.0 mU/L)

A computed tomography scan confirmed the diagnosis, and an appropriate therapy was planned. Which of the following was most likely the patient's disease?

A. Hashimoto thyroiditis
B. Graves disease
C. Myxedema
D. Pituitary tumor
E. Thyroid cancer

Difficulty level: Easy

25. A 24-year-old woman with Hashimoto thyroiditis was 6 weeks' pregnant. The only medication she was taking was levothyroxine. Laboratory test results showed free thyroxine (FT$_4$) 0.6 ng/dL (normal 0.7–1.9 ng/dL) and thyroid-stimulating hormone (TSH) 4.8 mU/L (normal 0.5–5.0 mU/L). The physician decided to increase her daily dose of levothyroxine by about 30%. Which of the following best explains the

primary reason for careful adjustment of the levothyroxine dose during pregnancy?

A. To avoid maternal preeclampsia
B. To control maternal weight gain
C. To avoid maternal myxedema coma
D. To maintain normal fetal brain development
E. To counteract the TSH activity of human chorionic gonadotropin

Difficulty level: Easy

26. A 43-year-old man was undergoing surgery to remove a very large nontoxic goiter, apparently due to iodide deficiency. A short course of potassium iodide was administered before surgery. Which of the following statements best explains why this drug was given to the patient?

A. To stimulate thyroid hormone synthesis before surgery
B. To overcome iodine deficiency after surgery
C. To reduce the size and vascularity of the thyroid gland
D. To decrease the risk of hypothyroidism after surgery
E. To inhibit the excessive secretion of thyroid-stimulating hormone (TSH, T_4) from the pituitary

Difficulty level: Medium

27. A 57-year-old woman was admitted to the hospital with restlessness, insomnia, tremor, and pronounced exophthalmos. The woman, who had been suffering from Graves disease for 3 months, had been treated with propylthiouracil, but the drug had been discontinued a few days earlier because of the appearance of neutropenia. Which of the following agents would be most appropriate for the longterm management of the patient at this time?

A. Methimazole
B. Radioactive iodine
C. Propranolol
D. Prednisone
E. Potassium iodide

Difficulty level: Easy

28. A 53-year-old woman who had undergone total thyroidectomy started replacement therapy with levothyroxine. Which of the following pharmacological properties best explains why the levo isomer of the hormone is currently used instead of a racemic mixture for replacement therapy in thyroid disorders?

A. Longer half-life
B. Less frequent adverse effects
C. Higher affinity for thyroid receptors
D. Better gastrointestinal absorption
E. Higher volume of distribution

Difficulty level: Medium

29. A 50-year-old woman complained to her physician of sleepiness, fatigue, cold intolerance, weigh gain, and constipation. Medical history was significant for a reentrant supraventricular tachycardia presently treated with amiodarone and for type 2 diabetes presently treated with metformin. Further exams led to the diagnosis of mild hypothyroidism, and an adequate treatment was planned. Which of the following would be the most appropriate initial therapeutic step for this patient?

A. Start oral levothyroxine.
B. Start oral potassium iodide.
C. Start oral liothyronine.
D. Withdraw metformin.
E. Withdraw amiodarone.

Difficulty level: Easy

30. A 75-year-old woman complained to her physician of very dry skin and constipation, which she treated with milk of magnesia. She had no other medical problems and took no other medications. A blood analysis gave the following results:

Free triiodothyronine (FT_3): 0.3 ng/dL (normal 0.23–0.42 ng/dL)

Free thyroxine (FT_4): 0.9 ng/dL (normal 0.8–2.7 ng/dL)

Thyroid-stimulating hormone (TSH, thyrotropin): 15 mU/L (normal 0.5–5.0 ng/dL)

Thyroperoxidase antibodies: 28 IU/L (normal < 0.8 IU/L)

Which of the following drugs would be appropriate for this patient?

A. Potassium iodide
B. Propranolol
C. Methimazole
D. Loperamide
E. Levothyroxine
F. Diltiazem

Questions: V-3 Corticosteroids and Antagonists

Directions for questions **1–5**

Match each corticosteroid or antagonist with the appropriate description (each lettered option can be selected only once).

- **A.** Aminoglutethimide
- **B.** Aldosterone
- **C.** Desoxycorticosterone
- **D.** Dexamethasone
- **E.** Fludrocortisone
- **F.** Hydrocortisone
- **G.** Ketoconazole
- **H.** Mifepristone
- **I.** Prednisone
- **L.** Spironolactone

Difficulty level: Easy

1. A glucocorticoid devoid of salt-retaining activity

Difficulty level: Easy

2. A mineralocorticoid antagonist

Difficulty level: Easy

3. A mineralocorticoid used to treat adrenal insufficiency

Difficulty level: Easy

4. This drug blocks the conversion of cholesterol to pregnenolone.

Difficulty level: Easy

5. This drug blocks the cytoplasmic glucocorticoid receptors.

Difficulty level: Easy

6. A 66-year-old man complained to his physician of heartburn and a weight gain of 15 lb (6.8 kg). The patient, who was suffering from myasthenia gravis, had been receiving a multiple drug treatment for 3 months. Lab results showed serum calcium of 7.4 mg/dL (normal 8.5–10.5 mg/dL) and fasting blood glucose of 160 mg/dL (normal 70–110 mg/dL). Which of the following drugs most likely caused the patient's signs and symptoms?

- **A.** Fludrocortisone
- **B.** Edrophonium
- **C.** Azathioprine
- **D.** Neostigmine
- **E.** Testosterone
- **F.** Dexamethasone

Difficulty level: Easy

7. A 57-year-old man suffering from severe dermatomyositis had been receiving high-dose prednisone for 6 months. Which of the following laboratory results would be most likely to occur in this patient?

- **A.** Hyponatremia
- **B.** Hypocalcemia
- **C.** Hyperkalemia
- **D.** Hypoglycemia
- **E.** Hyperchloremia

Difficulty level: Easy

8. A 74-year-old woman with a long history of rheumatoid arthritis has been receiving prednisone for the past 3 months. She also has been receiving captopril to treat her hypertension. Which of the following laboratory results would be most likely to occur in this patient?

- **A.** Hyponatremia
- **B.** Hypercalcemia
- **C.** Hypokalemia
- **D.** Hyperglycemia
- **E.** Hypocholesterolemia

Difficulty level: Easy

9. A 42-year-old woman, recently diagnosed with lupus erythematosus, started a therapy with high-dose dexamethasone. Which of the following best explains why synthetic glucocorticoids are usually preferred over cortisol in the therapy of nonendocrine disorders?

- **A.** Lack of ulcerogenic activity
- **B.** Less prone to induce salt and water retention
- **C.** Less prone to induce myopathy
- **D.** Less prone to induce opportunistic infections
- **E.** Lack of diabetogenic effects

Difficulty level: Medium

10. A 45-year-old man complained to his physician of severe shoulder pain. Further exams led to the diagnosis of acute bursitis, and intra-articular injections of dexamethasone were prescribed. Which of the following actions most likely contributed to the therapeutic efficacy of the drug in the patient's disease?

- **A.** Inhibition of adrenocorticotropic hormone (ACTH) release
- **B.** Increased catabolism of prostaglandins
- **C.** Increased postcapillary permeability
- **D.** Increased release of interleukin-1
- **E.** Induction of lipocortin synthesis

Difficulty level: Easy

11. A 55-year-old woman was admitted to the hospital because of increasing muscle weakness, anxiety, and loss of emotional control. The patient was diagnosed with polymyositis 5 months ago and had been receiving an appropriate therapy since then. Physical examination showed a patient with face and trunk obesity and thin and easily bruised skin. Vital signs were blood pressure 168/98 mm Hg, pulse 84 bpm, respirations 18/min. A bone x-ray revealed diffuse osteoporosis. Which of the following drugs most likely caused the patient's signs and symptoms?

A. Methotrexate
B. Azathioprine
C. Fludrocortisone
D. Cyclophosphamide
E. Dexamethasone
F. Mifepristone

Difficulty level: Hard

12. A 46-year-old obese woman was brought unconscious to the emergency department. The woman had been suffering from asthma usually controlled with inhaled albuterol. Oral prednisone was added to the therapeutic regimen 3 weeks ago because of an exacerbation of her disease. Vital signs on admission were blood pressure 130/85 mm Hg, heart rate 120 bpm, respirations 22/min. Physical examination showed a patient unresponsive to verbal stimuli, withdrawn to pain, and with pupils equal and reactive. Pertinent laboratory findings on admission were fasting blood glucose 900 mg/dL (normal 70–110 mg/dL), serum osmolality 500 mOsm/L (normal < 350 mOsm/L). Urinalysis: specific gravity 1.030, glucose 4+, no proteins, no ketones. Which of the following disorders most likely caused the patient's signs and symptoms?

A. Prednisone-precipitated hyperosmolar coma
B. Albuterol-precipitated diabetic ketoacidosis
C. Prednisone-induced diabetic ketoacidosis
D. Albuterol-induced ventricular tachycardia
E. Albuterol-induced cerebral edema

Difficulty level: Easy

13. A 42-year-old man complained to his physician of progressive loss of vision. The man, diagnosed with rheumatoid arthritis 6 months ago, had been receiving a high dose of a drug since then. An ophthalmic examination revealed early cataract formation. Which of the following drugs most likely caused the patient's signs and symptoms?

A. Mifepristone
B. Prednisone
C. Fludrocortisone
D. Methotrexate
E. Azathioprine
F. Cyclophosphamide

Difficulty level: Easy

14. A 65-year-old man complained to his physician of epigastric distress, muscle weakness, hypertension, and white plaques in his mouth. The patient, diagnosed with polyarteritis nodosa 8 months ago, had been receiving an appropriate therapy since then. Laboratory values showed fasting blood glucose of 135 mg/dL (normal 70–110 mg/dL) and blood urea nitrogen (BUN) of 40 mg/dL (normal 7–18 mg/dL). Which of the following drugs most likely caused the patient's signs and symptoms?

A. Indomethacin
B. Ketoconazole
C. Fludrocortisone
D. Spironolactone
E. Prednisone
F. Ibuprofen

Difficulty level: Medium

15. A 57-year-old woman complained to her physician of muscle weakness, recurrent epigastric distress, and dull, aching back pain. The woman, recently diagnosed with severe ulcerative colitis, had been taking an appropriate therapy for 5 months. Laboratory values showed a decreased number of lymphocytes and an increased number of neutrophils. Which of the following drugs most likely caused the patient's signs and symptoms?

A. Prednisone
B. Mesalamine
C. Loperamide
D. Azathioprine
E. Infliximab
F. Metronidazole

Difficulty level: Medium

16. A 33-year-old woman suffering from lupus erythematosus was admitted to the hospital because of fever (101.1°F, 38.5°C), cough, dyspnea, and thoracic pain aggravated by breathing. She had been receiving high doses of oral prednisone for 3 months to treat a flare-up of the disease. Chest x-rays confirmed the diagnosis of pleural effusion, and a sputum test showed acid-fast rods. The patient did not smoke, and past history for pulmonary disease was unremarkable. Which of the following disorders most likely caused the patient's signs and symptoms?

A. Pneumococcal pneumonia
B. Chronic obstructive pulmonary disease
C. Pulmonary tuberculosis
D. Mycoplasmal pneumonia
E. Pulmonary fibrosis
F. Acute pericarditis

Difficulty level: Easy

17. A 49-year-old woman underwent a blood test during a routine clinic visit. The woman, recently diagnosed with lupus erythematosus, had been receiving high-dose prednisone for 3 weeks. Which of the following changes in the patient's blood cell concentration most likely occurred as a result of her therapy?

 A. Decreased neutrophils
 B. Decreased erythrocytes
 C. Increased basophils
 D. Decreased lymphocytes
 E. Increased eosinophils

Difficulty level: Easy

18. A 12-year-old boy, recently diagnosed with acute lymphoblastic leukemia, received a multidrug treatment that included prednisone. The therapeutic effect of the drug is most likely mediated by the drug–receptor complex binding to which of the following molecular targets?

 A. Final sequence on peptidyl RNA
 B. Specific nucleotide sequences on DNA
 C. Final sequence on ribosomal RNA
 D. Phospholipase A$_2$
 E. Interleukin-6
 F. Cyclooxygenase-2

Difficulty level: Easy

19. A 72-year-old man complained to his physician of large purple blotches on his arms that did not seem to disappear in a reasonable amount of time. The man, recently diagnosed with dermatomyositis, had started an appropriate therapy 3 weeks earlier. Which of the following drugs most likely caused the adverse effect reported by the patient?

 A. Warfarin
 B. Prednisone
 C. Heparin
 D. Methotrexate
 E. Azathioprine
 F. Cyclosporine

Difficulty level: Medium

20. A 54-year-old man was admitted to the hospital because of a 1-month history of hypertension, heartburn, paresthesias, and transient paralysis. Serum values on admission were Na$^+$ 150 mEq/L (normal 136–145 mEq/L), K$^+$ 2.4 mEq/L (normal 3.5–5.0 mEq/L), pH 7.5, and decreased plasma renin activity. A computed tomography scan showed hypertrophy of both adrenal glands. Which of the following drugs would be appropriate to treat the patient's disease?

 A. Minoxidil
 B. Furosemide
 C. Prednisone
 D. Spironolactone
 E. Fludrocortisone
 F. Testosterone

Difficulty level: Medium

21. A 57-year-old woman had been receiving high-dose betamethasone for 6 months to treat severe relapsing polychondritis. Because of the ongoing therapy, the patient was most likely at increased risk of which of the following disorders?

 A. Exertional angina
 B. Osteoporosis
 C. Rheumatoid arthritis
 D. Agranulocytosis
 E. Ulcerative colitis

Difficulty level: Medium

22. A 41-year-old woman was preparing to undergo surgery to remove a biliary calculus. The woman had suffered from T-cell lymphoma treated successfully with a four-drug combination that included prednisone. The therapy ended 6 months previously. The physician prescribed a course of prednisone treatment before the upcoming surgery. Which of the following was most likely the primary goal for restarting prednisone treatment in this patient?

 A. To avoid adrenal insufficiency after surgery
 B. To speed up surgical wound healing
 C. To avoid opportunistic infections after surgery
 D. To promote gallbladder relaxation before surgery
 E. To decrease adrenocorticotropic hormone (ACTH) release before surgery

Difficulty level: Easy

23. A 46-year-old woman suffering from polyarteritis nodosa, an autoimmune disease, had been receiving high-dose dexamethasone. Which of the following actions most likely contributed to the therapeutic effect of the drug in the patient's disease?

 A. Inhibition of catabolism of prostaglandins
 B. Inhibition of liver protein synthesis
 C. Increased proliferation of B cells
 D. Increased activation of complement system
 E. Inhibition of catabolism of interleukin-1
 F. Inhibition of synthesis of tumor necrosis factor (TNF)

Difficulty level: Medium

24. A 40-year-old woman was admitted to the hospital complaining of nausea and vomiting, weight loss, fatigue, and weakness. She also reported a persistent feeling of faintness on

standing and decreased tolerance to cold. Physical examination showed a patient in moderate distress with increased pigmentation around the nipples, absence of axillary and pubic hair, and diffuse tanning of exposed portions of the body. Significant serum levels on admission were Na⁺ 130 mEq/L (normal 136–145 mEq/L), K⁺ 6.2 mEq/L (normal 3.5–5.0 mEq/L), fasting blood glucose 42 mg/dL (normal 70–110 mg/dL). Which of the following pairs of drugs would be appropriate for this patient?

A. Mifepristone and prednisone
B. Danazol and cortisol
C. Fludrocortisone and spironolactone
D. Cortisol and prednisone
E. Fludrocortisone and cortisol

Difficulty level: Medium

25. A 43-year-old man was admitted unconscious to the emergency department. The man had been suffering from bronchogenic carcinoma for 8 months. Vital signs on admission were blood pressure 90/50 mm Hg, pulse 95 bpm, respirations 10/min. Physical examination revealed signs of increased intracranial pressure, and a computed tomography scan disclosed diffuse cerebral edema due to brain metastases. The appropriate emergency treatment of this patient should include which of the following drugs?

A. Epinephrine
B. Albuterol
C. Dexamethasone
D. Nitroglycerin
E. Diltiazem
F. Nifedipine

Difficulty level: Medium

26. A 29-year-old woman was admitted to the hospital because of fever (102.7°F, 39.2°C), chills, and worsening dyspnea that required intubation and mechanical ventilation just after admission. A chest radiograph showed bilateral patchy alveolar infiltrates. The patient was given erythromycin and cefepime for presumed bacterial pneumonia, but 24 hours later a repeat chest radiograph showed progression of the infiltrates. A bronchoscopy with bronchoalveolar lavage was performed, and a differential cell count of a lavage specimen showed 33% eosinophils. Which of the following drugs would be appropriate for this patient?

A. Vancomycin
B. Acyclovir
C. Prednisone
D. Ketoconazole
E. Piperacillin
F. Gentamicin

Difficulty level: Hard

27. A 63-year-old man with known metastatic prostate cancer was admitted to the hospital because of sudden onset of low back pain that progressed over 24 hours. He also noted that his legs were weaker than usual. Neurologic exam on admission showed hyperreflexia, and magnetic resonance imaging (MRI) demonstrated spinal cord compression at the T12 vertebra. A drug was administered to reduce spinal cord edema. The following day, both the back pain and the hyperreflexia were substantially decreased. Which of the following drugs was most likely given?

A. Fludrocortisone
B. Ibuprofen
C. Prednisone
D. Ketorolac
E. Furosemide
F. Spironolactone

Difficulty level: Easy

28. A 54-year-old man, recently diagnosed with immunologic thrombocytopenic purpura, started treatment with a large dose of an appropriate drug. The molecular mechanism of action of that drug involved binding to a receptor–heat shock protein complex in the cytoplasm. Which of the following drugs was most likely prescribed?

A. Fludrocortisone
B. Azathioprine
C. Norethindrone
D. Prednisone
E. Calcitriol
F. Ethinyl estradiol

Difficulty level: Medium

29. A 43-year-old man presented to the hospital complaining of weight gain, mild but continuing facial acne, and decreased muscle strength. On physical examination, the patient was found to be plethoric, red-faced with violaceous pigmented striae on a protuberant abdomen, and with relatively thin extremities. On admission, serum K⁺ levels were 4.5 mEq/L (normal 3.5–5.0 mEq/L). A computed tomography scan disclosed an adrenal adenoma in the left adrenal gland, and the patient was scheduled for surgery. Which of the following drugs would be appropriate to give to this patient during and after surgery?

A. Fludrocortisone
B. Spironolactone
C. Cortisol
D. Aminoglutethimide
E. Mifepristone
F. Ketoconazole

Difficulty level: Easy

30. A 53-year-old woman complained to her physician of weight gain, mild but continuing facial acne, and pigmented striae on her abdomen. Further exams led to the diagnosis of Cushing syndrome, and a pharmacotherapy was prescribed. Which of the following drugs would be most appropriate to treat the patient's disease?

A. Prednisone
B. Fludrocortisone
C. Ketoconazole
D. Spironolactone
E. Methimazole
F. Triamterene

Difficulty level: Easy

31. A 24-year-old woman complained to her physician that she had to go to the bathroom several times at night. Two weeks earlier, the woman had started a treatment with spironolactone for excessive hair on her face and arms. Which of the following molecular actions most likely mediated the patient's nocturia?

A. Competitive blockade of α_1 receptors of the bladder internal sphincter
B. Activation of M_3 receptors on the detrusor muscle
C. Osmotic action on the thin descending loop of Henle
D. Competitive blockade of aldosterone receptors
E. Blockade of Na^+/Cl^- symport in the early distal tubule

Difficulty level: Easy

32. A 52-year-old man with Addison disease presented to the hospital complaining of episodic weakness, paresthesias, and constipation. He had been taking cortisol and fludrocortisone for several months. On admission, his blood pressure was 160/98 mm Hg, and an electrocardiogram showed prolongation of the Q-T interval. Lab results revealed a K^+ serum level of 2.5 mEq/L (normal 3.5–5.0 mEq/L). Which of the following events best explains the patient's syndrome?

A. Cortisol-induced hyperglycemia
B. Fludrocortisone excess
C. Inadequate therapy of adrenal insufficiency
D. Cortisol-induced myopathy
E. Essential hypertension

Difficulty level: Medium

33. A 45-year-old man complained to his physician of increasing anorexia and malaise. The man also noted that his urine was frothy. Medical history and physical examination of the patient were unremarkable. Urinalysis of a 24-hour urine collection showed 3.8 g of protein. Which of the following drugs would be appropriate to treat the patient's disease?

A. Indomethacin
B. Erythromycin
C. Danazol
D. Octreotide
E. Betamethasone
F. Mifepristone

Difficulty level: Easy

34. A 22-year-old man was admitted to the emergency department because of dyspnea, pruritus, and erythema that developed soon after receiving an ampicillin injection. On admission, the man was wheezing and had prominent swelling of the face, eyelids, lips, and tongue. A diagnosis of drug anaphylaxis was made, and an injection of epinephrine was given. Which of the following drugs should also be administered to the patient?

A. Aspirin
B. Prednisone
C. Phenylephrine
D. Acetaminophen
E. Atenolol
F. Dopamine

Difficulty level: Medium

35. A 45-year-old woman suffering from Crohn disease had been receiving high doses of oral prednisone to treat a severe flare-up. Which of the following actions was most likely to contribute to the therapeutic effect of the drug in the patient's disease?

A. Increased catabolism of prostaglandins
B. Decreased number of circulating neutrophils
C. Increased proliferation of T cells
D. Increased activation of complement system
E. Inhibition of lymphocyte-mediated production of interleukin-2

Difficulty level: Medium

36. A 44-year-old woman complained to her physician of hazy vision, black floating spots, and severe pain in both eyes. After an ophthalmoscopic evaluation, a diagnosis of acute iridocyclitis was made, and a local drug treatment was prescribed. Which of the following drugs would be appropriate for the patient's disease?

A. Indomethacin
B. Apraclonidine
C. Timolol
D. Dexamethasone
E. Latanoprost
F. Pilocarpine

Difficulty level: Medium

37. A 61-year-old man suffering from non-Hodgkin lymphoma was hospitalized for his first cycle of chemotherapy. A pharmacotherapy was prescribed to prevent chemotherapy-induced nausea and vomiting. The drug regimen most likely included ondansetron, aprepitant, and which of the following drugs?

    A. Dexamethasone
    B. Scopolamine
    C. Diphenhydramine
    D. Loperamide
    E. Diazepam
    F. Omeprazole

Difficulty level: Hard

38. A 45-year-old man, HIV positive, was admitted to the emergency department because of persistent epistaxis. Physical examination revealed fever (103.2°F, 39.6°C) and altered mental status. Laboratory results on admission showed renal failure, hemolytic anemia, and severe consumptive thrombocytopenia. A diagnosis of thrombotic thrombocytopenic purpura was made, and a therapy with repeated plasmapheresis was started. Which of the following drugs would be appropriate to add to the ongoing treatment?

    A. Fludrocortisone
    B. Alteplase
    C. Aspirin
    D. Iron dextran
    E. Prednisone
    F. Sargramostim

Difficulty level: Easy

39. A 33-year-old woman, 29 weeks' pregnant, was admitted to the obstetrical unit with ruptured membranes. The patient was treated with nifedipine to delay premature labor and with another drug to accelerate maturation of the fetal lungs, thus decreasing the incidence of neonatal respiratory distress syndrome. Which of the following drugs was most likely administered?

    A. Indomethacin
    B. Acetaminophen
    C. Dexamethasone
    D. Ergonovine
    E. Dinoprostone
    F. Ondansetron

Difficulty level: Easy

40. A 32-year-old woman suffering from ulcerative colitis had been receiving an appropriate treatment that included oral prednisone for 3 months. Which of the following reasons best explains why this drug was used in the treatment of the patient's disease?

    A. To induce a general depressive effect on intestinal functions
    B. To elicit antiinflammatory and immunosuppressive effects
    C. To control nausea and vomiting, which are prominent in this disease
    D. To induce an analgesic effect that can abolish abdominal pain
    E. To prevent the risk of colorectal cancer

Difficulty level: Easy

41. An 8-year-old boy with mild persistent asthma was in the chest clinic for follow-up of his disease. He had been only moderately well controlled on inhaled albuterol "as needed." Physical examination showed diffuse expiratory wheezes, and pulmonary function testing revealed a peak expiratory flow rate 60% of predicted. The physician decided to add inhaled beclomethasone to the therapy, but the boy's mother was concerned about the adverse effects of glucocorticoids. The physician told the mother that systemic adverse effects of inhaled beclomethasone are extremely rare. Which of the following statements best explains the reason for this low toxicity?

    A. The drug is completely metabolized by the lung.
    B. The drug is quickly eliminated by the kidney.
    C. The dose reaching the systemic circulation is very small.
    D. The drug is completely eliminated with the exhaled air.
    E. Beclomethasone is the least toxic of glucocorticoid drugs.

Difficulty level: Medium

42. A 63-year-old woman complained to her physician of a recent progressive loss of vision. The patient had been suffering from myasthenia gravis for 6 months and was being treated with prednisone, azathioprine, and neostigmine. Other medications taken by the patient included omeprazole for gastroesophageal reflux disease and lovastatin for hyperlipidemia. Further exams of the eye led to the diagnosis of glaucoma. Which of the drugs taken by the patient would be relatively contraindicated at this time?

    A. Azathioprine
    B. Omeprazole
    C. Prednisone
    D. Neostigmine
    E. Lovastatin

Difficulty level: Medium

43. A 40-year-old man complained to his physician that the drug he was taking caused an abnormal increase in the size of his breasts. Medical history of the patient was negative for past diseases or use of alcohol or drugs. Two weeks earlier, the man was diagnosed with bilateral adrenal hyperplasia and had started an appropriate treatment. Which of the following drugs most likely caused the adverse effect in this patient?

   A. Ketoconazole

   B. Cimetidine

   C. Ethinyl estradiol

   D. Spironolactone

   E. Oxandrolone

   F. Omeprazole

Difficulty level: Medium

44. A 59-year-old man was admitted to the emergency department because of a 1-week history of nausea, vomiting, and lower abdominal cramps. The man had recently been diagnosed with Cushing syndrome and had started an appropriate therapy 3 weeks earlier. Physical examination revealed an afebrile, jaundiced, and cachectic patient with clouded mentation. Pertinent lab exam results on admission were aspartate aminotransferase 510 U/L, alanine aminotransferase 392 U/L (normal 8–20 U/L), alkaline phosphatase 660 U/L (normal 25–100 U/L), total bilirubin 3 mg/dL (normal 0.1–1.0 mg/dL). Which of the following drugs most likely caused the patient's disorder?

   A. Metyrapone

   B. Acetaminophen

   C. Ketoconazole

   D. Indomethacin

   E. Valproic acid

   F. Lovastatin

Questions: V-4 Drugs for Gonadal Disorders

Directions for questions **1–5**

Match each drug used in gonadal disorders with the appropriate description (each lettered option can be selected only once, more than once, or not at all).

   A. Anastrozole

   B. Clomiphene

   C. Danazol

   D. Dihydrotestosterone

   E. Finasteride

   F. Flutamide

   G. Fulvestrant

   H. Mifepristone

   I. Norgestrel

   J. Oxandrolone

   K. Tamoxifen

Difficulty level: Easy

1. An inhibitor of the enzyme that catalyzes the conversion of androgens to estrogens

Difficulty level: Easy

2. A selective estrogen receptor modulator

Difficulty level: Easy

3. An inhibitor of the enzyme that catalyzes the conversion of testosterone to dihydrotestosterone

Difficulty level: Easy

4. A drug able to block estrogen receptors in all target tissues

Difficulty level: Easy

5. A competitive antagonist at androgen receptors

Difficulty level: Easy

6. A 56-year-old woman complained to her gynecologist of persistent vaginal burning and vaginal pain during intercourse. One year earlier, the woman had undergone total hysterectomy because of a large leiomyoma. Physical examination showed dryness and atrophy of the vagina. A vaginal cream was prescribed. Which of the following drugs would be appropriate for local therapy in this patient?

   A. Ethinyl estradiol

   B. Norgestrel

   C. Anastrozole

   D. Tamoxifen

   E. Finasteride

Difficulty level: Easy

7. A 61-year-old woman complained to her physician of increasing tiredness, a dry cough, and a lump in her right breast. The woman had a history of a hormone-positive carcinoma of her left breast 15 months earlier, for which she had a mastectomy and 3 months of chemotherapy. She had been taking tamoxifen daily since ending the chemotherapy. Magnetic resonance imaging revealed multiple pulmonary and liver metastases. Which of the following drugs would be appropriate to treat the metastatic cancer of this patient?

- **A.** Anastrozole
- **B.** Flutamide
- **C.** Mifepristone
- **D.** Norethindrone
- **E.** Ethinyl estradiol
- **F.** Finasteride

Difficulty level: Easy

8. A 63-year-old woman was admitted to the hospital because of severe thoracic pain after a fall at home. Medical history was significant for mastectomy for breast cancer 8 years ago. An x-ray showed fracture of three ribs and diffuse and advanced osteoporosis. An appropriate therapy was started that included a drug that could lead to an increase in the bone mass index and could also decrease the risk of breast cancer reactivation. Which of the following drugs was most likely administered?

- **A.** Anastrozole
- **B.** Alendronate
- **C.** Raloxifene
- **D.** Testosterone
- **E.** Norgestrel

Difficulty level: Easy

9. During her annual checkup, a 32-year-old woman was found to have mild hypertension (160/90 mm Hg). The woman, otherwise healthy, had started an oral contraceptive (ethinyl estradiol and norgestrel) 2 months earlier. The physician decided to change her contraceptive pill and prescribed ethinyl estradiol and drospirenone. An increased excretion of which of the following ions most likely occurred in this patient after a few days of therapy?

- **A.** Potassium
- **B.** Sodium
- **C.** Magnesium
- **D.** Calcium
- **E.** Bicarbonate

Difficulty level: Medium

10. A 16-year-old girl was seen by her physician because of primary amenorrhea. Physical examination showed a short girl (height 135 cm, 53.15 in.) with a broad chest, poor breast development, and normal external genitalia. Subsequent exams revealed rudimentary ovaries, and cytogenetic analysis showed a 45,X karyotype. A diagnosis was made, and an

appropriate therapy was prescribed. Which of the following drugs would be most appropriate for this patient?

- **A.** Diethylstilbestrol
- **B.** Oxandrolone
- **C.** Anastrozole
- **D.** Mifepristone
- **E.** Danazol
- **F.** Ethinyl estradiol

Difficulty level: Easy

11. A 40-year-old woman complained to her gynecologist of heavy and painful menstruation over the past 3 months. Further exams led to the diagnosis of uterine fibroids, and the patient was scheduled for surgery. Which of the following drugs would be appropriate to decrease the patient's symptoms before surgery?

- **A.** Ethinyl estradiol
- **B.** Flutamide
- **C.** Finasteride
- **D.** Mifepristone
- **E.** Medroxyprogesterone

Difficulty level: Easy

12. A 23-year-old woman asked her physician for a postcoital contraceptive 2 days following unprotected intercourse. Which of the following drugs would be most appropriate for this purpose?

- **A.** Clomiphene
- **B.** Leuprolide
- **C.** Levonorgestrel
- **D.** Fulvestrant
- **E.** Tamoxifen
- **F.** Danazol

Difficulty level: Medium

13. A 34-year-old woman complained to her physician of swelling and pain in her left ankle. The woman was otherwise healthy, and the only medication she had been taking was a combined oral contraceptive. Further exams confirmed the diagnosis of venous thrombosis that the physician believed to be caused by the contraceptive pill. Which of the following actions most likely contributed to the adverse effect of the drug in this patient?

- **A.** Increased antithrombin III synthesis
- **B.** Decreased platelet aggregation
- **C.** Increased synthesis of protein C
- **D.** Increased synthesis of clotting factors
- **E.** Decreased plasminogen synthesis

Difficulty level: Medium

14. A 26-year-old woman asked her family physician for a hormonal contraceptive. She refused other methods of contraception. Past history of the woman indicated disseminated intravascular coagulation that followed an abortion due to placental abruptio. Which of the following would be the most appropriate hormonal contraceptive preparation for this woman?

A. Diethylstilbestrol
B. Ethinyl estradiol and norethindrone
C. Mestranol and norethindrone
D. Mifepristone
E. Ethinyl estradiol and levonorgestrel
F. Levonorgestrel

Difficulty level: Easy

15. A 39-year-old obese woman was admitted to the hospital because of a severe pain in her right calf. Medical history included chronic bronchial asthma, currently treated with inhaled albuterol, and mild type II diabetes, currently treated with chlorpropamide and metformin. She had been taking combined oral contraceptives for 2 years. Physical examination showed a red, swollen, and tender right calf. A duplex ultrasonography confirmed the diagnosis of deep venous thrombosis. Which of the following drugs most likely caused the patient's disorder?

A. Norethindrone
B. Albuterol
C. Ethinyl estradiol
D. Chlorpropamide
E. Metformin
F. Diethylstilbestrol

Difficulty level: Easy

16. A 68-year-old man with a long history of chronic cardiac failure presented to his physician complaining of urinary hesitancy and frequent need to urinate during the night. An examination revealed an enlarged prostate, and further exams confirmed the diagnosis of benign prostatic hyperplasia. Finasteride was included as part of his therapeutic regimen. Which of the following actions most likely mediated the therapeutic effect of the drug in the patient's disease?

A. Inhibition of follicle-stimulating hormone (FSH) and luteinizing hormone (LH) release
B. Inhibition of gonadotropin-releasing hormone (GnRH) release
C. Inhibition of 5α-reductase enzyme
D. Blockade of progesterone receptors
E. Blockade of testosterone receptors

Difficulty level: Easy

17. A 20-year-old woman started using a hormonal contraceptive with a monophasic combination of ethinyl estradiol and norethindrone. The primary contraceptive mechanism of action of this contraceptive preparation most likely includes decreased secretion of a hormone from which of the following organs or tissues?

A. Ovary
B. Adrenals
C. Posterior pituitary
D. Endometrium
E. Hypothalamus

Difficulty level: Medium

18. A 43-year-old woman recently diagnosed with endometriosis started a treatment with medroxyprogesterone, one tablet daily. Which of the following effects most likely occurred after a few days of therapy?

A. Decreased body temperature
B. Increased estrogen secretion by the ovary
C. Increased ventilatory response to carbon dioxide
D. Decreased kidney excretion of sodium and water
E. Increased circulating levels of amino acids

Difficulty level: Easy

19. A 21-year-old woman started using a combined oral contraceptive pill (ethinyl estradiol and norethindrone). Which of the following cell structures is the primary site of action of both drugs?

A. Nucleus
B. Membrane
C. Mitochondria
D. Ribosomes
E. Golgi apparatus

Difficulty level: Easy

20. A 45-year-old woman complained to her physician that for the past month she had frequent episodes of developing a sudden feeling of warmth over her chest accompanied by a patchy flushing of her skin. She stated that these symptoms were extremely disturbing. She had been having irregular menstrual periods for the past year, often skipping two or three periods at a time. Which of the following preparations would be most appropriate for short-term hormonal replacement therapy in this woman?

A. Oral ethinyl estradiol
B. Transdermal estradiol
C. Oral norethindrone
D. Subcutaneous implant of levonorgestrel
E. Oral ethinyl estradiol–norgestrel combination
F. Parenteral medroxyprogesterone

Difficulty level: Medium

21. A 26-year-old woman came to her physician complaining of hyperpigmentation of her face. Physical examination revealed a poorly defined, blotchy, masklike zone of facial pigmentation with almost equal involvement of her cheeks, temples, and forehead. Skin biopsy showed increased melanin pigment in basal layers. The woman had been taking a hormonal contraceptive for 6 years. She was a long-distance runner and admitted the use of oxandrolone, erythropoietin, and methamphetamine while training. Which of the following drugs most likely caused the hyperpigmentation in this woman?

- **A.** Ethinyl estradiol
- **B.** Oxandrolone
- **C.** Erythropoietin
- **D.** Norethindrone
- **E.** Methamphetamine

Difficulty level: Easy

22. A 59-year-old woman diagnosed with metastatic breast cancer started a treatment that included anastrozole. Which of the following molecular actions most likely mediated the therapeutic effect of the drug in the patient's disease?

- **A.** Activation of estrogen catabolism
- **B.** Competitive blockade of estrogen receptors
- **C.** Competitive blockade of progesterone receptors
- **D.** Inhibition of conversion of androgens to estrogens
- **E.** Inhibition of conversion of progesterone to androgens

Difficulty level: Easy

23. A 32-year-old woman had been taking a combined oral contraceptive pill for the past 5 years. However, she recently developed a disorder that prompted her physician to withdraw the pill and to recommend other forms of contraception. Which of the following disorders most likely occurred to this patient?

- **A.** Rheumatoid arthritis
- **B.** Vein thrombosis
- **C.** Vaginal infection
- **D.** Acne
- **E.** Anorexia

Difficulty level: Easy

24. A 54-year-old woman was admitted to the hospital because of increasing shortness of breath. Five years earlier, the woman had been diagnosed with hormone-positive breast cancer and underwent radical mastectomy and six cycles of chemotherapy. She had been receiving hormonal therapy with tamoxifen since then. A computed tomography scan showed multiple lung metastases. Tamoxifen was stopped,

and a therapy with a competitive estrogen receptor antagonist was initiated. Which of the following drugs was most likely given?

- **A.** Anastrozole
- **B.** Danazol
- **C.** Leuprolide
- **D.** Fulvestrant
- **E.** Mifepristone

Difficulty level: Easy

25. A 52-year-old woman presented to her physician complaining of hot flushes and night sweats that disturbed her sleep. Her last menstrual period was 6 months ago. The physician prescribed a hormone replacement therapy with a combined contraceptive pill (ethinyl estradiol and norethindrone). This therapy might carry a small increase in the risk of which of the following diseases?

- **A.** Osteoporosis
- **B.** Breast cancer
- **C.** Colon cancer
- **D.** Ovarian cancer
- **E.** Endometrial cancer

Difficulty level: Easy

26. A 27-year-old woman who was having trouble trying to conceive started a cycle of therapy with clomiphene. Eight weeks later, she had a positive pregnancy test. Which of the following was most likely the primary site of action of the drug that led to the woman's successfully becoming pregnant?

- **A.** Corpus luteum
- **B.** Hypothalamus
- **C.** Uterine tube
- **D.** Posterior pituitary
- **E.** Ovary
- **F.** Endometrium

Difficulty level: Easy

27. A 22-year-old woman started using a combination hormonal contraceptive (ethinyl estradiol and norethindrone). Synthetic estrogens and progestins are currently used in most contraceptive formulations instead of natural hormones mainly because of which of the following pharmacological advantages?

- **A.** Much lower incidence of adverse effects
- **B.** Greater oral bioavailability
- **C.** Higher hormonal efficacy
- **D.** Higher inhibition of gonadotropin secretion
- **E.** Lower teratogenic activity

Difficulty level: Easy

28. A 24-year-old man complained to his physician of erectile dysfunction. Further exams led to the diagnosis of adult-onset hypogonadism, and a therapy with a testosterone patch was started. Which of the following effects most likely occurred after a few days of therapy?

A. Enhanced luteinizing hormone (LH) secretion

B. Decreased synthesis of clotting factors

C. Decreased growth of bone marrow stem cells

D. Enhanced erythropoietin synthesis

E. Increased high-density lipoprotein (HDL) levels

Difficulty level: Easy

29. A 30-year old man, who was a long-distance runner, had been using large doses of anabolic steroids for more than 10 years to increase his athletic performance. The man was most likely at increased risk of developing which of the following diseases?

A. Osteoporosis

B. Angioneurotic edema

C. Hemolytic anemia

D. Hepatic tumors

E. Kidney failure

F. Gastric ulcer

Difficulty level: Easy

30. A 16-year-old girl complained to her physician that her periods were very irregular, with intervals between 22 days and 4 months. She also noticed increased hair growth on her face, extremities, abdomen, and breasts. Further exams led to the diagnosis of polycystic ovary syndrome, and an appropriate treatment was prescribed. Which of the following pairs of drugs would be appropriate for this patient?

A. Ethinyl estradiol and mifepristone

B. Danazol and norgestrel

C. Ethinyl estradiol and danazol

D. Danazol and mifepristone

E. Mifepristone and norgestrel

F. Ethinyl estradiol and norgestrel

Difficulty level: Easy

31. A 23-year-old woman asked her physician for a contraceptive pill. Because the woman had suffered in the past from deep venous thrombosis, the physician prescribed a progestin-only oral contraceptive (the mini pill). Which of the following actions most likely contributed to the contraceptive effect of the prescribed drug?

A. Activation of progestin receptors in the corpus luteum

B. Stimulation of follicle-stimulating hormone (FSH) release from the pituitary

C. Increased viscosity of the cervical mucus

D. Increased frequency of gonadotropin-releasing hormone (GnRH) pulse generator

E. Stimulation of contraction of the myometrium

Difficulty level: Easy

32. A 54-year-old woman had been receiving tamoxifen for 1 year following surgery for breast cancer. Which of the following drug classes best defines this drug?

A. Estrogen receptor antagonist

B. Progestin receptor agonist

C. Progestin receptor antagonist

D. Selective estrogen receptor modulator

E. Aromatase synthesis inhibitor

F. Androgen receptor agonist

Difficulty level: Hard

33. A 15-year-old boy was admitted to the hospital because of a sudden swelling in his arms, legs, abdomen, lips, tongue, and throat. Past history of the patient indicated that his father had had a similar episode in his youth. An emergency therapy was started, and further exams indicated very low levels of C_1 esterase inhibitor. A few days later, the patient was discharged with a suitable therapy. Which of the following drugs would be appropriate to prevent further attacks in this patient?

A. Flutamide

B. Octreotide

C. Clomiphene

D. Medroxyprogesterone

E. Danazol

F. Mifepristone

Difficulty level: Medium

34. A 63-year-old man came to his physician complaining of a persistent backache. Rectal examination revealed a single, hard, irregular nodule within his prostate. Subsequent exams found his prostate-specific antigen (PSA) level to be 100 ng/mL (normal < 3.0 ng/mL), and a computed tomography scan showed several enlarged pelvic lymph nodes and multiple sclerotic lesions in his spine. Which of the following pairs of drugs would be most appropriate for the patient at this time?

A. Paclitaxel and cisplatin

B. Vincristine and prednisone

C. Leuprolide and flutamide

D. Tamoxifen and anastrozole

E. Vincristine and actinomycin

Difficulty level: Easy

35. A 19-year-old woman started using daily norethindrone pills as a hormonal contraceptive. Which of the following adverse effects would be most likely associated with this method of contraception?

A. Increased skin pigmentation
B. Megaloblastic anemia
C. Retinal thrombosis
D. Breakthrough bleeding
E. Galactorrhea

Difficulty level: Medium

36. A 21-year-old woman complained to her physician of recurrent nausea lasting most of the day. The woman had been suffering from a urinary tract infection presently being treated with ciprofloxacin and from gastroesophageal reflux disease presently being treated with omeprazole. She also routinely took ibuprofen during her menstrual period. One week ago, she started taking a contraceptive pill (ethinyl estradiol and norgestrel). Which of the following drugs most likely caused the patient's nausea?

A. Ethinyl estradiol
B. Ciprofloxacin
C. Norgestrel
D. Omeprazole
E. Ibuprofen

Difficulty level: Easy

37. A young couple presented to the physician complaining that they have been trying for 2 years to conceive a second child but have not been successful. Their first child was a healthy 4-year-old girl. Lab tests revealed that the husband was severely oligospermic. On questioning, he admitted he had been taking some drugs to aid his athletic performance. Which of the following drugs most likely contributed to the oligospermia of this man?

A. Vitamin B_{12}
B. Danazol
C. Ferrous sulphate
D. Medroxyprogesterone
E. Erythropoietin
F. Oxandrolone

Difficulty level: Easy

38. A 38-year-old woman underwent a hysterectomy and bilateral oophorectomy because of acute pelvic peritonitis. One month later, a hormonal treatment was started. Which of the following drugs would be appropriate for this patient?

A. Leuprolide
B. Estradiol
C. Tamoxifen
D. Human chorionic gonadotropin
E. Norgestrel
F. Anastrozole

Difficulty level: Medium

39. A 37-year-old woman complained of severe pelvic pain during menstruation and mild to moderate pain on some nonmenstrual days. Physical examination of the patient revealed diffuse uterine and adnexal tenderness and multiple nodes palpated along the uterosacral ligament. Laparoscopic examination showed endometriotic lesions. Which of the following drug therapies would be most appropriate for this patient?

A. Anastrozole
B. Human chorionic gonadotropin
C. Lutropin alfa
D. Tamoxifen
E. Combined oral contraceptives
F. Urofollitropin

Difficulty level: Hard

40. A 22-year-old woman was admitted to the emergency department because of excruciating abdominal pain over the past 4 hours. The woman had been suffering from asthma, presently treated with albuterol and ipratropium, and from recurrent urinary tract infection, presently treated with ciprofloxacin and azithromycin. A few days earlier, she had started using a combined oral contraceptive for the first time. Physical examination showed a patient in obvious distress with pronounced muscle weakness. Bladder catheterization showed clear red urine. Further exams confirmed the diagnosis of an acute porphyric attack. Which of the following drugs most likely triggered the patient's disorder?

A. Albuterol
B. Norethindrone
C. Ipratropium
D. Ciprofloxacin
E. Azithromycin

Difficulty level: Medium

41. A 10-year-old boy was brought to the emergency department with the admitting diagnosis of bacterial meningitis. Further exams confirmed the diagnosis of meningococcal meningitis, and a drug was given prophylactically to all the heath personnel assisting the boy. The female personnel were instructed that hormonal contraceptives were not effective when taken with the given drug, as that drug was able to significantly reduce plasma concentration of estrogens and progestins. Which of the following was most likely the drug used to prevent the infection in close contacts of this boy?

A. Ceftriaxone
B. Ciprofloxacin
C. Erythromycin
D. Ketoconazole
E. Rifampin

Questions: V-5 Drugs for Bone Homeostasis

Directions for questions **1–5**

Match each drug affecting bone homeostasis with the appropriate description (each option can be selected more than once).

A. Alendronate
B. Calcipotriene
C. Calcitonin
D. Calcitriol
E. Calcium
F. Cholecalciferol
G. Cinacalcet
H. Denosumab
I. Fluoride
J. Paricalcitol
K. Teriparatide
L. Sevelamer

Difficulty level: Easy

1. This drug can induce osteoclast apoptosis.

Difficulty level: Easy

2. This drug is a recombinant human parathyroid hormone (1-34).

Difficulty level: Easy

3. This drug activates a calcium-sensing receptor on the parathyroid glands.

Difficulty level: Easy

4. This drug can inhibit the gene expression of parathyroid hormone.

Difficulty level: Easy

5. This hormone is secreted by the parafollicular cells of the thyroid gland.

Difficulty level: Easy

6. A 61-year-old woman, suffering from severe osteoporosis, sustained a tibial fracture, and her physician decided to add teriparatide to the current therapy. Which of the following actions most likely mediated the therapeutic effect of teriparatide in this patient?

A. Stimulation of osteoblast activity
B. Inhibition of osteoclast activity
C. Inhibition of renal phosphate excretion
D. Stimulation of bone collagen synthesis
E. Inhibition of renal synthesis of calcitriol

Difficulty level: Easy

7. A 76-year-old man complained to his physician of muscle aches. Further exams led to the diagnosis of vitamin D deficiency due to inadequate intake. A vitamin D supplementation was prescribed. Which of the following would be the most appropriate pharmacotherapy for this patient?

A. Cholecalciferol
B. Calcitriol
C. Teriparatide
D. Cinacalcet
E. Calcitonin

Difficulty level: Easy

8. A 49-year-old man suffering from chronic renal failure was admitted to the hospital because of a hip fracture. Further exams revealed a diffuse demineralization of bone. An appropriate therapy was started that included calcitriol. Which of the following actions most likely mediated the therapeutic efficacy of the drug in this patient?

A. Stimulation of liver hydroxylation of cholecalciferol
B. Stimulation of renal α_1 hydroxylase
C. Decreased intestinal phosphate absorption
D. Increased intestinal calcium absorption
E. Decreased renal phosphate reabsorption

Difficulty level: Easy

9. A 66-year-old woman suffering from osteoporosis and hypertension has been treated for the past year with raloxifene and calcium carbonate for osteoporosis and with hydrochlorothiazide for hypertension. Despite the therapy, a recent bone mineral density test showed a significant decrease in bone mass. Which of the following would be an appropriate change in the treatment plan of this patient?

A. Substitute hydrochlorothiazide with propranolol.
B. Substitute raloxifene with ethinyl estradiol.
C. Add calcitonin to the current regimen.
D. Increase the daily dose of calcium carbonate.
E. Add prednisone to the current regimen.
F. Add alendronate to the current regimen.

Difficulty level: Easy

10. A 50-year-old woman recently hospitalized because of worsening of her disease started a treatment that included sevelamer. Which of the following was most likely the clinical condition for which the drug was prescribed?

A. Liver cirrhosis
B. Lupus erythematosus
C. Crohn disease
D. Chronic heart failure
E. End-stage renal disease

Difficulty level: Easy

11. A 7-year-old Black boy was brought to the emergency department after he fell while playing in the yard. Physical examination revealed only minor skin scratches, but an x-ray showed two rib fractures, clearly demineralized bone, and widening and cupping of metaphyses with exaggerated normal concavity and irregular calcification. Pertinent serum values on admission were calcium 8.3 mg/dL (normal 8.5–10.5 mg/dL), phosphate 2.2 mg/dL (normal 3.0–4.5 mg/dL), and a two-fold increase in alkaline phosphatase. Which of the following drugs would be most appropriate for this boy?

A. Cholecalciferol
B. Calcitonin
C. Calcitriol
D. Teriparatide
E. Alendronate
F. Cinacalcet

Difficulty level: Easy

12. A 4-year-old boy recently diagnosed with rickets started a treatment with cholecalciferol. Which of the following molecular actions most likely mediated the therapeutic effect of the drug in the patient's disease?

A. Cholecalciferol-activated vitamin D receptor complex binds to RNA.
B. Cholecalciferol-activated vitamin D receptor complex binds to DNA.
C. Calcitriol-activated vitamin D receptor complex binds to RNA.
D. Calcitriol-activated vitamin D receptor complex binds to DNA.
E. Ergocalciferol-activated vitamin D receptor complex binds to RNA.
F. Ergocalciferol-activated vitamin D receptor complex binds to DNA.

Difficulty level: Easy

13. A 52-year-old woman complained to her physician of a persistent gastric pain every time she took a prescribed drug. The woman, recently diagnosed with severe osteoporosis, had started a therapy with oral alendronate 1 week earlier.

The physician suspended alendronate and prescribed intravenous administration of zoledronate, explaining to the patient that a single injection would be effective for at least 5 to 6 months. Zoledronate has a half-life of about 7 days. Which of the following best explains the reason for the exceptionally long efficacy of the drug?

A. Alteration of gene expression of bone osteoblasts
B. Incorporation into bone hydroxyapatite crystals
C. Repeated enterohepatic cycling of the drug
D. Very slow biotransformation to active intermediates
E. Irreversible binding to plasma proteins

Difficulty level: Medium

14. A 63-year-old man was admitted to the hospital because of altered mental status and dehydration. Six months earlier, the patient had undergone radical prostatectomy for prostate cancer. Physical examination showed a dehydrated man with fluctuating consciousness level and disoriented to time and place. Pertinent serum values on admission were calcium 16.5 mg/L (normal 8.5–10.5 mg/L), alkaline phosphatase 304 U/L (normal 20–90 U/L). Which of the following drugs should be included in the therapeutic management of this patient?

A. Sodium phosphate
B. Hydrochlorothiazide
C. Pamidronate
D. Mannitol
E. Fludrocortisone
F. Cinacalcet

Difficulty level: Medium

15. A 46-year-old man complained to his physician of muscle weakness, fatigue, constipation, nausea, and polyuria. Past medical history was unremarkable. Subsequent lab exams showed the following serum values: calcium 14.5 mg/dL (normal 8.5–10.5 mg/dL), phosphate 2.1 mg/dL (normal 3.0–4.5 mg/dL), and immunoreactive parathyroid hormone 142 pg/mL (normal 11–54 pg/mL). Which of the following drugs would be appropriate to include in the therapeutic management of this patient?

A. Calcitriol
B. Hydrochlorothiazide
C. Sodium fluoride
D. Triamterene
E. Teriparatide
F. Calcitonin

Difficulty level: Easy

16. A 51-year-old woman, recently diagnosed with Paget disease of bone, had been receiving alendronate for 1 week, but the drug had to be suspended because of a persistent abdominal pain. The physician decided to replace the alendronate with calcitonin. Which of the following actions most likely mediated the therapeutic effect of calcitonin in the patient's disease?

    A. Inhibition of osteoclast activity
    B. Stimulation of osteoblast activity
    C. Stimulation of renal calcium reabsorption
    D. Stimulation of renal phosphate reabsorption
    E. Inhibition of intestinal calcium absorption

Difficulty level: Medium

17. A 43-year-old man with a 25-year history of type 1 diabetes was evaluated at a regular clinic visit. Pertinent serum values determined were glucose 190 mg/dL, calcium 7.3 mg/dL (normal 8.5–10.5 mg/dL), phosphate 5.1 mg/dL (normal 3.0–4.5 mg/dL), creatinine 3.9 mg/dL. An x-ray exam revealed density changes in the bones that were consistent with renal osteodystrophy. Which of the following drugs should be included in the treatment plan for this patient?

    A. Alendronate
    B. Calcitonin
    C. Calcitriol
    D. Teriparatide
    E. Cinacalcet

Difficulty level: Easy

18. A 59-year-old woman with a long history of chronic kidney disease was recently diagnosed with secondary hyperparathyroidism and started a treatment that included cinacalcet. Which of the following molecular actions most likely mediated the therapeutic effect of the drug in the patient's disease?

    A. Activation of parathyroid hormone (PTH) receptors
    B. Blockade of PTH receptors
    C. Activation of calcium-sensing receptors
    D. Blockade of calcium-sensing receptors
    E. Activation of calcitriol receptors
    F. Blockade of calcitriol receptors

Difficulty level: Medium

19. A 54-year-old homeless man with a 15-year history of alcoholism was brought to the hospital by the police, who had found him lying on the street. Physical examination showed a disheveled, confused, and cachectic man with prominent veins on a very tense abdomen. Pertinent serum values on admission were calcium 5.5 mg/L (normal 8.5–10.5) and alanine aminotransferase 300 U/L (normal 8–35). An x-ray

disclosed diffuse demineralization of bones. An appropriate therapy was ordered. Which of the following drugs should be included in the therapeutic management of this patient?

    A. Teriparatide
    B. Cholecalciferol
    C. Alendronate
    D. Calcitriol
    E. Calcipotriene

Difficulty level: Easy

20. A 64-year-old woman complained to her physician of persistent back pain for the past 3 days. Dual-energy x-ray absorptiometry showed diffuse osteoporosis of the spine and hips. The physician prescribed calcium and vitamin D supplementation and alendronate, one tablet daily. Which of the following actions most likely mediated the therapeutic effect of alendronate in the patient's disease?

    A. Stimulation of osteoblast activity
    B. Stimulation of intestinal calcium absorption
    C. Inhibition of renal calcium excretion
    D. Inhibition of osteoclast activity
    E. Inhibition of renal synthesis of calcitriol

Difficulty level: Medium

21. A 61-year-old woman suffering from osteoporosis had been receiving alendronate and vitamin D supplementation for 2 years. Recent dual-energy x-ray absorptiometry showed a big decrease in bone density. The patient's history was significant for a femur fracture 2 months earlier and a rib fracture 1 month earlier. Which of the following drugs is most likely to increase bone density in this patient?

    A. Teriparatide
    B. Ethynil estradiol
    C. Pamidronate
    D. Calcitonin
    E. Paricalcitol

Difficulty level: Easy

22. A 56-year-old woman complained to her physician of frequent heartburn and pain in the substernal region. The woman had started an appropriate therapy for osteoporosis 2 weeks earlier. Which of the following drugs most likely caused the patient's symptoms?

    A. Prednisone
    B. Calcitonin
    C. Raloxifene
    D. Teriparatide
    E. Cholecalciferol
    F. Alendronate

Difficulty level: Hard

23. A 57-year-old man complained to his physician of occasional bone pain, which was accentuated at night, and decreasing auditory acuity. The patient had a long history of gastroesophageal reflux disease currently treated with omeprazole. Physical examination revealed skull enlargement, a hobbling gait, and anterolateral bowing of the legs with warmth and periosteal tenderness. Plain x-rays showed increased bone density, cortical thickening, and bony enlargement. Laboratory results showed alkaline phosphatase of 230 IU/L (normal 20–90 IU/L). Which of the following drugs would be appropriate for this patient?

A. Parenteral calcitonin
B. Oral alendronate
C. Parenteral teriparatide
D. Oral cinacalcet
E. Oral raloxifene
F. Parenteral calcitriol

Difficulty level: Easy

24. A 49-year-old woman was admitted to the hospital because of tetanic muscle spasms and paresthesias following a recent thyroidectomy. Which of the following drugs given intravenously could rapidly reverse the patient's symptoms?

A. Vitamin D
B. Calcitonin
C. Sodium phosphate
D. Calcium gluconate
E. Hydrocortisone
F. Alendronate

Difficulty level: Easy

25. A 69-year-old woman was admitted to the emergency department with prominent skeletal muscle weakness, drowsiness, emotional lability, confusion, dizziness, nausea, and constipation. The patient's medications on admission included losartan and furosemide for chronic heart failure, teriparatide for osteoporosis, and timolol and dorzolamide for glaucoma. Lab tests revealed a serum calcium level of 14 mg/dL (normal 8.5–10.5 mg/dL). Which of the drugs taken by the patients most likely caused her hypercalcemia?

A. Losartan
B. Furosemide
C. Timolol
D. Teriparatide
E. Dorzolamide

Difficulty level: Medium

26. A 62-year-old woman suffering from severe osteoporosis started a therapy with teriparatide, a subcutaneous injection

daily. Which of the following actions most likely occurred after the administration of this drug?

A. Increased renal phosphate reabsorption
B. Increased renal calcium reabsorption
C. Decreased renal calcitriol production
D. Increased bone resorption
E. Increased parathyroid hormone secretion

Difficulty level: Easy

27. A 58-year-old woman suffering from increasingly worsening osteoporosis recently had denosumab added to her pharmacotherapeutic regimen. Which of the following actions most likely mediated the therapeutic effect of the drug in the patient's disease?

A. Enhancement of osteoblast apoptosis
B. Inhibition of parathyroid hormone biosynthesis
C. Inhibition of osteoclast formation
D. Enhancement of intestinal absorption of vitamin D
E. Enhancement of calcitonin biosynthesis

Difficulty level: Easy

28. A 42-year-old man suffering from advanced renal insufficiency was scheduled for kidney transplant. A recent laboratory test showed the following serum values: calcium 6.9 mg/dL (normal 8.5–10.5 mg/dL), phosphate 6.1 mg/dL (normal 3.0–4.5 mg/dL). Which of the following drugs would be appropriate to include in the current pharmacotherapy of this patient?

A. Alendronate
B. Sevelamer
C. Calcitonin
D. Furosemide
E. Cholecalciferol

Difficulty level: Medium

29. A 49-year-old man presented to his physician complaining of recurring skin lesions most prominent over the scalp, extensor surfaces of the elbows and knees, buttocks, and penis. The man also complained of increasing pain in his left hand and left hip. Physical examination showed oval erythematous plaques covered with thick, silvery, shiny scales. The distal interphalangeal joints of digits 2 and 3 of the left hand were swollen and tender. A diagnosis was made, and a topical drug treatment was prescribed. Which of the following drugs would be appropriate for this patient?

A. Fludrocortisone
B. Calcitonin
C. Calcipotriene
D. Erythromycin
E. Alendronate
F. Cinacalcet

Difficulty level: Easy

30. A 63-year-old man with a long history of chronic kidney disease was admitted to the hospital because of increasing anorexia, nausea and vomiting, and weight loss. Pertinent serum values on admission were creatinine 3.4 mg/dL, calcium 8.6 mg/dL (normal 8.5–10.5 mg/dL), phosphate 4.9 mg/dL (normal 3.0–4.5 mg/dL). A diagnosis of severe renal insufficiency was made, and an appropriate therapy was started that included cinacalcet. Which of the following was most likely the main site of action of this drug for treating the patient's condition?

A. Lung
B. Kidney
C. Parathyroid glands
D. Small intestine
E. Bone

Questions: V-6 Drugs for Diabetes Mellitus

Directions for questions **1–7**

Match each antidiabetic drug with the appropriate description (each lettered option can be selected once, more than once, or not at all).

A. Chlorpropamide
B. Exenatide
C. Insulin glargine
D. Glyburide
E. Insulin lispro
F. Metformin
G. Miglitol
H. NPH insulin
I. Regular insulin
L. Repaglinide
M. Pioglitazone
N. Sitagliptin

Difficulty level: Easy

1. An insulin preparation with a very fast onset of action

Difficulty level: Easy

2. Insulin preparation that can be used for intravenous administration

Difficulty level: Easy

3. A dipeptidyl peptidase inhibitor

Difficulty level: Easy

4. An inhibitor of an enzyme located on the brush border of the intestinal epithelium

Difficulty level: Easy

5. This noninsulin drug regulates transcription of several insulin-responsive genes.

Difficulty level: Easy

6. A drug used to treat both diabetes mellitus and diabetes insipidus

Difficulty level: Easy

7. Insulin preparation with no peak effect

Difficulty level: Easy

8. A 44-year-old man with type 1 diabetes started an intensive therapy to achieve a tight control of his diabetes. Which of the following complications will the man be at greatest increased risk of experiencing?

A. Loss of vision
B. Hypertension
C. Nephropathy
D. Hypoglycemia
E. Weigh loss
F. Allergic reactions

Difficulty level: Easy

9. A 22-year-old woman with type 1 diabetes was brought unconscious to the emergency department. Her blood glucose level was 395 mg/dL (normal 70–110 mg/dL). An intravenous infusion of insulin was started, and 6 hours later the patient's blood glucose decreased to a normal level. Which of the following molecular actions most likely contributed to the therapeutic effect of the drug in the patient's disorder?

A. Inhibition of glucose transporters in pancreas cell membranes
B. Phosphorylation of a tyrosine kinase–linked receptor
C. Activation of adenosine triphosphate (ATP)–sensitive K^+ channels in target cells
D. Stimulation of hormone-sensitive lipase
E. Inhibition of liver glucokinase

Difficulty level: Hard

10. A 17-year-old girl was admitted to the emergency department following a motor vehicle accident. She was obtunded and responded only to pain. Medical history obtained from her mother was unremarkable. Physical examination showed a patient with contusions on her face and arms but no signs of cranial trauma. Vital signs were temperature 97°F (36.1°C), blood pressure 105/70 mm Hg, pulse 112 bpm, respirations 22/min. Pertinent serum values were bicarbonate 6 mEq/L (normal 22–28 mEq/L), glucose 847 mg/dL (normal 70–110 mg/dL), creatinine 1.1 mg/dL (normal 0.6–1.2 mg/dL). Urinalysis showed the following: specific gravity 1.036, glucose 4+, ketones 4+. Which of the following correctly pairs the most likely patient disorder with the appropriate emergency treatment?

A. Diabetic hyperosmolar coma/intravenous (IV) regular insulin

B. Acute renal failure/furosemide

C. Posttraumatic liver failure/IV acetylcysteine

D. Respiratory acidosis/IV bicarbonate infusion

E. Diabetic ketoacidosis/IV regular insulin

Difficulty level: Easy

11. A 24-year-old obese woman in her 26th week of pregnancy was diagnosed with gestational diabetes mellitus after a positive glucose tolerance test. She was otherwise healthy, and her past medical history was unremarkable. Dietary management failed to control the blood glucose, and her physician decided to prescribe antidiabetic therapy. Which of the following drugs would be most appropriate for the patient at this time?

A. Glyburide

B. Metformin

C. Repaglinide

D. Insulin

E. Sitagliptin

Difficulty level: Easy

12. A 60-year-old woman with a long history of severe type 2 diabetes had been taking multiple daily injections of insulin, including an insulin glargine preparation. Which of the following sets of properties (from A to E) best describes the time course of effects of this preparation?

Set	Onset of Effect (h)	Peak Effect (h)	Duration of Effect (h)
A	1–2	6–10	12
B	0.25	2–3	3–5
C	0.25	No peak	3–5
D	1–4	6–10	12
E	1–4	No peak	24

Difficulty level: Easy

13. A 7-year-old boy was brought to the emergency department by his parents because of nausea, vomiting, and persistent abdominal pain secondary to the flu. Medical history of the patient was unremarkable. Pertinent serum values on admission were fasting blood glucose 300 mg/dL (70–110 mg/dL), glycosuria 3+. Which of the following drugs would be appropriate for this patient?

A. Regular insulin

B. Metformin

C. Pioglitazone

D. Repaglinide

E. Miglitol

F. Glyburide

Difficulty level: Medium.

14. An 11-year-old boy recently diagnosed with type 1 diabetes started insulin therapy. Which of the following insulin regimens (from A to E) would be appropriate for the chronic therapy of this boy?

Regimen	Before			
	Breakfast	Lunch	Supper	Bedtime
A	Lispro	Lispro	Lispro	Glargine
B	Regular	–	–	Lispro
C	NPH	Lispro	NPH	Lispro
D	Lispro	Regular	–	Regular
E	Glargine	–	–	–

Abbreviation: NPH, neutral protamine Hagedorn, or isophane insulin.

Difficulty level: Medium

15. A 42-year-old woman recently diagnosed with lupus erythematosus started a treatment with a high daily dose of prednisone. The woman had a history of type 1 diabetes currently controlled with two daily administrations of premixed insulin. Which of the following changes in the patient's antidiabetic regimen should be made at this time?

A. Decrease the daily insulin dosage.

B. Increase the daily insulin dosage.

C. Add glyburide to the antidiabetic regimen.

D. Add exenatide to the antidiabetic regimen.

E. Add sitagliptin to the antidiabetic regimen.

Difficulty level: Easy

16. A 16-year-old boy suffering from type 1 diabetes was admitted to the emergency department with the chief complaint of severe right-sided chest pain. Two hours earlier, he felt feverish and experienced a teeth-chattering chill. The patient's diabetes was well controlled on two daily administrations of premixed insulin. The patient was also very compliant with his prescribed diet. After physical examination and laboratory tests, a diagnosis of atypical pneumonia was made. Which of the following changes in the patient's treatment should be appropriate at this time?

A. Increase the daily insulin dosage.

B. Start a course of ampicillin therapy.

C. Add a daily administration of chlorpropamide.

D. Start a course of vancomycin therapy.

E. Add a daily administration of metformin.

Difficulty level: Easy

17. A 55-year-old woman suffering from type 2 diabetes had started treatment with metformin, but the drug was poorly tolerated, and her physician decided to shift to repaglinide. Which of the following actions most likely mediated the therapeutic effect of repaglinide in the patient's disease?

A. Decreased glucose absorption from the gastrointestinal tract

B. Blockade of glucagon receptors

C. Blockade of β_2 receptors in the liver

D. Blockade of somatostatin receptors in the pancreas

E. Stimulation of insulin release

F. Regulation of transcription of genes involved in glucose utilization

Difficulty level: Easy

18. An 8-year-old girl diagnosed with type 1 diabetes began treatment with insulin. Which of the following actions on lipid metabolism most likely occurred in this patient after starting the therapy?

A. Increased lipid breakdown by the liver

B. Decreased triglyceride storage in fat tissue

C. Increased triglyceride synthesis

D. Decreased synthesis of lipoprotein lipase

E. Increased activity of hormone-sensitive lipase

Difficulty level: Easy

19. A 59-year-old man suffering from type 2 diabetes had been receiving an oral antidiabetic therapy that included a drug that closes adenosine triphosphate (ATP)–sensitive K+ channels on pancreatic β-cell membranes. Which of the following drugs most likely uses this mechanism of action?

A. Acarbose

B. Insulin

C. Glyburide

D. Metformin

E. Exenatide

F. Pioglitazone

Difficulty level: Medium

20. A 78-year-old man was brought to the emergency room exhibiting bizarre behavior and paranoid ideation. He complained of headache, mental confusion, weakness, dizziness, and blurred vision. The man was suffering from type 2 diabetes, which was being treated with an oral antidiabetic drug. Pertinent serum values on admission were creatinine 1.8 mg/dL (normal 0.6–1.2 mg/dL), glucose 50 mg/dL (normal 70–110 mg/dL). Which of the following drugs most likely caused the patient's signs and symptoms?

A. Metformin

B. Pioglitazone

C. Glyburide

D. Acarbose

E. Exenatide

Difficulty level: Easy

21. A 52-year-old alcoholic man was brought unconscious to the emergency department. On admission, the patient was sweating, his body temperature was 94.5°F (34.7°C), and his cardiac pulse was 135 bpm. Shortly after admission, the patient developed a tonic-clonic seizure. His wife reported the man was a diabetic on insulin therapy. Which of the following disorders most likely caused the patient's syndrome?

A. Hyperglycemia due to insulin resistance

B. Hypoglycemia due to alcohol consumption

C. Ketoacidosis due to insufficient insulin therapy

D. Hyperglycemia due to alcohol withdrawal

E. Anaphylactic reaction to insulin

F. Hyperosmolar coma due to alcohol overdose

Difficulty level: Easy

22. A 12-year-old boy diagnosed with type 1 diabetes started a treatment with insulin. Which of the following sets of effects on the liver most likely contributed to the therapeutic effect of the drug in the patient's disease?

Set	Glycolysis	Gluconeogenesis	Glycogenolysis
A	↑	0	↓
B	↑	↓	↓
C	↓	0	0
D	0	↑	↑
E	↑	↑	↓

Note: ↑, increased; ↓, decreased; 0, no change.

Difficulty level: Easy

23. A 56-year-old man was found to have the following serum values during a routine clinic visit: fasting blood glucose 146 mg/dL (normal 70–110 mg/dL), glycated hemoglobin (HbA1c) 7.4% (normal 6%), total cholesterol 160 mg/dL (normal < 200 mg/dL). The patient had been suffering from type 2 diabetes for 6 years, and his disease was well controlled with diet and metformin until the most recent visit. The patient was otherwise healthy, and physical examination was unremarkable. All tests were confirmed in a second exam. Which of the following would be the most appropriate next step in the management of the patient's disease?

A. Add glyburide to the current regimen.
B. Substitute metformin with pioglitazone.
C. Substitute metformin with repaglinide.
D. Substitute metformin with insulin.
E. Add lovastatin to the current regimen.

Difficulty level: Easy

24. A 59-year-old woman recently diagnosed with type 2 diabetes started a therapy with diet and metformin. Which of the following actions most likely mediated the therapeutic effect of the drug in the patient's disease?

A. Blockade of adenosine triphosphate (ATP)–sensitive K⁺ channels
B. Blockade of glucagon receptors
C. Activation of glucagon-like polypeptide-1 (GLP-1) receptors
D. Activation of adenosine monophosphate (AMP)–activated protein kinase
E. Inhibition of metabolism of incretin hormones

Difficulty level: Easy

25. A 56-year-old woman was recently diagnosed with type 2 diabetes. Her medical history was significant for a serious allergic reaction to sulfamethoxazole and for recurrent urinary tract infections presently treated with ciprofloxacin. An appropriate therapy was prescribed that included a strict diet and an oral antidiabetic drug. Which of the following drugs would be contraindicated for this patient?

A. Glyburide
B. Metformin
C. Repaglinide
D. Acarbose
E. Pioglitazone

Difficulty level: Easy

26. A 78-year-old woman with type 2 diabetes was brought unconscious to the emergency department. Her husband stated that the woman took several pills of her antidiabetic medication in a suicide attempt. On admission, vital signs were blood pressure 134/90, pulse 80 bpm, respirations 22/min. Laboratory data showed an anion gap of 24 mmol/L (normal < 12 mmol/L), plasma lactate of 6 mmol/L (normal 0.5–1.5 mmol/L), creatinine 3.2 mg/dL (normal 0.6–1.2.0 mg/dL), and arterial blood pH 7.24 (normal 7.35–7.45). Which of the following drugs most likely caused the patient's signs and symptoms?

A. Glucagon
B. Metformin
C. Repaglinide
D. Insulin
E. Glyburide
F. Pioglitazone

Difficulty level: Medium

27. A 57-year-old obese man was diagnosed with type 2 diabetes mellitus. The patient had been suffering from chronic obstructive pulmonary disease for 5 years and from hypertension for 3 years. His current therapy included ipratropium and captopril. Which of the following antidiabetic drugs would be relatively contraindicated in this patient?

A. Acarbose
B. Metformin
C. Sitagliptin
D. Repaglinide
E. Glyburide

Difficulty level: Easy

28. A 51-year-old man with a long history of severe type 2 diabetes had been on a pharmacotherapy that involved two different insulin formulations. Several available insulin formulations differ from one another primarily because of which of the following pharmacokinetic properties?

A. Rate of absorption
B. Elimination half-lives
C. Total clearance
D. Volume of distribution
E. Oral bioavailability

Difficulty level: Easy

29. A 66-year-old man suffering from type 2 diabetes had been receiving a combination therapy with metformin and glyburide, but 2 months later lab exams indicated that the control of his diabetes was inadequate. His physician decided to add pioglitazone to the treatment regimen. Which of the following molecular actions most likely mediated the therapeutic effect of the added drug in the patient's disease?

A. Slowing glucose absorption from the gastrointestinal tract
B. Blockade of K⁺ channels in pancreatic β-cell membranes
C. Inhibition of incretin hormone metabolism
D. Activation of glucagon-like polypeptide-1 (GLP-1) receptors
E. Activation of adenosine monophosphate (AMP)–activated protein kinase
F. Regulation of transcription of genes related to glucose utilization

Difficulty level: Easy

30. A 54-year-old man complained to his physician of an annoying dry cough over the past few days and an unexpected weight gain over the past few weeks. The patient had been suffering from type 2 diabetes for 3 years, presently controlled with a combination of oral antidiabetic agents. Physical examination showed evident peripheral edema, mild jugular venous distention, and rales on both lungs. Which of the following drugs most likely caused the patient's signs and symptoms?

A. Acarbose
B. Metformin
C. Glyburide
D. Pioglitazone
E. Exenatide

Difficulty level: Easy

31. A 65-year-old obese man was in his physician's office for a routine visit. The patient had been suffering from type 2 diabetes for 1 year, and the disease was reasonably well controlled with diet and metformin. Physical examination showed that body mass index was increased about 40% from the last visit, and abdominal obesity was evident. Vital signs of the patient were blood pressure 150/90 mm Hg, pulse 85 bpm, respirations 14/min. Further laboratory tests showed the following serum values: fasting glucose 155 mg/dL (normal 70–110 mg/dL), fasting insulin 60 IU/mL (normal 5–20 IU/mL), total cholesterol 340 mg/dL (normal > 200 mg/dL). The patient was most likely suffering from which of the following pathologic conditions?

A. Lactic acidosis
B. Hypoglycemic reaction
C. Unstable angina
D. Diabetic ketoacidosis
E. Insulin resistance

Difficulty level: Medium

32. A 70-year-old man was admitted to the hospital because of anorexia, nausea and vomiting, and an unpleasant taste in his mouth for the past 12 hours. The man had been suffering from type 2 diabetes for 10 years and was being treated with metformin and sitagliptin. He also had a long history of hypertension and hypercholesterolemia, currently controlled with losartan, nifedipine, and lovastatin. Pertinent laboratory serum levels on admission were fasting blood glucose 115 mg/dL (normal 70–110), creatinine 3.4 mg/dL (normal 0.6–1.2 mg/dL), blood urea nitrogen (BUN) 42 mg/dL (normal 7–18 mg/dL), high-density lipoprotein (HDL) cholesterol 85 mg/dL (normal < 100 mg/dL). Taking into account the patient's history and symptoms, which of the following drugs should be removed from his current therapeutic regimen?

A. Losartan
B. Nifedipine
C. Lovastatin
D. Sitagliptin
E. Metformin

Difficulty level: Easy

33. A 47-year-old obese woman was found to have the following serum levels during a routine clinic visit: fasting blood glucose 122 mg/dL (normal 70–110 mg/dL), triglycerides 390 mg/dL (normal < 150 mg/dL), total cholesterol 220 mg/dL (normal < 200 mg/dL), glycated hemoglobin (HbA1c) 6.1% (normal < 6%). Past history of the patient was unremarkable, and the woman had no significant symptoms. Which of the following would be the most appropriate pharmacotherapy for this patient?

A. Insulin
B. Metformin
C. Miglitol
D. Glyburide
E. Exenatide

Difficulty level: Easy

34. A 7-year-old boy diagnosed with type 1 diabetes started a treatment with insulin. Which of the following actions on glucose metabolism most likely occurred in this patient after starting the therapy?

A. Increased liver glucose uptake
B. Increased glycogen synthase activity
C. Decreased glucose-6-phosphate synthesis
D. Decreased glucokinase activity
E. Decreased glycerol synthesis

Difficulty level: Easy

35. A 62-year-old woman recently diagnosed with type 2 diabetes started a therapy that included acarbose. Inhibition of which of the following enzymes most likely mediated the therapeutic effect of the drug in the patient's disease?

A. Pyruvate carboxylase
B. Alpha-glucosidase
C. Glucokinase
D. Hormone-sensitive lipase
E. Acyltransferase

Difficulty level: Easy

36. A 50-year-old obese woman with type 2 diabetes was found to have inadequate control of her disease 2 months after starting therapy with metformin and glyburide. The physician decided to add exenatide to the treatment regimen. Which of the following molecular actions most likely mediated the therapeutic effect of the added drug in the patient's disease?

A. Inhibition of dipeptidyl peptidase-4
B. Inhibition of α-glucosidase
C. Activation of adenosine monophosphate (AMP)–activated protein kinase
D. Activation of glucagon-like polypeptide-1 (GLP-1) receptors
E. Activation of adenosine triphosphate (ATP)–sensitive K⁺ channels
F. Phosphorylation of tyrosine kinase receptor

Difficulty level: Easy

37. A 13-year-old boy with type 1 diabetes received his morning injection of a mixture of insulin lispro and glargine. A few hours later, he was found unconscious in his room. His heart rate was 120 bpm and body temperature 94.7°F (34.8°C), and tetanic contractions of skeletal muscles were present. Which of the following would be the immediate appropriate treatment for this patient?

A. Regular insulin intravenous
B. Oral glucose
C. Glucagon intramuscular (IM)
D. Oral metformin
E. Exenatide IM
F. Epinephrine IM

Difficulty level: Easy

38. A 63-year-old obese man complained to his physician of flatulence, belching, diarrhea, and abdominal pain soon after starting an appropriate oral therapy for type 2 diabetes. The disease was diagnosed after the man was found to have a fasting blood glucose level of 170 mg/dL, and subsequent lab exams revealed decreased glucose tolerance and fasting hyperglycemia. Which of the following drugs most likely caused the patient's symptoms?

A. Regular insulin
B. Glyburide
C. Miglitol
D. Metformin
E. Repaglinide
F. Pioglitazone

Difficulty level: Easy

39. A 48-year-old obese man complained of frequent thirst and polyuria. His past history included serious angioedema apparently due to an allergic reaction to sulfonamide therapy. In the past he tried many times to control his diet without success. A fasting plasma glucose level was found to be 180 mg/dL (normal 70–110 mg/dL). Which of the following would be an appropriate treatment for this patient?

A. Strict dietary control
B. Chlorpropamide
C. Metformin
D. NPH (neutral protamine Hagedorn) insulin
E. Insulin lispro

Difficulty level: Easy

40. A 6-year-old girl diagnosed with type 1 diabetes started a treatment with insulin. Which of the following actions on protein metabolism most likely occurred in this patient after starting the therapy?

A. Stimulation of protein synthesis in the liver
B. Stimulation of protein catabolism in the liver
C. Inhibition of protein synthesis in muscle cells
D. Increased conversion of keto acids into amino acids
E. Decreased amino acid transport into cells

Answers and Explanations: V-1 Drugs for Hypothalamic and Pituitary Disorders

Questions 1–6

1. **C**
2. **F**
3. **J**
4. **H**
5. **G**
6. **B**

Learning objective: Explain the molecular mechanism of action of oxytocin.

7. **B** Oxytocin causes sustained contraction of uterine smooth muscle. Because calcium is needed to contract muscle cells, the activated signaling pathway must lead to increased intracellular calcium. This is brought about by a receptor-mediated activation of phospholipase C that splits by hydrolysis the phosphatidylinositol 4,5-biphosphate into two second messengers, inositol triphosphate (IP_3) and diacylglycerol (DAG). IP_3 triggers the release of calcium from storage vesicles, whereas DAG activates protein kinase C, an enzyme with a vast array of physiological effects, including smooth muscle contraction.

A, C–E Although the activation of these signaling pathways can in some cases cause increased intracellular calcium, the activation of the phosphoinositide pathway remains the most important trigger for intracellular calcium increase in smooth muscle cells.

Learning objective: Identify the site of action of octreotide.

8. **B** Octreotide is a somatostatin analogue that acts by activating receptors located in several organs, including the pituitary, pancreas, and gastrointestinal tract, and some types of tumors. In this patient, octreotide activates receptors located on somatotroph cells of the pituitary. This activation decreases the release of growth hormone, thus improving the patient's signs and symptoms.

A, D, E See correct answer explanation.

C Somatostatin receptors are also located on these cells, and their activation can inhibit the secretion of thyrotropin, but this inhibition is not the reason for the therapeutic effect of the drug in this patient.

Learning objective: Identify the drugs used for controlled ovarian hyperstimulation.

9. **C** Controlled ovarian hyperstimulation is used to stimulate the development of multiple ovarian follicles during a single cycle, resulting in the release of a larger than normal number of eggs that can be used for in vitro fertilization. In most cases,

a follicle-stimulating hormone (FSH) preparation is administered for 7 to 12 days, starting the third day after menstruation. Spontaneous ovulation during the cycle is typically prevented by daily subcutaneous injection of leuprolide or daily nasal application of nafarelin.

A, B, D, E See correct answer explanation.

Learning objective: Describe the adverse effects of leuprolide.

10. **D** Pharmacologic therapy and surgery are both effective in relieving most symptoms of endometriosis. Oral contraceptives or nonsteroidal antiinflammatory drugs are recommended as first-line therapy, but gonadotropin-releasing hormone (GnRH) agonists can be employed in women for whom the first-line agents are inadequate. Leuprolide, goserelin, and nafarelin are GnRH agonists approved by the U.S. Food and Drug Administration for this purpose. Continuous administration of these drugs inhibits the release of follicle-stimulating hormone (FSH) and luteinizing hormone (LH) from the pituitary, resulting in a hypoestrogenic state. Adverse effects of the GnRH therapy are similar to those of menopause, and hot flushes are very common (more than 80% with leuprolide).

A–C, E These are all adverse effects of estrogens. Therefore, they are unlikely in a hypoestrogenic patient.

Learning objective: Identify the drug used to control flushing in carcinoid syndrome.

11. **D** Carcinoid syndrome develops in some people with endocrinologically active malignant tumors that develop from enterochromaffin cells located mostly in the ileum, and (rarely) in other organs. Carcinoid syndrome is characterized by cutaneous flushing, abdominal cramps, and diarrhea. Flushing is the most common and often the earliest sign, occurring in more than 90% of patients. The syndrome results from vasoactive substances, including serotonin, bradykinin, histamine, and prostaglandins, secreted by the tumor. Resection of primary lung carcinoid is often curative. Somatostatin can reduce symptoms caused by a variety of hormone-secreting tumors, and octreotide, a long-acting somatostatin analogue, is a first-line agent to control flushing in carcinoid syndrome. Octreotide given before surgery is also the best drug to avoid carcinoid crisis, a dangerous condition that can occur during surgery, likely due to manipulation of the tumor. It is characterized by a profound drop in blood pressure, causing shock, sometimes accompanied by prolonged severe flushing, bronchospasm, and hemodynamic instability.

A–C, E See correct answer explanation.

Learning objective: Outline the therapeutic use of cabergoline in acromegaly.

12. **D** The woman was most likely suffering from acromegaly, as high serum levels of insulin-like growth factor 1 (IGF-1) are highly specific for acromegaly and correlate with clinical indexes of disease activity. Radiation therapy was contraindicated in this patient because modern pacemakers using metal oxide conductors are sensitive to radiation. Dopamine D_2 agonists such as cabergoline have been shown to reduce IGF-1 and growth hormone levels in about 50% of patients with acromegaly, when given alone, even in patients with normal prolactin levels. Moreover, they enhance the action of somatostatin analogues such as octreotide. Therefore, they are often added when octreotide alone is not fully effective, as in this case (see high levels of IGF-1). The reason for the effectiveness of D_2 agonists in acromegaly is still uncertain, but it is notable that dopamine appears to inhibit growth hormone–releasing hormone (GH-RH) release, and also that of the anterior pituitary hormones, growth hormone is most similar to prolactin.

    A–C, E See correct answer explanation.

Learning objective: Outline the diagnostic uses of thyrotropin-releasing hormone.

13. **B** The signs and symptoms of the patient suggest she was affected by hypothyroidism, which is confirmed by the low free thyroxine (FT_4) serum levels. The fact that thyroid-stimulating hormone (TSH) was low suggests that hypothyroidism was not primary (i.e., due to failure of the thyroid itself) but secondary (i.e., due to pituitary failure) or tertiary (i.e., due to hypothalamic failure). A thyrotropin-releasing hormone (TRH) test can be useful to clarify the diagnosis, although it is not often done. After TRH challenge, TSH will be increased if the source is hypothalamic failure, whereas it will not be increased in pituitary failure.

    A, C These diseases would cause primary hypothyroidism, as the thyroid itself cannot synthesize thyroid hormones.

    D Graves disease causes hyperthyroidism, not hypothyroidism.

    E See correct answer explanation.

Learning objective: Outline the diagnostic uses of adrenocorticotropic hormone (ACTH).

14. **C** The signs and symptoms of the patient suggest the diagnosis of Addison disease, which in the United States is mainly due to idiopathic atrophy of the adrenal cortex, probably caused by autoimmune processes. ACTH is currently used to establish the diagnosis by demonstrating failure to increase serum cortisol levels upon administration of the hormone.

    A, B, D–F See correct answer explanation.

Learning objective: Outline the therapeutic uses of vasopressin.

15. **E** The patient was likely suffering from liver cirrhosis, which caused an acute variceal hemorrhage secondary to portal hypertension. Esophageal varices represent a consequence of collaterals that develop in cirrhosis to shunt blood from the portal system (which is obstructed, usually at the level of sinusoids) into the systemic circulation. A consequence of this is that the perfusion pressure of the hepatic artery is partly transmitted into the portal vein, thus increasing the portal pressure. Endoscopic sclerotherapy is the procedure of choice to control acute bleeding. Pharmacologic agents can also be administered to decrease portal pressure. Most experience has been with vasopressin, a nonselective, very powerful vasoconstrictor that directly constricts mesenteric arterioles and decreases portal venous inflow, thereby reducing portal pressure. Other drugs used for the same purpose are nonselective β-blockers and octreotide.

    A, B Adrenaline and albuterol are β_2 stimulants. The β_2 receptor–mediated vasodilation would increase, not decrease, hepatic blood flow.

    C, D Nifedipine and prazosin can reduce the systemic blood pressure but would have unpredictable effects on the perfusion pressure of liver arterial vessels.

Learning objective: Explain the mechanism of action of octreotide.

16. **B** The diagnosis of pituitary adenoma and the high level of insulin-like growth factor 1 indicate that the patient was most likely suffering from acromegaly. Octreotide is a somatostatin analogue that effectively inhibits the secretion of growth hormone and represents a common treatment of acromegaly when radiation therapy is contraindicated or not effective, as in this case.

    A, D, E Somatostatin does not have these effects

    C Somatostatin can inhibit insulin release, but this is not the cause of the therapeutic effect of the drug in acromegaly.

Learning objective: Describe the adverse effects of somatropin.

17. **A** Arthralgias are the most common adverse effects of somatropin therapy in adults, being present in up to 23% of patients. They are likely related to the stimulation of chondrogenesis and skeletal growth that is mediated by insulin-like growth factor 1.

    B–E Growth hormone tends to cause actions opposite to those listed.

Learning objective: Explain the mechanism of action of chorionic gonadotropin when used to treat oligospermia.

18. **A** Human chorionic gonadotropin (hCG) is produced by human placenta and extracted from the urine of pregnant women. The structure and actions of hCG are practically identical to those of luteinizing hormone, the hormone that in men stimulates the Leydig cell secretion of testosterone, which is needed for normal growth and division of germinal cells in forming sperm.

    B The drug is not a testosterone agonist.

    C The hypothalamic secretion of gonadotropin-releasing hormone is inhibited by testosterone.

    D The production of prostatic fluid is stimulated by dihydrotestosterone.

    E The mitotic activity of Sertoli cells is stimulated by follicle-stimulating hormone.

Learning objective: Outline the therapeutic uses of goserelin.

19. **B** Goserelin is a synthetic analogue of naturally occurring gonadotropin-releasing hormone (GnRH). The hormone is physiologically released in pulses that vary in frequency in different phases of the menstrual cycle and control the synthesis and release of follicle-stimulating hormone (FSH) and luteinizing hormone (LH) in both women and men. Because the release of GnRH is pulsatile, the secretion of FSH and LH is also pulsatile, which is essential for the maintenance of normal ovulatory menstrual cycles and the normal production of sperm. However, when given continuously (or as a depot preparation), GnRH inhibits the release of FSH and LH in both men and women. This inhibition causes suppression of ovulation in women and cessation of testicular androgen synthesis in men. The synthetic analogues of GnRH are currently used alone or in combination with an antiandrogen in the pharmacotherapy of advanced prostate cancer.

    A, C–E See correct answer explanation.

Learning objective: Outline the adverse effects of octreotide.

20. **A** A major undesirable effect that can occur as a result of octreotide therapy is reduction of bile production and gallbladder contractility, which leads to increased viscosity of bile and increased incidence of gallstones. This can occur in up to 30% of patients after 6 months of treatment.

    B The drug does not efficiently cross the blood–brain barrier, so drowsiness is unlikely.

    C Because the drug can inhibit insulin secretion, hypoglycemia is rare.

    D The drug can inhibit thyrotropin secretion, which can lead to hypothyroidism. This in turn can lead to cold, not heat, intolerance.

    E In patients with carcinoid tumor, the drug can effectively reduce, not cause, flushing.

Learning objective: Identify the drug to be used to treat precocious puberty.

21. **F** True precocious puberty is the most frequent endocrine symptom of hypothalamic disease. The pathophysiology of the disorder is related to an activation of the hypothalamic-pituitary-gonadal axis. The therapy is to suppress pituitary gonadotropin secretion until an appropriate age for normal puberty to begin. Continuous administration of a gonadotropin-releasing hormone (GnRH) analogue such as leuprolide (intravenous infusion or depot formulation) inhibits follicle-stimulating hormone and luteinizing hormone secretion (due to receptor desensitization or downregulation) and will shut down the stimulation of ovarian function. The treatment is fully reversible, and normal function will resume when therapy is stopped.

    A–E See correct answer explanation.

Learning objective: Identify the drug that acts as a gonadotropin-releasing hormone (GnRH) antagonist.

22. **A** Degarelix is a synthetic decapeptide that functions as competitive antagonist at GnRH receptors. It reduces concentrations of gonadotropins and androgens more rapidly than GnRH agonists and avoids the initial testosterone surge seen with those drugs. Degarelix is approved for the treatment of symptomatic advanced prostate cancer.

    B–E See correct answer explanation.

Learning objective: Identify the drug used to treat Turner syndrome.

23. **B** Treatment with growth hormone (somatropin) has been shown to have a strong beneficial effect on final height in girls with Turner syndrome, the most common sex chromosome anomaly in females. Continuous chronic treatment of these girls can increase the mean stature by 10 to 12 cm.

    A Oxandrolone can increase the growth rate in girls with Turner syndrome, but the increase is limited (5 cm), and the drug is not currently used to treat Turner syndrome.

    C–F All of these drugs are useless, or even dangerous, in Turner syndrome.

Learning objective: Outline the therapeutic uses of mecasermin.

24. **C** Laron syndrome (also called Laron dwarfism) is an autosomal recessive disorder characterized by growth hormone insensitivity (also referred to as primary insulin-like growth factor 1 [IGF-1] deficiency) caused by a variant of growth hormone receptor. Because of this, growth hormone serum levels are normal or increased, but the hormone is ineffective. A major consequence of this insensitivity is extremely low serum levels of IGF-1, leading to severe impairment of growth. Recently, recombinant IGF-1 (mecasermin) was

approved by the U.S. Food and Drug Administration for dwarfism due to growth hormone insensitivity. Although the number of children treated with the drug is low (the disease is very rare), all data show a good increment of growth rate with mecasermin during the first year of treatment.

A, B, D, E See correct answer explanation.

Learning objective: Outline the therapeutic uses of antidiuretic hormone (ADH) antagonists.

25. **E** The patient was most likely suffering from syndrome of inappropriate antidiuretic hormone secretion (SIADH), a disorder characterized by low serum osmolality, high urine osmolality with respect to serum, and hypervolemic (or sometimes normovolemic) hyponatremia. SIADH is caused by an increased secretion of ADH, which is associated with a myriad of disorders, including malignancy, intracranial pathology (encephalitis, meningitis, subarachnoid hemorrhage, etc.), hormonal deficiency states (adrenal and thyroid insufficiency), and metabolic diseases (acute intermittent porphyria). The exact mechanism whereby these disorders provoke an increase in concentration of ADH is uncertain, but this patient was suffering from small-cell lung cancer, which is known to synthesize ADH de novo. Treatment modalities of SIADH depend on the underlying cause. In cases where this cause is untreatable, water restriction and ADH antagonists (conivaptan and tolvaptan) are the treatment of choice. These drugs block vasopressin receptors, causing reversible nephrogenic diabetes insipidus.

A, B These diuretics tend to cause hyponatremia and are therefore contraindicated in SIADH.

C ADH agonists (vasopressin and desmopressin) are contraindicated, as the syndrome is caused by an excessive ADH secretion.

D Glucocorticoids are useless, as SIADH secretion is not due to adrenal insufficiency (see the normal serum levels of K^+).

Learning objective: Describe the therapeutic use of octreotide in acromegaly.

26. **D** The patient's signs and symptoms indicate that he was affected by acromegaly due to pituitary adenoma, which is the cause of the disease in virtually all patients affected by acromegaly. Somatostatin can reduce growth hormone (GH) levels and symptoms in acromegaly, and octreotide (a somatostatin analogue) is frequently used for this purpose. The drug is 40 times more potent than somatostatin in blocking GH secretion but only twice as potent in blocking insulin secretion, and is therefore more suitable than the natural hormone to treat acromegaly.

A–C, E See correct answer explanation.

Learning objective: Outline the therapeutic uses of pegvisomant.

27. **A** The high serum levels of insulin-like growth factor 1 (IGF-1) are highly specific for acromegaly and correlate with clinical indices of disease activity. They are the simplest way to monitor the response to therapy, as they do not fluctuate like growth hormone levels do. The fact that IGF-1 levels are still elevated in this patient indicates that the therapy with octreotide was not completely effective. Pegvisomant is a growth hormone receptor antagonist. The drug is particularly useful in patients resistant to somatostatin analogues because it has been shown that it can normalize the high serum levels of IGF-1 in these patients.

B–E See correct answer explanation.

Learning objective: Identify the drug used to treat prolactinoma.

28. **F** The signs and symptoms of the patient indicate that she is most likely affected by prolactinoma, the most common secretory tumor in the pituitary. Dopamine agonists such as cabergoline and bromocriptine are widely used as first-line agents. By activating D_2 receptors in the pituitary, these drugs mimic the effect of dopamine to inhibit the secretion of prolactin. They can restore abnormal menstrual function in up to 90% of women, shrink prolactinomas, and improve galactorrhea and tumor-associated headache.

A–E See correct answer explanation.

Learning objective: Identify the enzyme whose synthesis is promoted by follicle-stimulating hormone (FSH).

29. **E** Follitropin alfa is recombinant follicle-stimulating hormone (FSH). It activates specific receptors that act via the adenylyl cyclase pathway to stimulate the granulosa cells of the ovary to produce aromatase. This enzyme (also called estrogen synthase) is a key step in biosynthesis of estrogens. It converts androstenedione to estrone and testosterone to estradiol. A "step-up" protocol of ovulation induction mimics the natural menstrual cycle. Increasing doses of FSH are given during the first half of the cycle to promote follicular development. Then an injection of human chorionic gonadotropin is administered to simulate the luteinizing hormone surge that naturally occurs in midcycle and triggers ovulation.

A–D See correct answer explanation.

Learning objective: Describe the therapeutic use of octreotide in vipoma tumor.

30. **D** Octreotide is a somatostatin analogue. When given in pharmacological amounts, somatostatin inhibits virtually all exocrine and endocrine secretions of the pancreas (insulin, glucagon, and pancreatic enzymes), stomach (gastrin), and intestine (secretin, motilin, vasoactive intestinal polypeptide [VIP], gastric inhibitory polypeptide [GIP], and serotonin), as well as secretion of growth hormone, thyroid-stimulating hormone, parathyroid hormone, calcitonin, and adrenocorticotropic hormone. Because of this, octreotide is used to reduce symptoms caused by a variety of hormone-secreting tumors. Vipoma is a rare VIP-secreting tumor of non-β pancreatic islet cells, causing a syndrome of prolonged, massive watery diarrhea, hypokalemia, and achlorhydria (WDHA syndrome). Octreotide effectively controls the diarrhea in most patients, but large doses may be needed.

A–C, E, F See correct answer explanation.

Learning objective: Outline the therapeutic uses of desmopressin.

31. **C** Polyuria and nocturia, with low urine osmolality, suggest the diagnosis of diabetes insipidus (DI). The previous basal skull fracture indicates that the DI is most likely related to a trauma of the pituitary stalk, and the undetectable serum antidiuretic hormone (ADH) levels confirms that the DI is neurogenic in nature. Desmopressin is the agent of choice in this disease. Unlike vasopressin, its vasoconstricting activity is negligible, as it activates only V_2 receptors.

A Thiazide diuretics paradoxically reduce polyuria both in central and nephrogenic DI (likely because of volume contraction, leading to enhanced proximal reabsorption), but they are not used in central DI, where a much better therapeutic choice exists.

B Amiloride is effective only in lithium-induced DI.

D, E Carbamazepine and chlorpropamide are ADH-releasing drugs used only when ADH secretion is not completely abolished (partial neurogenic DI) or when the patient cannot tolerate exogenous ADH.

Learning objective: Identify the main site of distribution of somatropin.

32. **C** Somatropin is a peptide hormone that is usually administered subcutaneously. Its molecular weight indicates that it is sufficiently small to be absorbed from the injection site by bulk flow transport and to leave the blood by the same transport system. However, it is too big to cross cell membranes. Therefore, it distributes primarily in the extracellular fluid. This is also indicated by the volume of distribution of the drug that is about 12 L.

A, B, D, E See correct answer explanation.

Learning objective: Describe the use of vasopressin in the treatment of vasodilatory shock.

33. **E** The patient's poor response to norepinephrine suggests that she was most likely suffering from septic shock that was catecholamine-resistant. Septic shock is a vasodilatory shock, and sepsis is a common cause of the disorder. Vasodilatory shock is characterized by low arterial blood pressure due to decreased systemic vascular resistance. Catecholamines are first-line agents for the therapy of vasodilatory shock, but loss of adrenergic sensitivity can occur due to multiple mechanisms, including downregulation of adrenoceptors, impairment of postreceptor signal pathways, and excessive production of nitric oxide and other inflammatory mediators. Mortality rates of vasodilatory shock are excessively high, and if the shock becomes catecholamine-resistant, mortality can be near 100%. Recently, several investigators have demonstrated that vasopressin can successfully stabilize hemodynamics even in advanced vasodilatory shock, and current guidelines suggest that vasopressin should be reserved for patients in whom adequate hemodynamic stabilization cannot be achieved with conventional therapy, as in this case.

A, C, D Because the shock is catecholamine-resistant, the use of these drugs may be dangerous by causing significant catecholamine toxicity.

B Desmopressin has negligible vasoconstricting activity because it activates only V_2 receptors.

DRUGS FOR HYPOTHALAMIC AND PITUITARY DISORDERS Answer key		
1. C	6. B	11. D
2. F	7. B	12. D
3. J	8. B	13. B
4. H	9. C	14. C
5. G	10. D	15. E
16. B	21. F	26. D
17. A	22. A	27. A
18. A	23. B	28. F
19. B	24. C	29. E
20. A	25. E	30. D
		31. C
		32. C
		33. E

Answers and Explanations: V-2 Drugs for Thyroid Disorders

Questions 1–3

1. **A**
2. **F**
3. **D**

Learning objective: Identify the serum level of free thyroxine (FT_4) and thyroid-stimulating hormone (TSH, thyrotropin) in a patient without functional thyroid after a few days of triiodothyronine treatment.

4. **D** Myxedema coma is a rare but serious consequence of long-standing uncorrected hypothyroidism. Despite aggressive therapy with large doses of thyroid hormones, mortality rates of 60 to 70% are common. Whether levothyroxine or triiodothyronine (T_3) is the drug of choice in myxedema coma is controversial. Although triiodothyronine is potentially more cardiotoxic, it is sometimes preferred because its more rapid onset can reverse coma faster and because deiodinase activity is markedly reduced in myxedema, thus impairing conversion of T_4 to T_3. In this patient, after a few days of triiodothyronine therapy, serum T_4 levels are low because of the disease, and thyrotropin (TSH) levels are low because of triiodothyronine negative feedback.

   A–C See correct answer explanation.

Learning objective: Identify the drug used first to treat levothyroxine poisoning.

5. **B** The patient's symptoms and the lab results indicated that he was suffering from drug-induced severe hyperthyroidism. A leading cause of death in thyroid hormone excess is related to the cardiovascular effects that can cause arrhythmias and acute myocardial ischemia due mainly to thyroid hormone–induced increased sensitivity of the sympathetic nervous system. Administration of a β-blocker can promptly counteract cardiovascular symptoms and may be lifesaving.

   A, C, D All of these drugs are used in severe thyroid hormone excess from any cause, but the administration of a β-blocker must be done first.

   E Radioactive iodine is not an emergency therapy.

Learning objective: Identify the correct percentage of levothyroxine (T_4) bound to plasma proteins.

6. **E** Most circulating T_3 and T_4 are bound to plasma proteins (about 75% to thyroxine-binding globulin, the rest to prealbumin and albumin). Only 0.4% T_3 and 0.04% T_4 are free. Therefore, the bound hormones represent a huge reservoir, which explains why, in a person with the thyroid gland destroyed by radioactive iodine, it takes 3 months to 1 year after radioactive treatment before hypothyroidism occurs, even though radioactive iodine disrupts hormone synthesis in a few days.

   A–D See correct answer explanation.

Learning objective: Identify the drug used in a newborn baby with neonatal hypothyroidism.

7. **C** The signs and symptoms of the baby suggest that he is suffering from neonatal hypothyroidism, which occurs in about 1/4000 live births. The most frequent cause is congenital absence of the thyroid gland, which requires lifelong therapy. Treatment with levothyroxine must be started immediately and closely monitored.

   A, B, D–F See correct answer explanation.

Learning objective: Identify the drug used in thyroid storm in an asthmatic patient.

8. **A** The signs and symptoms of the patient and the lab exams indicate that she is suffering from thyroid storm, a life-threatening syndrome characterized by the abrupt onset of the more florid symptoms of hyperthyroidism. An emergency treatment is mandatory and usually includes propranolol to control hypertension and tachycardia. When propranolol is contraindicated, as in this case, calcium channel blockers with cardiac activity (diltiazem or verapamil) can be used.

   B Radioactive iodine can be used for the long-term management of the disease but is not a drug for the emergency treatment of thyroid storm.

   C–F See correct answer explanation.

Learning objective: Describe the treatment of thyrotoxicosis during pregnancy.

9. **E** The patient's FT_4 (free thyroxine) and TSH (thyrotropin) levels indicate that she was suffering from thyrotoxicosis. Either surgery or thioamide is the treatment of choice for hyperthyroidism in a pregnant patient. When antithyroid drug therapy must be used during pregnancy, propylthiouracil is the preferred thioamide during the first trimester because it crosses the placenta much less than methimazole does, and because a rare embryopathy was associated with methimazole. Subsequently, methimazole should be prescribed to avoid the rare but serious potential hepatic damage associated with propylthiouracil.

   A Radioactive iodine is contraindicated during pregnancy.

   B Octreotide is a somatostatin analogue. It is used only in rare cases of hyperthyroidism due to a pituitary adenoma secreting TSH (thyrotropinoma). This is not the case in this patient, as TSH was very low.

   C Iodine compounds are not used for routine treatment of hyperthyroidism. Low doses of iodine have been used in pregnancy, but only when all other approaches are contraindicated.

   D Methyldopa is used during pregnancy only in hypertensive patients.

   F Beta-blockers are used in hyperthyroidism, but esmolol has a very short half-life and therefore is not suited for chronic use.

Learning objective: Explain the mechanism of action of levothyroxine.

10. **C** Levothyroxine (T_4) can activate a specific thyroid hormone (TH) receptor that is located in the nucleus of most body cells. This action in turn leads to activation or repression of transcription of specific genes, which ultimately mediate excitatory or inhibitory responses.

    A, E By definition, an agonist is a drug that binds to a receptor and activates it. Levothyroxine does not activate thyroid-stimulating hormone (TSH) or thyrotropin-releasing (TRH) receptors.

    B, D, F By definition, a receptor antagonist is a drug that binds to a receptor and blocks receptor actions. Levothyroxine does not block TH, TSH, or TRH receptors.

Learning objective: Identify the cell target of thyroid hormones.

11. **D** Thyroid hormones are transported into the target cells by a specific transport system. Within the cytoplasm, levothyroxine (T_4) is converted to T_3 and moves into the nucleus, where it binds to the thyroid receptor. The binding displaces a bound corepressor and binds a coactivator to the receptor complex. The receptor–coactivator complex modulates gene transcription.

    A–C, E, F See correct answer explanation.

Learning objective: Identify the drug that can cause agranulocytosis in a patient with hyperthyroidism.

12. **C** The patient's very low white blood cell count indicates that she was suffering from agranulocytosis, a potentially lethal adverse effect of thioamide antithyroid drugs, such as methimazole and propylthiouracil. Agranulocytosis occurs in 0.3 to 0.6% of patients treated with these drugs, but the risk is increased in older patients. The mechanism of agranulocytosis is still unknown, and both allergic and toxic-type reactions have been suggested. The disease is usually rapidly reversible if the drug is promptly discontinued, and colony-stimulating factors may hasten the recovery of granulocytes.

    A, B, D, E These drugs have a negligible risk of agranulocytosis.

Learning objective: Identify the drug that causes toxic hepatitis.

13. **C** The patient's history, signs, and symptoms suggest that she was most likely suffering from propylthiouracil-induced toxic hepatitis. More than 900 drugs have been implicated in causing liver injury, but propylthiouracil, isoniazid, halothane, valproate, and certain antipyretics (acetaminophen, diclofenac, and indomethacin) are among the drugs most frequently involved in acute hepatocellular toxicity. Propylthiouracil-induced toxic hepatitis occurs in about 1% of treated patients, is always severe, and can be lethal. The U.S. Food and Drug Administration has added a black box warning to the label of propylthiouracil.

    A Methimazole-induced liver injury is extremely rare. In addition, propylthiouracil is preferred over methimazole in the first trimester of pregnancy because it crosses the placenta much less than methimazole.

    B, D, E Liver injury with these drugs is negligible.

Learning objective: Explain the mechanism of action of thioamide antithyroid drugs.

14. **E** Methimazole and propylthiouracil are thioamides used as antithyroid agents. These drugs inhibit thyroid peroxidase, the enzyme that catalyzes the following three steps in thyroid hormone biosynthesis:

    - Oxidation of iodide to iodine
    - Iodination of tyrosine residues within thyroglobulin (iodide organification)
    - Combination of two diiodotyrosines (DITs), leading to T_4, and combination of monoiodotyrosine (MIT) and DIT, which leads to T_3.

    By blocking the enzyme, the synthesis of thyroid hormones is blocked.

    In addition, propylthiouracil and, to a lesser extent, methimazole inhibit the peripheral deiodination of T_4 and T_3.

    A–D See correct answer explanation.

Learning objective: Identify the signs and symptoms of hyperthyroidism.

15. **C** The patient's history and the low thyroid-stimulating hormone (TSH) value indicate that the patient was suffering from subclinical hyperthyroidism, which is defined as a low level of TSH in conjunction with normal thyroid hormone levels. The disorder can occur in many patients taking levothyroxine because of inappropriate adjustment of the daily hormone dose. Patients with subclinical hyperthyroidism are usually asymptomatic or present only a few specific symptoms (i.e., insomnia), as in this case. An excess of thyroid hormones can cause significant alteration in cardiovascular function. At rest, peripheral vascular resistance is decreased, which explains the decreased diastolic pressure, whereas systolic pressure is increased due to increased heart rate and cardiac output.

A, B, D–F Levothyroxine excess tends to cause effects opposite to those listed.

Learning objective: Describe the adverse effects of excessive doses of levothyroxine.

16. **B** Atrial fibrillation is the most common cardiac complication of hyperthyroidism, affecting 10 to 25% of hyperthyroid patients. The disorder seems to be due, at least in part, to hyperthyroidism-induced increased sensitivity of the autonomic nervous system. Both sympathetic and parasympathetic impulses can increase automaticity and conduction in atrial myocytes, thus triggering atrial fibrillation. Because it is known that cardiac fibrosis (which increases with age) is the most common cause of atrial fibrillation, the disorder is seen more frequently in elderly hyperthyroid patients, as in this case.

A, C–E All of these disorders can cause tachyarrhythmias, but they are very rarely associated with hyperthyroidism.

Learning objective: Identify the enzyme that is inhibited by thioamides such as methimazole.

17. **D** Thioamides such as methimazole inhibit thyroid peroxidase, the enzyme that oxidizes iodide to a reactive intermediate that couples with tyrosine in the initial step of thyroid hormone synthesis (iodide organification). The enzyme also catalyzes monoiodotyrosine and diiodotyrosine coupling to form T_3 and T_4.

A This enzyme catalyzes the proteolysis of thyroglobulin.

B This enzymes catalyzes the relaxation of supercoiled RNA.

C This enzyme converts some T_4 into T_3 in the follicular cell.

E This enzyme is a glycolytic enzyme found mainly in thyroid tumors.

Learning objective: Identify the drug and administration route used to treat myxedema coma.

18. **D** The signs and symptoms of the patient suggest she is affected by myxedema coma, a life-threatening complication of long-standing hypothyroidism. Factors that can precipitate the disorder are exposure to cold, illness, trauma, and drugs that are central nervous system depressants, as in this case. Emergency treatment is imperative, as the condition is rapidly fatal. A large dose of T_4 (levothyroxine) or T_3 (triiodothyronine) should be given intravenously.

A, B, E These drugs are absolutely contraindicated in hypothyroidism.

C T_4 can be given, but the intravenous route is mandatory.

Learning objective: Describe the main symptoms of drug-induced hypothyroidism.

19. **E** Thioamide antithyroid drugs such as methimazole are currently used to treat hyperthyroidism, but excessive doses of these drugs can shift a hyperthyroid patient to a hypothyroid one, as in this case. Constipation is a common symptom of hypothyroidism.

A–D All of these are symptoms of hyperthyroidism and therefore unlikely after an excessive dose of methimazole.

Learning objective: Explain the mechanism of action of thyroid hormones.

20. **A** Most of the effects of thyroid hormones appear to be mediated by activation of nuclear receptors that lead to activation or repression of transcription of specific genes. Large numbers of thyroid hormone receptors are found in most tissues. Although genomic actions of thyroid hormones predominate, nongenomic actions of thyroid hormones have also been observed, including enhancement of mitochondrial oxidative phosphorylation, as well as actions on ion channels, second messengers, and protein kinases.

B–D Thyroid hormones have actions opposite to those listed.

E Plasma catecholamine levels are not changed by thyroid hormones, but these hormones raise the sensitivity of tissues to the action of catecholamines.

Learning objective: Identify the drug used in treating hypothyroidism.

21. **C** The patient's signs and symptoms indicate that she was most likely suffering from hypothyroidism, and lab results confirmed that the disorder was due to Hashimoto thyroiditis. In most cases, high levels of antibodies to thyroid peroxidase are diagnostic for this disease. Hashimoto thyroiditis is likely the most common cause of hypothyroidism in North America. The treatment usually requires lifelong replacement therapy with thyroid hormones.

A, B, D, E See correct answer explanation.

Learning objective: Outline the emergency pharmacotherapy of thyroid storm.

22. **E** Thyroid storm (also called thyrotoxic crisis) is a life-threatening syndrome due to a sudden increase in all of the symptoms of hyperthyroidism. The management of thyroid storm must be aggressive and fast. Treatment includes four drugs: propylthiouracil (which blocks hormone synthesis and the peripheral conversion of T_4 to T_3), potassium iodide (which blocks hormone synthesis and inhibits the release of hormones from the thyroid gland), hydrocortisone (which protects the patient against shock and inhibits the peripheral conversion of T_4 to T_3), and propranolol (which antagonizes the severe cardiovascular manifestations of the syndrome). The treatment can restore the normal concentration of triiodothyronine in 24 to 48 hours.

    A, D Methimazole can be used (although propylthiouracil is a better choice, because methimazole does not block the conversion of T_4 to T_3), but diltiazem, atenolol, esmolol, and verapamil are useless, as the patient was receiving propranolol.

    B Because fever is almost always present in thyroid storm, antipyretics are indicated, but salicylates should be avoided because they compete with T_3 and T_4 for binding to thyroxine-binding globulin, thus increasing free hormone levels.

    C Radioactive iodine is contraindicated because it can increase thyroid hormone release from degenerating follicles in the first days after treatment. Dexamethasone is useless, as the patient was receiving a glucocorticoid.

Learning objective: Identify the transporter that carries iodide ions through the apical membrane of thyroid follicular cells.

23. **C** Iodide ions are carried through the apical membrane of thyroid follicular cells by a secondary active Cl^-/iodide antiporter called pendrin that exchanges one iodide ion with a chlorine ion.

    A, B, D, E See correct answer explanation.

Learning objective: Identify the most likely disease in a patient with low thyroid-stimulating hormone (TSH) and low thyroid hormones.

24. **D** The low levels of both thyroid hormones and TSH indicate that the patient was suffering from secondary hypothyroidism, which occurs when the pituitary produces insufficient TSH or the hypothalamus produces insufficient thyrotropin-releasing hormone (TRH; this insufficiency is sometimes termed tertiary hypothyroidism).The fact that a computed tomography scan confirmed the diagnosis indicates that the patient's hypothyroidism was due to a pituitary tumor that caused TSH deficiency.

A, C, E In hypothyroidism due to diseases of the thyroid, such as Hashimoto thyroiditis, myxedema, or papillary thyroid cancer, TSH levels are usually high, not low.

B In Graves disease, thyroid hormone levels are high, not low.

Learning objective: Explain why it is essential to maintain maternal euthyroidism during pregnancy.

25. **D** Congenital hypothyroidism, abnormal fetal development, and impaired cognitive development in the newborn have been attributed to maternal hypothyroidism. A delay in both mental and motor development was observed in children who were born to mothers with low circulating thyroid hormone levels but normal thyroid-stimulating hormone (TSH, thyrotropin) levels during the first trimester of pregnancy. This is because early development of the fetal brain depends on maternal levothyroxine. Most women with primary hypothyroidism will require about 30 to 50% increment in hormone dosage to maintain euthyroidism during pregnancy. Explanations for this increment include the pregnancy-induced increase in thyroid-binding proteins and an increased volume of distribution during pregnancy.

    A–C Maternal hypothyroidism can be associated with excessive weight gain, preeclampsia, or even myxedema coma, but these are very rare events, and to avoid these disorders is not the main reason for the increased dosage of thyroid hormone during pregnancy.

    E Human chorionic gonadotropin has significant TSH activity, but this has nothing to do with the reason for the increased dosage of thyroid hormone during pregnancy.

Learning objective: Outline the therapeutic uses of potassium iodide.

26. **C** Potassium iodide is often used for the preoperative preparation of patients undergoing thyroidectomy because it decreases the vascularity and fragility of a hyperplastic gland.

    When there is chronic iodine deficiency, more iodine needs to go to the thyroid to maintain production of thyroid-stimulating hormone (T_4) at the required levels. To do this, the blood flow to the gland must be increased, and the thyroid cells must increase in number. These actions are promoted by TSH, whose production is increased, making the gland hyperplastic. When iodine supply is restored, the feedback mechanism is no longer needed, and vascularity and fragility of the gland decrease. There is convincing evidence of decreased thyroid blood flow from iodine treatment. However, whether this decrease results in any additional benefits at surgery is still controversial.

    A, B, D, E See correct answer explanation.

Learning objective: Identify the drug used for thyroid ablation.

27. **B** Treatment of hyperthyroidism includes antithyroid drugs, surgical thyroidectomy, or destruction of the gland with radioactive iodine. When antithyroid drugs are contraindicated, as in this case, or when the disease is severe, radioactive iodine is currently the treatment of choice.

A Thioamide antithyroid drugs (propylthiouracil and methimazole) can cause neutropenia and agranulocytosis and are therefore contraindicated in this patient because of propylthiouracil-induced neutropenia.

C–E These drugs can be used to control symptoms of hyperthyroidism but are not suitable for the long-term management of the disease.

Learning objective: Explain why levothyroxine is used instead of a racemic mixture in thyroid replacement therapy.

28. **C** The use of the levo isomer of thyroxine is an example of the stereo selectivity of drugs. More than one half of all useful drugs are chiral molecules. Chirality (also called stereoisomerism) means that drugs can exist as enantiomer pairs; that is, they have asymmetric centers. A racemic mixture is a mixture of these enantiomers. In most cases, one of these enantiomers (dextro or levo) has greater affinity for the receptors than its mirror image; it fits better to the receptor molecule. However, most studies of clinical efficacy of drugs have been carried out with racemic mixtures of the drug rather than with separate enantiomers. Therefore, only a small percentage of the chiral drugs used clinically are marketed as the active isomers. The receptor affinity of levothyroxine is about 25 times higher than that of dextrothyroxine, and this is the reason why the levo isomer is used clinically.

A, B, D, E See correct answer explanation.

Learning objective: Describe the appropriate therapeutic management of a hypothyroid patient on amiodarone therapy.

29. **E** Chronic treatment with amiodarone can cause hyper- or (more often) hypothyroidism because the drug is rich in iodine. When amiodarone is metabolized by the liver, iodine molecules are released and can exert pharmacological effects. In general, the resulting hypothyroidism is mild, as in this case, and it disappears in a few days when the drug is withdrawn.

A, C When hypothyroidism is caused by drugs, the first procedure is to stop the offending agent. Thyroid hormones can be given later if symptoms persist.

B Potassium iodide can block thyroid hormone release. Therefore, it is contraindicated in hypothyroidism.

D Metformin does not affect thyroid function.

Learning objective: Identify the drug used to treat subclinical hypothyroidism.

30. **E** The woman was most likely affected by subclinical hypothyroidism, which is defined as elevated thyroid-stimulating hormone (TSH) in the presence of normal thyroid hormone levels. The prevalence of subclinical hypothyroidism is 4 to 10% but can increase to 26% in the elderly population, particularly women. The risk of developing overt hypothyroidism is related to the level of TSH and is increased in patients with positive antibodies, as in this case. Treatment of subclinical hypothyroidism is controversial, but thyroid replacement appears reasonable in asymptomatic patients with levels greater than 10 mU/L and in those with positive thyroid antibodies.

A–D, F See correct answer explanation.

DRUGS FOR THYROID DISORDERS Answer key					
1.	A	6.	E	11.	D
2.	F	7.	C	12.	C
3.	D	8.	A	13.	C
4.	D	9.	E	14.	E
5.	B	10.	C	15.	C
16.	B	21.	C	26.	C
17.	D	22.	E	27.	B
18.	D	23.	C	28.	C
19.	E	24.	D	29.	E
20.	A	25.	D	30.	E

Answers and Explanations: V-3 Corticosteroids and Antagonists

Questions 1–5

1. **D**
2. **L**
3. **E**
4. **A**
5. **H**

Learning objective: Describe the long-term adverse effects of glucocorticoids.

6. **F** Myasthenia gravis is an autoimmune disease that destroys acetylcholine receptors at the neuromuscular junction. Therapy includes cholinesterase inhibitors to relieve symptoms and corticosteroids, immunosuppressive drugs, and thymectomy to interfere with autoimmune pathogenesis. The patient's signs and symptoms indicate that his treatment most likely included a glucocorticoid, such as dexamethasone. Glucocorticoids can cause heartburn (because of the increased gastric secretion and decreased prostaglandin biosynthesis), hypocalcemia (by decreasing intestinal absorption and increasing renal Ca^{2+} excretion), and hyperglycemia (by stimulating glycogen synthesis and gluconeogenesis).

    A, E Fludrocortisone and testosterone are not used for treating myasthenia gravis.

    B–D Edrophonium, azathioprine, and neostigmine are used for treating myasthenia gravis, but they do not cause the symptoms reported by the patient.

Learning objective: Describe the long-term effects of glucocorticoids on serum ion values.

7. **B** Glucocorticoids lower Ca^{2+} absorption by the gut and increase Ca^{2+} excretion by the kidney. Therefore hypocalcemia is an expected adverse effect of long-term therapy with these drugs.

    A, C–E Glucocorticoids tend to produce actions opposite to those listed.

Learning objective: Describe the effects of glucocorticoids on serum glucose levels.

8. **D** Glucocorticoids can lead to hyperglycemia by causing simulation of gluconeogenesis, decreased glucose utilization by cells, and increased glucagon secretion. These effects are dose-dependent, and hyperglycemia can occur even with a low dose of daily prednisone.

    A, B, E Glucocorticoids tend to cause effects opposite to those listed.

    C Glucocorticoids can cause hypokalemia, but this is rare with synthetic drugs that have very low mineralocorticoid activity, such as prednisone. Moreover, the patient was receiving captopril, which tends to cause hyperkalemia, thus balancing the possible hypokalemic effect of prednisone.

Learning objective: Explain why synthetic glucocorticoids are usually preferred over cortisol in the therapy of nonendocrine disorders.

9. **B** Synthetic glucocorticoids are usually preferred over natural hormones for the treatment of nonendocrine disorders because they are less prone to induce salt and water retention when given at equivalent antiinflammatory doses.

    A, C–E All of these effects of glucocorticoids are dose-related and closely parallel their antiinflammatory effect.

Learning objective: Explain the mechanisms of the antiinflammatory action of glucocorticoids.

10. **E** Acute bursitis results from the inflammation of a fluid-filled sac, the bursa, which is located between two surfaces that rub together when moving. The inflammation has a rapid onset and can be very uncomfortable. Intra-articular injections of glucocorticoids provide rapid relief because of their powerful antiinflammatory activity. This effect is mediated by a vast array of actions, including the induction of the synthesis of lipocortins. These enzymes act as inhibitors of phospholipase A_2, the enzyme that catalyzes the release of arachidonic acid from membrane phospholipids. Because arachidonic acid is the precursor of eicosanoids, the corticosteroid-induced induction of lipocortins leads to an inhibition of phospholipase A_2 and, in turn, to an inhibition of biosynthesis of all eicosanoids, which are proinflammatory compounds.

    A Glucocorticoids inhibit adrenocorticotropic hormone (ACTH) release, but this has nothing to do with their antiinflammatory action.

    B Glucocorticoids do not affect the catabolism of prostaglandins.

    C, D Glucocorticoids decrease post capillary permeability (due to inhibition of histamine release and kinin activity) and decrease the synthesis of most proinflammatory interleukins, such as IL-6.

Learning objective: Describe glucocorticoid-induced osteoporosis.

11. **E** The patient's signs and symptoms indicate that she was suffering from Cushing syndrome, most likely due to high-dose glucocorticoid therapy. Polymyositis is a chronic autoimmune disease of unknown cause characterized by inflammatory and degenerative changes in the muscles. High-dose glucocorticoid is usually the treatment of choice. Drugs with high potency and negligible salt-retaining activity, such as dexamethasone, are commonly the preferred agents.

    A, B, D Methotrexate, azathioprine, and cyclophosphamide are sometimes used to treat polymyositis, but they do not cause the syndrome shown by the patient.

C, F Fludrocortisone and mifepristone are not used to treat polymyositis.

Learning objective: Describe prednisone-precipitated hyperosmolar coma.

12. **A** The neurologic signs, together with the huge glycemic value, the high-serum osmolality, and the absence of urinary ketones, suggest the diagnosis of hyperglycemic, hyperosmolar coma. The syndrome typically occurs in elderly type 2 diabetics, but occasionally it may be the initial presentation of previously latent diabetes mellitus. It is frequently precipitated by comorbid conditions or by certain drugs, including glucocorticoids, thiazides, and phenytoin.

B Beta-2 stimulants such as albuterol can cause hyperglycemia by stimulating liver gluconeogenesis. Therefore, they could precipitate diabetic ketoacidosis if given at high doses. However, inhaled albuterol rarely causes significant hyperglycemia, and diabetic ketoacidosis is unlikely, mainly because of the absence of urinary ketones.

C See correct answer explanation.

D, E The signs and symptoms of ventricular tachycardia and cerebral edema are not the ones exhibited by the patient.

Learning objective: Describe glucocorticoid-induced subcapsular cataract.

13. **B** The patient's history and symptoms indicate that he was most likely suffering from steroid-induced cataract development. Long-term therapy with a high dose of glucocorticoids has been associated with the development of posterior subcapsular cataracts, which occur in about 20% of patients treated for 1 year or more.

A, C Mifepristone and fludrocortisone are not used to treat rheumatoid arthritis, nor do they cause cataracts.

D–F Methotrexate, azathioprine, and cyclophosphamide are sometimes used to treat rheumatoid arthritis, but they do not cause cataract formation.

Learning objective: Describe the long-term effects of glucocorticoids on glucose and blood urea nitrogen (BUN) levels.

14. **E** The patient's signs and symptoms indicate he was suffering from adverse effects of chronic glucocorticoid therapy. Polyarteritis nodosa is a connective tissue disorder of unknown cause that is usually treated with high doses of glucocorticoids. Chronic treatment with these drugs can cause epigastric distress because of increased peptic acid secretions and inhibition of prostaglandin synthesis, muscle weakness because of muscle wasting, hypertension (mechanism still uncertain), and candidiasis (oral white plaques) because of the immunosuppressive effect that increases the probability of opportunistic infections. These drugs can also cause hyperglycemia (due to increased gluconeogenesis, decreased glucose utilization, and increased glucagon secretion) and increased BUN because of protein wasting.

A–D, F These drugs do not cause the syndrome presented by the patient and are not currently used in the therapy of polyarteritis nodosa.

Learning objective: Describe the effects of glucocorticoids.

15. **A** The patient's signs and symptoms indicate that she was most likely suffering from the adverse effects of chronic glucocorticoid therapy. Glucocorticoids such as prednisone are currently used to treat severe cases of ulcerative colitis. They can cause muscle weakness (because of skeletal muscle wasting, so-called steroid myopathy) and epigastric distress (because of increased peptic acid secretions and inhibition of prostaglandin synthesis). Osteoporosis is a frequent serious complication of long-term glucocorticoid therapy and can explain the dull, aching back pain of the patient. Glucocorticoids decrease the number of lymphocytes (due to increased efflux from blood to the lymphoid tissue) and increase the number of neutrophils (due both to increased efflux from bone marrow and to decreased migration from the blood vessels).

B–F All of these drugs are used to treat ulcerative colitis, but they do not cause the signs and symptoms shown by the patient.

Learning objective: Identify the opportunistic infections that can be triggered by chronic glucocorticoid therapy.

16. **C** High-dose glucocorticoid therapy increases the risk of opportunistic infections because they lower the resistance of the host. The signs and symptoms of the patient indicate that she was most likely affected by pulmonary tuberculosis, one of the most common diseases that can be triggered or reactivated by high-dose glucocorticoid therapy.

A, D These pneumonias can be triggered by high-dose glucocorticoid therapy, but offending organisms are not acid-fast bacilli.

B, E, F All of these diseases can have some of the symptoms exhibited by the patient, but they are not triggered by glucocorticoid therapy.

Learning objective: Describe the effects of glucocorticoids on the hematopoietic system.

17. **D** Glucocorticoids decrease the concentration of lymphocytes, monocytes, eosinophils, and basophils (due to increased efflux from blood to the lymphoid tissue and to increased apoptosis). They also increase the concentration of neutrophils (due to increased efflux from bone marrow and to decreased migration from blood vessels) and the concentration of red blood cells and platelets.

A–C, E See correct answer explanation.

Learning objective: Explain the molecular mechanism of action of glucocorticoids.

18. **B** Glucocorticoids cross the membrane of the target cell by passive diffusion. In the cytoplasm, the drug binds to a glucocorticoid receptor (GR)–heat shock protein complex in the cytoplasm. The heat shock protein is released, and the hormone receptor complex is transported into the nucleus, where it binds to specific nucleotide sequences along the DNA, called glucocorticoid response elements (GREs). Binding of ligand-activated GRs at GREs regulate (up or down) transcription of genes coding for specific proteins. Changes in the rate of synthesis of specific proteins carry out most biologic actions of the hormones.

    A, C See correct answer explanation.

    D–F Glucocorticoids can decrease the activity of these enzymes, but this is not due to a blockade of the enzymes following their direct binding to the drug-receptor complex, but to an inhibition of the enzyme synthesis due to subsequent downstream effects of gene regulation by the drug-receptor complex.

Learning objective: Describe the long-term adverse effects of glucocorticoids on the hematopoietic system.

19. **B** Ecchymoses and easy bruisability are common side effects of prolonged glucocorticoid use. They occur most often in the elderly and are dose-related. Steroids such as prednisone destroy the collagen support of small blood vessels, resulting in leakage of blood into surrounding tissue. Moreover, their antiinflammatory effects reduce the normal resorption of blood leakage, making the bruise last longer.

    A, C Warfarin and heparin can cause bruises, but they are not used to treat dermatomyositis.

    D–F Methotrexate, azathioprine, and cyclosporine are used to treat dermatomyositis, but they do not cause bruises.

Learning objective: Outline the use of spironolactone in treating adrenal hyperplasia.

20. **D** The patient's symptoms and the laboratory values indicate that he was most likely suffering from primary hyperaldosteronism due to bilateral adrenal hyperplasia. Surgical therapy of the disease is not recommended because most patients remain hypertensive even after bilateral adrenalectomy. Hyperaldosteronism in these patients can usually be controlled by spironolactone, a competitive antagonist at mineralocorticoid receptors.

    A About one half of patients with primary hyperaldosteronism need additional antihypertensive treatment, but minoxidil is an antihypertensive rarely used today because of its toxicity.

    B, C, E, F These drugs are useless, or even dangerous, in primary hyperaldosteronism.

Learning objective: Identify the risk of osteoporosis in a patient under glucocorticoid therapy.

21. **B** Glucocorticoids are first-line agents to treat relapsing polychondritis, an episodic, destructive disorder involving various cartilages of the body. The disease is fatal after 5 years in about 30% of cases. Glucocorticoids or immunosuppressants can relieve symptoms, but they do not affect mortality. Osteoporosis is a frequent, serious complication of glucocorticoid therapy and is related to dosage and duration of treatment. These drugs decrease bone density by multiple mechanisms, including inhibition of intestinal absorption and increased renal excretion of Ca^{2+} with secondary increase of parathyroid hormone, thereby increasing bone resorption. In addition, glucocorticoids inhibit osteoblast activity and lead to uncoupling of bone formation and resorption. Osteoporosis occurs in patients of all ages but is more frequent when additional risk factors (sex and postmenopausal age) occur, as in this case.

    A, C–E The risk of these diseases is not increased by glucocorticoid therapy.

Learning objective: Describe the use of glucocorticoids under stressful conditions in a patient with latent adrenal insufficiency.

22. **A** When glucocorticoids are discontinued in patients who had been treated with high doses of these drugs for long periods, adrenal insufficiency can occur for some time. During chronic glucocorticoid therapy, a negative feedback mechanism inhibits corticotropin-releasing hormone (CRH) and adrenocorticotropic hormone (ACTH) secretion, resulting in atrophy of the adrenal cortex and decreased secretion of cortisol. The amount and the duration of adrenal insufficiency depend on the dose of glucocorticoids and the duration of the steroid treatment. Following long-term therapy, this insufficiency can last up to 1 year. When the insufficiency is not pronounced, the adrenal cortex can secrete enough cortisol under normal conditions, but this secretion may be insufficient under stressful conditions, such as surgery, which may require up to a 10-fold increase in cortisol secretion. It is a common therapeutic practice to resume the glucocorticoid treatment in patients previously treated with chronic, high-dose glucocorticoids when the patient is under stressful conditions (including surgery), as in this case.

    B, C Glucocorticoids would cause effects opposite to those listed.

    D Glucocorticoids can cause general depressive effects on intestinal functions (after high doses), but this is not the reason for restarting prednisone treatment in this patient.

    E Glucocorticoid treatment can cause a decrease of ACTH release, but this is not the reason for restarting prednisone treatment in this patient.

Learning objective: Explain the mechanisms of the immunosuppressive action of glucocorticoids.

23. **F** Polyarteritis nodosa is a systemic vasculitis consisting of segmental inflammation and necrosis of medium-size vascular arteries with secondary tissue ischemia. The cause is unknown, but immune mechanisms appear to be involved. Untreated, the disease is usually fatal, often ending in failure of the heart, kidneys, or other vital organs. High-dose glucocorticoids may prevent progression and induce partial or near-complete remission in about 30% of patients, likely because of their powerful immunosuppressive action, which includes the inhibition of macrophage-mediated production of interleukins, including tumor necrosis factor (TNF).

    A Glucocorticoids do not affect catabolism of leukotrienes.

    B–E Glucocorticoids have effects opposite to those listed.

Learning objective: Outline the pharmacotherapy of Addison disease.

24. **E** The patient's signs and symptoms indicate that she was most likely suffering from Addison disease, a progressive hypofunctioning of the adrenal cortex. Mineralocorticoid deficiency results in increased excretion of Na^+ and decreased excretion of K^+, whereas glucocorticoid deficiency contributes to postural hypotension and causes severe insulin sensitivity. Gluconeogenesis is impaired, and hypoglycemia results. Decreased blood cortisol causes increased pituitary adrenocorticotropic hormone (ACTH) production and increased blood β-lipotropin, which has melanocyte-stimulating activity. Both ACTH and β-lipotropin cause hyperpigmentation of the skin and mucous membranes characteristic of Addison disease. The rational pharmacotherapy of the disease is to provide both mineralo- and glucocorticoid treatment. Fludrocortisone is preferred over aldosterone because of its long duration of action and its powerful salt-retaining activity. It is the only drug used for mineralocorticoid supplementation. Cortisol or a synthetic steroid are used for glucocorticoid supplementation.

    A–D See correct answer explanation.

Learning objective: Outline the therapeutic uses of glucocorticoids.

25. **C** Cerebral edema is an excessive accumulation of water in the intra- or extracellular space of the brain due to a breakdown of tight endothelial junctions that make up the blood–brain barrier. This allows excess fluid to penetrate into cerebral extracellular space. This type of edema, called vasogenic, is seen in response to trauma, tumors, focal inflammation, late stages of cerebral ischemia, and hypertensive encephalopathy. Because the edema occurs in an enclosed space, the brain is compressed, and the condition can be rapidly fatal. Glucocorticoids are of value for the reduction or prevention of cerebral edema associated with cerebral infections or neoplasms because of their powerful antiinflammatory action. However, they are of no value in case of cerebral edema due to trauma or ischemic stroke.

    A, B, D–F These drugs are contraindicated in this patient because they could decrease the already low diastolic pressure.

Learning objective: Outline the therapeutic uses of glucocorticoids.

26. **C** In the right clinical setting, an increased number of eosinophils in the bronchoalveolar lavage is diagnostic for acute eosinophilic pneumonia. The disorder can be a cause of acute respiratory failure, as in this case. Although the pathogenesis of this disorder is unknown, a hypersensitivity reaction to some unidentified inhaled antigen is thought to play an etiologic role. Unlike chronic eosinophilic pneumonia, which requires long treatment with high doses of glucocorticoids, a short course of glucocorticoids causes a complete resolution of symptoms in most cases of acute eosinophilic pneumonia.

    A, B, D–F Eosinophilic pneumonia is not an infectious disease, so all the listed drugs are useless.

Learning objective: Outline the uses of glucocorticoids to treat spinal cord edema.

27. **C** Spinal cord involvement with cancer metastases occurs most commonly in patients with cancers of the lung, breast, and prostate. Cord compression usually results from vertebral erosion with tumor extension into the epidural space. Glucocorticoids are administered to all patients with documented or suspected cord compression to reduce the edema due to compression and the tumor-induced inflammatory reaction.

    A, F Mineralocorticoids such as fludrocortisone and mineralocorticoid receptor antagonists such as spironolactone are practically devoid of antiinflammatory properties.

    B, D Nonsteroidal antiinflammatory drugs (NSAIDs) such as ibuprofen and ketorolac can reduce edema due to the inflammatory reaction but are much less effective than glucocorticoids.

    E Diuretics such as furosemide can reduce edema due to conditions that directly or indirectly affect renal or circulatory function (i.e., cardiac failure, renal failure, and liver disease) but have only marginal effects in localized edema due to the inflammatory reaction.

Learning objective: Explain the molecular mechanism of action of glucocorticoids.

28. **D** In most adults, immunologic thrombocytopenic purpura is a chronic disorder that results from development of an antibody directed against a structural platelet antigen. Treatment in the adult usually begins with a large dose of an oral glucocorticoid, such as prednisone. The mechanism of action of all steroid drugs involves binding to a receptor–heat shock protein complex in the cytoplasm.

    A, C, E, F The mechanism of action of these drugs also involves binding to a receptor–heat shock protein complex in the cytoplasm, but these drugs are not used in autoimmune diseases.

    B Azathioprine is an immunosuppressant drug sometimes used in immunologic thrombocytopenic purpura, but its mechanism of action is different from the one described above.

Learning objective: Outline the therapeutic uses of glucocorticoids.

29. **C** The patient's signs and symptoms indicate that he was suffering from Cushing syndrome due to production of cortisol by an adrenocortical adenoma. These neoplasms are treated by surgical removal, and patients must receive supplementary cortisol during surgery and the postoperative period, as the adrenal cortex of the nontumor gland is atrophic and suppressed. The suppressed adrenal may require up to 18 months' recovery, and glucocorticoid therapy should be tapered but not discontinued until that recovery has been documented.

    A The normal potassium levels indicate that the aldosterone secretion is not affected, so there is no need for a mineralocorticoid administration.

    B, D–F These drugs are useless, or even dangerous, in this disease.

Learning objective: Outline the pharmacotherapy of Cushing syndrome.

30. **C** In patients with Cushing syndrome, the main goal of pharmacotherapy is to block glucocorticoid secretion. Ketoconazole is an antifungal agent. In doses higher than those employed in antifungal therapy, the drug inhibits cytochrome P-450 enzymes, thus blocking several steps of steroidogenesis. As a result, the drug is the most effective inhibitor of steroid biosynthesis. Another drug that can be used in Cushing syndrome to inhibit steroid biosynthesis is aminoglutethimide, which inhibits CYP11A, the enzyme that catalyzes the conversion of cholesterol to pregnenolone, the rate-limiting step in steroid biosynthesis.

    A, B, D–F These drugs are useless, or even dangerous, in treating Cushing syndrome.

Learning objective: Explain the molecular mechanism of action of spironolactone.

31. **D** Spironolactone is a competitive antagonist of aldosterone. By blocking aldosterone receptors, the drug inhibits the aldosterone-mediated production of Na^+, K^+, and water channels in the collecting tubules. The excretion of Na^+ and water increases, which explains the patient's nocturia. Spironolactone is used as a diuretic and sometimes to inhibit hirsutism in women due to its action as an androgen receptor antagonist.

    A–C, E Spironolactone does not elicit these actions.

Learning objective: Describe the adverse effects of mineralocorticoid excess.

32. **B** In the patient being treated for adrenal insufficiency, the high blood pressure, the low K^+ levels, and the electrocardiogram data suggest that his signs and symptoms are due to an excessive dose of fludrocortisone, a mineralocorticoid currently used as part of the therapy for Addison disease.

    A, D Hyperglycemia or myopathy induced by cortisol excess would not cause the patient's signs and symptoms.

    C, E Neither of these situations is consistent with the patient's signs and symptoms.

Learning objective: Outline the use of glucocorticoids to treat nephrotic syndrome.

33. **E** The patient's symptoms and the lab results indicate that he was most likely suffering from nephrotic syndrome. In fact, the finding of more than 3 g urinary proteins in a 24-hour urine collection is diagnostic. The syndrome can be a primary glomerular disease (minimal change disease, etc.) or secondary to a vast array of disorders, including various infections, diabetes, cancer, or immunologic disorders. Proteinuria results from damage of the kidney glomerulus that causes it to lose its filtrating capacity. Because the patient was otherwise healthy, the syndrome was most likely due to minimal change disease (also called lipoid nephrosis). Spontaneous remission of the disease occurs in about 40% of cases, but most patients are given glucocorticoids, such as betamethasone.

    A–D These drugs are not used to treat minimal change disease.

Learning objective: Outline the therapeutic uses of glucocorticoids.

34. **B** Epinephrine is the cornerstone of treatment of anaphylaxis and should be given immediately. Glucocorticoids such as prednisone cannot control the immediate symptoms (due to their slow onset of action) but are usually given to alleviate or prevent later recurrence of bronchospasm,

hypotension, and urticaria because of their powerful immunosuppressive effects.

A, C–F These drugs are useless, or even contraindicated, in anaphylaxis.

Learning objective: Explain the mechanism of the antiinflammatory action of glucocorticoids.

35. **E** Crohn disease is a chronic inflammatory bowel disease of unknown origin. A consensus hypothesis is that in genetically predisposed individuals, both exogenous factors and endogenous host factors interact to cause a chronic state of dysregulated mucosal immune function. The antiinflammatory effect of glucocorticoids, which may dramatically reduce fever, diarrhea, and abdominal pain in the acute stage of the disease, has multiple components, including inhibition of lymphocyte-mediated production of interleukin-2. This cytokine induces proliferation of B and T cells (including cytotoxic T cells) and activation of natural killer cells; therefore, it plays a central role in the immune response.

A Glucocorticoids have no effect on the catabolism of prostaglandins.

B–D Glucocorticoids have effects opposite to those listed.

Learning objective: Outline the therapeutic uses of glucocorticoids.

36. **D** Glucocorticoids are frequently used to suppress inflammation in the eye. They are administered topically into the conjunctival space when the inflammation occurs in the anterior segment of the eye (e.g., in conjunctivitis, keratitis, iritis, or iridocyclitis), but systemic administration is required for inflammation of the posterior segment of the eye (e.g., in uveitis and optic neuritis).

A Although indomethacin is an antiinflammatory drug, it is not used topically in the eye.

B, C, E, F These drugs are used to treat glaucoma, not inflammatory diseases of the eye.

Learning objective: Outline the use of glucocorticoids in treating chemotherapy-induced nausea and vomiting.

37. **A** The best and most common regimen to prevent chemotherapy-induced nausea and vomiting is a three-drug combination of a serotonin 5-HT$_3$ receptor antagonist, a glucocorticoid such as dexamethasone, and aprepitant. This combination prevents acute emesis in 80 to 90% of patients and delayed emesis in more than 70% of patients. The mechanism of the antiemetic action of glucocorticoids is still unknown, but it is likely mediated by their inhibition of prostaglandin biosynthesis in the central nervous system.

B, C These antiemetic drugs are poorly effective in chemotherapy-induced nausea and vomiting

D Loperamide is an antidiarrheal, not an antiemetic, drug.

E Benzodiazepines such as diazepam have no direct antiemetic effect. They are sometimes added to the main regimen because their antianxiety effect could reduce the anticipatory component of nausea and vomiting.

F Omeprazole is an inhibitor of gastric acid secretion, not an antiemetic drug.

Learning objective: Outline the therapeutic uses of glucocorticoids.

38. **E** Thrombotic thrombocytopenic purpura is an acute, potentially fatal disorder characterized by the pentad of

- Severe thrombocytopenia (platelets are utilized in the formation of diffuse microthrombi)
- Neurologic signs and symptoms
- Manifestation of ischemic changes in multiple organs
- Fever
- Microangiopathic hemolytic anemia

The disorder is associated with many conditions, including HIV infection, and is almost always fatal if untreated. The etiology is unknown. Repeated plasmapheresis has dramatically changed the prognosis, and now about 85% of patients recover completely. The use of immunosuppressive drugs such as rituximab or glucocorticoids, in addition to plasmapheresis, has further increased survival and decreased the frequency of relapse.

A Mineralocorticoids such as fludrocortisone are of no value in this disease.

B Thrombolytic drugs such as alteplase are contraindicated in hemorrhagic diseases.

C Antiplatelet drugs have been given to some patients with very questionable benefit.

D Because the anemia of thrombotic thrombocytopenic purpura is not due to iron deficiency, iron preparations are useless.

F The thrombocytopenia in thrombotic thrombocytopenic purpura is not due to myelosuppression; thus, a myeloid growth factor such as sargramostim is not useful.

Learning objective: Outline the therapeutic uses of glucocorticoids.

39. **C** Glucocorticoids are used frequently in the setting of premature labor to prevent infant respiratory distress syndrome (RDS). The main cause of RDS is pulmonary surfactant deficiency. Without an adequate amount of surfactant, the surface tension within the alveoli is so great that the alveoli collapse, resulting in poor gas exchange. In the fetus, endogenous cortisol stimulates the synthesis and secretion of surfactant at 30 to 32 weeks' gestational age. Maternal administration of glucocorticoids can accelerate fetal lung maturation and decrease the incidence and severity of RDS.

A, B, D–F See correct answer explanation.

Learning objective: Outline the therapeutic uses of glucocorticoids.

40. **B** Glucocorticoid therapy is indicated in selected patients with inflammatory bowel diseases, such as ulcerative colitis. The cause of inflammatory bowel diseases is unclear, but one hypothesis includes autoimmunity. Under normal conditions, the immune system of the intestinal mucosa interacts with luminal antigens and bacteria to ensure an appropriate immune response to these antigens. In inflammatory bowel diseases, this immune response is perpetuated, and an autoimmune cascade occurs. The beneficial effect of glucocorticoids most likely results from their prominent anti-inflammatory and immunosuppressive properties.

A Glucocorticoids have general depressive effects on intestinal functions when given at high doses, but this is not the primary reason for their use in ulcerative colitis.

C Glucocorticoids have antiemetic properties, but this is not the main reason for their use in ulcerative colitis.

D Glucocorticoid actions can contribute to pain relief, but this is not the main reason for their use in ulcerative colitis.

E Patients with ulcerative colitis have an increased risk of colon cancer, but the prevention of cancer is not the main reason for the use of glucocorticoids in ulcerative colitis.

Learning objective: Describe the pharmacokinetics of inhaled glucocorticoids

41. **C** The reason for the low toxicity of inhaled glucocorticoids is related to their special pharmacokinetics. Approximately 80 to 90% of an inhaled dose is deposited in the oropharynx, swallowed, and subsequently absorbed from the gastrointestinal tract. This fraction undergoes first-pass metabolism in the liver, which is quite high (the oral bioavailability of beclomethasone is about 10 to 20%).Ten to 20% of an inhaled dose enters the lung. This fraction exerts the therapeutic effect and is then absorbed into the systemic circulation. Therefore, when given by inhalation, the drug can achieve a concentration in the lung that is adequate for the local therapeutic effect but too small for systemic adverse effects.

A, B, D, E See correct answer explanation.

Learning objective: Describe the main contraindications of glucocorticoids

42. **C** Corticosteroids are well known to cause cataracts and to exacerbate glaucoma during long-term administration. They are therefore contraindicated, or should be used very cautiously, in patients with glaucoma.

A, B, D, E See correct answer explanation.

Learning objective: Identify the drug that can cause gynecomastia in a patient affected by bilateral adrenal hyperplasia.

43. **D** The patient's bilateral adrenal hyperplasia most likely caused primary hyperaldosteronism, a disorder that is usually controlled by spironolactone. Gynecomastia is a well-known adverse effect of this drug; the overall prevalence is about 10%. Spironolactone is a competitive aldosterone receptor antagonist, but it can bind to other steroid receptors. The blockade of androgen receptors is most likely the primary mechanism of spironolactone-induced gynecomastia.

A–C, E, F All of these drugs can cause gynecomastia, but they are not used to treat primary hyperaldosteronism.

Learning objective: Identify the drug that can cause liver failure in a patient treated for Cushing syndrome

44. **C** The patient's symptoms and laboratory exams indicate that he was most likely suffering from liver failure. Ketoconazole is a drug currently used to treat Cushing syndrome because it inhibits cytochrome P-450 enzymes, thus blocking several steps of steroidogenesis. Serious hepatotoxicity, including cases with a fatal outcome or requiring liver transplantation, has occurred with the use of oral ketoconazole. These cases occurred both in patients receiving high doses for short treatment durations and in patients receiving low doses for long durations.

A Metyrapone is used to treat Cushing syndrome, but its liver toxicity is exceedingly rare.

A, B, D–F These drugs can cause liver toxicity but are not used to treat Cushing syndrome.

CORTICOSTEROIDS AND ANTAGONISTS Answer key							
1.	D	6.	F	11.	E	16.	C
2.	L	7.	B	12.	A	17.	D
3.	E	8.	D	13.	B	18.	B
4.	A	9.	B	14.	E	19.	B
5.	H	10.	E	15.	A	20.	D
21.	B	26.	C	31.	D	36.	D
22.	A	27.	C	32.	B	37.	A
23.	F	28.	D	33.	E	38.	E
24.	E	29.	C	34.	B	39.	C
25.	C	30.	C	35.	E	40.	B
						41.	C
						42.	C
						43.	D
						44.	C

Answers and Explanations: V-4 Drugs for Gonadal Disorders

Questions 1–5

1. **A**
2. **K**
3. **E**
4. **G**
5. **F**

Learning objective: Identify the drug to be used locally in case of vaginal atrophy.

6. **A** Total hysterectomy includes removal of the ovaries. Vaginal dryness and atrophy due to estrogen deficiency is a common cause of dyspareunia (painful vaginal intercourse) and can be cured with estrogen administration. Topical forms of estrogens (creams, vaginal tablets, etc.) are as effective as or more effective than oral forms for this indication and are usually preferred. When estrogen cream is used, women with a uterus are also given a progestin, which is not needed following hysterectomy, as in this case.

   B–E See correct answer explanation.

Learning objective: Identify the drug used in a patient with a metastatic breast cancer resistant to tamoxifen.

7. **A** Early-stage breast cancer is curable. However, if the patient develops metastases, the goal of treatment shifts from cure to palliation and stabilization of disease.

   Anastrozole is a selective inhibitor of aromatase, the enzyme that converts androgens to estrogens. The low levels of estrogens in postmenopausal women are produced by aromatization of adrenal and ovarian androgens. Aromatase inhibitors cause almost a total suppression of estrogen levels. They are used in postmenopausal women with a hormone receptor–positive breast cancer when tamoxifen is contraindicated or has proven ineffective, as in this case.

   B–F See correct answer explanation.

Learning objective: Identify the drug that can decrease both the risk of breast cancer and the degree of osteoporosis in postmenopausal women.

8. **C** Raloxifene is a selective estrogen receptor modulator. Such drugs can have estrogenic effects in bone but estrogen antagonist action on breast and uterine receptors. Raloxifene is approved both for the treatment of postmenopausal osteoporosis and for breast cancer risk reduction, and therefore can be appropriate therapy in a subset of women with postmenopausal osteoporosis who are at risk of breast cancer, as in this case.

A Anastrozole can reduce the risk of breast cancer but has no effect or a negative effect (due to further decrease in estrogen levels) on bone mass.

B Alendronate can increase the bone mass index more than raloxifene, but has not proven to reduce breast cancer risk. Bisphosphonates are used to treat bone metastases of breast cancer. It has been suggested that bisphosphonate therapy may decrease the risk of developing breast cancer, but the effectiveness for either prevention or treatment of breast cancer has not yet been proven.

D, E Androgens and progestins are not used to treat postmenopausal osteoporosis.

Learning objective: Describe the pharmacological effects of drospirenone.

9. **B** Drospirenone is the only progestin drug with definite antihypertensive properties. It is structurally related to spironolactone and acts as an aldosterone receptor antagonist. Therefore, it causes an increased renal sodium excretion, which can account for its diuretic and antihypertensive effects.

   A Potassium excretion is decreased, not increased, by aldosterone antagonists.

   C–E The renal excretion of these ions is minimally affected by drospirenone.

Learning objective: Identify the drug used to induce puberty in girls with Turner syndrome.

10. **F** The patient's signs and lab exams indicate that the girl was affected by Turner syndrome, a sex chromosome abnormality in which there is a complete or partial absence of one of the two sex chromosomes, producing a phenotypic female. The phenotype varies from that of the typical Turner syndrome to normal. Failure to go to puberty and begin menses occurs in 90% of affected persons, as in this case. Replacement with female hormones will bring on puberty in most cases.

    A Diethylstilbestrol is a synthetic estrogen but is not used in replacement therapy because of the risk of adenocarcinoma in the offspring.

    B–E These drugs are of no value in replacement therapy.

Learning objective: Identify the drug used to decrease menometrorrhagia due to uterine fibroid.

11. **E** Uterine fibroid, a benign uterine tumor, is the most common pelvic tumor, occurring in about 70% of women. It frequently causes abnormal vaginal bleeding and pelvic pain, as in this case. Fibroids tend to enlarge during reproductive years, when estrogen production is high, because they have estrogen receptors. Asymptomatic fibroids do not require treatment. For symptomatic fibroids, medical options are focused on suppression of estrogen stimulation, but results are limited. Progestins such as medroxyprogesterone can partially suppress estrogen stimulation, which in turn can decrease fibroid growth and vaginal bleeding. Danazol, an androgen agonist, can also suppress fibroid growth but has a high rate of adverse effects and is less frequently used.

    A Estrogens such as ethinyl estradiol are contraindicated in uterine fibroids because they stimulate uterine growth and bleeding.

    B, C Finasteride inhibits dihydrotestosterone synthesis, and flutamide is an androgen receptor antagonist. By decreasing androgen activity, these drugs can indirectly enhance estrogen actions and are therefore contraindicated in uterine fibroids.

    D Mifepristone is a progestin antagonist and therefore is contraindicated in uterine fibroids.

Learning objective: Identify the drug effective as a contraceptive within 3 days of unprotected intercourse.

12. **C** Levonorgestrel, a progestin compound, is an effective postcoital contraceptive. The effectiveness is most likely due to a combination of effects of interaction with progesterone receptors and the time of the cycle. Among the contraceptive actions are inhibition of ovulation, alterations in cervical mucus production, and decreased fallopian tube motility, all of which can hinder fertilization and/or disrupt development of an endometrium suitable for implantation. Ulipristal, a selective progesterone receptor modulator, is also effective and appears to be even more effective at preventing ovulation.

    A, B, D–F See correct answer explanation.

Learning objective: Explain the mechanism of the thromboembolic effect of oral contraceptives.

13. **D** Estrogens enhance the coagulability of blood because they
    - Increase plasma levels of coagulation factors II, VII, VIII, IX, X, and XII (the main action)
    - Decrease plasma levels of antithrombin III
    - Increase platelet production and aggregation

These actions augment the risk of thromboembolic disease in women taking combined oral contraceptives about threefold compared to women taking no hormones.

A–C, E Estrogens tend to cause actions opposite to those listed.

Learning objective: Identify the best hormonal contraceptive for a woman with an abnormal coagulation history.

14. **F** Progestin alone (daily progestin tablets or implantable preparation) is the best hormonal contraceptive for women with an abnormal coagulation history, as in this case. In fact, estrogens must be avoided because they increase blood coagulability.

    A–C, E See correct answer explanation.

    D Mifepristone is not currently available as a regular contraceptive preparation.

Learning objective: Identify the drug that most likely caused deep venous thrombosis in a patient taking multiple medications.

15. **C** The estrogens contained in the contraceptive pill can contribute to thromboembolic events by several mechanisms. They increase plasma levels of factors II, VII, VIII, IX, X, and XII, decrease plasma levels of antithrombin III, and increase platelet production and aggregation in a manner similar to that seen late in pregnancy.

    A Progestins play a minimal role, if any, in thromboembolism risk.

    B, D, E These drugs do not cause or favor thromboembolism.

    F This estrogen is not used in contraceptive preparations.

Learning objective: Explain the mechanism of action of finasteride.

16. **C** Finasteride is a competitive inhibitor of 5α-reductase, the enzyme that converts testosterone to dihydrotestosterone. Dihydrotestosterone is the principal androgen responsible for stimulation of prostatic growth. The definitive therapy of benign prostatic hyperplasia is surgical, but drugs can be used when surgery is contraindicated, as in this case.

    A, B, D, E See correct answer explanation.

Learning objective: Explain the molecular mechanism of action of combination hormonal contraceptives.

17. **E** Combination hormonal contraceptives act mainly through inhibition of ovulation most likely due to the following mechanisms:
    - In the brain, activation of estrogen and progestin receptors located on arcuate hypothalamic nuclei inhibits the secretion of gonadotropin-releasing hormone (GnRH).

In current low-dose preparations, the primary hypothalamic effect of the estrogen component may be to increase expression of progesterone receptors. The progestin component acts to disrupt the normal cyclical pulsatility of GnRH release.

- Activation of estrogen receptors in the anterior pituitary gland mainly inhibits follicle-stimulating hormone (FSH) secretion.
- Activation of progestin receptors in the anterior pituitary gland mainly inhibits luteinizing hormone (LH) secretion.

When combination hormonal contraceptives are given daily, the midcycle surge of LH is absent, and ovulation fails to occur.

A Although combined oral contraceptives do result in decreased ovarian hormone secretion, this effect is not part of the contraceptive action

B, D Activation of receptors on these organs does not decrease the secretion of a hormone involved in the contraceptive effect of estrogens.

C Activation of receptors located in the anterior, not posterior, pituitary inhibits the secretion of FSH and LH.

Learning objective: Describe the pharmacological actions of progesterone.

18. **C** Medroxyprogesterone is a synthetic progesterone derivative that is about 15 times more potent and has the same pharmacological properties of the parent compound. Progesterone increases the sensitivity of the respiratory center to carbon dioxide, thus leading to an increased ventilatory response. This can explain the measurable reduction of arterial and alveolar carbon dioxide that occurs during pregnancy.

A, B, D, E Progesterone actually exhibits actions opposite to those listed.

Learning objective: Identify the cell site of action of estrogen and progestins.

19. **A** All gonadal steroid hormones act primarily via intracellular receptors to regulate gene transcription, which occurs in the nucleus of target cells, where the ligand-activated receptor binds to specific estrogen response elements or progestin response elements in the DNA of regulated genes.

B–E See correct answer explanation.

Learning objective: Outline the therapeutic uses of combination hormonal contraceptives.

20. **E** Although the exact triggering mechanism of hot flushes is unknown, it has been shown that there is a clear association between the development of hot flushes and the wide swings in circulating estrogen levels that can occur during perimenopause. Hormonal replacement therapy is indicated for perimenopausal (and sometimes postmenopausal) women who complain of overt menopausal symptoms that disrupt their lives, as in this case. Women with an intact uterus should receive estrogen–progestin therapy to decrease the risk of endometrial and ovarian cancers. The therapy can often be slowly withdrawn once the woman's system has progressed to established menopause.

A, B Estrogens alone are not indicated because of the increased risk of endometrial and ovarian cancers.

C, D, F Progestins alone are not effective in reducing hot flushes.

Learning objective: Describe the adverse effects of oral contraceptives.

21. **A** The patient's history and signs indicate that she was affected by chloasma, an increased skin pigmentation characterized by extensive brown patches of irregular shape and size. Chloasma occurs in 5% of women after 1 year and in 40% of women after 8 years of oral contraceptive use. It is similar to the so-called mask of pregnancy that sometimes occurs in pregnant women. The hyperpigmentation usually fades slowly when the hormone is withdrawn.

B–E These drugs do not cause skin hyperpigmentation.

Learning objective: Explain the molecular mechanism of action of anastrozole.

22. **D** Anastrozole and letrozole are selective inhibitors of aromatase, the enzyme responsible for the conversion of androgens to estrogens, including the extra-adrenal synthesis of estrogen from androstenedione, which takes places in several tissues, including breast. Aromatase inhibitors are considered second-line agents for hormone-dependent breast cancers, but they are increasingly used in this disease in postmenopausal women, in whom they cause an almost total suppression of estrogen synthesis.

A–C, E Aromatase inhibitors such as anastrozole are devoid of these actions.

Learning objective: Describe the contraindications to combination hormonal contraceptives.

23. **B** Estrogens increase plasma levels of factors II, VII, VIII, IX, X, and XII and are therefore absolutely contraindicated in thromboembolic diseases. Progestin-only contraceptives may be used in women with thromboembolic diseases.

A, C–E These disorders do not contraindicate the use of hormonal contraceptives.

Learning objective: Identify a drug indicated for metastatic breast cancer in women resistant to tamoxifen.

24. **D** Hormonal therapy in the metastatic breast cancer setting can provide long progression-free survival in patients. If the patient responds to a hormonal agent for a long period of time, the likelihood of response to another hormonal agent is high. Because the patient was well controlled with tamoxifen for 5 years, another hormonal agent is a reasonable choice. Fulvestrant, a competitive estrogen receptor antagonist, has been approved for patients who have become resistant to tamoxifen, as in this case.

    A Anastrozole is used in metastatic breast cancer but is an aromatase inhibitor, not an estrogen receptor antagonist.

    B, C, E These drugs are not used in the therapy of breast carcinoma.

Learning objective: Outline the risk of breast cancer associated with hormone replacement therapy in postmenopausal women.

25. **B** Hormone replacement therapy is the most effective treatment option for alleviating vasomotor symptoms in postmenopausal women. The risk of malignant tumors in women taking hormonal contraceptives is probably the major concern for the use of these medications in perimenopausal women. Although the issue is still controversial, it appears that there is a small duration-related increase in the risk of breast cancer. This prompted the U.S. Food and Drug Administration to mandate the addition of new safety warnings to the labels of all systemic estrogens, including estrogen-only and combined estrogen–progestin products. The labels caution that the use of estrogen-containing hormone therapy regimens by postmenopausal women may be associated with an increased risk of breast cancer, myocardial infarction, stroke, and thromboembolism.

    A, C–E The risk of these diseases is actually decreased in postmenopausal women on hormonal estrogen plus progestin therapy.

Learning objective: Identify the site of action of clomiphene when given to treat infertility.

26. **B** Clomiphene is an estrogen receptor antagonist in most target tissues. Blockade of estrogen receptors in the hypothalamus counteracts the estrogen-induced negative feedback on the hypothalamic-pituitary-ovarian axis. This effect often allows normal pulsatility of gonadotropin-releasing hormone (GnRH) release from the hypothalamus to occur, stimulating a normal pattern of follicle-stimulating hormone (FSH) and luteinizing hormone (LH) release from the anterior pituitary, resulting in ovulation. The drug has been used for more than 25 years to treat infertility when other causes have been ruled out. However, clomiphene may exhibit negative effects, including an increased incidence of multiple births, ovarian cysts, and ovarian hyperstimulation syndrome.

    A, C–F See correct answer explanation.

Learning objective: Identify the main reason for the preference of synthetic estrogens and progestins over natural compounds.

27. **B** Synthetic estrogens and progestins are often preferred over natural hormones mainly because they have greater oral bioavailability due to lower first-pass metabolism. The slower metabolism of these drugs also accounts for their longer half-life (i.e., estradiol 1 to 2 hours, ethinyl estradiol 8 to 24 hours).

    A, C–E Synthetic compounds do not differ significantly from natural hormones in their hormonal efficacy, inhibition of gonadotropin secretion, incidence of adverse effects, or teratogenic activity.

Learning objective: Describe the pharmacological effects of testosterone.

28. **D** Several disorders can cause erectile dysfunction, but when this is due to hypogonadism, androgen replacement therapy is indicated. Androgens can increase erythropoietin synthesis in the kidney, and this can explain the increased erythropoiesis that occurs with these hormones. Because of this, in the past, high doses of testosterone were used in the treatment of certain types of anemia, but today the direct administration of erythropoietin is largely preferred.

    A–C, E Androgens tend to cause effects opposite to those listed.

Learning objective: Describe the adverse effects of anabolic steroids.

29. **D** Hepatocellular adenoma and carcinoma, although rare, are clearly associated with the use of both oral contraceptives and alkylated anabolic steroids. The relative risk in those exposed for more than 10 years is 100-fold higher than that of patients not receiving these drugs. The risk may be even higher for athletes than for patients using hormones for other purposes, as relatively very high doses are taken to increase athletic performance.

    A–C, E, F The risk of these diseases is not increased by the use of anabolic steroids.

Learning objective: Outline the use of hormonal contraceptives to treat polycystic ovary syndrome.

30. **F** Polycystic ovary syndrome is the most common form of chronic anovulation associated with androgen excess. It occurs in 5 to 10% of women of reproductive age, making it the leading cause of infertility and the most common endocrine abnormality for this age group. The primary defect leading to the disease is unknown, but there are at least three potential mechanisms that act synergistically:

   - Inappropriate gonadotropin secretion: there is an increased frequency of gonadotropin-releasing hormone (GnRH) secretion leading to an increased luteinizing hormone (LH) pulse frequency and amplitude; thus no dominant follicle develops, and no ovulation occurs.
   - Excessive androgen production in the theca cell of the ovary leads to hyperandrogenism.
   - Insulin resistance with compensatory hyperinsulinemia

   Estrogen–progestin therapy with a combination hormonal contraceptive preparation is the first-line treatment for women seeking regular menstrual cycles and relief from androgenic symptoms. The hormones suppress the hypothalamic-pituitary-ovarian axis, including decreasing LH secretion, thus decreasing androgen production. The pills also provide "replacement therapy," and a cycle of 21 days of active pills followed by 7 days of inactive pills usually normalizes the menstrual cycle.

   A–E Mifepristone and danazol are useless in polycystic ovary syndrome

Learning objective: Identify the main mechanism of contraceptive action of daily progestin tablets.

31. **C** The doses of progestin in mini pills are sufficient to block ovulation in only 60 to 80% of cycles. The effectiveness of these preparations is thought to be mainly related to a combination of effects, including: increased viscosity of cervical mucus, which decreases sperm penetration; a decrease in fallopian tube motility (estrogens increase but progestins decrease tube motility); and endometrial alterations that impair implantation.

   A The corpus luteum is formed from the rupture of ovarian follicle and produces a large amount of progesterone and estrogens. Activation of progesterone receptors in the corpus luteum has nothing to do with the contraceptive effect.

   B Progestins do not enhance follicle-stimulating hormone (FSH) release; if they did, this effect would favor, not inhibit, ovulation.

   D Progestins decrease, not increase, the frequency and increase the amplitude of pulsatile gonadotropin-releasing hormone (GnRH) release.

   E Progestins inhibit, not increase, the contractility of the myometrium.

Learning objective: Identify the drug class to which tamoxifen belongs.

32. **D** Tamoxifen is a common hormonal adjunct therapy for breast cancer because it has been shown that 5-year treatment reduces annual odds of death by about 25% in both pre- and postmenopausal women regardless of axillary lymph node involvement. Tamoxifen is classified as a selective estrogen receptor modulator (SERM). SERMs such as tamoxifen and raloxifene bind to estrogen receptors, but they have different allosteric modulation effects than estrogen. The result is that the conformational change following SERM binding allows them to be agonists in the modulation of some genes in some target tissues and antagonists in the modulation of expression of other genes. Furthermore, each SERM has a different spectrum of actions. For example, tamoxifen acts as an estrogen antagonist in breast tissue but as an agonist in bone and endometrial tissue, whereas raloxifene is an antagonist in both breast and endometrium tissue but an agonist in bone.

   A–C, E, F See correct answer explanation.

Learning objective: Outline the therapeutic uses of danazol.

33. **E** The signs and symptoms of the patient suggest that he was affected by hereditary angioedema, a disease caused by hereditary impairment of C_1 esterase inhibitor, a protein that regulates activation of the complement, contact, and fibrinolytic systems. C_1 inhibitor is one of the major inhibitors of plasma kallikrein, the contact system protease that cleaves kininogen and releases bradykinin. Presumably, uncontrolled activation of the contact system allows for the release of kinin-like mediators, resulting in edema of subcutaneous or submucosal tissues. The disease is estimated to occur in 1 in 50,000 to 150,000 individuals, with a mortality rate estimated at 15 to 33%, resulting from laryngeal edema and asphyxiation.

   Chronic androgenic treatment of patients with hereditary angioedema effectively prevents the attacks. Androgens most likely act by stimulating the hepatic synthesis of C_1 esterase inhibitor. Danazol is the drug most frequently used for this purpose.

   A–D, F See correct answer explanation.

Learning objective: Outline the therapeutic use of leuprolide and flutamide.

34. **C** The patient's signs and symptoms suggest prostate cancer, and the exam results confirm the diagnosis of metastasized prostatic carcinoma. Prostate-specific antigen (PSA) is the most used lab test for early detection of prostate cancer, and spine metastases with prevalent necrotic lesions are the most common metastases of prostatic carcinoma. The mainstay of treatment for metastasized prostate cancer is hormonal therapy. Because the cancer is testosterone-dependent, hormonal manipulation focuses on reducing testosterone levels. Leuprolide is a synthetic gonadotropin-releasing hormone (GnRH) analogue. When administered daily (or as a depot preparation) to maintain stable blood levels, it inhibits the release of follicle-stimulating hormone (FSH) and luteinizing hormone (LH), likely due to downregulation of pituitary receptors. This inhibition strongly reduces testicular androgen synthesis. Flutamide is an androgen receptor antagonist. Combined treatment with these drugs reduces symptoms in 70 to 80% of patients, causes an appreciable regression of established metastases, and prolongs survival. In contrast, cytotoxic chemotherapy has failed to prolong survival in patients with advanced prostate cancer.

    A This is a therapy for advanced ovarian cancer.

    B This is a therapy for acute lymphoblastic leukemia.

    D These drugs are used in hormone receptor–positive breast cancer.

    E These drugs are used in Wilms tumor.

Learning objective: Identify the most common adverse effect of progestin-only hormonal contraceptives.

35. **D** Some women experience breakthrough bleeding while taking oral contraceptives, but breakthrough bleeding is the most common problem (in up to 25% of patients) in women using the progestin-only pill. It is more frequently encountered in women taking a low dose of progestins and often resolves on its own. If it persists for more than 3 months, the best strategy is to switch to a combined oral contraceptive with a higher ratio of estrogen to progestin.

    A–C, E All of these adverse effects can occur with combination oral contraceptives but are due mainly to the estrogen component of the preparation, and the risk is therefore minimal with a progestin-only oral contraceptive.

Learning objective: Describe the main adverse effect of estrogens.

36. **A** Many drugs can cause nausea and vomiting in sensitive patients. However, the woman was most likely suffering from nausea due to the contraceptive preparation, as she had been taking the other drugs for some time without adverse effects. Nausea from a combined oral contraceptive can generally be attributed to the estrogen component (ethinyl estradiol). It was a common adverse effect and was one of the main reasons for discontinuing use of combined contraceptives. Today, with the use of low-dose contraceptive pills, this adverse effect is much less common.

    B–E See correct answer explanation.

Learning objective: Describe the adverse effects of anabolic steroids.

37. **F** High doses of androgens or anabolic steroids, used by athletes to improve competitive performance, can produce oligospermia and reduction in testicular size. This is the consequence of negative feedback by androgen on the hypothalamus that inhibits the secretion of gonadotropin-releasing hormone (GnRH), which in turn causes a corresponding decrease in both follicle-stimulating and luteinizing hormones.

    A–E See correct answer explanation.

Learning objective: Outline the therapeutic uses of estrogens.

38. **B** Estrogen replacement therapy is definitely indicated to postpone menopause in young women who undergo ablation of the ovary. Some risks associated with estrogen replacement therapy (endometrial and ovarian cancer) cannot occur in this case because the organs are no longer present. Other risks of this therapy (breast cancer and thromboembolic disorders) are also minimal in this case, because the therapy simply restores the physiological levels of estrogens.

    A, C–F See correct answer explanation.

Learning objective: Outline the noncontraceptive uses of combined oral contraceptives.

39. **E** The patient is most likely suffering from endometriosis, an estrogen-dependent inflammatory disease in which functioning endometrial tissue is present outside the uterine cavity. The incidence of the disorder is high, as it is commonly found in 10 to 15% of women between the ages of 25 and 45 who are actively menstruating. Medical therapy of endometriosis usually involves medical suppression of ovarian function to arrest the growth and the activity of endometrial implants. Endometriosis is estrogen-dependent. Low-dose oral contraceptives are appropriate initial therapy, with the goal of suppressing the endogenous production of estrogen. The low dose provided by the pill may offer some protection against bone loss without significantly promoting endometrial tissue formation. Depot injections of gonadotropin-releasing hormone (GnRH) agonists are an alternative therapy for endometriosis. Danazol is also approved for this use, but the adverse effect profile is considered to be worse than that of low-dose combined oral contraceptives or GnRH analogues.

    A Although anastrozole may be useful in treating postmenopausal endometriosis by blocking peripheral conversion of androgens to estrogens, it is not able to fully suppress estrogen production in premenopausal women and is not effective when used as monotherapy in premenopausal women; it has been proposed to use anastrozole in combination with a GnRH agonist, such as leuprolide.

B, C, F These drugs provide luteinizing hormone–like (human chorionic gonadotropin and lutropin alfa) and follicle-stimulating hormone (urofollitropin) activity and would not be useful in the treatment of endometriosis; furthermore, they potentially could be counterproductive.

D Tamoxifen is a selective estrogen receptor modulator that has estrogen-like actions on endometrial tissues and would be contraindicated in this situation.

Learning objective: Identify the drug that can trigger an acute porphyric attack in a genetically predisposed patient.

40. **B** The patient was most likely suffering from acute intermittent porphyria that manifests as intermittent attacks of abdominal, mental, or neurologic symptoms. Porphyrias result from genetic deficiencies of enzymes in the heme biosynthetic pathway. A large number of drugs, especially those that can induce hepatic aminolevulinic acid (ALA) synthase and cytochrome P-450 enzymes, can precipitate a porphyric attack in predisposed patients. These include barbiturates, phenytoin, valproate, sulfonamides, rifampin, progesterone, and synthetic progestins. Therefore, it is most likely that the progestin of the contraceptive pill (norethindrone) was the drug that triggered the attack in this patient.

A, C–E The administration of these drugs is considered safe in a patient affected by porphyrias.

Learning objective: Describe the interaction between rifampin and oral contraceptives.

41. **E** The drug currently used to prevent infection in close contacts of patients with meningococcal meningitis is rifampin. Historically, several cases of unexpected pregnancies were reported among women taking rifampin, and now it is well known that this occurs because rifampin can strongly reduce the plasma concentration of estrogens and progestins by inducing their metabolism.

A, B Ceftriaxone and ciprofloxacin are used to prevent infection in close contacts of patients with meningococcal meningitis, but they are not metabolism inducers.

C, D Erythromycin and ketoconazole are metabolism inhibitors, not inducers, and they are not used for meningococcal prophylaxis.

DRUGS FOR GONADAL DISORDERS Answer key			
1. A	6. A	11. E	16. C
2. K	7. A	12. C	17. E
3. E	8. C	13. D	18. C
4. G	9. B	14. F	19. A
5. F	10. F	15. C	20. E
21. A	26. B	31. C	36. A
22. D	27. B	32. D	37. F
23. B	28. D	33. E	38. B
24. D	29. D	34. C	39. E
25. B	30. F	35. D	40. B
			41. E

Answers and Explanations: V-5 Drugs for Bone Homeostasis

Questions 1–5

1. **A**
2. **K**
3. **G**
4. **D**
5. **C**

Learning objective: Explain the mechanism of action of teriparatide.

6. **A** Teriparatide is a recombinant analogue of parathyroid hormone (PTH) with physiological actions equal to those of the natural hormone. PTH targets osteoblasts, with the net effect on bone being dose-dependent. The effect of excess of PTH is a net increase in bone resorption (removal of bone mineral and matrix). However, intermittent low doses of PTH increase bone formation by increasing osteoblast number and activity without stimulating bone resorption. This has led to the approval of teriparatide for the treatment of osteoporosis. It is currently recommended that teriparatide be reserved for those who have proven refractory to other therapies and/or patients with a high risk of fractures, as in this case.

B, C, E PTH induces effects opposite to those listed.

D Collagen synthesis is not involved in bone turnover of mature bone.

Learning objective: Describe the pharmacological effects of vitamin D.

7. **A** Cholecalciferol (vitamin D$_3$), which is a prodrug, is the most appropriate therapy for vitamin D deficiency in anyone with normal renal function. Cholecalciferol is metabolized to 25(OH)D by the liver and circulates bound to vitamin D–binding protein, making it available for conversion to calcitriol. For the regulation of calcium homeostasis, the renal conversion of calcitriol plays a major role in stimulating intestinal calcium absorption, thus adding calcium to the system. Conversion in other tissues contributes to noncalcemic effects of calcitriol, such as muscle strength and support of the innate immune system.

    B Administration of calcitriol as a drug is reserved for cases where the body is unable to make calcitriol, as in renal failure, because of the risk of hypercalcemia.

    C–E None of these drugs would address vitamin D deficiency.

Learning objective: Explain the primary mechanism of action of calcitriol.

8. **D** Intestinal calcium absorption is potently augmented by calcitriol, and this is most likely the main action that mediates the therapeutic efficacy of calciferols in osteomalacia. There is little evidence that calcitriol directly promotes bone mineralization. Rather, it is the increased serum calcium level that indirectly promotes bone mineralization by decreasing parathyroid hormone–mediated bone resorption.

    A–C, E See correct answer explanation.

Learning objective: Outline the therapeutic uses of alendronate.

9. **F** Bisphosphonates are first-line therapy for osteoporosis, and adding alendronate to the current regimen is a rational choice, as the ongoing therapy failed to prevent the decrease in bone mass.

    A This option is irrational. Hydrochlorothiazide is useful in osteoporosis because it decreases the renal excretion of calcium.

    B Selective estrogen receptor modulators are today preferred over estrogens for the therapy of osteoporosis because they do not increase the risk of breast and endometrial cancer.

    C Calcitonin is much less effective than bisphosphonates in the therapy of osteoporosis.

    D The dose of calcium taken by the patient is the standard for calcium supplementation in postmenopausal women. It is unlikely that a larger dose would add benefit.

    E Glucocorticoids are contraindicated in osteoporosis because they counteract the effects of vitamin D to stimulate intestinal calcium absorption.

Learning objective: Outline the therapeutic uses of sevelamer.

10. **E** The patient was most likely suffering from end-stage renal disease, a condition commonly associated with hyperphosphatemia. Sevelamer is a nonabsorbable, calcium- and aluminum-free, polymeric amine that binds dietary phosphate within the gastrointestinal tract, thereby preventing phosphate absorption. It has been approved for the management of hyperphosphatemia in patients with end-stage renal disease.

    A–D These diseases are not associated with hyperphosphatemia.

Learning objective: Identify the drug used to treat rickets.

11. **A** The patient's signs and symptoms, together with the lab results, suggest that he was suffering from rickets, a disease that can affect children. Dark-skinned are at greater risk, because skin pigmentation blocks ultraviolet irradiation needed for synthesis of vitamin D. Rickets is due to vitamin D deficiency, which in turn causes deficient mineralization of epiphyseal cartilage and osteoid matrix. Vitamin D deficiency tends to cause hypocalcemia. When this occurs, parathyroid hormone (PTH) production is increased. Thus, the serum level of calcium is restored to nearly normal, but hypophosphatemia persists (due to PTH-mediated increase in renal secretion of phosphate), and mineralization of bone is impaired. The elevated alkaline phosphatase reflects the increased osteoblast activity. Cholecalciferol (vitamin D$_3$) supplementation with adequate calcium and phosphate intake is the standard therapy for rickets.

    C Although calcitriol is the active form of vitamin D$_3$, it is not used for rickets, as its action is short, and it can cause hypercalcemia in about 30% of patients. With adequate cholecalciferol, the body can regulate the production of appropriate levels of calcitriol.

    B, D–F See correct answer explanation.

Learning objective: Explain the mechanism of action of cholecalciferol.

12. **D** Both cholecalciferol (vitamin D$_3$) and ergocalciferol (vitamin D$_2$) are prodrugs and need to be transformed in the body into active metabolites. The primary active metabolite of these vitamins is calcitriol, which binds to vitamin D receptors within target cells. The calcitriol–vitamin D receptor complex binds to specific recognition sites on DNA to modify gene transcription.

    A–C, E, F See correct answer explanation.

Learning objective: Describe the reason for the long duration of action of bisphosphonates.

13. **B** Bisphosphonates in bones are often retained for months or years, and a single injection of zoledronate can be effective for up to 1 year in the treatment of osteoporosis. The reason for this exceptionally long duration of action is because these drugs are incorporated into the hydroxyapatite crystals of bone in place of pyrophosphate, thus altering the structure of the crystal. When bisphosphonates are released from resorbed bone mineral, they cause apoptosis of the osteoclasts, thus reducing the rate of bone resorption and decreasing the net bone loss that characterizes osteoporosis.

A, C–E See correct answer explanation.

Learning objective: Outline the therapeutic uses of pamidronate in bone metastases.

14. **C** The patient's signs and symptoms, along with the elevated alkaline phosphatase, indicated that he was most likely suffering from hypercalcemia due to metastatic prostate cancer. In fact, hyperparathyroidism and cancer, with or without metastases, are the two major causes of hypercalcemia, accounting for over 90% of cases. The disorder occurs in 10 to 20% of all adults with cancer. Rehydration with saline and diuresis with furosemide are the first step in the treatment of severe hypercalcemia. Bisphosphonates such as pamidronate have been approved for the acute treatment of hypercalcemia of malignancy. Because they have a slow onset of activity, calcitonin is frequently given concomitantly.

A Intravenous (IV) sodium phosphate is probably the fastest way to lower serum calcium level, but it is a hazardous procedure because of the risk involved (sudden hypocalcemia, ectopic calcification, hypotension, and acute renal failure). In light of satisfactory responses to other agents, IV sodium phosphate is used only after other methods of treatment have failed to control hypercalcemia.

B Hydrochlorothiazide increases, not decreases, serum calcium level.

D Osmotic diuretics such as mannitol are absolutely contraindicated in dehydrated patients.

E Fludrocortisone is used only when dehydration is caused by adrenal insufficiency.

F Cinacalcet decreases parathyroid hormone (PTH) secretion by activating calcium-sensing receptors in the parathyroid gland. It can decrease PTH-mediated hypercalcemia but not cancer-mediated hypercalcemia. The reason is that the main humoral factor associated with cancer-related hypercalcemia is PTH-related peptide, whose production is not under the control of calcium-sensing receptors.

Learning objective: Outline the therapeutic uses of calcitonin.

15. **F** The patient's symptoms, together with the high calcium, low phosphorus, and high parathyroid hormone (PTH) levels, are consistent with the diagnosis of primary hyperparathyroidism. In fact, PTH values are elevated in more than 90% of parathyroid-related causes of hypercalcemia, undetectable or low in malignancy-related hypercalcemia, and undetectable or normal in high bone turnover causes of hypercalcemia. The approach to medical treatment of hypercalcemia varies with its severity. Mild hypercalcemia (< 12 mg/dL) can be managed by hydration. More severe hypercalcemia (> 13–14 mg/dL) must be managed aggressively because, above those levels, it can be life-threatening. Therefore, the more severe the hypercalcemia, the greater the number of combined therapies that should be used. The mainstay of treatment in patients with normal renal function is to increase renal calcium excretion with intravenous saline and furosemide, which inhibits calcium reabsorption in the thick ascending limb of Henle. Bisphosphonates, which are long-lasting inhibitors of bone resorption, have become first-line agents for the antiresorptive treatment of hypercalcemia. However, they have a slow onset of action (1 or 2 days). Calcitonin has a rapid, albeit short-lived, blockade of bone resorption. An effect on serum calcium is observed within 4 to 6 hours and lasts 6 to 10 hours. Therefore, an addition of both calcitonin and pamidronate is the standard treatment.

A Calcitriol is contraindicated in this case because it tends to increase serum calcium level; also, calcitriol levels may be elevated in this patient secondary to the hyperparathyroidism.

B Thiazides are contraindicated because they enhance calcium reabsorption in the distal convolute tubule.

C Fluoride stimulates bone formation, but the doses that cause hypocalcemia are toxic, and the drug is not used for this purpose.

D Potassium-sparing diuretics have low efficacy and are contraindicated in this case, as they tend to enhance calcium reabsorption in the distal convolute tubule.

E Teriparatide is an analogue of parathyroid hormone and therefore is contraindicated in a patient with hyperparathyroidism.

Learning objective: Explain the mechanism of action of calcitonin.

16. **A** Calcitonin is a hormone secreted by the parafollicular cells of the thyroid. The principal action of the hormone is a direct inhibition of osteoclastic bone resorption. This action is mediated by the activation of calcitonin receptors located on osteoclasts, which in turn causes a profound decrease in the ruffled border of these cells, thereby inhibiting bone resorption. Calcitonin is not a first-line agent in the treatment of Paget disease of bone, but it can be used as an alternative drug when bisphosphonates are not tolerated, as in this case.

   B Although calcitonin may decrease apoptosis of osteoblasts, Paget disease is mainly characterized by uncontrolled osteoclastic bone resorption. Therefore, inhibition of osteoclast activity, not stimulation of osteoblast activity, is the main action that mediates the therapeutic effect of the drug in Paget disease.

   C, D Calcitonin causes actions opposite to those listed.

   E Calcitonin does not directly affect intestinal calcium absorption.

Learning objective: Identify the drug used to treat renal osteodystrophy.

17. **C** The patient's high creatinine level points out that he was most likely suffering from chronic renal failure, presumably due to diabetic nephropathy (the most common cause of renal failure in the United States). Chronic renal failure can cause renal osteodystrophy, a term used to describe collectively all the skeletal changes in chronic renal disease. Renal osteodystrophy is due to several factors, including loss of calcitriol production because the damaged kidney no longer contains sufficient renal α_1 hydroxylase to convert $25(OH)D_3$ into calcitriol. This contributes to secondary hyperparathyroidism due to the resulting hypocalcemia (also, calcitriol suppresses parathyroid hormone gene expression). The combination of hyperparathyroidism and calcitriol deficiency leads to the development of renal osteodystrophy, which has features of both osteomalacia and osteoporosis. In chronic renal failure, calcitriol can help alleviate both the hypocalcemia and the bone disease.

   A, B, D, E See correct answer explanation.

Learning objective: Explain the molecular mechanism of action of cinacalcet.

18. **C** Cinacalcet is the first representative of a new class of drugs that activate the calcium-sensing receptor. This receptor is widely distributed but has its greatest concentration in the parathyroid gland. By activating this receptor cinacalcet inhibits parathyroid hormone (PTH) secretion. Cinacalcet lowers serum PTH levels in patients with normal or reduced renal function. The drug is approved for the treatment of secondary hyperparathyroidism due to chronic kidney disease and for patients with hypercalcemia associated with parathyroid carcinoma.

   A, B, D, E See correct answer explanation.

Learning objective: Identify the drug used to treat hypocalcemia in a patient with liver cirrhosis.

19. **D** The symptoms, the lab results, and the history of the patient indicate that he was most likely suffering from alcoholic cirrhosis. The bone demineralization and low calcium levels suggest that liver disease caused an impaired synthesis of $25(OH)D$ with the final outcome of osteomalacia. Calcitriol is the most effective agent for hypocalcemia in a patient with impaired liver function because it bypasses the impaired synthesis of the precursor essential for production of calcitriol. Clinically, severe calcitriol deficiency as a consequence of liver disease is rare because the degree of hepatic destruction necessary to impair 25-hydroxylation is incompatible with long-term survival. However, it is not rare when the patient also has vitamin D deficiency, which frequently occurs in homeless people because of a poor diet.

   A Patients with hypocalcemia already have an increased production of parathyroid hormone (PTH). Teriparatide, a PTH analogue, can add very little to the therapy.

   B Vitamin D_3 would be only marginally effective because of the impairment of liver 25-hydroxylation.

   C Bisphosphonates are absolutely contraindicated in patients with hypocalcemia.

   E Calcipotriene, a vitamin D analogue, is used only locally.

Learning objective: Explain the mechanism of action of alendronate.

20. **D** Bisphosphonates are drugs of choice in osteoporosis. They are incorporated into the bone mineral and inhibit the activity of osteoclasts in a dose-dependent manner. The mechanism of this inhibition is still incompletely understood and likely multifactorial. Amino bisphosphonates such as alendronate inhibit an enzyme, farnesyl pyrophosphate synthase, in the mevalonate pathway that appears to be critical for osteoclast survival. Therefore, promotion of osteoclast apoptosis or death seems an important mechanism of the inhibition of osteoclast activity.

   A–C, E See correct answer explanation.

Learning objective: Explain the mechanism of action of teriparatide.

21. **A** Teriparatide is a recombinant analogue of parathyroid hormone (PTH) with physiological actions equal to those of the natural hormone. PTH exerts both catabolic and anabolic effects on bone. Catabolic effects prevail with chronically elevated PTH; there is a net increase in bone resorption. Anabolic effects prevail with intermittent low doses of PTH; there is a net increase in bone formation (by increasing

osteoblast number and activity) without stimulating bone resorption. This has led to the approval of teriparatide for the treatment of osteoporosis. The drug is reserved for advanced osteoporosis when bisphosphonate therapy has failed, extreme bone loss has already occurred, and/or fracture has already occurred, as in this case. Teriparatide is the only currently available therapy that results in net bone deposition.

B Estrogens are used for prevention, not for treatment, of osteoporosis only in postmenopausal women who need estrogen treatment for the management of menopausal symptoms.

C Because alendronate was not effective, the use of another bisphosphonate would be irrational. Bisphosphonates are considered antiresorptive agents as opposed to bone anabolic agents.

D Calcitonin does not consistently decrease hip fracture risk and does not increase bone density.

E Paricalcitol is an analogue of calcitriol, used for the treatment of secondary hyperparathyroidism in specific stages of chronic kidney disease.

Learning objective: Describe the adverse effects of alendronate.

22. **F** When administered orally, bisphosphonates (mainly alendronate) frequently cause esophageal and gastric irritation. Because of this, patients are instructed to take the medication early in the morning on an empty stomach with a large glass of water and then to stay quiet and upright for 30 minutes to reduce the chance of esophageal irritation.

A Glucocorticoids can cause gastric irritation, but they are contraindicated in osteoporosis.

B–E These drugs are used for osteoporosis, but their risk of esophageal and gastric irritation is very low.

Learning objective: Outline the therapeutic uses of calcitonin.

23. **A** The patient's signs and symptoms indicate that he was most likely affected by Paget disease of bone, a chronic disorder of the adult skeleton characterized by uncontrolled osteoclastic bone resorption with secondary increase in poorly organized bone formation. The disease is fairly common, affecting about 3% of adults over age 40. It is often asymptomatic and usually progresses slowly. Pharmacological therapy is indicated (even in the absence of symptoms) when alkaline phosphatase is more than 2 to 3 times the normal levels, as in this case. Bisphosphonates are first-line agents for this disease. Calcitonin is an alternative to bisphosphonates when these drugs are contraindicated, as in this case (see answer explanation B).

B Oral bisphosphonates are relatively contraindicated in patients with gastrointestinal reflux disease, esophagitis, gastritis, and peptic ulcer, as they can cause esophageal and gastric irritation.

C–F These drugs are useless in Paget disease.

Learning objective: Outline the therapeutic uses of calcium.

24. **D** The symptoms and history of the patient indicate that she was suffering from severe hypocalcemia secondary to hypoparathyroidism, likely due to accidental damage of parathyroid glands or their circulation during thyroidectomy. The treatment of severe hypocalcemia can be best accomplished with slow infusion of calcium gluconate (the preferred calcium salt for intravenous therapy because it is less irritating to the vein).

A Vitamin D can increase calcium levels, but its onset of action is too slow for an emergency therapy.

B, C, E, F All of these drugs are actually contraindicated because they decrease serum calcium levels.

Learning objective: Describe the adverse effects of teriparatide.

25. **D** Teriparatide is a recombinant analogue of parathyroid hormone (PTH) with physiological actions equal to those of the natural hormone. It is used in patients with advanced osteoporosis and previous bone fractures. Although hypercalcemia is not a common adverse effect, the hormone acts like the natural PTH; it increases renal reabsorption of calcium and the efflux of calcium from bone into the serum. Several cases of teriparatide-induced hypercalcemia have been reported in the literature.

B Furosemide actually decreases serum calcium levels.

A, C, E These drugs do not affect serum calcium levels.

Learning objective: Describe the pharmacological effects of teriparatide.

26. **B** Teriparatide is a recombinant analogue of parathyroid hormone (PTH) with physiological actions equal to those of the natural hormone. The drug has been approved for the treatment of osteoporosis. The primary function of PTH is to maintain a constant concentration of Ca^{2+} and phosphate in the extracellular fluid. The principal processes regulated by the hormone are renal Ca^{2+} (elevated) and phosphate (decreased) reabsorption and mobilization of bone Ca^{2+}. Administration of teriparatide will transiently increase the renal reabsorption of Ca^{2+} after each dose.

A, C The drug causes actions opposite to those listed.

D PTH exerts both catabolic and anabolic effects on bone. Chronically elevated PTH enhances bone resorption by increasing osteoclast activity, but intermittent exposure to low levels of the hormone (as occurs with daily injection of low doses of teriparatide) increases bone formation without causing net bone resorption.

E The transient increase in serum Ca^{2+} after each dose would decrease, not increase, PTH secretion.

Learning objective: Explain the mechanism of action of denosumab.

27. **C** Denosumab is a monoclonal antibody with affinity for receptor activator of nuclear factor κ_B ligand (RANKL). In bone, osteoclast formation is regulated by an osteoclast receptor protein called RANK (receptor activator of nuclear factor κ_B). The natural ligand of RANK, called RANKL, is a soluble protein produced by osteoblasts. On binding to RANK, RANKL induces osteoclast formation.

   Denosumab binds and neutralizes RANKL. In this way, osteoclast formation and bone turnover are decreased. The drug is at least as effective as bisphosphonates in inhibiting bone resorption.

   A, B, D, E None of these processes is affected by denosumab.

Learning objective: Outline the therapeutic uses of sevelamer.

28. **B** The laboratory results show a pronounced hyperphosphatemia, most likely due to advanced renal insufficiency. Sevelamer is a nonabsorbable, calcium- and aluminum-free, polymeric amine. The drug binds dietary phosphate within the gastrointestinal tract, thereby preventing phosphate absorption. It has been approved for use as an oral agent for the management of hyperphosphatemia in patients with end-stage renal disease, as in this case.

   A, C, D These drugs tend to reduce serum calcium levels and are therefore contraindicated in hypocalcemia.

   E Vitamin D is useless in this case because the kidney has lost the ability to transform the drug into the active metabolite.

Learning objective: Identify a drug used to treat plaque psoriasis.

29. **C** The patient's signs and symptoms indicate that he was most likely affected by plaque psoriasis, a common skin disorder that affects 1 to 5% of the population worldwide. The disease is diagnosed most often by clinical appearance and distribution of lesions. Arthritis develops in up to 30% of patients, as in this case (see the swollen and tender joints). Calcitriol analogues were discovered to be effective in the treatment of psoriasis. However, oral calcitriol has limited usefulness due to hypercalcemia associated with the large doses often needed for therapy. Topical calcipotriene, a calcitriol analogue, provides a safe and effective alternative to oral calcitriol. It induces normal keratinocyte proliferation and differentiation. Marked improvement of psoriasis is generally noted following 2 weeks of therapy, with continued improvement for up to 8 weeks of treatment in up to 70% of patients, although lesions can recur within 2 to 3 months following discontinuance of treatment. Clinical trials comparing calcipotriene with other antipsoriatic agents have demonstrated that calcipotriene is at least as effective as topical glucocorticoids.

   A Glucocorticoids, not mineralocorticoids, are used for psoriasis.

   B, D, E, F See correct answer explanation.

Learning objective: Identify the site of action of cinacalcet.

30. **C** The patient was diagnosed with severe renal insufficiency. Virtually all patients with renal failure have secondary hyperparathyroidism to some degree. These patients usually have a low-normal calcium level and high phosphate level, as in this case. Alternatively, phosphate levels are usually low when secondary hyperparathyroidism is due to vitamin D deficiency. Cinacalcet is the first representative of a new class of drugs that activate the calcium-sensing receptor. This receptor is widely distributed but has its greatest concentration in the parathyroid gland and in the kidney. By activating the calcium-sensing receptor, cinacalcet inhibits parathyroid hormone secretion. Cinacalcet is approved for the treatment of secondary hyperparathyroidism due to chronic kidney disease. Because the drug can rapidly cause hypocalcemia, it should not be used for patients with a serum calcium level below 8.4 mg/dL.

   A, B, D, E See correct answer explanation.

DRUGS FOR BONE HOMEOSTASIS Answer key		
1. A	6. A	11. A
2. K	7. A	12. D
3. G	8. D	13. B
4. D	9. F	14. C
5. C	10. E	15. F
16. A	21. A	26. B
17. C	22. F	27. C
18. C	23. A	28. B
19. D	24. D	29. C
20. D	25. D	30. C

Answers and Explanations: V-6 Drugs for Diabetes Mellitus

Questions 1–7

1. **E**

2. **I**

3. **N**

4. **G**

5. **M**

6. **A**

7. **C**

Learning objective: Identify the main risk for a diabetic patient under tight glycemic control.

8. **D** A large, long-term study has shown that tight control of blood glucose using multiple insulin injections or an insulin pump is associated with a lower incidence of long-term complications from diabetes. However, intensively treated patients had a threefold greater risk of hypoglycemia.

A, C These pathologic conditions are decreased, not increased, in patients with tight control of blood glucose.

B Hypertension is not affected by tight control of blood glucose. Another study, however, has shown that a tight control of hypertension has a beneficial effect on diabetic microvascular complications.

E Tightly controlled diabetic patients have an increased risk of weight gain, not weight loss.

F Allergic reactions to insulin are not dose-dependent, so it is unlikely that they are affected by tight control of blood glucose.

Learning objective: Describe the molecular mechanism of action of insulin.

9. **B** Insulin binds to a specific transmembrane, tyrosine kinase–linked receptor located in the cell membranes of most tissues. The receptor consists of two α subunits linked to two β subunits. Insulin binding to the α subunits causes the activation of the β-receptor subunit, which contain tyrosine kinase. The enzyme is phosphorylated, which in turn activates a cascade of downstream signaling events that ultimately lead to a hypoglycemic effect.

A, C–E All of these actions would increase, not decrease, blood glucose levels.

Learning objective: Outline the therapy of diabetic ketoacidosis.

10. **E** Metabolic conditions may be the result of recent injuries, or they may be the cause of altered consciousness leading to the traumatic event, as in this patient. Most likely the girl had undetected diabetes that led to her involvement in the accident. The marked hyperglycemia, glycosuria, and ketosis indicate that the patient has diabetic ketoacidosis and therefore must receive intravenous (IV) regular insulin at once.

A Latent diabetes can lead to hyperosmolar coma, which should be treated with IV regular insulin. However, the patient was not unconscious, and the ketotic bodies in the urine indicate that the most likely diagnosis is diabetic ketoacidosis.

B Acute renal failure can result from a motor accident. However, the lab results do not indicate kidney insufficiency.

C Acute liver failure can occur after trauma, but the patient has no signs or symptoms of acute liver failure.

D Even if the patient is acidotic (see the very low bicarbonate level), acidosis is due to diabetes and therefore is metabolic, not respiratory. In fact, respiratory frequency is increased in this patient.

Learning objective: Identify the appropriate drug to treat gestational diabetes.

11. **D** Gestational diabetes mellitus is defined as any glucose intolerance that develops or is recognized during pregnancy, regardless of severity or time of onset. Gestational diabetes affects about 4% of all pregnancies in the United States and is the most common maternal medical complication during pregnancy. Because gestational diabetes carries several risks for both the mother and the offspring, treatment is mandatory. Most gestational diabetics can control their glucose level with diet and regular exercise; drug therapy is needed only if these procedures are failing, as in this case. Insulin is the hypoglycemic drug of choice during pregnancy because it does not cross the placenta and has an established safety record for both mother and fetus.

A–C, E Although recent evidence suggests that glyburide or metformin can be effective in diabetes during pregnancy, most authorities believe that oral antidiabetic agents should be used during pregnancy only in the setting of approved clinical trials.

Learning objective: Describe the pharmacokinetics of different insulin preparations.

12. **E** Insulin glargine is a long-acting insulin analogue that was designed to provide a broad plasma concentration plateau. It has an onset of action of 1 to 4 hours, achieves a maximum effect after 4 to 6 hours, and can maintain this effect for over 24 hours. It is usually given once daily to provide basal levels of insulin.

A–D See correct answer explanation.

Learning objective: Identify the drug used in a child with new-onset type 1 diabetes.

13. **A** The age, symptoms, lab values, and history of the patient indicate that he was most likely suffering from type 1 diabetes. An acute viral illness can trigger autoimmune destruction of the pancreas in genetically susceptible individuals. Because of the markedly diminished insulin levels associated with type 1 diabetes, insulin is crucial to the survival of these patients.

B–F Oral hypoglycemic agents are not useful in type 1 diabetes.

Learning objective: Describe the main daily insulin regimens for type 1 diabetes.

14. **A** Endocrinologists have developed a variety of insulin regimens that are intended to mimic the release of insulin from the pancreas. The general goal of these insulin regimens is to provide a basal level of insulin over 24 hours and to supply additional mealtime insulin coverage. This can be done by administering a rapid-acting insulin at meals and a long-acting insulin at bedtime to ensure basal coverage for the following 24 hours.

    B A regular insulin at breakfast cannot supply a basal level of insulin over 24 hours. Moreover, rapid-acting insulins such as lispro are given to control postprandial hyperglycemia; administration at bedtime is irrational.

    C NPH (neutral protamine Hagedorn) insulin at breakfast and lunch can supply a basal level of insulin over 24 hours but cannot control postprandial hyperglycemia.

    D This regimen cannot provide a basal level of insulin over 24 hours.

    E Insulin glargine alone cannot control postprandial hyperglycemia.

Learning objective: Explain the mechanism of insulin–glucocorticoid interaction.

15. **B** In a diabetic patient on insulin therapy, the daily dose of insulin is often increased when a new therapy is started with a drug that can cause hyperglycemia, especially if the new drug is given in high doses, as in this case.

    A See correct answer explanation.

    C–E These drugs are approved for type 2 diabetes, as they can increase insulin synthesis and release. They are of very little value in type 1 diabetes, where the insulin synthesis is already severely decreased or absent.

Learning objective: Outline the appropriate therapy for a diabetic patient on insulin treatment, when an acute infection supervenes.

16. **A** Insulin requirement always increases in the presence of stressful situations, including acute illnesses. This is, at least in part, because of hyperglycemia brought about by the high plasma cortisol levels associated with stress.

    B, D These antibiotics are not effective against *Mycoplasma pneumoniae* or *Chlamydia pneumoniae*, the most frequent causative agents of atypical pneumonia.

    C, E Because insulin requirement is increased, the best course of action is to increase the daily insulin dosage, not to add an oral antidiabetic agent.

Learning objective: Explain the mechanism of action of repaglinide.

17. **E** Repaglinide is a meglitinide derivative with mechanisms of action very close to those of sulfonylureas. The main mechanism is stimulation of insulin release, most likely due to the drug-induced closure of adenosine triphosphate (ATP)–dependent K^+ channels. This causes a membrane depolarization, which in turn opens voltage-gated Ca^{2+} channels, allowing Ca^{2+}-mediated exocytosis of insulin.

    A–D, F All of these actions would decrease the hyperglycemia, but they are not elicited by repaglinide.

Learning objective: Describe the actions of insulin on lipid metabolism.

18. **C** Insulin influences lipid metabolism in both the liver and adipose tissue. In the liver, insulin favors esterification of fatty acids with glycerol, thus forming triglycerides. In adipose tissue, insulin affects lipid metabolism by the following actions:

    - It promotes the breakdown of glucose to α-glycerol phosphate that is used to synthesize triglycerides.
    - It inhibits the activity of hormone-sensitive triglyceride lipase, the enzyme that mediates the conversion of stored triglycerides to fatty acids.
    - It increases the synthesis of lipoprotein lipase, the enzyme that is transferred to endothelial cells where it cleaves triglycerides into glycerol and fatty acids.

    A, B, D, E Insulin elicits actions opposite to those listed.

Learning objective: Explain the mechanism of action of glyburide.

19. **C** Sulfonylureas such as glyburide act by binding to a specific receptor that is closely linked to the adenosine triphosphate (ATP)–sensitive K^+ channels in pancreatic β-cell membranes. This causes a blockade of the efflux of K^+, which in turn leads to membrane depolarization. Voltage-gated Ca^{2+} channels open in response to depolarization, thus increasing intracellular Ca^{2+} concentrations. This increased concentration ultimately stimulates the release of insulin by exocytosis.

    A, D, F Acarbose, metformin, and pioglitazone can be used in the treatment of type 2 diabetes, but none of them have the described mechanism of action.

    B, E Insulin and exenatide are not orally active.

Learning objective: Identify the oral antidiabetic drug that can cause hypoglycemia in a diabetic patient.

20. **C** The low glucose level indicates that the behavior and symptoms of the patient are due to hypoglycemia; that is, they are neuroglycopenic symptoms. These symptoms are more frequent in older patients under antidiabetic treatment. In fact, sulfonylureas account for almost all cases of drug-induced hypoglycemia in individuals older than 60.

    A, B, D These drugs are considered euglycemic, not hypoglycemic, because they do not cause hypoglycemia when given alone.

E Exenatide is a glucagon-like polypeptide 1 (GLP-1) receptor agonist. It is a peptide and therefore is given by the parenteral route only. Moreover, it does not cause hypoglycemia when given alone.

Learning objective: Describe hypoglycemic coma due to excessive alcohol consumption in a diabetic patient.

21. **B** The patient's signs (unconsciousness, sweating, hypothermia, tachycardia, and tonic-clonic seizure) and his history (alcoholic and insulin treatment) indicate that he was suffering from hypoglycemic coma. Hypoglycemia often occurs in alcoholics, likely due to a combination of starvation and impaired liver gluconeogenesis. In this case, the insulin treatment most likely made the patient even more sensitive to the hypoglycemic effects of alcohol, thus precipitating the hypoglycemic coma.

    A, C, D Signs of hyperglycemia and ketoacidosis are different (often opposite) to those shown by the patient.

    E Signs of an anaphylactic reaction are different from those shown by the patient.

    F Hyperosmolar coma can follow an excessive dose of alcohol. Signs of this coma are different from those shown by the patient.

Learning objective: Describe the pharmacological actions of insulin.

22. **B** Insulin increases glycolysis and decreases glycogenolysis and gluconeogenesis in the liver. The final effect is a decrease of glucose production and an increase of glucose utilization.

    A, C–E See correct answer explanation.

Learning objective: Outline the addition of a second antidiabetic agent in type 2 diabetes when a single agent fails to control the disease.

23. **A** The patient's serum values indicate that the control of his diabetes was no longer adequate. When a single oral antidiabetic agent fails to control the disease, a second oral agent should be added to the therapy. Many combinations of antidiabetic agents can be used. The key is that they should have different mechanisms of action. Because the patient was on metformin, the addition of a sulfonylurea is appropriate.

    B, C Substitution of an oral antidiabetic agent with another usually does not produce any significant change in glycemic control.

    D Diabetes is a progressive condition, and most patients with type 2 diabetes eventually require insulin. However, insulin is usually added to, not substituted for, oral agents when diabetic control is not achieved.

    E Because the patient's total cholesterol is low, lovastatin is not needed.

Learning objective: Explain the molecular mechanism of action of metformin.

24. **D** Biguanides such as metformin cause activation of adenosine monophosphate (AMP)–activated protein kinase, an enzyme that acts as a sensor of cellular energy status in all eukaryotic cells. The enzyme is activated when cellular energy stores are reduced or when biguanide drugs are administered. Its activation in turn causes

    • Inhibition of gluconeogenesis and lipogenesis
    • Stimulation of glucose uptake and utilization (glycolysis)
    • Stimulation of fatty acid oxidation
    • Reduction of plasma glucagon levels

    The net result is increased glycogen storage in skeletal muscle, decreased glucose production by the liver, and decreased hyperglycemia.

    A–C, E All of these actions would decrease hyperglycemia, but they are not elicited by metformin.

Learning objective: Outline the main contraindications to sulfonylureas.

25. **A** Glyburide is a sulfonylurea-derivative antidiabetic drug. Sulfonylureas are sulfa drugs (i.e., they have a sulfur group in their molecule), and are therefore contraindicated in patients with a history of previous severe allergic reaction to sulfonamides, as in this case.

    B–E These oral antidiabetic agents are not sulfa drugs.

Learning objective: Describe the adverse effects of metformin.

26. **B** The patient's symptoms and the lab data indicate that she was suffering from lactic acidosis, a serious adverse effect of biguanides. Lactic acidosis is extremely rare, but it can result from metformin overdose, especially in patients with renal insufficiency (the drug is all eliminated by the kidney), as in this case. The syndrome is highly lethal (50% mortality) and seems to be due to drug-induced inhibition of gluconeogenesis, which in turn impairs the hepatic uptake of lactic acid.

    A, C–F Overdose of these drugs does not cause lactic acidosis.

Learning objective: Describe the main contraindications to the use of metformin.

27. **B** Biguanides can cause lactic acidosis and therefore are relatively contraindicated in all conditions that predispose to acidosis. This patient is suffering from chronic obstructive pulmonary disease and is under treatment with an angiotensin-converting enzyme (ACE) inhibitor. The respiratory disease predisposes to respiratory acidosis, and ACE inhibitors predispose to metabolic acidosis because they lower aldosterone serum levels.

    A, C–E None of these drugs are contraindicated in this patient.

Learning objective: Describe the pharmacokinetics of different insulin formulations.

28. **A** Insulin formulations differ one from another in the absorption rate of the drug from subcutaneous tissue, which in turn affects the duration of action of the drug. The variation in absorption is accomplished in the following ways:

    - Modification of the insulin molecule (by recombinant technology)
    - Conjugation of insulin with protamine in a low soluble complex. After injection, proteolytic enzymes degrade protamine, allowing absorption of insulin.
    - Combination of insulin with zinc to form zinc salts. After injection, the salt precipitates, and insulin is slowly released.

    B, C These properties refer to the elimination of the drug and therefore are not affected by variations in the rate of absorption.

    D The distribution of a drug is not affected by variation in absorption.

    E The oral bioavailability of all insulin preparations is zero.

Learning objective: Explain the molecular mechanism of action of pioglitazone.

29. **F** Pioglitazone is a thiazolidinedione derivative. Thiazolidinediones act by binding to a nuclear receptor called peroxisome proliferator activated receptor gamma (PPAR-γ), which is located mainly in adipose tissue, skeletal muscle, and liver. The receptor regulates the transcription of several insulin-responsive genes. The overall effect is an enhancement of tissue sensitivity to insulin (i.e., a reduction in insulin resistance). Therefore, the need for exogenous insulin is reduced. Because of this, they are called insulin sensitizers.

    A This is the mechanism of miglitol.

    B This is the mechanism of sulfonylureas.

    C This is the mechanism of sitagliptin.

    D This is the mechanism of exenatide.

    E This is the mechanism of metformin.

Learning objective: Describe the main adverse effects of thiazolidinediones.

30. **D** The patient's signs and symptoms indicated that he was suffering from edema, weight gain, and initial heart failure. Pioglitazone is a thiazolidinedione derivative. Most common adverse effects of these drugs are edema (up to 27%), weight gain (up to 14%), and upper respiratory tract infections (up to 15%). In addition, they can cause heart failure, mainly in at-risk patients; these patients should be closely monitored.

    A–C, E These drugs do not cause all of the signs and symptoms reported by the patient.

Learning objective: Describe the insulin resistance in a diabetic patient.

31. **E** The simultaneous elevation of blood glucose and insulin levels is strongly suggestive of insulin resistance. Insulin resistance can develop especially in diabetics who have a clustering of cardiovascular risk factors, including hypertension, abdominal obesity, and dyslipidemia. The association of insulin resistance with the above-mentioned clustering has been referred to by a variety of names, including insulin resistance syndrome, metabolic syndrome, and dysmetabolic syndrome. The prevalence of this syndrome is more than 30% in the US population. An estimated 75% of patients with type 2 diabetes have metabolic syndrome, as in this case. The syndrome is strongly associated with an increased risk of cardiovascular diseases.

    A Metformin can cause lactic acidosis, but symptoms of this disorder (vomiting, lethargy, hyperventilation, hypotension) are absent in this patient.

    B Because the patient has hyperglycemia and insulin resistance, a hypoglycemic reaction is quite unlikely.

    C The patient is at increased risk of unstable angina, but symptoms of unstable angina are absent in this patient.

    D The signs and symptoms of ketoacidosis are absent in this patient.

Learning objective: Describe the main contraindications to the use of metformin.

32. **E** The patient's symptoms and serum values indicate that he was most likely suffering from kidney failure (see high creatinine and blood urea nitrogen [BUN] values), a frequent complication of long-standing diabetes and hypertension. Metformin is excreted as such by the kidney and is therefore absolutely contraindicated in a patient with renal failure.

    A–D These drugs are not contraindicated in renal failure.

Learning objective: Outline the appropriate pharmacotherapy to treat a prediabetic state with high cholesterol and triglycerides.

33. **B** The absence of subjective symptoms and the values of fasting blood glucose and glycated hemoglobin (HbA1c; both are in the prediabetic range) indicate that the patient was most likely suffering from prediabetes, a state in which some, but not all, of the diagnostic criteria for diabetes are met. Prediabetes is also called impaired glucose tolerance (IGT) or impaired fasting glucose (IFG), depending on the test used to measure blood glucose levels. Having prediabetes puts the patient at higher risk for developing type 2 diabetes. People with prediabetes are also at increased risk for developing cardiovascular disease. Newly diagnosed prediabetic states are normally managed with diet and physical activity, but

when dyslipidemia is also present, a pharmacotherapy is usually administered. Metformin can decrease serum triglycerides by 15 to 20% and serum cholesterol by 10%. In addition, it can decrease body weight and is therefore appropriate for obese patients, as in this case.

A, C–E See correct answer explanation.

Learning objective: Describe the actions of insulin on glucose metabolism.

34. **B** Insulin influences glucose metabolism mainly in liver, adipose tissue, and muscle. In liver and muscle, the hormone increases glycogen synthase activity, thus increasing glycogen synthesis.

A Glucose enters the hepatocyte from the blood through glucose transporter 2 (GLUT2), whose activity is not influenced by insulin.

C–E Insulin elicits actions opposite to those listed.

Learning objective: Explain the mechanism of action of acarbose.

35. **B** Acarbose and miglitol are inhibitors of α-glucosidase, an enzyme located on the brush border of intestinal cells that is involved in the breakdown of starches and disaccharides into simple sugars. Inhibition of this enzyme slows the absorption of carbohydrates from the gastrointestinal tract and blunts the rate of rise of postprandial glucose.

A This is a liver enzyme that catalyzes the first step in gluconeogenesis.

C This is a liver enzyme that phosphorylates glucose to glucose-6-phosphate.

D, E These are adipocyte enzymes involved in lipid metabolism.

Learning objective: Explain the molecular mechanism of action of exenatide.

36. **D** Exenatide is a glucagon-like polypeptide-1 (GLP-1) receptor agonist. GLP-1 is one of the so-called incretin hormones, a group of small intestinal peptides that are released after meals and stimulate "glucose-activated" insulin secretion. This ultimately decreases fasting and postprandial glucose excursions, thus avoiding the risk of hyper- or hypoglycemia. Other useful effects of the drug are suppression of glucagon secretion, slowing gastric emptying (thus slowing the rate of glucose entry into the circulation), and decreased appetite, which in turn can cause weight loss. Exenatide is therefore especially useful in obese diabetic patients, as in this case.

A–C, E, F See correct answer explanation.

Learning objective: Outline the therapeutic uses of glucagon.

37. **C** The patient's history and symptoms indicate that he was suffering from hypoglycemic coma. Hypoglycemia is a serious and often life-threatening complication of diabetes management, especially in children. The major use of glucagon is for emergency treatment of severe hypoglycemic reactions when unconsciousness precludes oral feeding and intravenous glucose is not available, as in this case. The drug is usually given intramuscularly, most frequently by a patient's family member who is trained to administer the drug. Because the action of glucagon is transient, patients should be given glucose as soon they regain consciousness.

A, B, D–F See correct answer explanation.

Learning objective: Describe the adverse effects of α-glucosidase inhibitors.

38. **C** Miglitol is an α-glucosidase inhibitor. These drugs are approved for people with type 2 diabetes as monotherapy and in combination with other oral antidiabetic drugs. The patient's symptoms are classic adverse effects of α-glucosidase inhibitors, which occur in more than 50% of subjects at the start of the therapy. These drugs decrease the absorption of monosaccharides from the duodenum and upper jejunum by inhibiting the enzyme that is involved in the breakdown of starches into simple sugars. The adverse effects are due to fermentation of unabsorbed carbohydrates in the small intestine.

A, B, D–F These drugs do not cause the collection of symptoms reported by the patient.

Learning objective: Outline the therapeutic uses of metformin.

39. **C** The symptoms of the patient and the lab results indicate that he his most likely suffering from type 2 diabetes mellitus, which is characterized by defects in insulin secretion, resistance to insulin action, and increased hepatic glucose production. Obese individuals constitute 60 to 90% of the type 2 diabetic population. A stepped care approach to type 2 diabetes mellitus indicates lifestyle modifications in case of a fasting plasma glucose less than 240 mg/dL and no or mild symptoms. If this goal is not achieved, monotherapy should be initiated with any oral antidiabetic drug. Metformin is the first-line agent for type 2 diabetes. Moreover, the serious allergic reaction to sulfonamides contraindicates the use of sulfonylureas in this patient.

A To try strict dietary control would be useless in this patient because of the history of repeated past failures.

B See correct answer explanation.

D, E Insulin should be used in type 2 diabetes only when control is not achieved with oral antidiabetic drugs.

Learning objective: Describe the actions of insulin on lipid metabolism.

40. **A** Insulin stimulates the synthesis of proteins and simultaneously reduces the degradation of proteins within the liver. The general mechanisms of these effects are still not well defined, but they are most likely mediated by the following insulin actions:

- Increased amino acid transport into cells
- Phosphorylation of several insulin receptor substrate docking proteins (IRSs) in cell cytosol

B–E Insulin elicits actions opposite to those listed.

ANTIDIABETIC DRUGS Answer key							
1.	E	6.	A	11.	D	16.	A
2.	I	7.	C	12.	E	17.	E
3.	N	8.	D	13.	A	18.	C
4.	G	9.	B	14.	A	19.	C
5.	M	10.	E	15.	B	20.	C
21.	B	26.	B	31.	E	36.	D
22.	B	27.	B	32.	E	37.	C
23.	A	28.	A	33.	B	38.	C
24.	D	29.	F	34.	B	39.	C
25.	A	30.	D	35.	B	40.	A

VI Respiratory, Gastrointestinal, and Hematopoietic Systems

Questions: VI-1 Drugs for Bronchospastic Disorders

Directions for questions **1–4**

Match each respiratory drug with the appropriate description (each lettered option can be selected once, more than once, or not at all).

- **A.** Acetylcysteine
- **B.** Albuterol
- **C.** Beclomethasone
- **D.** Codeine
- **E.** Dextromethorphan
- **F.** Dornase alfa
- **G.** Ipratropium
- **H.** Omalizumab
- **I.** Salmeterol
- **J.** Theophylline
- **K.** Zafirlukast
- **L.** Zileuton

Difficulty level: Easy

1. A long-acting β_2 adrenoceptor agonist

Difficulty level: Easy

2. An opioid derivative with no addiction liability, used as an antitussive

Difficulty level: Easy

3. A bronchodilator drug that can block Nn acetylcholine receptors

Difficulty level: Easy

4. A drug that blocks high-affinity immunoglobulin E (IgE) receptors of sensitized mast cells

Difficulty level: Medium

5. A 51-year old man was admitted to the hospital with an asthmatic attack. The man had been suffering from seasonal asthma for 1 year. On questioning, he reported that he took two aspirin tablets the previous evening for a headache. A diagnosis of drug hypersensitivity was made, an appropriate therapy was instituted, and later he was discharged from the hospital. Which of the following treatments would be most appropriate for his postdischarge therapy?

- **A.** Oral zafirlukast
- **B.** Oral triamcinolone
- **C.** Parenteral ipratropium
- **D.** Oral theophylline
- **E.** Parenteral salmeterol

Difficulty level: Medium

6. A 34-year-old woman who has been suffering from persistent asthma for 4 years was admitted to the emergency department because of impending respiratory failure. She was treated with oxygen, nebulized albuterol, intravenous (IV) theophylline, and IV hydrocortisone. A half hour later, a substantial clinical improvement was noted. Blockade of which of the following receptors most likely contributed to the bronchodilating effect of theophylline in this patient?

- **A.** M_3 cholinergic
- **B.** Adenosine A_1
- **C.** Leukotriene B_4
- **D.** Thromboxane A_2
- **E.** Beta-2 adrenergic
- **F.** Prostaglandin I_2

Difficulty level: Medium

7. A 34-year-old asthmatic man was brought to the emergency department with a severe asthma exacerbation. The patient's forced expiratory volume in 1 second (FEV_1) did not improve upon administration of inhaled albuterol, and the attending physician decided to administer parenteral triamcinolone. Which of the following would be the most likely benefit provided by parenteral glucocorticoids in this setting?

- **A.** Direct bronchodilation
- **B.** Decreased sympathetic tone of airway smooth muscle
- **C.** Increased mucociliary clearance
- **D.** Increased bronchial responsiveness to albuterol
- **E.** Improved diaphragmatic performance

Difficulty level: Easy

8. A 51-year-old woman with a long history of chronic obstructive pulmonary disease was admitted to the hospital for an acute exacerbation of her disease. The patient's medications on admission were inhaled ipratropium and oral theophylline. Which of the following molecular actions on bronchial smooth muscle most likely contributed to the bronchodilating effect of theophylline in this patient?

A. Inhibition of phosphodiesterase 4 (PDE_4)
B. Inhibition of catecholamine release
C. Stimulation of nitric oxide release
D. Activation of β_2 adrenoceptors
E. Activation of adenosine receptors

Difficulty level: Medium

9. A 3-day-old baby girl born after 30 weeks of pregnancy had five episodes of apnea. The episodes lasted about 30 seconds and required oxygen administration. Between apneic spells, the neonate appeared well, and physical examination and lab tests were normal for gestational age. An appropriate therapy was started that included intravenous administration of theophylline. Which of the following actions most likely mediated the therapeutic effect of the drug in this patient?

A. Bronchodilation
B. Inhibition of mucociliary clearance
C. Stimulation of the medullary respiratory center
D. Stimulation of diaphragm contractility
E. Inhibition of catecholamine release

Difficulty level: Easy

10. A 69-year-old man complained to his physician of a cough that had been increasing over the past few days. The man had a 40-pack-year history of cigarette smoking and had been suffering from chronic obstructive pulmonary disease for 10 years. He was currently on ipratropium and albuterol. The physician decided to add theophylline to the regimen, but he knew that in this patient the clearance of theophylline would probably be increased. Which of the following factors most likely caused an increased theophylline clearance in this patient?

A. Chronic lung diseases
B. Age over 65
C. Concomitant albuterol treatment
D. Smoking
E. Concomitant ipratropium treatment

Difficulty level: Easy

11. A 43-year-old woman with a long history of severe persistent asthma was admitted to the emergency department with serious labored respiration. Physical examination showed a distressed patient with dyspnea and severe cyanosis. Vital signs were blood pressure 140/90 mm Hg, heart rate 130 bpm, respirations 30/min. The patient's cyanosis indicated a serious ventilation/perfusion mismatch, and inhaled albuterol, given immediately, was able to improve cyanosis and to decrease dyspnea. Which of the following actions most likely mediated these drug effects in the patient's disorder?

A. Increased bronchial secretions
B. Decreased pulmonary perfusion
C. Increased pulmonary ventilation
D. Decreased pulmonary artery pressure
E. Increased mucociliary clearance

Difficulty level: Easy

12. A 45-year-old man had been suffering from chronic obstructive pulmonary disease that was not adequately controlled by inhaled salmeterol and ipratropium. His physician decided to add a third drug that is thought to act by multiple mechanisms, including inhibition of phosphodiesterase 4 in inflammatory cells and enhancement of histone deacetylation. Which of the following drugs was most likely added to the patient's therapeutic regimen?

A. Ipratropium
B. Salmeterol
C. Zileuton
D. Zafirlukast
E. Theophylline

Difficulty level: Medium

13. A 59-year-old man with a long history of chronic obstructive pulmonary disease recently had theophylline added to his therapeutic regimen. Which of the following actions most likely occurred during the first days of the new therapy?

A. Decreased cardiac contractility
B. Dilation of cerebral blood vessels
C. Decreased diuresis
D. Increased gastric secretion
E. Depression of the respiratory center

Difficulty level: Hard

14. A 45-year-old man with a long history of chronic severe asthma was admitted to the emergency department with extreme dyspnea and wheezing. His medical history was significant for a recently diagnosed duodenal ulcer. Current medications included inhaled albuterol, beclomethasone, and ipratropium on a chronic basis. Vital signs were heart rate

130 bpm, blood pressure 140/90 mm Hg, respirations 30/min. An electrocardiogram showed sinus tachycardia with occasional premature ventricular contractions. Which of the following two events most likely contributed to the patient's arrhythmia?

A. Ipratropium dosage and the hypertensive effect of beclomethasone
B. Duodenal ulcer and the hypertensive effect of beclomethasone
C. Albuterol dosage and duodenal ulcer
D. Ipratropium dosage and the disease-induced hypoxemia
E. Albuterol dosage and the disease-induced hypoxemia

Difficulty level: Easy

15. A 54-year-old woman with chronic obstructive pulmonary disease (COPD) was diagnosed with an upper respiratory tract infection, and erythromycin was prescribed. Her COPD was reasonably well controlled on oral theophylline and inhaled albuterol. Which of the following would be an appropriate change in the patient's therapeutic regimen at this time?

A. Add inhaled dexamethasone.
B. Add inhaled ipratropium.
C. Increase the dose of albuterol.
D. Decrease the dose of theophylline.
E. Add inhaled salmeterol.

Difficulty level: Easy

16. A 60-year-old man was admitted to the emergency department because of nausea, vomiting, headache, tremor, nervousness, tinnitus, and atrial tachycardia for the past 4 hours. The man, who had been suffering from chronic obstructive pulmonary disease for 3 years, recently had a new drug added to his therapeutic regimen. Which of the following drugs most likely caused the patient's adverse effects?

A. Albuterol
B. Prednisone
C. Ipratropium
D. Zileuton
E. Theophylline

Difficulty level: Easy

17. A 58-year-old woman complained to her physician of increasing dyspnea and cough over the past few days. The woman had a 22-pack-year history of cigarette smoking and had been suffering from chronic obstructive pulmonary disease for 5 years. She was currently on inhaled ipratropium and albuterol. Her physician decided to add a drug that acts by selectively inhibiting phosphodiesterase 4 in bronchial muscle. Which of the following drugs was most likely prescribed?

A. Zafirlukast
B. Zileuton
C. Roflumilast
D. Beclomethasone
E. Omalizumab

Difficulty level: Medium

18. A 30-year-old woman recently diagnosed with moderate intermittent asthma started a treatment with inhaled albuterol as needed. Which of the following effects on pulmonary function testing most likely occurred soon after drug administration?

A. Increased total lung capacity
B. Decreased peak expiratory flow
C. Decreased forced vital capacity
D. Increased residual volume
E. Increased forced expiratory volume

Difficulty level: Hard

19. A 78-year-old female resident of a rehabilitation center exhibited Cheyne–Stokes breathing from time to time and suffered from urge urinary incontinence and spasticity in her left limb. The woman had suffered from an ischemic stroke 2 months earlier. Which of the following drugs should be included in the pharmacological therapy of this patient?

A. Neostigmine
B. Theophylline
C. Albuterol
D. Ipratropium
E. Metoclopramide
F. Bromocriptine

Difficulty level: Medium

20. A 15-year-old boy with a 10-year history of asthma was admitted to the hospital for evaluation. The patient complained of increasing respiratory difficulty and awakening from sleep five to seven times per night. Present medications were high-dose inhaled fluticasone and salmeterol. Pulmonary function testing indicated a forced expiratory volume (FEV_1) 30% of predicted, and laboratory exams showed total serum immunoglobulin E (IgE) level of 615 IU/mL (normal > 120 IU/mL). Which of the following would be appropriate to add to the patient's treatment at this time?

A. Inhaled albuterol
B. Inhaled beclomethasone
C. Oral zileuton
D. Oral zafirlukast
E. Subcutaneous omalizumab

Difficulty level: Easy

21. A 46-year-old man with a long history of chronic severe asthma was admitted to the hospital with extreme dyspnea and impending respiratory failure. Emergency therapy was started with inhaled albuterol, glucocorticoids, and oxygen, but the patient's response to the treatment was poor. It was decided to initiate intravenous theophylline. The goal was to reach an immediate therapeutic plasma concentration of 15 mg/L. Knowing that the volume of distribution of theophylline is about 0.5 L/kg, which of the following loading doses (in milligrams) was most likely given?

   A. 525
   B. 435
   C. 110
   D. 600
   E. 85

Difficulty level: Medium

22. A 50-year old man was admitted to the hospital because of severe dyspnea and coughing that had been increasing over the past few days. The man had been suffering from persistent severe asthma for 10 years and from diabetes for 8 years. Current medications included insulin, inhaled beclomethasone, and inhaled ipratropium. Spirometry showed a forced expiratory volume (FEV_1) 40% of the predicted value. The patient was intubated and was given high-dose albuterol therapy by continuous nebulization. Which of the following adverse effects would most likely be associated with this treatment?

   A. Hypertension
   B. Sleepiness
   C. Bradycardia
   D. Hypoglycemia
   E. Hypokalemia

Difficulty level: Medium

23. A 25-year-old woman was seen at a clinic because of episodes of shortness of breath and cough that had occurred almost every day since she had an upper respiratory infection 2 months earlier. The woman also stated that several times weekly she awoke at night with the same symptoms. Spirometry showed a forced expiratory volume (FEV_1) 62% of the predicted value. Which of the following drugs would be most appropriate to be included in the patient's treatment at this time?

   A. Theophylline
   B. Isoproterenol
   C. Salmeterol
   D. Propranolol
   E. Aspirin

Difficulty level: Medium

24. A 52-year-old woman had been on a ventilator for 5 days because of ventilatory failure due to polymyositis when the physician noted increasing endotracheal secretions and decreased oximetry. A bronchoscopy showed abundant mucus plugs filling the bronchial lumen. Suctioning of the bronchial tree was performed, and a drug was given to improve mucociliary clearance. Which of the following drugs was most likely administered?

   A. Epinephrine
   B. Albuterol
   C. Ipratropium
   D. Zileuton
   E. Dexamethasone
   F. Zafirlukast

Difficulty level: Easy

25. A 57-year-old man complained to his physician that his chronic mucoid cough had gotten worse, and he had increasing breathing difficulty. The man had a long history of smoking and currently smoked one pack daily. Spirometry showed a forced expiratory volume (FEV_1) of 50% the predicted value. The physician decided to start a therapy with a drug that can block acetylcholine-mediated increase in Ca^{2+} availability in bronchial smooth muscle. Which of the following drugs was most likely administered?

   A. Beclomethasone
   B. Ipratropium
   C. Theophylline
   D. Albuterol
   E. Atropine

Difficulty level: Medium

26. A 44-year-old man presented to his physician complaining of increasing cough producing yellow sputum and moderate shortness of breath on exertion. The man had a long history of heavy cigarette smoking and had suffered from an episode of sustained ventricular tachycardia 1 year ago. Physical examination showed a patient with shallow breathing and a barrel chest. Auscultation demonstrated wheezing and distant heart sounds. An inhalation therapy was prescribed. A drug with which of the following mechanisms of action would be most appropriate for this patient?

   A. Activation of adenosine receptors
   B. Inhibition of phospholipase A_2
   C. Activation of β_2 adrenoceptors
   D. Blockade of Nn and M_3 acetylcholine receptors
   E. Blockade of leukotriene receptors

Difficulty level: Medium

27. A 63-year old woman complained to her physician of recurrent wheezing that caused frequent nocturnal awakening. She also noted that wheezing occurred when she was anxious and tense. The woman had been suffering from allergic rhinitis for 4 years and from atrial fibrillation for 1 year. A diagnosis of mild allergic asthma was made. Which of the following drug treatments would be most appropriate for relief of her bronchospasm?

A. Oral glucocorticoids
B. Oral theophylline
C. Inhaled ipratropium
D. Inhaled salmeterol
E. Oral zileuton

Difficulty level: Easy

28. A 13-year-old boy recently diagnosed with asthma started a therapy that included inhaled fluticasone. Which of the following molecular actions most likely contributed to the therapeutic effect of the drug in the patient's disease?

A. Blockade of M_3 acetylcholine receptors
B. Blockade of leukotriene receptors
C. Inhibition of phospholipase A_2
D. Activation of β_1 adrenoceptors
E. Activation of α_2 adrenoceptors
F. Inhibition of lipocortin biosynthesis

Difficulty level: Easy

29. A 43-year-old woman with mild persistent asthma started a daily treatment with low-dose inhaled glucocorticoids. Which of the following adverse effects was most likely to occur in this patient?

A. Hypokalemia
B. Weight gain
C. Oral candidiasis
D. Restlessness
E. Increased heart rate
F. Osteoporosis

Difficulty level: Medium

30. A 21-year-old man with severe persistent asthma had been on daily inhaled salmeterol, inhaled beclomethasone, and oral zafirlukast for 2 months, with inhaled albuterol as needed. However, his asthma was poorly controlled, and his physician decided to add another drug to the current treatment. Which of the following drugs would be most appropriate for the patient at this time?

A. Oral triamcinolone
B. Oral ipratropium
C. Inhaled omalizumab
D. Inhaled theophylline
E. Oral zileuton

Difficulty level: Easy

31. An 11-year-old boy was recently diagnosed with mild seasonal asthma. The boy was otherwise healthy and was a member of his school basketball team. Which of the following drugs would be most appropriate for the initial treatment of the patient's disease?

A. Inhaled albuterol
B. Oral triamcinolone
C. Inhaled ipratropium
D. Oral zafirlukast
E. Inhaled salmeterol

Difficulty level: Medium

32. A 45-year-old man with moderate persistent asthma was in the chest clinic for evaluation of his clinical state. His asthma was only partially controlled on daily inhaled salmeterol and beclomethasone. Recently, zafirlukast was added to the therapy with significant improvement of the disease, but it was withdrawn 10 days later because of the appearance of a severe headache. Physical examination showed diffuse expiratory wheezes, and pulmonary function testing revealed a peak expiratory flow rate 70% of predicted. Which of the following drugs would be appropriate to add to the patient's regimen at this time?

A. Inhaled albuterol
B. Oral zileuton
C. Inhaled theophylline
D. Parenteral omalizumab
E. Oral montelukast

Difficulty level: Easy

33. A 9-year-old girl with a long history of cystic fibrosis presented to the hospital because of worsening of respiratory symptoms. An appropriate therapy was prescribed that included inhaled dornase alfa. Which of the following best explains the mechanism of action of dornase alfa in the patient's disease?

A. Supports bactericidal activity against *Pseudomonas aeruginosa*
B. Releases nitric oxide from airway epithelium
C. Depolymerizes the DNA of purulent airways secretions
D. Stimulates the cystic fibrosis transmembrane regulator
E. Inhibits the neutrophil migration into lung tissue

Difficulty level: Medium

34. A 43-year-old man complained to his physician that the therapy he was taking improved his breathing, but that he still had an annoying cough from time to time. He asked the physician for a cough suppressant. Two weeks earlier, the man was diagnosed with moderate persistent asthma and started a therapy with inhaled albuterol and fluticasone. Which of the following drugs would be appropriate to treat the patient's cough?

A. Codeine
B. Theophylline
C. Dextromethorphan
D. Ipratropium
E. Dornase alfa
F. Fentanyl

Questions: VI-2 Drugs for Gastrointestinal Disorders

Directions for questions **1–8**

Match each gastrointestinal drug with the appropriate description (each lettered option can be selected once, more than once, or not at all).

A. Bisacodyl
B. Calcium carbonate
C. Castor oil
D. Docusate
E. Erythromycin
F. Loperamide
G. Meclizine
H. Mesalamine
I. Metoclopramide
J. Methylcellulose
K. Magnesium hydroxide
L. Mineral oil
N. Misoprostol
O. Omeprazole
P. Aprepitant
Q. Sucralfate

Difficulty level: Easy

1. An antacid that also has laxative properties

Difficulty level: Easy

2. An antiemetic drug used primarily for chemotherapy-induced vomiting

Difficulty level: Easy

3. A prostaglandin E$_1$ analogue that can have a cytoprotective effect on gastric mucosa

Difficulty level: Easy

4. An antiulcer agent that binds to necrotic peptic ulcer tissue, thus acting as a barrier to gastric juice

Difficulty level: Easy

5. An antiulcer agent that can inhibit 24-hour gastric acid secretion up to 95%

Difficulty level: Easy

6. A drug that can increase intestinal peristalsis by activating motilin receptors

Difficulty level: Easy

7. An opioid drug used to treat diarrhea

Difficulty level: Easy

8. A salicylate derivative used in inflammatory bowel diseases

Difficulty level: Easy

9. A 45-year-old woman had been self-medicating for heartburn. The preparation she was using was a combination of magnesium hydroxide and aluminum hydroxide. Which of the following reasons best explains why many antacid preparations on the market contain a combination of these two antacids instead of a single product?

A. To achieve a bactericidal effect on *Helicobacter pylori*
B. To avoid antacid overdose toxicity
C. To avoid interaction with other drugs given concomitantly
D. To facilitate gastric emptying
E. To decrease the occurrence of constipation or diarrhea

Difficulty level: Hard

10. A 76-year-old woman who underwent surgery to remove a colon polyp complained of epigastric pain the day after the operation. Her general condition rapidly deteriorated, and she was transferred to the intensive care unit because of septic shock. Which of the following therapeutic regimens would be appropriate to prevent stress-related mucosal bleeding in this patient?

A. Metoclopramide by intravenous (IV) infusion
B. Ondansetron by IV infusion
C. Sucralfate by nasogastric tube
D. Bismuth salicylate by nasogastric tube
E. Misoprostol by nasogastric tube
F. Famotidine by IV infusion

Difficulty level: Easy

11. A 61-year-old man with newly diagnosed lung cancer was scheduled to receive his first course of chemotherapy. A prophylactic antiemetic treatment was planned that included ondansetron. Which of the following brain regions represent a site of the antiemetic action of the drug?

A. Nucleus tractus solitarius
B. Putamen
C. Locus ceruleus
D. Nucleus accumbens
E. Medial forebrain bundle

Difficulty level: Easy

12. A 70-year-old woman complained to her physician of obstinate constipation. The physician prescribed a laxative that acts in the colon by absorbing water into the fecal contents, thus promoting peristalsis about 1 or 2 days after administration. Which of the following drugs was most likely prescribed?

A. Castor oil
B. Docusate
C. Sodium phosphate
D. Magnesium sulfate
E. Methylcellulose

Difficulty level: Medium

13. A 58-year-old alcoholic man suffering from hepatic cirrhosis was admitted to the hospital because of drowsiness and disorientation in time and place. Further exams led to the diagnosis of portal-systemic encephalopathy. Which of the following drugs would be appropriate to eliminate toxic enteric products in this patient?

A. Omeprazole
B. Lactulose
C. Loperamide
D. Sucralfate
E. Aprepitant
F. Ranitidine

Difficulty level: Easy

14. A 65-year-old woman suffering from chronic heartburn was routinely taking a large amount of an antacid preparation containing aluminum hydroxide. Lab exams of this patient would most likely show which of the following results?

A. Hyperglycemia
B. Hypercalcemia
C. Hypernatremia
D. Hypokalemia
E. Hypophosphatemia

Difficulty level: Easy

15. A 45-year-old woman presented to her physician because of a 2-week history of painless diarrhea that was urgent and usually occurred during meals. After physical examination, lab tests, and colonoscopy, a diagnosis of irritable bowel syndrome was made, and the woman was prescribed an appropriate therapy that included loperamide. Direct activation of which of the following receptors most likely mediated the therapeutic effect of the drug in this patient?

A. Beta-2 adrenergic
B. Nn cholinergic
C. 5-HT$_3$ serotonergic
D. Alpha-2 adrenergic
E. Mu opioid
F. M$_3$ cholinergic

Difficulty level: Medium

16. A 74-year old man was admitted to the hospital because of persistent epigastric pain and tarry stools. The patient had been suffering from hypertension for 5 years and was being treated with hydrochlorothiazide and losartan. Past history was significant for a serious hypersensitivity reaction to omeprazole taken 1 year ago for heartburn. Pertinent laboratory results on admission were red blood cell count $3.5 \times 10^6/mm^3$ (normal 4.5–$5.5 \times 10^6/mm^3$), hemoglobin 9 g/dL (normal 14–16 g/dL), creatinine 4.5 mg/dL (normal 0.9–1.3 mg/dL). Endoscopy disclosed a large gastric ulcer. Therapy with famotidine was started, but the standard dose was reduced by one half. Which of the following was the most likely reason for the use of a reduced dose of famotidine in this patient?

A. The patient's anemia
B. The patient's hypertension
C. The patient's age
D. The patient's renal insufficiency
E. The patient's hypersensitivity to omeprazole

Difficulty level: Easy

17. An 18-year-old man traveling on vacation in Mexico noted some mild abdominal cramps and three or four unformed stools over the past 24 hours. No blood was seen in the stool. Which of the following drugs would be appropriate to treat the patient's diarrhea?

    A. Magnesium sulfate
    B. Bismuth subsalicylate
    C. Vancomycin
    D. Erythromycin
    E. Metoclopramide
    F. Sucralfate

Difficulty level: Medium

18. A 45-year-old man recently diagnosed with mild colonic Crohn disease had been receiving sulfasalazine for 4 weeks, but remission was not achieved. Prednisone was added for another 2 weeks, but improvement was negligible, and the gastroenterologist decided to add a third drug to the therapy. Which of the following drugs would be appropriate for the patient at this time?

    A. Mesalamine
    B. Daclizumab
    C. Dexamethasone
    D. Amikacin
    E. Infliximab

Difficulty level: Easy

19. A 43-year-old man suffering from heartburn had been using antacid preparations as needed. Which of the following best describes the mechanism of action of antacids?

    A. Inhibition of pepsin and hydrochloric acid secretion
    B. Stimulation of bicarbonate secretion by epithelial cells
    C. Reaction with hydrochloric acid in the stomach lumen
    D. Binding to necrotic ulcer tissue
    E. Reaction with pepsin in the stomach lumen

Difficulty level: Hard

20. A 30-year-old man went to his physician because of 1 month of worsening intermittent abdominal pain, bloating, diarrhea, and rectal bleeding. Vital signs were normal, and physical examination disclosed only diffuse abdominal pain. Sigmoidoscopy showed erythematous mucosa in the rectum and sigmoid and distal descending colon. The mucosa had areas of fine granular appearance with some focal hemorrhage and ulcerations. Biopsies demonstrated abnormal crypt abscesses. A diagnosis was made, and a therapy was prescribed. Which of the following drugs would be most appropriate for the patient at this time?

    A. Metronidazole
    B. Clarithromycin
    C. Loperamide
    D. Ondansetron
    E. Prednisolone

Difficulty level: Medium

21. A 50-year-old woman complained to her physician of regurgitation of foul-tasting fluid into her mouth and occasional nausea and vomiting. The physician prescribed a drug that can both prevent nausea and vomiting and promote upper gastrointestinal motility. Blockade of which of the following receptors most likely contributed to the therapeutic effect of the drug in the patient's disease?

    A. M_3 cholinergic
    B. Nn cholinergic
    C. Beta-2 adrenergic
    D. H_2 histaminergic
    E. D_2 dopaminergic

Difficulty level: Medium

22. A 61-year-old man was seen at a clinic because of heartburn and abdominal pain for the past month. He had self-medicated with various over-the-counter preparations, but he got only temporary relief. All routine laboratory tests were within normal limits except the serum gastrin level, which was 3240 pg/mL (normal < 100 pg/mL). Radiographic and endoscopic studies demonstrated one gastric and two duodenal ulcers, and magnetic resonance imaging showed a small pancreatic tumor. A drug with which of the following mechanisms of action would be most appropriate for this patient?

    A. Blockade of H_2 receptors in gastric parietal cells
    B. Activation EP_3 receptors in gastric epithelial cells
    C. Coating the gastric ulcer craters
    D. Neutralization of hydrochloric acid in the stomach lumen
    E. Inhibition of H^+/K^+ ATPase in gastric parietal cells

Difficulty level: Easy

23. A 61-year-old woman with newly diagnosed ovarian cancer was scheduled to receive her first course of chemotherapy. A prophylactic antiemetic medication was planned. A drug from which of the following classes would be most appropriate to include in the antiemetic therapy of this patient?

    A. Serotonergic antagonists
    B. Dopaminergic agonist
    C. Muscarinic antagonists
    D. Gabaergic agonists
    E. Adrenergic agonists

Difficulty level: Medium

24. A 44-year-old man who has been receiving his first course of chemotherapy for a non-Hodgkin lymphoma still complains of recurrent nausea and vomiting despite antiemetic medication with ondansetron, dexamethasone, and aprepitant. Which of the following drugs would be appropriate to add to the patient's antiemetic regimen at this time?

- **A.** Famotidine
- **B.** Omeprazole
- **C.** Loperamide
- **D.** Dronabinol
- **E.** Triamcinolone
- **F.** Meclizine

Difficulty level: Medium

25. A 64-year-old woman suffering from episodic heartburn routinely took an over-the-counter medication as needed. The drug acts by inhibiting the action of an endogenous compound released from enterochromaffin-like cells of the stomach. Which of the following drugs did the patient most likely take?

- **A.** Ondansetron
- **B.** Loperamide
- **C.** Metoclopramide
- **D.** Famotidine
- **E.** Loratadine
- **F.** Sucralfate

Difficulty level: Medium

26. A 36-year-old man complained to his physician of dizziness and drowsiness. The man, recently diagnosed with gastroesophageal reflux disease, had started an appropriate treatment 2 weeks earlier. Laboratory findings showed an increase of the patient's prolactin levels. Which of the following drugs could have caused the signs and symptoms of this patient?

- **A.** Ranitidine
- **B.** Omeprazole
- **C.** Aluminum hydroxide
- **D.** Calcium carbonate
- **E.** Sucralfate
- **F.** Metoclopramide

Difficulty level: Easy

27. A 51-year-old man complained to his physician of indigestion. He described a burning sensation and some belching, often associated with foul-tasting acid in his mouth, especially after large or spicy meals. If meals were too close to his bedtime, the burning kept him awake at night. He would like to have a treatment that prevents meal-related symptoms. Which of the following drugs would be most appropriate for this patient?

- **A.** Famotidine
- **B.** Atropine
- **C.** Ondansetron
- **D.** Dronabinol
- **E.** Erythromycin
- **F.** Bismuth

Difficulty level: Easy

28. A 60-year-old man suffering from recurrent heartburn routinely took large quantities of different antacid preparations. Which of the following antacids had the highest risk of metabolic alkalosis in this patient?

- **A.** $NaHCO_3$
- **B.** $CaCO_3$
- **C.** $Al(OH)_3$
- **D.** $Mg(OH)_2$
- **E.** $Ca(OH)_2$

Difficulty level: Medium

29. A 67-year-old man complained to his physician of nervousness, insomnia, palpitations, and stomach ache. The man had a long history of chronic obstructive pulmonary disease currently treated with inhaled ipratropium and oral theophylline. He told the physician that he had started taking cimetidine for heartburn 3 days ago. Which of the following best explains the reason for the patient's current complaints?

- **A.** Cimetidine increased the clearance of theophylline.
- **B.** Cimetidine decreased the clearance of theophylline.
- **C.** Cimetidine increased the clearance of ipratropium.
- **D.** Theophylline increased the clearance of cimetidine.
- **E.** Theophylline decreased the clearance of cimetidine.

Difficulty level: Easy

30. A 71-year-old man with terminal metastatic lung cancer had been hospitalized for 3 months. His renal function had deteriorated, and laboratory results showed serum creatinine 4.5 mg/dL (normal 0.9–1.2 mg/dL) and blood urea nitrogen (BUN) 75 mg/dL (normal 6–20 mg/dL). Because of poor food intake, immobility, and requirement for an opioid analgesia, the patient was severely constipated and required daily laxative therapy. Which of the following would be a suitable laxative for this patient?

- **A.** Lactulose
- **B.** Castor oil
- **C.** Magnesium hydroxide
- **D.** Sodium phosphate
- **E.** Mineral oil

Difficulty level: Easy

31. A 74-year-old patient suffering from chronic constipation complained of very loose stools after a treatment with bisacodyl, one tablet daily for 1 week. Which of the following would be the best advice to give to this patient?

A. There is no cause for alarm; the situation is self-limiting.

B. Continue bisacodyl, but take the medication with a small snack.

C. Continue bisacodyl, and add lactulose.

D. Discontinue bisacodyl, and increase fiber and fluid intake.

E. Discontinue bisacodyl, and switch to castor oil.

Difficulty level: Easy

32. A 43-year-old man recently diagnosed with testicular cancer was in the hospital for his second cycle of chemotherapy. A three-drug combination was given to prevent chemotherapy-induced nausea and vomiting. The combination included a drug that blocks NK_1 neurokinin receptors in the area postrema. Which of the following drugs has this molecular mechanism of action?

A. Ondansetron

B. Dronabinol

C. Aprepitant

D. Metoclopramide

E. Diphenhydramine

Difficulty level: Easy

33. A 57-year-old man complained to his physician of epigastric pain that was stronger at night and was temporarily relieved by food. Upper gastrointestinal endoscopy showed two small gastric ulcers, and a urease breath test was positive for *Helicobacter pylori* infection. The physician prescribed a triple therapy with omeprazole, clarithromycin, and metronidazole for 14 days, followed by omeprazole daily for 6 weeks. Which of the following statements best explains why this drug regimen is the first-line therapy for *H. pylori*–associated ulcers?

A. Omeprazole is rapidly bactericidal against *H. pylori*.

B. The regimen almost completely eliminates the risk of ulcer recurrence.

C. Clarithromycin greatly enhances the bactericidal activity of omeprazole.

D. Metronidazole greatly enhances the bactericidal activity of omeprazole.

E. The regimen can cure the ulcer in up to 70% of cases.

Difficulty level: Medium

34. A 34-year-old hospitalized male patient complained of torticollis, grimacing, and spasm of the ocular muscles 1 day after surgery. The man had received an intravenous drug soon after surgery to treat nausea and vomiting. Which of the following antiemetic drugs most likely caused the patient's symptoms?

A. Ondansetron

B. Scopolamine

C. Dexamethasone

D. Metoclopramide

E. Dronabinol

Difficulty level: Easy

35. A 59-year-old woman suffering from chronic constipation routinely self-administered milk of magnesia (magnesium hydroxide) daily. Which of the following actions most likely mediated the laxative effect of the drug?

A. Inhibition of cholecystokinin release

B. Retention of water in the vessels by osmosis

C. Lubrication of fecal material

D. Stretching of the intestinal wall

E. Formation of a bulky emollient gel

Difficulty level: Easy

36. A 41-year-old woman complained to her physician of increasing frequency and urgency of bowel movements that she attributed to increased stress at work. The woman was diagnosed with spastic colon 4 years ago but was able to tolerate the symptoms until recently, when she noted the increasing frequency of bowel movements. A drug from which of the following classes could be appropriate to treat the patient's disorder?

A. Opioid agonists

B. Serotonergic agonists

C. Muscarinic agonists

D. H_1 agonists

E. Adrenergic antagonists

F. Gabaergic antagonists

Difficulty level: Easy

37. A 46-year-old man recently diagnosed with a duodenal ulcer started a treatment that included daily sucralfate. Which of the following mechanisms most likely mediates the therapeutic efficacy of the drug in the patient's disease?

A. Acting as a barrier to acid by binding to necrotic ulcer tissue

B. Reacting with gastric hydrochloric acid to form salt and water

C. Inhibiting hydrochloric acid secretion

D. Stimulating bicarbonate secretion by antral parietal cells

E. Exerting a bactericidal effect against *Helicobacter pylori*

Difficulty level: Easy

38. A 24-year-old woman in her second trimester of pregnancy complained of constipation at a routine prenatal visit. The physician instructed the woman to maintain bowel function by drinking plenty of water, increasing bulk in the diet with vegetables, and taking a laxative daily. Which of the following laxatives would be most appropriate for this patient?

A. Castor oil

B. Bisacodyl

C. Senna

D. Docusate

E. Magnesium hydroxide

F. Sodium sulfate

Difficulty level: Medium

39. A 64-year-old man complained to his physician of burning and substernal pain for about 3 weeks. The pain usually occurred after dinner when he was lying on the couch watching television and was sometimes accompanied by regurgitation of foul-tasting fluid into his mouth. The man had been suffering from Parkinson disease for 1 year and was currently receiving pramipexole and selegiline. Which of the following drugs would be most appropriate to treat the patient's symptoms?

A. Atropine

B. Misoprostol

C. Ondansetron

D. Omeprazole

E. Metoclopramide

F. Cimetidine

Difficulty level: Hard

40. A 63-year-old man suffering from a small cell carcinoma of the lung was hospitalized for his first cycle of chemotherapy. Which of the following three-drug regimens would be the best to prevent nausea and vomiting in this patient?

A. Ranitidine, diazepam, dexamethasone

B. Scopolamine, dexamethasone, ondansetron

C. Ondansetron, aprepitant, dexamethasone

D. Aprepitant, scopolamine, loperamide

E. Diphenhydramine, prochlorperazine, dronabinol

F. Prochlorperazine, ranitidine, loperamide

Difficulty level: Easy

41. A 34-year-old-man with a 2-year history of AIDS was admitted to the hospital for evaluation. The patient's only complaint was a poor appetite that had gotten progressively worse over the past 3 weeks. He was currently taking a highly active antiretroviral therapy (HAART) with lamivudine, stavudine, and atazanavir. Physical examination and laboratory exams showed that the patient was in stable condition except for decreasing body weight. Which of the following drugs would be appropriate to treat the patient's anorexia?

A. Metoclopramide

B. Omeprazole

C. Famotidine

D. Dronabinol

E. Loperamide

F. Meclizine

Difficulty level: Easy

42. A 53-year-old woman complained to her physician that the drug she was taking did not work and that she was still suffering from obstinate constipation. The woman had a long history of irritable bowel syndrome and took several drugs in the past with limited success. She was presently taking lactulose. The physician decided to try another drug recently approved for irritable bowel syndrome with constipation in adult women. The drug is a prostanoid derivative that acts by opening type 2 chloride channels in the small intestine. Which of the following drugs was most likely prescribed?

A. Ondansetron

B. Dronabinol

C. Lubiprostone

D. Metoclopramide

E. Diphenhydramine

F. Sorbitol

Questions: VI-3 Drugs for Hematopoietic Disorders

Directions for questions **1–6**

Match each hematopoietic drug with the appropriate description (each lettered option can be selected once, more than once, or not at all).

- **A.** Cyanocobalamin
- **B.** Deferoxamine
- **C.** Erythropoietin
- **D.** Ferrous sulfate
- **E.** Filgrastim
- **F.** Folic acid
- **G.** Iron dextran
- **H.** Iron sucrose
- **I.** Leucovorin
- **J.** Oprelvekin
- **K.** Sargramostim

Difficulty level: Easy

1. This drug is sometimes used to prevent transfusional iron overload.

Difficulty level: Easy

2. An endogenous compound synthesized by the kidney in response to hypoxia

Difficulty level: Easy

3. There is a lifetime requirement for this drug in patients who have undergone gastrectomy.

Difficulty level: Easy

4. A recombinant form of interleukin 11

Difficulty level: Easy

5. A multilineage myeloid growth factor

Difficulty level: Easy

6. This drug is absorbed through the distal ileum by a process of receptor-mediated endocytosis.

Difficulty level: Medium

7. A 62-year-old man presented to his physician complaining of tiredness and abdominal pain. Medical history revealed that the man had been taking two tablets of naproxen twice daily for arthritic pain for the past 3 months. Pertinent lab results on admission were red blood cell count (RBC) $3.1 \times 10^6/mm^3$ (normal, male $4.3–5.9 \times 10^6/mm^3$), hemoglobin 8.5 g/dL (normal, male > 13.5 g/dL), mean corpuscular volume 70 fL (normal 80–100 fL), serum ferritin 6 ng/mL (normal: 30–300). An appropriate therapy was prescribed. Which of the following actions most likely mediated the therapeutic effect of the prescribed drug?

- **A.** Activation of specific receptors on RBC progenitors
- **B.** Replacement of a chemical whose stores are severely depleted
- **C.** Increased life span of RBCs
- **D.** Stimulation of erythropoietin production by the kidney
- **E.** Stimulation of transferrin production by the liver

Difficulty level: Easy

8. A 22-year-old woman in her first week of pregnancy started on daily folic acid supplementation. The therapy was given to decrease the risk of which of the following congenital abnormalities?

- **A.** Atrial septal defect
- **B.** Spina bifida
- **C.** Tetralogy of Fallot
- **D.** Esophageal atresia
- **E.** Congenital cataract
- **F.** Cryptorchidism

Difficulty level: Easy

9. A 58-year-old man recently diagnosed with iron deficiency anemia was found to have a severe depletion of total body iron stores. Which of the following compounds represents the most important store for iron?

- **A.** Transferrin
- **B.** Ferroportin
- **C.** Ferritin
- **D.** Myoglobin
- **E.** Hemoglobin

Difficulty level: Medium

10. A 71-year-old man complained to his physician of tiredness, breathlessness, and fatigue. Four years earlier, the patient had undergone total gastrectomy for advanced Zollinger–Ellison syndrome. A blood analysis showed megaloblastic anemia. Which of the following statements best explains why folic acid supplementation would be contraindicated in this patient?

- **A.** The drug would mask hematologic signs of vitamin B_{12} deficiency.
- **B.** The drug would block vitamin B_{12} actions in the central nervous system.
- **C.** The drug may increase vitamin B_{12} metabolism.
- **D.** Older patients are especially at risk of folic acid toxicity.
- **E.** Gastrectomy completely prevents folic acid absorption.

Difficulty level: Medium

11. A 32-year-old woman in her second trimester of pregnancy presented to the clinic for a check-up. The patient had a 5-year history of excessive alcohol intake and had been using cocaine frequently for the past 3 years. She appeared malnourished and had lost 12 pounds during the first trimester, secondary to anorexia, nausea, and vomiting. Pertinent laboratory values were red blood cell count (RBC) $2.7 \times 10^6/mm^3$ (normal, female $3.5–5.5 \times 10^6/mm^3$), mean corpuscular volume 112 fL (normal 80–100 fL), serum vitamin B_{12} 350 pg/mL (normal > 280 pg/mL), serum ferritin 200 ng/mL (normal 30–300 ng/mL). Blood stain showed macro-ovalocytic RBCs and hypersegmentation of neutrophils. Which of the following drugs would be most appropriate for this patient?

   A. Cyanocobalamin
   B. Folic acid
   C. Ferrous sulfate
   D. Iron dextran
   E. Erythropoietin

Difficulty level: Medium

12. A 34-year-old woman was seen at a clinic because of severe weakness and dizziness for the past several months. The woman had a long history of menorrhagia and of chronic headaches for which she had been using several analgesic medications on a daily basis. Physical examination revealed a pale, lethargic female appearing older than her stated age. Notable signs were a sore tongue, spooning of the nails, and splenomegaly. Pertinent laboratory values were red blood cell count $2.3 \times 10^6/mm^3$ (normal, female $3.5–5.5 \times 10^6/mm^3$), mean corpuscular volume 72 fL (normal 80–100 fL), hemoglobin 5 g/dL (normal, female > 12 g/dL), serum ferritin 7 ng/mL (normal 30–300 ng/mL). Which of the following drugs would be most appropriate for this patient?

   A. Ferrous sulfate
   B. Folic acid
   C. Erythropoietin
   D. Iron sucrose
   E. Vitamin B_{12}
   F. Filgrastim

Difficulty level: Hard

13. A 22-year-old man complained to his physician of increasing fatigue, anorexia, and irritability over the past 2 months. The man had been suffering from gluten enteropathy since his infancy. Physical examination revealed pallor, glossitis, paresthesias, and muscle weakness. Pertinent laboratory values were red blood cell count (RBC) $3.4 \times 10^6/mm^3$ (normal, male $4.3–5.9 \times 10^6/mm^3$), mean corpuscular volume 116 fL (normal 80–100 fL), serum vitamin B_{12} 330 pg/mL (normal > 280 pg/mL), serum ferritin 200 ng/mL (normal 30–300 ng/mL). Blood stain showed macro-ovalocytic red blood cells and hypersegmentation of neutrophils. An appropriate drug was started, and 10 days later, the RBC was normal. Which of the following actions most likely mediated the therapeutic effect of the drug in the patient's disease?

   A. Increased conversion of homocysteine to methionine
   B. Increased synthesis of tetrahydrofolate
   C. Increased absorption of iron from duodenal mucosa
   D. Decreased erythrocyte destruction
   E. Increased synthesis of erythropoietin

Difficulty level: Easy

14. A 34-year-old woman recently diagnosed with iron deficiency anemia started a treatment with ferrous sulfate. Which of the following mechanisms was most likely involved in the delivery of iron to the patient's erythroblasts?

   A. Lipid diffusion
   B. Facilitated diffusion
   C. Aqueous diffusion
   D. Receptor-mediated endocytosis
   E. Bulk flow transport

Difficulty level: Medium

15. A 53-year-old man recently diagnosed with pernicious anemia started a treatment with vitamin B_{12}. Which of the following molecular actions most likely mediated the antianemic effect of the drug in this patient?

   A. Formation of succinyl–coenzyme A (CoA)
   B. Hydroxylation of folic acid
   C. Demethylation of N_5-methyltetrahydrofolate
   D. Hydroxylation of dihydrofolic acid
   E. Glycine formation from serine

Difficulty level: Medium

16. A 66-year-old woman was admitted to the hospital because of tiredness, breathlessness, and fatigue over the past 3 weeks. Two years ago, she underwent gastrectomy for severe non-healing ulcers. The only medication the patient was taking was cyanocobalamin, intramuscularly, once a month. Pertinent laboratory values on admission were red blood cell count $2.8 \times 106/mm^3$ (normal, female $3.5–5.5 \times 106/mm^3$), mean corpuscular volume 60 fL (normal 80–100 fL), hemoglobin 8.6 g/dL (normal, female > 12 g/dL), hematocrit 32% (normal 36–46%). Which of the following drugs given orally would most likely improve the patient's condition?

A. Vitamin B_{12}
B. Folic acid
C. Iron dextran
D. Sargramostim
E. Erythropoietin
F. Ferrous sulfate

Difficulty level: Medium

17. A 65-year-old man was seen at a clinic because of muscle weakness, emotional instability, burning of the tongue, and alternating constipation and diarrhea. Physical examination showed a pale man with red tongue, loss of vibratory sense in the lower extremities, and ataxia. Pertinent blood values were red blood cell count $3.4 \times 106/mm^3$ (normal, male $4.3–5.9 \times 106/mm^3$), mean corpuscular volume 110 fL (normal 80–100 fL), vitamin B_{12} 96 pg/mL (normal > 280 pg/mL), serum ferritin 250 ng/mL (normal 30–300 ng/mL). Which of the following drugs would be most appropriate for this patient?

A. Folic acid
B. Ferrous sulfate
C. Deferoxamine
D. Iron dextran
E. Cyanocobalamin

Difficulty level: Easy

18. A 54-year-old woman recently diagnosed with iron deficiency anemia started a treatment with oral ferrous sulfate. Which of the following mechanisms was most likely involved in the patient's intestinal absorption of the drug?

A. Aqueous diffusion
B. Lipid diffusion
C. Facilitated diffusion
D. Active transport
E. Exocytosis

Difficulty level: Hard

19. A 33-year-old malnourished woman in her eighth month of pregnancy presented to the clinic complaining of extreme lethargy. The woman was multiparous and living in a poor suburban area with her two daughters. Pertinent laboratory values on admission were red blood cell (RBC) count $2.9 \times 106/mm^3$ (normal, female $3.5–5.5 \times 106/mm^3$), mean corpuscular volume 90 fL (normal 80–100 fL), hemoglobin 7 g/dL (normal, female > 12 g/dL), serum ferritin 8 µg/dL (normal 30–300 µg/dL), serum vitamin B_{12} 350 pg/mL (normal > 280 pg/mL), RBC folate 45 ng/mL (normal 150–800 ng/mL). Blood stain demonstrated both micro- and macrocytic erythrocytes and blood hypochromia. Which of the following pairs of drugs would represent an appropriate treatment for this patient?

A. Cyanocobalamin and ferrous sulfate
B. Erythropoietin and hydroxocobalamin
C. Folic acid and ferrous sulfate
D. Iron dextran and filgrastim
E. Folic acid and erythropoietin

Difficulty level: Easy

20. A 6-year-old boy recently diagnosed with thalassemia major was started on whole blood transfusion therapy. Which of the following drugs was most likely given during the transfusion to prevent transfusional iron overload?

A. Ferritin
B. Folic acid
C. Filgrastim
D. Erythropoietin
E. Sargramostim
F. Deferoxamine

Difficulty level: Hard

21. A 72-year-old man was admitted to the hospital with a 2-week history of weakness, decreased appetite, and exercise intolerance. Pertinent laboratory values on admission were red blood cell count $3.0 \times 10^6/mm^3$ (normal, male $4.3–5.9 \times 10^6/mm^3$), mean corpuscular volume 96 fL (normal 80–100 fL), hemoglobin 6 g/dL (normal, male > 13.5 g/dL), serum iron 45 µg/dL (normal 50–150 µg/dL), serum creatinine 4.7 mg/dL (normal 0.6–1.2 mg/dL). Which of the following pairs of drugs would be most appropriate to treat the patient's disease?

A. Cyanocobalamin and ferrous sulfate
B. Erythropoietin and ferrous sulfate
C. Erythropoietin and filgrastim
D. Cyanocobalamin and iron dextran
E. Folic acid and oprelvekin
F. Folic acid and iron dextran

Difficulty level: Easy

22. A 42-year-old man suffering from diffuse non-Hodgkin lymphoma was in the hospital for autologous bone marrow transplantation. Which of the following drugs should be administered after transplantation to hasten neutrophil recovery?

A. Leucovorin
B. Filgrastim
C. Oprelvekin
D. Ondansetron
E. Cyanocobalamin
F. Allopurinol

Difficulty level: Easy

23. A 65-year-old man suffering from lung cancer was admitted to the hospital for a cycle of chemotherapy. After completion of the cycle, a treatment with oprelvekin was started. The therapeutic effect of the drug is most likely mediated by activation of specific receptors located mainly on which of the following cells?

A. Neutrophils
B. Lymphocytes
C. Macrophages
D. Monocytes
E. Megakaryocytes
F. Platelets

Difficulty level: Easy

24. A 33-year-old woman recently diagnosed with severe microcytic anemia felt uneasy and became agitated and flushed soon after the first intravenous injection of an antianemic drug. She also complained of palpitations, coughing, urticaria, and difficulty in breathing. Within 5 minutes, cardiovascular collapse developed. Which of the following drugs most likely caused the patient's syndrome?

A. Leucovorin
B. Ferrous sulfate
C. Iron dextran
D. Cyanocobalamin
E. Filgrastim
F. Sargramostim

Difficulty level: Medium

25. A 51-year-old man undergoing ambulatory hemodialysis for end-stage renal disease had been receiving erythropoietin for normochromic normocytic anemia. A blood analysis showed the following results: red blood cell count 4.4 × 10^6/mm³ (nor-

mal, male 4.3–5.9 × 10^6/mm³), mean corpuscular volume 98 fL (normal 80–100 fL), hemoglobin 14 g/dL (normal, male > 13.5 g/dL). The patient was most likely at greater risk of which of the following drug-related adverse effects?

A. Thrombotic complications
B. Hypotension
C. Angioedema
D. Hypokalemia
E. Adynamic ileus

Difficulty level: Medium

26. A 66-year-old woman complained to her physician of bleeding gums. The woman had been receiving her third cycle of chemotherapy for metastatic ovarian cancer. A blood analysis showed the following results: red blood cell count 3.2 × 10^6/mm³ (normal, female 3.5–5.5 × 10^6/mm³), mean corpuscular volume 96 fL (normal 80–100 fL), hemoglobin 9 g/dL (normal, female > 12 g/dL), neutrophil count 4600/mm³ (normal 3000–7000/mm³), platelet count 7000/mm³ (normal 130,000–400,000/mm³). A hematopoietic agent was administered intravenously. Which of the following drugs would be appropriate for this patient?

A. Filgrastim
B. Erythropoietin
C. Cyanocobalamin
D. Leucovorin
E. Folic acid
F. Oprelvekin

Difficulty level: Easy

27. A 2-year-old boy was brought to the emergency department after suffering two episodes of brownish vomit containing pills, followed by a large hematemesis. The mother, who was pregnant, suspected her son had ingested several tablets of her medication. Physical examination showed a lethargic and cyanotic child complaining of abdominal pain. Vital signs were blood pressure 80/50 mm Hg (normal for 2 years 100/65 mm Hg), pulse 130 bpm (normal for 2 years 115 bpm) respirations 30/min (normal at 2 years 24/min). Laboratory values indicated severe metabolic acidosis. Which of the following drugs would be most appropriate for this child?

A. Iron dextran
B. Deferoxamine
C. Folic acid
D. Ferrous sulfate
E. Cyanocobalamin
F. Erythropoietin

Difficulty level: Easy

28. A 13-year-old boy suffering from acute lymphoblastic leukemia was admitted to the hospital for the third cycle of anticancer therapy, which included high-dose methotrexate. Which of the following drugs should be given to the patient to counteract methotrexate toxicity?

   A. Folic acid
   B. Cyanocobalamin
   C. Leucovorin
   D. Ferrous sulfate
   E. Oprelvekin
   F. Filgrastim

Difficulty level: Medium

29. A 39-year-old male AIDS patient has had recent episodes of cytomegalovirus esophagitis. The man was being treated with a zidovudine, lamivudine, efavirenz combination for AIDS and with ganciclovir for cytomegalovirus prophylaxis. His last blood analysis revealed the following: red blood cell count 4.1×10^6/mm^3 (normal, male 4.3–5.9 $\times 10^6$/mm^3), white blood cell count 1.5×10^3/mm^3 (normal 4.5–11.0 $\times 10^6$/mm^3), neutrophil count 250/mm^3 (normal 3000–7000/mm^3). Which of the following drugs would be appropriate to add to the patient's therapeutic regimen at this time?

   A. Erythropoietin
   B. Saquinavir
   C. Cyanocobalamin
   D. Filgrastim
   E. Ferrous sulfate

Difficulty level: Medium

30. A 15-year-old girl was seen at a clinic because of easy fatigue, irritability, and decreased mental alertness over the past month. The girl was a strict vegetarian and reported heavy menstrual periods since her menarche. Pertinent lab results on admission were red blood cell count 3.1×10^6/mm^3 (normal, female 3.5–5.5 $\times 10^6$/mm^3), hemoglobin 9 g/dL (normal, female > 12 g/dL), mean corpuscular volume 71 fL (normal 80–100 fL), serum ferritin 5 ng/mL (normal 30–300 ng/mL). Which of the following drugs would be most appropriate for this patient?

   A. Folic acid
   B. Erythropoietin
   C. Iron dextran
   D. Sargramostim
   E. Ferrous sulfate
   F. Iron sucrose

Answers and Explanations: VI-1 Drugs for Bronchospastic Disorders

Questions 1–4
1. **I**
2. **E**
3. **G**
4. **H**

Learning objective: Describe the main therapeutic uses of zafirlukast.

5. **A** Leukotriene inhibitors and antagonists have demonstrated the important role of leukotrienes in aspirin-induced asthma. Some asthmatic patients are very sensitive to aspirin as well as to all nonsteroidal antiinflammatory drugs, and even small doses can cause profound bronchoconstriction, flushing, and abdominal cramping. The syndrome is not allergic in nature but seems to be related to the inhibition of cyclooxygenase, which most likely causes

   • A shift of arachidonic acid metabolism to the leukotriene pathway; leukotrienes are powerful bronchoconstricting agents.

   • Decreased synthesis of prostaglandin E_2 (PGE$_2$), which is an endogenous bronchodilator, very important in maintaining airway patency for most asthmatics

   Leukotriene antagonists such as zafirlukast and montelukast are the drugs most frequently used for maintenance therapy in patients with aspirin-induced asthma.

   B, D Systemic glucocorticoids and theophylline are used only in case of severe asthma that is resistant to other pharmacotherapies.

   C, E These drugs are used only by inhalation.

Learning objective: Describe the proposed molecular mechanisms of the bronchodilating action of theophylline.

6. **B** The molecular basis for the antiasthmatic action of methylxanthines is still uncertain. Although the primary mechanism of the bronchodilating effect most likely involves the inhibition of phosphodiesterase enzymes, an additional mechanism seems related to the blockade of adenosine A$_1$ receptors. Adenosine acts as both an autacoid and a transmitter with

myriad biological actions, including bronchoconstriction, mainly in patients with bronchospastic disease.

A, C–F Theophylline does not block these receptors.

Learning objective: Describe the interaction between β_2 adreno-ceptor agonists and glucocorticoids in the treatment of asthma.

7. **D** Systemic corticosteroids are given in cases of severe asthma exacerbation for two main reasons:

- They improve the responsiveness of β_2 receptors.
- They inhibit many phases of the inflammatory responses.

The antiinflammatory activity of corticosteroids is delayed for 4 to 6 hours after administration. However, the restoration of responsiveness to endogenous catecholamines, as well as to exogenous β_2 agonists, occurs within 1 hour of glucocorticoid administration in severe chronic asthmatics. This restoration is therefore the main potential benefit of intravenous administration of corticosteroids to a patient with severe asthma exacerbation under treatment with β_2 agonists.

A–C, E Corticosteroids do not have these effects.

Learning objective: Describe the proposed molecular mechanisms of the bronchodilating action of theophylline.

8. **A** The molecular basis for methylxanthine actions is still uncertain, but the bronchodilating action seems to be primarily due to inhibition of phosphodiesterase enzymes, mainly phosphodiesterase 4 (PDE_4). The inhibition causes a rise in the intracellular cyclic adenosine monophosphate (cAMP) and cyclic guanosine monophosphate (cGMP) concentrations, which in turn leads to smooth muscle relaxation.

B Methylxanthines stimulate, not inhibit, catecholamine release from adrenergic terminals.

C, D Methylxanthines do not cause these effects.

E See correct answer explanation.

Learning objective: Describe the main action mediating the therapeutic effect of theophylline in apnea of preterm infants.

9. **C** Methylxanthines, specifically theophylline and caffeine, are widely accepted as the initial pharmacological approach for the treatment of idiopathic apnea of prematurity. Methylxanthines stimulate the respiratory center in the medulla, increasing respiratory drive. These central effects may be mediated by adenosine receptor blockade. Adenosine is a known inhibitor of the respiratory center, and methylxanthines are competitive antagonists at adenosine receptors.

A, D These actions may contribute to the improvement of apneic episodes but are not the primary mechanism of the therapeutic effect of xanthines in infant apnea.

B, E Methylxanthines cause effects opposite to those listed.

Learning objective: List the main condition that can increase the clearance of theophylline.

10. **D** The clearance of theophylline can be affected by many conditions; some decrease the clearance, and some increase it. Factors that can increase clearance are smoking, and concomitant treatment with drugs that induce the P-450 system, such as barbiturates and rifampin. Theophylline clearance is also higher in children than in adults.

A, B These factors actually can decrease, not increase, the clearance of theophylline.

C, E These drugs do not affect theophylline clearance.

Learning objective: Describe the mechanism of the improvement of the ventilation/perfusion ratio by albuterol.

11. **C** In severe bronchospastic disorders, the ventilation/perfusion ratio is decreased because the narrowing of bronchial lumen decreases ventilation. By dilating the bronchial musculature, β_2 agonists such as albuterol increase ventilation, thus increasing the ratio. A high ratio increases the partial pressure of oxygen, which in turn decreases cyanosis and dyspnea.

A, E Beta-2 agonists can have these actions, but they are not the cause of the beneficial effect of albuterol in this patient.

B Because activation of β_2 receptors causes vasodilation, albuterol actually increases, not decreases, pulmonary perfusion.

D Albuterol-induced vasodilation can decrease pulmonary artery pressure, but this would decrease, not increase, the ventilation/perfusion ratio.

Learning objective: Describe the proposed mechanisms of anti-asthmatic action of theophylline.

12. **E** The antiasthmatic action of theophylline seems to result from both bronchodilating and nonbronchodilating actions. The inhibition of phosphodiesterase 4 (PDE_4) in smooth muscle most likely explains the bronchodilating activity. Proposed nonbronchodilating mechanisms involve inhibition of PDE_4 in inflammatory cells, which most likely reduces the release of inflammatory cytokines and enhances histone deacetylation (acetylation of histone is needed for activation of inflammatory gene transcription).

A, B Ipratropium and salmeterol are bronchodilators but are devoid of antiinflammatory actions.

C, D Zileuton and zafirlukast have antiinflammatory actions but are devoid of bronchodilating activity.

Learning objective: Describe the main adverse effects of theophylline.

13. **D** Methylxanthines stimulate gastric secretion, which can explain the abdominal discomfort that frequently occurs after the administration of theophylline. The effect on gastric secretion is most likely due to theophylline-induced inhibition of phosphodiesterase, which in turn increases intracellular cyclic adenosine monophosphate (cAMP), thus causing an activation of H^+/K^+ ATPase.

    A–C, E Theophylline causes effects opposite to those listed.

Learning objective: Explain the likely cause of arrhythmia in an asthmatic patient under albuterol therapy.

14. **E** The patient's severe asthma most likely caused hypoxemia, which by itself can predispose to arrhythmias. Moreover, the patient was likely receiving a high dose of β agonists, as the increased dyspnea prompted him to increase the number of puffs taken daily. Tachycardia is a common adverse effect of $β_2$ agonists, likely due to activation of $β_2$ receptors in the heart, as well as to reflex effects that stem from $β_2$ receptor-mediated vasodilation.

    A, B, D Ipratropium and glucocorticoids very seldom cause systemic effects when taken by the inhaled route.

    C Duodenal ulcer is not a risk factor for arrhythmias.

Learning objective: Describe the interaction between erythromycin and theophylline.

15. **D** Erythromycin has been reported to inhibit the cytochrome P-450-mediated metabolism of several drugs, including theophylline. Because theophylline has a narrow therapeutic index, it is appropriate to decrease the dosage of the drug for the duration of the erythromycin therapy to avoid overdose toxicity.

    A–C, E Because the patient's asthma is well controlled, there is no need to change the therapeutic regimen.

Learning objective: Describe the main adverse effects of theophylline.

16. **E** The signs and symptoms of the patient suggest theophylline overdose toxicity. Methylxanthine overdose can cause nausea and vomiting (likely due to stimulation of the chemoreceptor trigger zone), headache, tremor, nervousness, tinnitus (likely due to stimulation of many areas of the central nervous system), and tachycardia (likely due to increased cyclic adenosine monophosphate [cAMP] and blockade of adenosine receptors).

    A–D These drugs do not cause the effects from which the patient was suffering.

Learning objective: Explain the mechanism of action of roflumilast.

17. **C** Roflumilast is a selective phosphodiesterase 4 inhibitor in bronchial smooth muscle that has been approved by the U.S. Food and Drug Administration for chronic obstructive pulmonary disease. Inhibition of phosphodiesterase results in higher concentrations of intracellular cyclic adenosine monophosphate (cAMP). In comparison to theophylline, roflumilast has lower overdose toxicity and less potential for drug–drug interactions.

    A, B, D, E See correct answer explanation.

Learning objective: Describe the effects of albuterol on pulmonary function testing in asthmatics.

18. **E** Albuterol is a $β_2$ agonist currently used as a bronchodilator in treating asthma. By dilating the bronchial tree, all bronchodilators can increase the forced expiratory volume in 1 second (FEV_1). The FEV_1 is the most useful parameter in diagnosing and monitoring patients with obstructive pulmonary disease.

    A Total lung capacity (TLC) is the amount of air in the lungs after maximum inflation. TLC is normal or increased in obstructive disorders. Bronchodilators do not significantly affect TLC.

    B Peak expiratory flow (PEF) is the highest forced respiratory flow measured by a peak flow meter. PEF is decreased in obstructive respiratory disorders. All bronchodilators increase, not decrease, PEF.

    C Forced vital capacity (FVC) is the maximum amount of air forcibly expired after maximum inspiration. FVC is normal or decreased in obstructive respiratory disorders. All bronchodilators can increase, not decrease, FVC.

    D Residual volume (RV) can be expressed as

$$RV = TLC - FVC$$

RV is normal or increased in obstructive respiratory disorders. All bronchodilators decrease, not increase, RV.

Learning objective: Describe the main therapeutic uses of theophylline.

19. **B** Cheyne–Stokes breathing, which occurs in various disease states, including following stroke, is a type of periodic breathing in which periods of hyperpnea alternates with periods of apnea. Methylxanthines such as theophylline and caffeine have been shown to improve Cheyne–Stokes respiration, probably because of their stimulant effect on the respiratory center.

    A Neostigmine actually can worsen urge incontinence, because it increases urinary bladder contractility.

    C–F These drugs have no effect on Cheyne–Stokes breathing, urge urinary incontinence, or limb spasticity.

Learning objective: Explain the therapeutic uses of omalizumab.

20. **E** Omalizumab is a monoclonal anti–immunoglobulin E (IgE) antibody that binds to free IgE in the serum, preventing binding of IgE to high-affinity receptors on mast cells, blocking initiation of the allergic inflammatory cascade. Omalizumab is effective in reducing asthma exacerbations and the inhaled and oral dose requirement for glucocorticoids in patients with severe asthma. It is administered subcutaneously every 2 to 3 weeks. Potentially serious adverse effects include anaphylaxis, which can occur after any dose, even if previous doses had been well tolerated, and may occur as long as 1 day after administration.

   A, B The patient is already receiving a β agonist and a glucocorticoid, so the addition of other drugs with the same mechanism of action would be irrational.

   C, D, F These drugs are usually minimally effective in severe asthma.

Learning objective: Calculate the loading dose of theophylline, given sufficient data.

21. **A** The loading dose of a drug given intravenously can be calculated as follows:

$$LD = V_d \times C_p,$$

where LD = loading dose, V_d = volume of distribution, and C_p = plasma concentration. Because theophylline does not distribute into adipose tissue, the ideal body weight (70 kg) can be used to calculate the LD. Therefore,

$$LD = 0.5 \times 70 \times 15 = 525 \text{ mg}$$

   B–E See correct answer explanation.

Learning objective: Describe the main adverse effects of β_2 agonists.

22. **E** Beta-2 agonists promote the uptake of potassium into the cells, likely by stimulating Na^+/K^+ ATPase. High doses of these drugs can cause hypokalemia, and these drugs are sometimes used in the therapy of hyperkalemic states. In this case, hypokalemia is even more likely because of the earlier treatment with insulin (insulin tends to cause hypokalemia, as it promotes potassium entry into cells).

   A Both hypertension and hypotension can be adverse effects of albuterol, but in this patient, hypotension is more likely due to the hypokalemia.

   B–D Beta-2 agonists tend to cause effects opposite to those listed.

Learning objective: Describe the therapeutic uses of salmeterol.

23. **C** Forced expiratory volume (FEV_1) is one of the best indicators of the severity of a bronchospastic disorder. FEV_1 between 60 and 80% of the predicted value indicates moderate disease. Because the patient's symptoms occurred daily, her asthma can be classified as moderate persistent. The preferred treatment for moderate persistent asthma is a low to medium dose of inhaled corticosteroids and a long-acting inhaled β_2 agonist such as salmeterol daily, plus a short-acting inhaled β_2 agonist such as albuterol, as needed.

   A Theophylline is very rarely used today for the therapy of asthma.

   B This drug, used in the past, is now obsolete.

   D Beta-blockers are contraindicated in asthmatics.

   E Aspirin is relatively contraindicated in asthmatics.

Learning objective: Describe the main therapeutic actions of albuterol in bronchospastic disorders.

24. **B** A patient who is artificially ventilated cannot clear bronchial secretions, mainly because effective cough cannot be performed. Beta-2 agonist drugs improve mucociliary clearance and are therefore often given to patients on artificial ventilation to decrease airway resistance and to remove secretions from bronchial mucosa.

   A Epinephrine, by activating β_2 receptors, can improve mucociliary clearance but would cause several adverse effects in this patient due to its cardiovascular actions.

   C Ipratropium has bronchodilating activity but does not improve mucociliary clearance, although, unlike other anticholinergic drugs, it does not reduce bronchial secretions and therefore does not affect mucociliary clearance.

   D–F Corticosteroids and leukotriene pathway inhibitors have no effect on mucociliary clearance.

Learning objective: Explain the molecular mechanism of action of ipratropium.

25. **B** Ipratropium is an antimuscarinic drug. By blocking M_3 acetylcholine receptors in the bronchial tree, these drugs prevent the increased synthesis of inositol triphosphate, which in turn triggers the release of Ca^{2+} from storage vesicles.

   A, C, D These drugs do not block muscarinic receptors.

   E Like ipratropium, atropine can block M_3 acetylcholine receptors in the bronchial tree, thus counteracting the acetylcholine-mediated increase in Ca^{2+} availability. However, anticholinergics (except ipratropium and tiotropium) are usually contraindicated in bronchospastic disorders because they decrease bronchial secretion and mucociliary clearance.

Learning objective: Describe the mechanism of action of ipratropium.

26. **D** The patient's history and symptoms indicate that he was most likely suffering from chronic obstructive pulmonary disease (COPD). Ipratropium is a first-line agent in COPD because its action in these patients is equal or superior to that achieved by β_2 agonists. Ipratropium is a quaternary ammonium antimuscarinic drug. Unlike tertiary amines, quaternary ammonium antimuscarinic drugs mainly block muscarinic receptors but also have a significant blocking activity on nicotinic Nn receptors. Therefore, inhaled ipratropium can block both M_3 receptors on bronchial smooth muscle and Nn receptors located in small parasympathetic ganglia within the bronchial tree. Both actions can contribute to the final bronchodilating effect of the drug.

A This activation would cause bronchoconstriction, not bronchodilation.

B This is a mechanism of action of glucocorticoids. These drugs are not bronchodilators, and they are used only in patients with advanced COPD and frequent exacerbations.

C This is the mechanism of action of β_2 agonists. These drugs are contraindicated in this patient because of the history of ventricular tachycardia. Patients who have survived an episode of sustained ventricular tachycardia or ventricular fibrillation have an extraordinarily high risk of experiencing a recurrent arrhythmia.

E Leukotriene receptor blockers are not bronchodilators and are not used in COPD.

Learning objective: Describe the bronchodilating use of ipratropium when β_2 adrenoceptor agonists are contraindicated.

27. **C** Accepted guidelines for the treatment of asthma indicate a short-acting β_2 agonist as needed in all patients. In this case, however, the patient's atrial fibrillation contraindicates the use of β_2 agonists. In general, when drugs are given by inhalation, only 10 to 20% of the dose can reach the target site of action (lower airways); the rest is swallowed and can be absorbed by the intestine, causing systemic effects. Ipratropium is an effective bronchodilator agent, and the swallowed dose is not absorbed by the intestine (the drug is a quaternary ammonium compound). Moreover, in this patient

- The bronchospasm was triggered by emotional upset, and it has been shown that inhaled anticholinergic drugs can block this response.
- The nocturnal awakening indicates that the bronchospasm is triggered by a prevalence of the parasympathetic system (which is predominant during the night), so an antimuscarinic drug is appropriate.

A, E These drugs are not bronchodilators and cannot be used for relief of bronchospasm.

B Oral sustained-release theophylline is an effective bronchodilator, but it has the potential to cause more adverse effects, may interfere with sleep, and is less effective than ipratropium.

D See correct answer explanation.

Learning objective: Explain the mechanism of the antiasthmatic action of fluticasone.

28. **C** Current therapeutic strategies available for the treatment of asthma include inhibition of eicosanoid biosynthesis (glucocorticoids), inhibition of leukotriene biosynthesis (zileuton), activation of β_2 receptors (β_2 agonists), and blockade of leukotriene receptors (zafirlukast). The glucocorticoid-induced inhibition of eicosanoid biosynthesis is mediated by the inhibition of phospholipase A_2, the enzyme that releases arachidonic acid from membrane-bound phospholipids.

A This would be the mechanism of action of ipratropium.

B This would be the mechanism of action of zafirlukast.

D, E These receptors are not involved in bronchodilation.

F Activation (not inhibition) of lipocortin biosynthesis mediates the glucocorticoid-induced inhibition of phospholipase A_2.

Learning objective: Describe the main adverse effects of inhaled glucocorticoids.

29. **C** Local adverse effects of inhaled glucocorticoids include cough, dysphonia, and oral candidiasis. *Candida albicans* is a fungal organism that is a normal constituent of oral flora, but it can cause infection when cellular immunity is compromised due to corticosteroids.

A, B, D–F All of these adverse effects can occur with oral glucocorticoids but are extremely rare with inhaled glucocorticoids.

Learning objective: Describe the use of oral glucocorticoids in bronchospastic disorders.

30. **A** Oral steroids are usually administered to treat severe asthma that is not controlled by other antiasthmatic drugs. Corticosteroids have potent antiinflammatory activity, and although they are not direct bronchodilators, they can relieve bronchial obstruction by improving the responsiveness of β_2 receptors to β_2 agonists.

A Ipratropium is not administered by the oral route.

C Omalizumab is a monoclonal anti–immunoglobulin E (IgE) antibody approved for the treatment of allergic asthma. It is not given by inhalation.

D Theophylline is not given by inhalation.

E Because a leukotriene antagonist (zafirlukast) was not effective, it is unlikely that an inhibitor of leukotriene synthesis (zileuton) would be effective.

Learning objective: Choose the right drug for the therapy of mild seasonal asthma.

31. **A** Inhaled short-acting β_2 agonists are considered first-line drugs for the treatment of asthma. According to current guidelines, a short-acting β_2 agonist should be given as needed to all patients with asthma. Because the patient's asthma is mild, inhaled albuterol as needed is most likely the preferred drug.

B Oral steroids are administered only in case of severe asthma that is not controlled by other antiasthmatic drugs

C Ipratropium alone is not used for the treatment of asthma. It can be used with albuterol in severely ill patients where it has been shown to improve pulmonary function.

D Zafirlukast is an antiinflammatory, not a bronchodilating, drug. Therefore, it is never used alone to treat asthma.

E Salmeterol is a long-acting β_2 agonist. Monotherapy treatment of asthma with long-acting β_2 agonists is contraindicated because it was found that this therapy increases the risk of asthma-related events (i.e., asthma-related hospitalization, asthma-related intubation, and asthma-related death). A black box warning about monotherapy is required by the U.S. Food and Drug Administration. However, combination products containing a long-acting β_2 agonist with an inhaled steroid can retain current indications, including asthma, as an increased risk of asthma-related complications was not demonstrated with this combination.

Learning objective: Choose the appropriate drug as a substitute for zafirlukast when this drug has caused a disturbing adverse effect.

32. **B** The patient improved when zafirlukast was added to the therapy, but the drug caused a disturbing adverse effect. When a drug is effective but causes an adverse effect, a good therapeutic strategy is to change the drug with another that has a similar effect but different chemical structure. Zileuton is a lipoxygenase inhibitor. Its final effect is similar to that of zafirlukast (i.e., to decrease leukotriene activity), but its mechanism of action is different. The clinical use of zileuton is limited due to the potential for elevated liver enzymes and liver injury, and immediate-release tablets were discontinued in the United States. Extended-release tablets are still available and can be used in specific cases, as in this one.

A The patient was already using salmeterol. There is no need to add an inhaled β_2 agonist.

C Theophylline is not used by inhalation.

D Omalizumab is given only in cases of severe refractory asthma.

E Montelukast is close chemically to zafirlukast and has the same mechanism of action. Therefore, the risk of headache would be significant in this patient.

Learning objective: Explain the mechanism of action of dornase alfa.

33. **C** The principal source of DNA in the sputum of cystic fibrosis patients is from the nuclei of degenerating neutrophils that accumulate in the lung because of chronic bacterial infections. DNA is the principal factor that increases the viscosity of the sputum in these patients. Dornase alfa is a recombinant human deoxyribonuclease that is administered by inhalation. It degrades the DNA, which has been shown to significantly decrease the viscosity of the sputum, thus reducing obstruction and the severity of respiratory infections.

A, B, D, E See correct answer explanation.

Learning objective: Identify the appropriate drug to treat cough in an asthmatic patient.

34. **C** Opioids are among the most effective drugs available for the suppression of cough. Their action is primarily due to the depression of the respiratory neurons in the brainstem, but the receptors involved in the antitussive effect appear to differ from those associated with other actions of opioids. For example, dextromethorphan, a stereoisomer of a levorphanol derivative, has lost the analgesic, sedative, and addictive properties of the parent compound but is an effective cough suppressant with potency nearly equal to that of codeine. The drug can be an appropriate cough suppressant in asthmatic patients.

A Codeine is the most commonly used cough suppressant but is not indicated in asthmatic patients because opioids can cause respiratory depression even when given in subanalgesic doses. This respiratory depression does not occur with dextromethorphan.

B, D Theophylline and ipratropium are not used as antitussives.

E Dornase alfa is a mucolytic drug. Mucolytics can help the expectoration but cannot depress the respiratory neurons.

F Strong opioids are not used as antitussives.

DRUGS FOR BRONCHOSPASTIC DISORDERS Answer key					
1.	I	6.	B	11.	C
2.	E	7.	D	12.	E
3.	G	8.	A	13.	D
4.	H	9.	C	14.	E
5.	A	10.	D	15.	D
16.	E	21.	A	26.	D
17.	C	22.	E	27.	C
18.	E	23.	C	28.	C
19.	B	24.	B	29.	C
20.	E	25.	B	30.	A
				31.	A
				32.	B
				33.	C
				34.	C

Answers and Explanations: VI-2 Drugs for Gastrointestinal Disorders

Questions 1–8

1. **K**
2. **P**
3. **N**
4. **Q**
5. **O**
6. **E**
7. **F**
8. **H**

Learning objective: Explain why many antacid preparations on the market contain a combination of magnesium hydroxide and aluminum hydroxide.

9. **E** Because magnesium hydroxide tends to cause diarrhea, and aluminum hydroxide tends to cause constipation, a combination of the two can have a balanced effect on intestinal motility without any loss of antacid effectiveness.

   A Antacid preparations have no bactericidal effect on *Helicobacter pylori*.

   B Overdose toxicity is extremely rare because intestinal absorption of these drugs is negligible.

   C Interactions between antacids and other drugs given concomitantly is uncommon and is mainly due to the increase of the pH of intestinal contents, not to the specific salt used as an antacid.

   D Because magnesium hydroxide tends to increase gastric emptying, and aluminum hydroxide tends to do the opposite, the combination actually has little effect on gastric emptying.

Learning objective: Outline the use of H_2 antagonists in stress-induced peptic ulcer.

10. **F** Acute stress-related mucosal bleeding is a type of erosive gastritis that occurs in critically ill patients with severe psychological stress (surgery, trauma, sepsis, etc.). The patient was in septic shock, and her abdominal pain suggested that stress-related mucosal bleeding was impending. Therefore, she needed aggressive prophylactic treatment. H_2 antagonists are the most widely used drugs for prevention of stress ulcer. They must be given intravenously, and infusion is more effective than a single bolus in maintaining the gastric pH above 4. Although proton pump inhibitors (not listed) would appear to be the preferred option because of their greater ability to inhibit gastric acid secretion, there is very little evidence to confirm the clinical superiority to H_2 antagonists for stress ulcer prevention.

   A, B These drugs have no antiulcer properties.

   C–E These antiulcer drugs are much less effective than H_2 antagonists and are not suited for emergency treatment.

Learning objective: Identify the site of antiemetic action of ondansetron.

11. **A** Serotonergic antagonists such as ondansetron are currently considered to be first-line agents for prevention of chemotherapy-induced nausea and vomiting. Ondansetron and congeners block 5-HT_3 serotonin receptors located in the nucleus tractus solitarius (likely the main site of action), chemoreceptor trigger zone, and visceral afferent nerves. In this way, it is thought that they can prevent both peripheral and central stimulation of the vomiting center.

   B–E See correct answer explanation.

Learning objective: Explain the mechanism of action of methylcellulose.

12. **E** Methylcellulose is an indigestible hydrophilic polysaccharide polymer that absorbs water, forming a bulky gel that distends the intestine, thus stimulating peristaltic activity. It acts mainly in the colon and takes 1 or 2 days to work. The laxative effect is mild.

   A–D All of these laxatives act mainly in the small intestine.

Learning objective: Outline the use of lactulose in portal-systemic encephalopathy.

13. **B** Eliminating toxic enteric products (mainly fecal ammonia) is a therapeutic goal in portal-systemic encephalopathy. Patients with severe liver disease have an impaired capacity to detoxify ammonia coming from the colon, where it is produced by bacterial metabolism of fecal urea. Ammonia is an important cause of brain toxicity. Lactulose, in high doses, can lower colonic pH, which results in "trapping" of the ammonia by its conversion to polar ammonium ion, which is poorly absorbed.

   A, C–F See correct answer explanation.

Learning objective: Describe the effects of aluminum hydroxide on serum ions.

14. **E** Aluminum salts bind phosphate in the gut, preventing phosphate absorption. Moreover, they can induce a blood-to-gut phosphorus gradient that favors the elimination of circulating phosphate. In fact, chronic use of high doses of aluminum salts is one of the common causes of hypophosphatemia. The disorder is usually asymptomatic, but severe phosphorus depletion can cause anorexia, muscle weakness, and osteomalacia.

   A–D Aluminum salts usually do not cause this effect.

Learning objective: Explain the molecular mechanism of the anti-diarrheal action of loperamide.

15. **E** Loperamide is an opioid agonist that directly activates mu (μ) receptors in the enteric nervous system. This activation of enteric neurons and smooth muscle ultimately causes a decrease in contraction of intestinal longitudinal muscle and a marked increase in contraction of circular muscle. Therefore, propulsive peristaltic waves are diminished, and tone is increased, thus relieving diarrhea.

A–D, F Loperamide cannot bind these receptors.

Learning objective: Explain why the dose of H_2 histamine antagonists must be reduced in patients with renal insufficiency

16. **D** The high creatinine level indicates that the patient was suffering from chronic renal insufficiency. Famotidine is an H_2 histamine antagonist. All drugs of this class are cleared mainly by the kidney. Although the overdose toxicity of H_2 antagonists is quite low, the dosage should be reduced in elderly patients with renal insufficiency, as in this case.

A–C, E See correct answer explanation.

Learning objective: Outline the therapeutic uses of bismuth subsalicylate.

17. **B** The patient is most likely affected by travelers' diarrhea, which typically begins within 24 to 48 hours after eating fecally contaminated food. Several enterobacteriaceae can cause travelers' diarrhea, varying according to the area of travel. *Escherichia coli* is the most common in Central America. Bismuth subsalicylate is effective in patients with diarrhea caused by *E. coli, Helicobacter pylori, Campylobacter jejuni,* and *Salmonella* species and also inhibits enteric secretions.

A Magnesium sulfate is an osmotic laxative and therefore is contraindicated in the treatment of diarrhea.

C, D These antibiotics are not effective against enterobacteriaceae.

E, F These drugs have no antidiarrheal properties.

Learning objective: Outline the therapeutic use of infliximab in Crohn disease.

18. **E** Treatment of mild colonic Crohn disease can start with sulfasalazine or glucocorticoids. If remission is not achieved, infliximab, azathioprine, or methotrexate is added. An important proinflammatory cytokine in Crohn disease is tumor necrosis factor (TNF). Infliximab is a monoclonal antibody that binds to soluble and membrane-bound TNF with high affinity, thus preventing the binding of the cytokine to its receptors.

A, C To add these drugs is irrational, as prednisone and sulfasalazine were not effective.

B Daclizumab is a monoclonal antibody used only for treatment of acute organ rejection.

D Antibiotics have no role in remission induction. Metronidazole is sometimes used in fistulizing disease or in patients with abscesses, but amikacin is not effective against anaerobes, the prevalent bacteria in intestinal flora.

Learning objective: Explain the mechanism of action of antacids.

19. **C** Antacids are salts of sodium, calcium, magnesium, and/or aluminum. They react with the hydrochloric acid of the stomach to form chlorides, water, and carbon dioxide. In this way, they neutralize gastric acidity and raise the gastrointestinal pH sufficiently to relieve the pain of heartburn.

A Because antacids neutralize gastric acid, the gastric secretion of hydrochloric acid and pepsin is stimulated, not inhibited.

B, D, E Antacids do not cause these effects.

Learning objective: Outline the therapy for ulcerative colitis.

20. **E** The patient's symptoms, together with macroscopic and microscopic findings, suggest that he was most likely affected by ulcerative colitis. The limitation of the lesions to the superficial mucosa and crypt abscesses confirm the diagnosis (Crohn disease involves all layers of the bowel from mucosa to serosa). Remission induction in ulcerative colitis is usually accomplished with glucocorticoids. Their effects on inflammatory bowel disease are well documented, but the response in individual patients is variable. About 40% of patients are responsive, 40% have only partial response, and 20% are resistant.

A, B Antibiotics such as metronidazole and clarithromycin are used only as adjunctive treatment along with other medications.

C, D These drugs are not effective and may be dangerous in inflammatory bowel disease.

Learning objective: Identify the receptors that can be blocked by metoclopramide.

21. **E** Metoclopramide is a dopamine D_2 receptor antagonist, a serotonin 5-HT$_3$ receptor antagonist, and a serotonin 5-HT$_4$ receptor agonist. In the enteric nervous system, all of these molecular actions seem to contribute to the final effect that is related to an increased activity of cholinergic motor neurons. In this way, the drug exerts a prokinetic effect; that is, it increases the lower esophageal sphincter tone and enhances transit in the upper digestive tract. It has negligible effects on gastric secretion or motility of the large intestine. In addition, the blockade of D_2 receptors and 5-HT$_3$ receptors in the chemoreceptor trigger zone can explain the antiemetic activity of the drug.

A–D See correct answer explanation.

Learning objective: Outline the therapeutic uses of proton pump inhibitors.

22.　**E** The patient is most likely suffering from Zollinger–Ellison syndrome, a rare condition characterized by a triad of clinical findings, including severe recurrent peptic ulcer disease, significant hypersecretion of gastric acid, and a tumor of the pancreas (gastrinoma) that functions as an ectopic source of gastrin. This tumor is usually located in the pancreas but can be found in other regions, particularly the duodenum. Currently, most patients with gastrinomas can be effectively treated with high doses of a drug such as omeprazole that inhibits H^+/K^+ ATPase in gastric parietal cells.

　　A–D These are the mechanisms of action of H_2-receptor antagonists (A), misoprostol (B), sucralfate (C), and antacids (D). All of these antiulcer drugs are less effective than proton pump inhibitors in reducing gastric acid secretion and therefore are not first-line agents in Zollinger–Ellison syndrome.

Learning objective: Describe the drug classes used to treat chemotherapy-induced nausea and vomiting.

23.　**A** Serotonergic antagonists are currently considered first-line agents to prevent chemotherapy-induced nausea and vomiting. Ondansetron and congeners block $5-HT_3$ receptors located in the nucleus of the tractus solitarius (likely the main site of action), chemoreceptor trigger zone, and visceral afferent nerves. In this way, it is thought that they can prevent both peripheral and central stimulation of the vomiting center.

　　B, E These drugs can cause, not prevent, nausea and vomiting.

　　C, D These drugs have antiemetic properties but are much less effective than serotonergic antagonists in chemotherapy-induced nausea and vomiting.

Learning objective: Describe the antiemetic activity of dronabinol.

24.　**D** Dronabinol is a Δ^9-tetrahydrocannabinol, the most active cannabinoid from cannabis. Its mechanism of antiemetic action is still uncertain, but the drug likely activates specific cannabinoid receptors in the vomiting center. Because of the availability of more effective agents, dronabinol is uncommonly used in patients receiving cancer chemotherapy, but can be a useful addition when other antiemetic medications are not effective, as in this case.

　　A–C These drugs are devoid of antiemetic properties.

　　E It would be illogical to add a glucocorticoid drug when dexamethasone was not effective.

　　F Meclizine is an antihistamine agent useful in prevention of motion sickness–induced vomiting. Antihistamines are not effective in chemotherapy-induced vomiting.

Learning objective: Identify the drug that inhibits the action of a neurotransmitter released by enterochromaffin-like cells of the stomach.

25.　**D** Heartburn is caused by gastroesophageal reflux disease (GERD). Drugs for heartburn act by decreasing the secretion of or neutralizing hydrochloric acid in the stomach. They include antacids, H_2 antagonists, and proton pump inhibitors. H_2 antagonists such as famotidine block H_2 receptors, thus inhibiting the action of histamine that is released from enterochromaffin-like cells located on the stomach wall.

　　A–C, E, F See correct answer explanation.

Learning objective: Describe the adverse effects of metoclopramide.

26.　**F** Metoclopramide is an antagonist of D_2 and $5-HT_3$ receptors. Blockade of D_2 receptors in the central nervous system can cause dizziness and drowsiness, and blockade of D_2 receptors in the pituitary leads to hyperprolactinemia, a common adverse effect of metoclopramide.

　　A–E These drugs can be used for gastroesophageal reflux disease, but they do not cause hyperprolactinemia.

Learning objective: Outline the therapeutic use of H_2 blockers in gastroesophageal reflux disease (GERD).

27.　**A** The patient was most likely suffering from GERD. Because the patient requested a medication to specifically prevent meal-related symptoms, H_2 antagonists such as famotidine are appropriate. Their onset of symptom relief occurs within 30 to 45 minutes and persists up to 10 hours. They also have a beneficial effect of reducing nocturnal acid secretion, which is mainly histamine-dependent. Proton pump inhibitors (not listed) have an efficacy higher than that of H_2 antagonists with regard to symptom relief and duration of suppression, but their onset of activity is slower (2 to 3 hours), and complete relief may take up to 4 days of therapy.

　　B Atropine is actually contraindicated, as it may favor reflux by relaxing the lower esophageal sphincter.

　　C–E These drug are of no value in GERD.

　　F This drug would be indicated only in case of peptic ulcer, which is unlikely in this patient.

Learning objective: Identify the antacid with the greater risk of metabolic alkalosis.

28.　**A** All antacids can cause metabolic alkalosis, due to the spared endogenous bicarbonate that is secreted in the stomach under prostaglandin E_2 control. In addition, exogenous bicarbonate is readily and completely absorbed; therefore, the risk of metabolic alkalosis is higher than that of calcium, magnesium, and aluminum salts that have an oral bioavailability less than 30%.

　　B–E See correct answer explanation.

Learning objective: Describe the effects of cimetidine–theophylline interaction.

29. **B** The symptoms of the patient are most likely due to theophylline overdose. Cimetidine (and, to a lesser extent, ranitidine, but not other H_2 blockers) strongly inhibits the cytochrome P-450 system, decreasing the metabolism of several drugs, including theophylline. Because theophylline has a low therapeutic index, even a small increase in plasma drug concentration can cause symptoms of overdose toxicity.

　　A, C–E See correct answer explanation.

Learning objective: Identify the best laxative for a patient with renal insufficiency.

30. **A** Lactulose is a nonabsorbable sugar that is hydrolyzed in the colon to organic acids. These acids draw water into the lumen by osmotic forces, stimulating colonic propulsive motility by stretching the colonic wall. The laxative effect is mild.

　　B Castor oil is too strong a cathartic to be used regularly.

　　C, D Magnesium and phosphate preparations are contraindicated in renal insufficiency because the small amount of absorbed salt cannot be readily excreted, thus causing systemic toxicity (hypermagnesemia or hyperphosphatemia).

　　E Mineral oil has several adverse effects (interference with absorption of fat-soluble substances, elicitation of foreign-body reaction) that preclude its regular use.

Learning objective: Describe the best treatment in case of laxative-induced diarrhea.

31. **D** When diarrhea is experienced with the use of laxatives, the laxative should be discontinued until resolution of the diarrhea. A diet rich in fiber and abundant fluid intake usually helps to normalize the intestine.

　　A The situation is not self-limiting. Tolerance to bisacodyl is negligible.

　　B, C These options would maintain the drug-induced diarrhea.

　　E Castor oil is too strong a cathartic to be used regularly.

Learning objective: Explain the molecular mechanism of action of aprepitant.

32. **C** NK_1 neurokinin receptors are located in the nucleus of the tractus solitarius in the brainstem. Activation of these receptors by substance P and related substances causes an increase in firing to the vomiting center. Aprepitant is an NK_1-receptor antagonist that is able to cross the blood–brain barrier. It has antiemetic effects, especially in cases of delayed emesis, and it improves the efficacy of standard antiemetic regimens in patients receiving multiple cycles of chemotherapy.

　　A, B, D, E See correct answer explanation.

Learning objective: Explain the efficacy of a triple-drug regimen in the therapy of *Helicobacter pylori*–associated ulcers.

33. **B** For *H. pylori*–associated ulcers, there are two therapeutic goals: eradicate the *H. pylori* and heal the ulcer. The first goal is important because it has been shown that eradication of *H. pylori* almost completely eliminates the risk of ulcer recurrence. The most effective regimens for *H. pylori* eradication are combinations of two antibiotics and a proton pump inhibitor. After completion of triple-drug therapy, the proton pump inhibitor should be continued for 3 to 6 weeks to ensure complete ulcer healing.

　　A, C, D Omeprazole has no bactericidal activity against *H. pylori*. It only creates a hostile environment for *H. pylori* by increasing gastric pH.

　　E The triple-drug regimen can cure the ulcer in more than 90%, not up to 70%, of cases.

Learning objective: Describe the adverse effects of metoclopramide.

34. **D** The patient's symptoms suggest that he is suffering from acute dystonia, an extrapyramidal syndrome that can occur after treatment with neuroleptics and other drugs that block D_2 receptors in the basal ganglia. Young patients, especially males who receive these drugs intravenously, are at greater risk of this adverse effect, as in this case. Metoclopramide is a drug with antiemetic properties, probably due to its blocking activity on both D_2 and $5\text{-}HT_3$ receptors located in the chemoreceptor trigger zone and the nucleus of the tractus solitarius. It is often used to treat postoperative nausea and vomiting.

　　A–C, E These antiemetic drugs do not cause acute dystonias.

Learning objective: Explain the mechanism of action of saline laxatives.

35. **D** Saline laxatives such as magnesium salts (citrate and hydroxide) and phosphate salts are poorly absorbed and hold water in the intestine by osmotic forces. The increased volume of intestinal content stretches the intestinal wall, thus stimulating peristalsis.

　　A Magnesium salts stimulate, not inhibit, cholecystokinin release.

　　B The drug causes water retention in the intestinal lumen, not in the vessels.

　　C This is the mechanism of action of mineral oil.

　　E This is the mechanism of action of dietary fibers.

Learning objective: Describe the therapeutic uses of loperamide.

36. **A** The patient's symptoms suggest that she was most likely suffering from irritable bowel syndrome, a condition that affects 10 to 15% of the population in the United States. Many patients with this syndrome can be managed satisfactorily with simple medical counseling and supportive measures, including dietary restriction and fiber supplementation. The pharmacological treatment of bowel symptoms (either diarrhea or constipation) is symptomatic. In this case, an antidiarrheal drug is needed. Opioid agonists such as loperamide and diphenoxylate are commonly used. They have the advantage of negligible central nervous system (CNS) activity because penetration into the CNS is poor. Other drugs used for this purpose are muscarinic and 5-HT$_3$ antagonists.

    B–F Drugs from these classes would increase, not decrease, bowel movements.

Learning objective: Explain the mechanism of action of sucralfate.

37. **A** Sucralfate is a mucosal protective agent. In a strong acid environment (pH < 4), the negatively charged sucrose sulfate undergoes extensive cross-linking to positively charged proteins to produce a viscous, sticky polymer that adheres to epithelial cells and ulcer craters for up to 6 hours after a single dose.

    B, E Sucralfate does not have these effects.

    C, D Sucralfate may have cytoprotective effects, including stimulation of local production of prostaglandins, which in turn can inhibit acid secretion and stimulate bicarbonate secretion, but this is not the main mechanism of action of the drug.

Learning objective: Identify the most appropriate laxative used during pregnancy

38. **D** Up to 30% of women experience constipation during pregnancy. Laxatives must be used cautiously because they can increase motility and blood flow in the lower abdomen, and mild agents are preferred. A stool softener such as docusate or a bulk-producing product such as psyllium is commonly used.

    A–C, E, F Stimulant cathartics (castor oil, bisacodyl, and senna) and saline cathartics (magnesium hydroxide and sodium sulfate) are not recommended during pregnancy.

Learning objective: Identify the drug used to treat gastroesophageal reflux disease (GERD) in a patient with concomitant disorders.

39. **D** The substernal pain and reflux of gastric contents into the esophagus are classic symptoms of GERD, a disorder that affects 7% of the population in the United States. Proton pump inhibitors such as omeprazole are effective in the treatment of GERD, and a once-daily dose for 4 weeks will heal 60 to 80% of patients with severe esophagitis.

A Atropine is contraindicated, because it may favor reflux by relaxing the lower esophageal sphincter.

B, C These drugs are not effective in treating GERD.

E Metoclopramide is used in the treatment of GERD because it promotes gastric peristalsis and also increases the lower esophageal sphincter resting tone. However, it is contraindicated in patients with Parkinson disease because it is a D$_2$ antagonist.

F H$_2$ antagonists are currently used in GERD, but cimetidine is not appropriate in a patient taking other drugs because it can inhibit the metabolism of most drugs, including selegiline.

Learning objective: Identify the best drug regimen to prevent chemotherapy-induced nausea and vomiting.

40. **C** According to the guidelines for the use of antiemetics in oncology from the American Society of Clinical Oncology, the best regimen to prevent nausea and vomiting in patients undergoing chemotherapy is a three-drug combination of a 5-HT$_3$ receptor antagonist, a glucocorticoid, and aprepitant. This combination prevents acute emesis in 80 to 90% of patients and prevents delayed emesis in more than 70% of patients.

    A Benzodiazepines have no direct antiemetic effect. They are sometimes added to the main regimen because the anti-anxiety effect could reduce the anticipatory component of nausea and vomiting. Ranitidine has no antiemetic effect.

    B Anticholinergic drugs such as scopolamine are not effective in chemotherapy-induced nausea and vomiting.

    D Loperamide is not an antiemetic drug.

    E These drugs are used in chemotherapy-induced nausea and vomiting only when other antiemetic drugs are not effective.

    F See correct answer explanation.

Learning objective: Describe the use of dronabinol as an appetite stimulant in treating AIDS.

41. **D** Appetite-enhancing (also called orexigenic) drugs are a vast array of medications used to prevent undesired weight loss in the elderly and in patients suffering from such diseases as AIDS and cancer, which often result in wasting of the body's muscle tissue, as well as overall weight loss. Agents with orexigenic effects include 5-HT$_{2C}$ serotonin receptor antagonists (cyproheptadine), adrenergic antagonists (carvedilol and mirtazapine), anabolic steroids (oxandrolone and nandrolone), glucocorticoids (cortisol, prednisone, and dexamethasone), antidiabetic drugs (Insulin and glibenclamide), and cannabinoids. Dronabinol, the most active cannabinoid of cannabis, has been shown to stimulate appetite in patients with AIDS and is often used for this purpose.

    A–C, E, F These drugs are devoid of orexigenic properties.

Learning objective: Identify the prokinetic drug that acts by opening type 2 chloride channels in the small intestine.

42. **C** Lubiprostone is a prokinetic drug that acts in the small intestine. Several agents, commonly called laxatives, can stimulate intestinal motility in nonspecific or indirect ways, but the term *prokinetic* generally is reserved for agents that enhance intestinal transit through interaction with specific receptors. Lubiprostone is a prostaglandin E_1 derivative that appears to bind to prostaglandin E_4 receptors linked to activation of adenylyl cyclase. This in turn can open specific type 2 chloride channels in the luminal cells of the intestinal epithelium, increasing chloride-rich fluid secretion into the intestine. Clinically, lubiprostone alters stool consistency and promotes regular bowel movements. Signs and symptoms related to constipation, including abdominal bloating, abdominal discomfort, stool consistency, and straining, are improved, and long-term data suggest a sustained response over a 6- to 12-month treatment period.

A, B, D–F These drugs do not affect intestinal type 2 chloride channels.

DRUGS FOR GASTROINTESTINAL DISORDERS Answer key							
1.	K	6.	E	11.	A	16.	D
2.	P	7.	F	12.	E	17.	B
3.	N	8.	H	13.	B	18.	E
4.	Q	9.	E	14.	E	19.	C
5.	O	10.	F	15.	E	20.	E
21.	E	26.	F	31.	D	36.	A
22.	E	27.	A	32.	C	37.	A
23.	A	28.	A	33.	B	38.	D
24.	D	29.	B	34.	D	39.	D
25.	D	30.	A	35.	D	40.	C
						41.	D
						42.	C

Answers and Explanations: VI-3 Drugs for Hematopoietic Disorders

Questions 1–6

1. **B**
2. **C**
3. **A**
4. **J**
5. **K**
6. **A**

Learning objective: Explain the purpose of iron administration.

7. **B** The patient's history and lab results indicate that he was most likely suffering from iron deficiency anemia due to blood loss, which is the most common cause of the disease. In this case, the loss was most likely caused by naproxen therapy; the prevalence of endoscopically confirmed gastrointestinal ulcers in nonsteroidal antiinflammatory drug users is 15 to 30%. Iron is the standard therapy for iron deficiency anemia, and it acts only by replacing the severely depleted stores of the metal.

A There are no specific receptors for iron.

C–E Iron does not cause these effects.

Learning objective: Identify the risk associated with folic acid deficiency during pregnancy.

8. **B** It has been shown that neural tube defects are associated with folic acid deficiency during pregnancy. Folate supplementation during early pregnancy may substantially reduce the risk of neural tube defects, such as spina bifida and encephalocele.

A, C–F The risk of these congenital abnormalities is not related to folic acid deficiency.

Learning objective: Identify the most important body iron store.

9. **C** Iron not used for erythropoiesis is stored in two storage pools. The most important is ferritin, a heterogeneous family of proteins formed around an iron core. Ferritin is found in hepatocytes, liver, bone marrow, macrophages, red blood cells, and serum. The pool is very labile and readily available to meet any body requirement for iron. The second storage pool of iron is hemosiderin, which is located primarily in the liver and bone marrow.

A, B, D, E See correct answer explanation.

Learning objective: Explain why folic acid is contraindicated in megaloblastic anemias due to vitamin B_{12} deficiency.

10. **A** The patient's megaloblastic anemia was most likely due to vitamin B_{12} deficiency resulting from the previous total gastrectomy. Administration of folic acid can correct the anemia caused by vitamin B_{12} deficiency but does not prevent the potentially irreversible neurologic damage caused by vitamin B_{12} deficiency. In this patient, treatment with folic acid would mask the hematologic signs of anemia, thus increasing the risk of neurologic symptoms due to undiagnosed vitamin B_{12} deficiency.

B–E See correct answer explanation.

Learning objective: Outline the therapeutic uses of folic acid.

11. **B** The patient's lab values indicate that she was suffering from megaloblastic anemia. Because the serum vitamin B_{12} is normal, the anemia is most likely due to folic acid deficiency. The disorder is not rare in a pregnant woman with malnutrition and excessive alcohol intake, as in this case.

A, C–E See correct answer explanation.

Learning objective: Outline the use of parenteral iron preparation in case of severe iron deficiency anemia.

12. **D** The patient's signs and symptoms, together with lab values, indicate that she was suffering from severe iron deficiency anemia, probably related to chronic blood loss due to menorrhagia and overuse of nonsteroidal antiinflammatory drugs. Because the hemoglobin and ferritin levels are very low, parenteral iron therapy is mandatory. Iron sucrose is a preparation given by the parenteral route. It appears to be less likely than iron dextran to cause hypersensitivity reactions.

    A–C, E, F See correct answer explanation.

Learning objective: Explain the mechanism of action of folic acid.

13. **B** The patient's symptoms and lab exams indicate that he was most likely suffering from megaloblastic anemia. The normal serum vitamin B_{12} levels suggest that the anemia is due to folic acid deficiency, which can occur in people suffering from malabsorption syndromes, as in this case (see gluten enteropathy). Administration of folic acid can cure the anemia because folic acid is needed for the synthesis of tetrahydrofolate acid (THF). This molecule can subsequently be transformed into several THF cofactors that participate in many one-carbon unit transfer reactions. The reaction needed for purine and DNA synthesis transfers one carbon unit of N_5-N_{10}-methylenetetrahydrofolate to deoxyuridine monophosphate to form thymidine 5′-monophosphate. In rapidly proliferating tissues, considerable amounts of THF are consumed in the reaction, and continued DNA synthesis requires continued regeneration of THF. Therefore, in folate deficiency, thymidine 5′-monophosphate formation is decreased, which in turn decreases the synthesis of DNA. RNA synthesis continues, resulting in increased cytoplasmic mass and maturation. Therefore, cytoplasmic maturity is greater than nuclear maturity, and megaloblasts are produced in the bone marrow.

    A This is an action of vitamin B_{12} in the treatment of vitamin B_{12} deficiency, which was not the case in this patient.

    C This is an action of ferrous sulfate in the treatment of iron deficiency anemia, which was not the case in this patient.

    D The patient's anemia was not caused by hemolysis.

    E The patient's anemia was not caused by erythropoietin deficiency

Learning objective: Describe the transport of iron to maturing erythroid cells.

14. **D** Iron is transported in plasma bound to transferrin, a β globulin that specifically binds ferric iron. The complex binds to a specific receptor located on erythroblasts and other proliferating erythroid cells. The complex is then internalized by endocytosis, releasing iron within the cell, and transferrin and the receptors are recycled.

    A–C, E See correct answer explanation.

Learning objective: Explain the mechanism of antianemic action of vitamin B_{12}.

15. **C** Megaloblastic anemias (both folate and vitamin B_{12} deficiency anemias) are due to a decreased availability of tetrahydrofolate (THF). Vitamin B_{12} transfers a methyl group from N_5-methyltetrahydrofolate to homocysteine, forming methionine and THF. In vitamin B_{12} deficiency, N_5-methyltetrahydrofolate accumulates with associated depletion of THF (methylfolate trapping). The administration of vitamin B_{12} restores the demethylation of N_5-methyltetrahydrofolate, thus correcting the megaloblastic anemia.

    A This formation is another chemical reaction catalyzed by vitamin B_{12}, but the reaction is not needed for the synthesis of THF.

    B, D, E These reactions are not catalyzed by vitamin B_{12}.

Learning objective: Describe the therapeutic uses of ferrous sulfate.

16. **F** The patient's symptoms and lab results indicate that she was suffering from microcytic anemia, most likely secondary to iron deficiency due to total gastrectomy. Removal of the stomach leads to marked decrease in the production of gastric acid, which is necessary to convert dietary iron to a form that is readily absorbed by the duodenum. Iron deficiency anemia does not occur for a few years after gastrectomy because iron is stored in moderately large amounts in bone marrow. When anemia is caused by iron deficiency, oral iron supplementation is appropriate.

    A–E See correct answer explanation.

Learning objective: Outline the therapeutic uses of vitamin B_{12}.

17. **E** The patient's signs and symptoms are classic for pernicious anemia. The disease occurs equally in both genders, with an average onset of age 60. The anemia is caused by vitamin B_{12} malabsorption due to severe atrophy of the gastric glands with loss of parietal cells and inability to secrete intrinsic factor. The cause of the disease is unknown, but several findings point to an immunologic or inherited basis of the disease. Approximately 90% of patients have antibodies to parietal cells, and 2 to 10% of relatives of these patients exhibit similar antibodies. Parenteral cyanocobalamin should be given daily to replenish tissue stores, and a monthly maintenance dose should be given for life.

    A–D See correct answer explanation.

Learning objective: Describe the intestinal absorption of iron.

18. **D** Iron crosses the luminal membrane of duodenal mucosal cells by two mechanisms: active transport of ferrous iron by a carrier named divalent metal transporter 1 (DMT1) and absorption of iron complexed with heme.

    Because the patient received ferrous sulfate, the drug was actively transported by DMT1.

    A–C, E See correct answer explanation.

Learning objective: Outline the appropriate therapeutic treatment in case of mixed anemia.

19. **C** The patient's blood values indicate that the woman was most likely suffering from a mixed anemia, due to both iron and folate deficiency. The combination of both macro- and microcytic red blood cells offset each other to produce a normal mean corpuscular volume. There are many examples of situations in which mixed anemia occurs, including pregnancy, as both iron and folate requirements increase during gestation. When anemia is both microcytic and megaloblastic, treatment with iron and folic acid is indicated.

    A, B Vitamin B_{12} precursors are not needed because blood concentration of vitamin B_{12} is normal

    D, E See correct answer explanation.

Learning objective: Outline the therapeutic uses of deferoxamine.

20. **F** In thalassemic children with severe anemia, blood transfusions are necessary to maintain life and normal activity. To prevent iron overloading as a result of repeated blood transfusions, deferoxamine is often given during the transfusion. The drug can remove iron from hemosiderin, ferritin, and transferrin, but not iron from hemoglobin and cytochromes. Therefore, the drug can eliminate iron excess without affecting hemoglobin formation.

    A–E See correct answer explanation.

Learning objective: Outline the therapeutic treatment for hypoproliferative anemia due to renal insufficiency

21. **B** The patient's lab results indicate that he was most likely suffering from a hypoproliferative anemia due to renal insufficiency. Anemia usually occurs when creatinine clearance is less than 45 mL/min (which corresponds roughly to serum creatinine > 3 mg/dL in a normal man over age 70). When anemia is due to renal disease, erythropoietin is the treatment of choice. Iron supplements must also be given to achieve an adequate erythropoietin response.

    A, C–F See correct answer explanation.

Learning objective: Identify the myeloid growth factor that can stimulate proliferation and differentiation of neutrophil progenitor cells only.

22. **B** Bone marrow transplantation is associated with profound granulocytopenia due to the myeloablative preparative regimen. Filgrastim is a human granulocyte colony-stimulating factor that stimulates the production of granulocyte progenitor cells. Therefore, once engraftment occurs, hematopoietic recovery can be accelerated.

    A, C–F See correct answer explanation.

Learning objective: Identify the main location of oprelvekin receptors.

23. **E** Oprelvekin is the recombinant form of interleukin-11. The drug activates specific receptors located on megakaryocytes and megakaryocyte progenitors, thus stimulating the production of platelets. It is used clinically to prevent severe chemotherapy-induced thrombocytopenia and to reduce the need for platelet transfusions following chemotherapy for nonmyeloid malignancies.

    A–D, F See correct answer explanation.

Learning objective: Describe the anaphylactoid reaction to iron dextran.

24. **C** The signs and symptoms of the patient indicate that she was most likely suffering from an anaphylactoid reaction, which is a rare but potentially fatal adverse effect of iron dextran therapy. Other parenteral preparations, such as sodium ferric gluconate and iron sucrose, appear to cause fewer hypersensitivity reactions than iron dextran and are now preferred for parenteral iron therapy.

    A, D Leucovorin and cyanocobalamin do not cause anaphylactoid reactions and are not used to treat microcytic anemia.

    B Ferrous sulfate is given only by the oral route.

    E, F Filgrastim and sargramostim can cause anaphylactoid reactions, but they are not used to treat microcytic anemia.

Learning objective: Describe the adverse effects of erythropoietin.

25. **A** The most common adverse effects of erythropoietin are hypertension and thrombotic complications. The mechanism of the thrombotic effect is still uncertain but is likely related to an excessive increase of hemoglobin levels. Recently, the U.S. Food and Drug Administration issued a warning that patients with renal failure or cancer whose hemoglobin rises to more than 12 g/dL are at greater risk of thrombotic events, as in this case.

    B–E See correct answer explanation.

Learning objective: Outline the therapeutic uses of oprelvekin

26. **F** The patient's lab results indicate severe thrombocytopenia, likely due to cytotoxic anticancer chemotherapy. Oprelvekin, the recombinant form of interleukin-11, has been approved for treatment of severe thrombocytopenia due to chemotherapy for nonmyeloid malignancies.

    A Filgrastim is human granulocyte colony-stimulating factor that stimulates the production of granulocyte progenitor cells. The normal neutrophil count indicates that there is no granulocytopenia.

    B Erythropoietin is given when the anemia is hypoproliferative (i.e., due to a deficient response to cytokine humoral stimuli). There is no evidence that the patient's anemia is hypoproliferative.

    C–E These drugs are used for megaloblastic anemias. The normal mean corpuscular volume indicates that the patient's anemia is not megaloblastic.

Learning objective: Identify the drug used to treat iron poisoning.

27. **B** The large hematemesis and the pregnancy of the mother suggest the possible ingestion of iron tablets. The signs and symptoms of the patient are indicative of first-stage acute iron poisoning. As few as 10 to 12 prenatal multivitamin with iron tablets can cause serious illness in a young child. Deferoxamine is an iron-chelating compound that can bind iron that has already been absorbed. The iron–deferoxamine complex is not toxic and is excreted by the kidney.

    Deferoxamine therapy should be promptly initiated when severe symptoms of iron toxicity are prominent, as in this case.

    A, C–F See correct answer explanation.

Learning objective: Outline the therapeutic uses of leucovorin.

28. **C** Methotrexate inhibits dihydrofolate reductase, preventing the formation of tetrahydrofolate (THF), an essential factor for DNA synthesis. The blockade of this synthesis in cancer cells mediates the therapeutic action of the drug, but the blockade of the synthesis in normal cells causes methotrexate toxicity. Leucovorin bypasses the dihydrofolate reductase step in tetrahydrofolate synthesis, thus rescuing normal cells while cancer cells are less affected.

    A Folic acid is useless in this situation because it cannot be transformed to THF due to the dihydrofolate reductase inhibition.

    B, D–F See correct answer explanation.

Learning objective: Outline the therapeutic uses of filgrastim.

29. **D** The patient's lab results indicate a profound neutropenia, which can occur in AIDS patients taking zidovudine. Filgrastim is recombinant human granulocyte colony-stimulating factor that stimulates proliferation and differentiation of progenitors already committed to neutrophil lineage. It has been shown that zidovudine-induced neutropenia can be partially or completely reversed by filgrastim treatment.

    A–C, E See correct answer explanation.

Learning objective: Describe the therapeutic uses of ferrous sulfate.

30. **E** The patient's lab results indicate that she was suffering from microcytic anemia, most likely due to iron deficiency (see the vegetarian diet and heavy menstrual periods). Oral iron should correct the anemia rapidly and completely and therefore is the preferred starting therapy. Parenteral iron administration (iron dextran or iron sucrose) would most likely also be effective, but should be used only when clearly indicated, that is, when the anemia is very severe, or when oral therapy fails.

    A–D, F See correct answer explanation.

DRUGS FOR HEMATOPOIETIC DISORDERS Answer key					
1.	B	6.	A	11.	B
2.	C	7.	B	12.	D
3.	A	8.	B	13.	B
4.	J	9.	C	14.	D
5.	K	10.	A	15.	C
16.	F	21.	B	26.	F
17.	E	22.	B	27.	B
18.	D	23.	E	28.	C
19.	C	24.	C	29.	D
20.	F	25.	A	30.	E

VII Inflammation and Immunomodulation

Questions: VII-1 Histamine and Serotonin: Agonists and Antagonists

Directions for questions **1–3**

Match each histamine and serotonin receptor agonist and antagonist with the appropriate description (each lettered option can be selected once, more than once, or not at all).

- **A.** Cyproheptadine
- **B.** Ergonovine
- **C.** Loratadine
- **D.** Ondansetron
- **E.** Promethazine
- **F.** Sumatriptan

Difficulty level: Easy

1. An antihistamine drug with pronounced sedative properties

Difficulty level: Easy

2. A histamine and serotonin receptor antagonist sometimes used for treatment of intestinal hypermobility of carcinoid

Difficulty level: Easy

3. This drug can act as an agonist at serotonergic and α-adrenergic receptors.

Difficulty level: Medium

4. A 64-year-old man suffering from benign prostatic hyperplasia presented to his physician complaining of generalized itching. The problem began 1 week earlier, after an afternoon of prolonged sun exposure. The patient reported that the itching was distressing, especially during the night. Physical examination showed an enlarged prostate and no other evidence of ongoing disease. Which of the following drugs would be appropriate for this patient?

- **A.** Cyproheptadine
- **B.** Diphenhydramine
- **C.** Famotidine
- **D.** Loratadine
- **E.** Acetaminophen
- **F.** Ibuprofen

Difficulty level: Easy

5. A 46-year-old woman recently diagnosed with classic migraine had a headache attack at least once a week. Ergotamine was prescribed to prevent the impending attacks. Which of the following actions most likely contributed to the therapeutic effect of the drug in the patient's disorder?

- **A.** Constriction of cerebral vessels
- **B.** Extravasation of plasma into perivascular space
- **C.** Prostaglandin release from vascular endothelium
- **D.** Platelet aggregation in the cerebral vascular bed
- **E.** Increased firing of trigeminal neurons

Difficulty level: Easy

6. A 30-year-old man presented to the clinic with a 2-month history of right-side head pain recurring on a weekly basis. His headaches were usually preceded by unformed flashes of light, bilaterally, and were associated with nausea, vomiting, and photophobia. The headaches were not relieved by aspirin or ibuprofen and usually lasted all day unless he was able to sleep. A drug acting on which of the following receptors would be most appropriate to stop the migraine attack in this patient?

- **A.** Beta-2 adrenergic
- **B.** GABAergic
- **C.** M_1 cholinergic
- **D.** $5\text{-HT}_{1B/1D}$ serotonergic
- **E.** Alpha-2 adrenergic
- **F.** D_1 dopaminergic

Difficulty level: Easy

7. A 34-year-old woman underwent magnetic resonance imaging (MRI) to investigate an acoustic neurinoma. Because the woman had had a mild allergic reaction to contrast media in the past, she was given a prescription for drugs to be taken before the MRI. Which of the following drugs should be included in that prescription?

- **A.** Fludrocortisone
- **B.** Famotidine
- **C.** Zafirlukast
- **D.** Diphenhydramine
- **E.** Ondansetron
- **F.** Bromocriptine

Difficulty level: Easy

8. A 30-year-old primipara woman had visible vaginal bleeding within a few hours after delivering her baby. Uterine massage and infusion of oxytocin did not control the bleeding. Upon examination, it was felt that the hemorrhage was due to uterine atony. An intramuscular injection of ergonovine was given. Which of the following actions most likely mediated the therapeutic effect of the drug in this patient?

   A. Selective constriction of uterine arteries
   B. Endothelin release in the uterine vascular bed
   C. Platelet aggregation in the uterine vascular bed
   D. Activation of coagulation cascade in uterine capillaries
   E. Induction of powerful uterine contracture

Difficulty level: Easy

9. A 24-year-old woman experienced severe motion sickness whenever she traveled by air or sea. Diphenhydramine taken before a trip was effective in minimizing her symptoms. The therapeutic effect of the drug was most likely due to blockade of which of the following pairs of central receptors?

   A. Dopaminergic and β-adrenergic
   B. GABAergic and serotonergic
   C. Alpha-adrenergic and muscarinic
   D. Histaminergic and muscarinic
   E. Serotonergic and peptidergic

Difficulty level: Medium

10. A 33-year-old woman was hospitalized after 1 week of increasing pain, tenderness, and cyanosis in her legs. She admitted to taking several medications to relieve a migraine headache. Physical examination revealed that no pulses could be palpated below the femoral vessels, and an aortogram showed a pronounced constriction of the vessels distal to the iliac arteries. The vasoconstriction disappeared after 3 hours of nitroprusside intravenous infusion. Which of the following drugs most likely caused the vessel constriction?

   A. Aspirin
   B. Propranolol
   C. Ergotamine
   D. Acetaminophen
   E. Naproxen
   F. Diclofenac

Difficulty level: Easy

11. A 33-year-old man complained to his physician that the drug he was taking made him feel tightness in his chest and throat soon after the injection. The man, recently diagnosed with classic migraine, had started a treatment that included the subcutaneous administration of a drug to block an impending acute attack. Which of the following drugs most likely caused the patient's symptoms?

   A. Ibuprofen
   B. Propranolol
   C. Sumatriptan
   D. Valproic acid
   E. Diphenhydramine
   F. Aspirin

Difficulty level: Easy

12. A 25-year-old man suffering from hay fever started treatment with an over-the-counter antihistamine preparation. Which of the following statements best explains the molecular mechanism of action of the prescribed drug to treat this patient's hay fever?

   A. Reversible binding to H_3 receptors
   B. Irreversible binding to H_3 receptors
   C. Reversible binding to H_2 receptors
   D. Irreversible binding to H_2 receptors
   E. Reversible binding to H_1 receptors
   F. Irreversible binding to H_1 receptors

Difficulty level: Medium

13. A 34-year-old man presented to his physician complaining of dry mouth, constipation, and difficulty in urination. He also noticed an increase in appetite. The man had started a therapy with cyproheptadine 2 weeks earlier to treat cold-induced urticaria. Drug-induced blockade of which of the following pairs of receptors most likely mediated the patient's symptoms?

   A. Dopaminergic and α_1-adrenergic
   B. H_2-histaminergic and muscarinic
   C. H_2-histaminergic and α_1-adrenergic
   D. Serotonergic and GABAergic
   E. Muscarinic and serotonergic
   F. Dopaminergic and GABAergic

Difficulty level: Medium.

14. A 43-year-old man with a long history of exertional angina was recently diagnosed with migraine. Which of the following antimigraine drugs would be contraindicated in this patient?

   A. Aspirin
   B. Acetaminophen
   C. Sumatriptan
   D. Ibuprofen
   E. Propranolol

Difficulty level: Easy

15. A 40-year-old woman suffering from chronic classic migraine headaches took three sublingual tablets of ergotamine to abort an impending migraine attack. Which of the following adverse effects were most likely to occur in this patient?

   A. Visual hallucinations
   B. Postural hypotension
   C. Facial flushing
   D. Adynamic ileus
   E. Nausea and vomiting

Difficulty level: Easy

16. A 48-year-old woman suffering from allergic urticaria started a treatment with loratadine. The decreased synthesis of which of the following substances most likely mediated the therapeutic effect of the drug in the patient's disease?

   A. Cyclic adenosine monophosphate (cAMP)
   B. Cyclic guanosine monophosphate (cGMP)
   C. Inositol triphosphate
   D. Cyclooxygenase-1
   E. Cyclooxygenase-2

Difficulty level: Easy

17. A 10-year-old boy developed pruritus and skin wheals after eating fried eggs. He was diagnosed with food allergy, and loratadine was prescribed. Which of the following statements best explains why loratadine is used in several allergic disorders?

   A. It blocks the antigen-induced release of histamine from mast cells.
   B. It prevents the antigen–antibody reaction on the surface of mast cells.
   C. It elicits effects that are opposite to those elicited by histamine.
   D. It blocks muscarinic and adrenergic receptors in smooth muscle.
   E. It prevents many histamine-induced effects in peripheral tissues.

Difficulty level: Easy

18. A 33-year-old woman complained to her physician of numbness and tingling in her fingers and toes. The woman had been taking a drug for 1 month to abort headache. Which of the following drugs most likely caused the patient's symptoms?

   A. Ibuprofen
   B. Valproic acid
   C. Ergotamine
   D. Propranolol
   E. Acetaminophen
   F. Aspirin

Difficulty level: Easy

19. A 59-year-old man with a body mass index of 42 and a long history of poorly controlled hypertension was recently diagnosed with migraine headaches. Which of the following antimigraine drugs would be contraindicated in this patient?

   A. Aspirin
   B. Acetaminophen
   C. Ergotamine
   D. Ibuprofen
   E. Propranolol
   F. Verapamil

Difficulty level: Medium

20. A 29-year-old woman suffering from allergic rhinitis started treatment with loratadine. The drug can completely counteract the histamine-induced release of which of the following endogenous compounds?

   A. Pepsin
   B. Gastric acid
   C. Cyclic adenosine monophosphate (cAMP)
   D. Nitric oxide
   E. Bradykinin

Difficulty level: Hard

21. A 47-year-old man presented to the clinic complaining of a recent onset of repeating episodes of vertigo associated with nausea and vomiting. The patient was otherwise healthy and denied use of alcohol or illicit drugs. Physical examination was unremarkable, but a provocative test elicited severe vertigo. A diagnosis was made, and a pharmacotherapy was prescribed. Which of the following drugs would be appropriate for this patient?

   A. Diphenhydramine
   B. Ondansetron
   C. Dronabinol
   D. Ergotamine
   E. Loratadine
   F. Propranolol

Difficulty level: Medium

22. A 43-year-old woman complained to her physician of annoying daytime sleepiness. The woman, who was treated in the past with several drugs for generalized anxiety, had been receiving diazepam for the past month. One week ago, she started taking an over-the-counter preparation for seasonal allergic rhinitis. Which of the following drugs most likely precipitated the patient's daytime sleepiness?

A. Loratadine
B. Prednisone
C. Diphenhydramine
D. Zolpidem
E. Trazodone
F. Mirtazapine

Difficulty level: Hard

23. A 53-year-old man presented to the clinic complaining of itching, flushing, arthralgia, heartburn, and diarrhea. Further exams led to the diagnosis of systemic mastocytosis. Which of the following pairs of drugs should be included in the therapeutic treatment of this patient?

A. Aspirin and ergotamine
B. Misoprostol and ergotamine
C. Loratadine and famotidine
D. Loratadine and diphenhydramine
E. Aspirin and famotidine

Difficulty level: Easy

24. A 28-year-old woman who was 26 weeks' pregnant had been recently diagnosed with classic migraine. Which of the following drugs would be appropriate to reduce the frequency and severity of her migraine attacks?

A. Ergonovine
B. Propranolol
C. Ergotamine
D. Valproic acid
E. Sumatriptan

Difficulty level: Medium

25. A 66-year-old man suffering from benign prostatic hyperplasia was admitted to the hospital because of severe suprapubic pain and an inability to pass urine for the past 24 hours. On questioning, he said he had been taking diphenhydramine for a few days to relieve itching. Which of the following actions most likely mediated the adverse effect of the drug in this patient?

A. Relaxation of the detrusor muscle
B. Constriction of the bladder external sphincter
C. Constriction of the prostate capsule
D. Relaxation of the bladder internal sphincter
E. Increased diuresis

Difficulty level: Medium

26. A 48-year-old woman was admitted to the emergency department because of fever (103.1°F, 39.5°C), flushing, sweating, tremors, and altered consciousness. Medical history indicated that she had been suffering from depression for 8 years, currently treated with paroxetine, and for insomnia, currently treated with zolpidem. The patient also reported that 24 hours earlier, she had self-administered three tablets of a drug given to her by a friend to treat a severe headache. Further exams confirmed the preliminary diagnosis, and an appropriate treatment was started. Which of the following drugs most likely triggered the patient's disorder?

A. Acetaminophen
B. Sumatriptan
C. Ibuprofen
D. Zolpidem
E. Cyproheptadine
F. Diclofenac

Difficulty level: Medium

27. A 48-year-old man had a long history of classic migraine that was recently well controlled by sumatriptan. Which of the following parts of the central nervous system was most likely a primary site of therapeutic action of the drug in the patient's disease?

A. Nucleus accumbens
B. Trigeminal nerve
C. Vestibular nuclei
D. Chemoreceptor trigger zone
E. Olfactory nerve
F. Nucleus caudalis

Difficulty level: Medium

28. A 2-year-old boy was brought to the emergency department with high body temperature (104°F, 40°C), flushed and dry skin, and widely dilated pupils unresponsive to light. He was agitated and underwent a brief tonic-clonic convulsion. His mother stated that the boy apparently swallowed several tablets of her allergy medication. Which of the following drugs most likely caused the patient's poisoning?

A. Ibuprofen
B. Diphenhydramine
C. Phenylephrine
D. Celecoxib
E. Loratadine
F. Atropine

Difficulty level: Medium

29. A 54-year-old man at a scheduled ophthalmic check-up was found to have increased intraocular pressure. The man had been suffering from open-angle glaucoma for 2 years, but up until the current visit, the disease was found to be well controlled by local treatment with timolol and latanoprost. Drugs taken recently by the patient included over-the-counter preparations for episodic headache, heartburn, and insomnia. Which of the following drugs could have caused the patient's increased intraocular pressure?

A. Acetaminophen
B. Omeprazole
C. Ibuprofen
D. Diphenhydramine
E. Famotidine

Difficulty level: Medium

30. A 21-year-old woman suffering from seasonal allergic conjunctivitis started a treatment with eye drops of azelastine, a second-generation histamine H_1 antagonist. Second-generation H_1 antagonists are used locally in the conjunctiva instead of first-generation H_1 antagonists to provide which of the following therapeutic advantages?

A. Negligible effects on pupil size and accommodation
B. Negligible penetration into the central nervous system
C. Higher dilating activity on conjunctival vessels
D. Higher antibacterial activity against conjunctival infections
E. Higher blocking activity on lacrimal gland secretion

Difficulty level: Easy

31. An 8-year-old girl was diagnosed with seasonal allergic conjunctivitis triggered by exposure to airborne pollen. She started a topical therapy with cromolyn sodium. Which of the following actions most likely mediated the therapeutic effectiveness of cromolyn in this patient?

A. Blockade of H_1 receptors
B. Blockade of mediator release from mast cells
C. Inhibition of prostaglandin biosynthesis
D. Blockade of leukotriene receptors
E. Constriction of conjunctival vessels

Questions: VII-2 Eicosanoids: Agonists, Antagonists, and Inhibitors

Directions for questions **1–5**

Match each drug acting on the eicosanoid pathway with the appropriate description (each lettered option can be selected once, more than once, or not at all).

A. Alprostadil
B. Dinoprostone
C. Latanoprost
D. Misoprostol
E. Epoprostenol
F. Prednisone

Difficulty level: Easy

1. This drug can inhibit the biosynthesis of all eicosanoids.

Difficulty level: Easy

2. This drug is a synthetic prostaglandin I_2.

Difficulty level: Easy

3. This drug is a prostaglandin E_1 analogue.

Difficulty level: Easy

4. This drug is a prostaglandin $F_{2\alpha}$ analogue.

Difficulty level: Easy

5. This drug is a synthetic prostaglandin E_2.

Difficulty level: Medium

6. A 48-year-old man with open-angle glaucoma still had elevated intraocular pressure despite 1 month of treatment with timolol and dorzolamide. The ophthalmologist decided to add latanoprost to the therapeutic regimen. Which of the following effects on aqueous humor most likely mediated the therapeutic effect of the drug in the patient's disease?

A. Increased outflow through Schlemm canal
B. Decreased production by ciliary epithelium
C. Increased outflow through uveoscleral route
D. Decreased production by eye vessel constriction
E. Increased outflow through trabecular meshwork

Difficulty level: Easy

7. A 47-year-old man complained to his physician of an inability to maintain an erection. After a complete medical workup, he was prescribed intraurethral administration of alprostadil to be used before intercourse. Which of the following molecular mechanism of action most likely mediated the efficacy of the drug in the patient's erection disorder?

A. Activation of prostaglandin E_1 receptors
B. Blockade of α_1 adrenoceptors
C. Activation of muscarinic M_3 acetylcholine receptors
D. Blockade of thromboxane A_2 receptors
E. Activation of β_2 adrenoceptors
F. Release of nitric oxide

Difficulty level: Easy

8. A 22-year-old primipara woman was admitted to the obstetrical unit for labor induction because of a postdated pregnancy. Her obstetrical examination was normal, but her cervix was unfavorable for induction of labor with oxytocin. Which of the following drugs given intravaginally would be appropriately administered at this time?

A. Thromboxane A_2
B. Dinoprostone
C. Ergonovine
D. Diclofenac
E. Albuterol
F. Ibuprofen

Difficulty level: Easy

9. A 35-year-old woman at 24 weeks gestation was admitted to the obstetrical unit because of signs of severe fetal distress. Fetal death was diagnosed on admission, and induction of labor was planned. An oxytocin drip was initiated, and a vaginal suppository was inserted. Which of the following drugs was most likely given intravaginally?

A. Metoprolol
B. Albuterol
C. Bethanechol
D. Ergonovine
E. Dinoprostone

Difficulty level: Easy

10. A 22-year-old woman recently diagnosed with mild persistent asthma started treatment with albuterol as needed and oral zileuton daily. Which of the following molecular mechanisms of action most likely mediated the therapeutic effect of zileuton in the patient's disease?

A. Activation of β_2 receptors
B. Inhibition of 5-lipoxygenase
C. Competitive blockade of leukotriene receptors
D. Inhibition of cyclooxygenase-2
E. Competitive blockade of muscarinic M_3 receptors

Difficulty level: Easy

11. A 35-year-old woman presented to her physician complaining of recent onset of nausea and vomiting in the mornings. A pregnancy test confirmed she was pregnant. Past medical history was significant for chronic heart failure, necessitating a medical abortion. A drug treatment for abortion induction was prescribed. Which of the following drugs was most likely included in that treatment?

A. Quinidine
B. Ergonovine
C. Norgestrel
D. Clomiphene
E. Misoprostol

Difficulty level: Easy

12. A 2-day-old premature male baby, born by normal vaginal delivery, presented with severe cyanosis. Chest x-rays and echocardiography confirmed the diagnosis of congenital transposition of the great arteries, and the baby was scheduled for surgery. Which of the following drugs was most likely administered by intravenous infusion to the baby until surgery?

A. Indomethacin
B. Alprostadil
C. Dinoprostone
D. Latanoprost
E. Misoprostol

Difficulty level: Easy

13. A 35-year-old woman was seen at the clinic because of progressive exertional dyspnea and arthralgias. Further exams led to the diagnosis of primary pulmonary hypertension, and an intravenous infusion of epoprostenol was started. Which of the following molecular actions most likely mediated the therapeutic efficacy of the drug in the patient's disease?

A. Blockade of Ca^{2+} channels
B. Activation of β_2 adrenoceptors
C. Opening of K^+ channels
D. Blockade of α_1 adrenoceptors
E. Activation of prostaglandin I_2 receptors

Difficulty level: Easy

14. A 26-year-old man was brought to the emergency department because of a gunshot wound in his right leg. Physical examination showed a distressed patient with abundant hemorrhage from the wound. The synthesis and release of which of the following endogenous compounds was most likely increased in this patient?

A. Prostacyclin
B. Prostaglandin E_2
C. Bradykinin
D. Histamine
E. Adenosine
F. Thromboxane A_2

Difficulty level: Medium

15. A 64-year-old man recently diagnosed with open-angle glaucoma started a treatment with latanoprost. Which of the following sets of ocular effects (from A to E) most likely occurred after the administration of the drug?

Drug	Pupillary Diameter	Lens Curvature	Ocular Pressure
A	+	–	+
B	–	+	–
C	+	0	0
D	0	0	–
E	+	0	–

Note: +, increased; –, decreased; 0, negligible effect.

Difficulty level: Easy

16. A 42-year-old man was seen in the clinic with general malaise, fever (102.5°F, 39.2°C), cough, and dyspnea. Further exams led to the diagnosis of acute bronchitis. Which of the following enzymes was primarily involved in the patient's inflammatory disease?

A. Creatinine kinase
B. Cyclooxygenase-2
C. 5-lipoxygenase
D. Lactic dehydrogenase
E. 12-lipoxygenase
F. Cyclooxygenase-1

Difficulty level: Easy

17. A 13-year-old girl complained to her physician of painful menstruation accompanied by headache and nausea. She underwent menarche 6 months earlier, and dysmenorrhea had occurred since then. The physician prescribed ibuprofen to be started on the day prior to the expected start of menstruation. Inhibition of synthesis of which of the following endogenous compounds most likely mediated the therapeutic effect of ibuprofen in the patient's disorder?

A. Magnesium
B. Nitric oxide
C. Prostaglandin E_2
D. Epinephrine
E. Prostaglandin I_2

Difficulty level: Easy

18. A 64-year-old woman recently diagnosed with osteoarthritis started treatment with ibuprofen and misoprostol. Which of the following adverse effects is most likely expected from misoprostol treatment?

A. Peptic ulcer
B. Drowsiness
C. Hypertension
D. Diarrhea
E. Increased intraocular pressure

Difficulty level: Easy

19. A 54-year-old man complained to his physician that the alprostadil he was using before intercourse was able to improve his erectile dysfunction but caused penile pain. Which of the following actions most likely mediated the adverse effect of the drug?

A. Sensitization of substantia gelatinosa in the spinal cord
B. Decreased firing of corticospinal projection to the dorsal horn
C. Increased sensitivity of the brain periaqueductal area
D. Lowering threshold of nociceptive afferent neurons
E. Increased sensitivity of the frontal cortex

Difficulty level: Medium

20. A 59-year-old woman complained to her physician of persistent heartburn. She had been taking ibuprofen for osteoarthritis of the right hip for the past 2 months. She refused to stop the medication, which she said was very good for her pain. The physician prescribed another drug, to be taken together with ibuprofen, to prevent peptic ulcer formation. Which of the following actions most likely contributed to the preventive effect of the prescribed drug?

A. Binding to necrotic ulcer tissue, acting as a barrier for acid and pepsin
B. Blockade of muscarinic M_3 receptors on gastric parietal cells
C. Blockade of gastrin receptors on gastric parietal cells
D. Stimulation of bicarbonate and mucus secretion by superficial epithelial cells
E. Bactericidal effect against *Helicobacter pylori*

Questions: VII-3 Nonsteroidal Antiinflammatory Drugs

Directions for questions **1–7**

Match each drug with the appropriate description (each lettered option can be selected once, more than once, or not at all).

- **A.** Acetaminophen
- **B.** Aspirin
- **C.** Celecoxib
- **D.** Diclofenac
- **E.** Indomethacin
- **F.** Ketorolac
- **G.** Mesalamine
- **H.** Naproxen
- **I.** Piroxicam
- **J.** Salicylic acid

Difficulty level: Easy

1. An irreversible inhibitor of cyclooxygenase

Difficulty level: Easy

2. A salicylate derivative mainly used in inflammatory bowel disease

Difficulty level: Easy

3. A selective inhibitor of cyclooxygenase-2

Difficulty level: Easy

4. This drug follows zero-order kinetics when given at intermediate to high doses.

Difficulty level: Easy

5. This drug can inhibit both cyclooxygenase and phospholipase A_2.

Difficulty level: Easy

6. The analgesic effect of this drug is primarily mediated by central impairment of pain transmission.

Difficulty level: Easy

7. The long half-life of this drug (more than 50 hours) permits once-daily dosing.

Difficulty level: Easy

8. The mother of a 17-month-old girl took the baby to the pediatrician because she found that her daughter's rectal temperature was 103.1°F (39.5°C). After physical examination, the pediatrician said the fever was most likely due to a viral infection and prescribed ibuprofen. Which of the following molecular actions most likely mediated the antipyretic effect of the drug in this patient?

- **A.** Blockade of prostaglandin receptors in the hypothalamus
- **B.** Inhibition of phospholipase A_2 in the hypothalamus
- **C.** Decreased interleukin concentration in the hypothalamus
- **D.** Decreased concentration of prostaglandins in the hypothalamus
- **E.** Inhibition of cyclooxygenase in peripheral tissues
- **F.** Blockade of oxidative phosphorylation in skeletal muscle

Difficulty level: Medium

9. A 66-year-old man complained to his physician that he had urinated very little over the past 24 hours. The man was being treated with digoxin, furosemide, and captopril for congestive heart failure, and the therapy had improved his cardiac conditions. Two days ago, the patient had pain on movement of his left leg that got better with two ibuprofen tablets. The physician found no clinical signs of intravascular volume depletion and increased the dose of furosemide, but 6 hours later, urination was not improved. Which of the following actions most likely mediated the patient's oliguria?

- **A.** Ibuprofen-mediated decrease of the glomerular filtration rate
- **B.** Worsening of cardiac failure despite the therapy
- **C.** Furosemide-mediated decrease of renin secretion
- **D.** Digoxin-mediated decrease of the glomerular filtration rate
- **E.** Furosemide-induced hypokalemia

Difficulty level: Medium

10. A 45-year-old alcoholic woman, brought to the emergency department by her husband, was disoriented, combative, and complained of headache, vertigo, and "ringing in my ears." The husband reported that she recently said she wanted to commit suicide. Vital signs were temperature 103.8°F, pulse 108 bpm, respirations 6/min, blood pressure 85/60. Pertinent lab data on admission were arterial blood pH 7.25, creatinine 2.2 mg/dL (normal 0.9–1.2 mg/dL), bicarbonate 18 mEq/L (normal 22–26 mEq/L), glucose 170 mg/dL (normal 70–110 mg/dL). Arterial blood gases were P_aCO_2 48 mm Hg (normal 35–45 P_aCO_2), P_aO_2 75 mm Hg (normal > 80 P_aO_2). Which of the following drugs most likely caused the patient's poisoning?

- **A.** Ethanol
- **B.** Celecoxib
- **C.** Ibuprofen
- **D.** Propranolol
- **E.** Aspirin
- **F.** Diphenhydramine

Difficulty level: Medium

11. A 48-year-old woman was brought to the emergency department because of serious breathing difficulty. Two hours earlier, she had taken a drug for a headache. The patient had been suffering from sinusitis and nasal polyps for 6 months. Physical examination showed severe bronchospasm. Which of the following drugs most likely caused the patient's signs and symptoms?

A. Ergotamine

B. Acetaminophen

C. Acetylsalicylic acid

D. Sumatriptan

E. Cyproheptadine

Difficulty level: Easy

12. A 32-year-old man suffering from hemophilia had been recently diagnosed with tension headache. The headaches occurred two to four times weekly, usually toward the end of his workday. The pain was constant, dull in character, and usually lasted the rest of the day with variable intensity. Which of the following analgesic drugs would be appropriate for this patient?

A. Indomethacin

B. Acetaminophen

C. Aspirin

D. Ketorolac

E. Piroxicam

F. Naproxen

Difficulty level: Medium

13. A 20-year-old man, diagnosed with acute rheumatic fever, started high-dose salicylate treatment. A few days later, laboratory values indicated increased blood pH, decreased P_aCO_2, and decreased plasma bicarbonate content. Which of the following acid–base disturbances was most likely caused by salicylate treatment?

A. Respiratory acidosis

B. Respiratory alkalosis

C. Metabolic acidosis

D. Metabolic alkalosis

E. Mixed acidosis

Difficulty level: Hard

14. A 54-year-old man presented to the emergency department with nausea, headache, dizziness, tinnitus, difficulty in hearing, and sweating. His body temperature was 103.1°F (39.5°C). The patient was suffering from osteoarthritis and had been overtreating himself with aspirin for 4 days in an attempt to relieve severe pain in his right hip. Which of the following actions most likely mediated the drug-induced hyperthermia in this patient?

A. Resetting the hypothalamic thermostat

B. Inflammatory reaction in the joints

C. Increased release of interleukin-10

D. Uncoupling oxidative phosphorylation in skeletal muscle

E. Metabolic alkalosis

Difficulty level: Medium

15. A 42-year-old woman had been recovering from breast cancer surgery. Because her postoperative pain was severe, she received an intravenous injection of ketorolac that was able to reduce the pain. Which of the following molecular actions most likely mediated the analgesic effect of the drug?

A. Drug binding to prostaglandin receptors in the surgical area

B. Decreased concentration of prostaglandins in the surgical area

C. Decreased oxygen radical production in the surgical area

D. Inhibition of prostaglandin biosynthesis in the central nervous system

E. Lowering of anxiety, fear, and suffering evoked by pain

Difficulty level: Easy

16. A 60-year-old man recently diagnosed with osteoarthritis asked his physician for an analgesic drug because of intermittent pain in both hips. Past history of the patient was significant for myocardial infarction 2 years ago and for pronounced aspirin hypersensitivity. Which of the following would be the best advice to give to this patient at this time?

A. To use a propionic acid derivative like naproxen

B. To take only very low doses of aspirin

C. To take aspirin with misoprostol

D. To use indomethacin

E. To avoid all nonsteroidal antiinflammatory drugs

Difficulty level: Easy

17. A 28-year-old man was admitted to the emergency department because of persistent nausea and vomiting, general malaise, and diaphoresis for the past 6 hours. The man had been overtreating himself for 4 days with an analgesic medication to relieve severe pain from a neck injury. Two days earlier, he had gotten drunk at a party. Physical exam showed a slightly confused and dehydrated patient with icterus and a flapping tremor. Pertinent lab results on admission were alanine aminotransferase 300 U/L (normal 8–20 U/L), aspartate aminotransferase 480 U/L (normal 8–20 U/L). The patient had most likely taken an excessive dose of which of the following drugs?

A. Aspirin
B. Indomethacin
C. Acetaminophen
D. Ibuprofen
E. Ketorolac

Difficulty level: Easy

18. A 65-year-old man had been recently diagnosed with osteoarthritis. Six months ago, the patient suffered from peptic ulcer disease that healed after triple antiulcer therapy. Which of the following nonsteroidal antiinflammatory drugs would be most appropriate for this patient?

A. Ibuprofen
B. Piroxicam
C. Indomethacin
D. Ketorolac
E. Celecoxib
F. Aspirin

Difficulty level: Easy

19. A 32-year-old man called his physician because of fever (102.2°F, 39.0°C) for the past 4 hours. Past medical history of the patient was significant for a serious allergic reaction to sulfonamides. A diagnosis of flu was made. Which of the following antipyretic drugs would be contraindicated in this patient?

A. Aspirin
B. Celecoxib
C. Naproxen
D. Acetaminophen
E. Ibuprofen

Difficulty level: Hard

20. A 59-year-old obese woman presented to the emergency department because of severe colicky pain in the right lumbar region. The patient had a long history of osteoarthritis and experienced frequent episodes of strong arthritic pain for which she had been taking several different pain killers daily for the past year. Current medications included atorvastatin and ezetimibe for hyperlipidemia and hydrochlorothiazide for mild hypertension. A renal biopsy confirmed the diagnosis of papillary necrosis and tubulointerstitial inflammation of the kidney. Which of the following drugs most likely caused the patient's disease?

A. Codeine
B. Tramadol
C. Diclofenac
D. Hydrochlorotiazide
E. Atorvastatin
F. Ezetimibe

Difficulty level: Medium

21. A 32-year-old woman had been suffering severe pain during menses. The only relevant history was that she had undergone conization 6 months earlier for a fibroid of the cervix. Ibuprofen as needed was able to relieve the menstrual pain. Which of the following molecular actions most likely mediated the analgesic effect of the drug in the patient's disorder?

A. Binding of the drug to prostaglandin receptors in the myometrium
B. Decreased production of prostaglandins by the endometrium
C. Inhibition of prostaglandin biosynthesis in the spinal cord
D. Antiinflammatory action of the drug in the pelvic area
E. Decreased production of leukotrienes by the endometrium

Difficulty level: Medium

22. A 6-year-old boy suffering from influenza received an antipyretic drug for 4 days. On the fifth day, he lapsed into a coma and died. The autopsy disclosed diffuse microvescicular fatty infiltration of the liver, heart, and kidneys, as well as cerebral edema. Which of the following antipyretics most likely caused the patient's death?

A. Acetaminophen
B. Piroxicam
C. Ibuprofen
D. Indomethacin
E. Ketorolac
F. Aspirin

Difficulty level: Easy

23. A 58-year-old man complained to his physician of morning stiffness in the hip and knee and some joint stiffness after inactivity. Past medical history of the patient was significant for a myocardial infarction 6 months earlier. Further exams led to the diagnosis of osteoarthritis, and an analgesic pharmacotherapy was prescribed. Which of the following analgesic drugs would be contraindicated for this patient?

A. Ibuprofen
B. Piroxicam
C. Celecoxib
D. Acetaminophen
E. Diclofenac

Difficulty level: Easy

24. A 14-year-old girl was seen in the clinic because of severe abdominal pain secondary to her menstrual periods. The pain began with the onset of her menstrual flow and had occurred monthly since her first menstrual period at age 13. Her physical examination was unremarkable. A diagnosis of primary dysmenorrhea was made. Which of the following drugs would be most appropriate for this patient?

A. Acetaminophen
B. Albuterol
C. Dinoprostone
D. Ibuprofen
E. Misoprostol
F. Ergonovine

Difficulty level: Easy

25. A 10-year-old boy was brought to the clinic with fever (102.2°F, 39.0°C), general malaise, and the characteristic rash of a measles infection. Past medical history was significant for an episode of hemolytic anemia, most probably related to his congenital deficiency of red blood cell glutathione synthase. Which of the following drugs would be a suitable antipyretic for this boy?

A. Aspirin
B. Indomethacin
C. Acetaminophen
D. Ibuprofen
E. Prednisone
F. Sulfinpyrazone

Difficulty level: Hard

26. A 58-year-old man complained to his physician of dull, continuous bone pain that had been increasing over the past few days. The patient had been suffering from prostatic carcinoma for 2 years. Past history was significant for an episode of hemolytic anemia, ascribed to his congenital glucose-6-phosphate dehydrogenase (G6PD) deficiency, and for

erythema multiforme, apparently due to an allergic reaction to naproxen. Which of the following would be an appropriate analgesic drug for this patient?

A. Aspirin
B. Acetaminophen
C. Piroxicam
D. Ibuprofen
E. Amitriptyline

Difficulty level: Easy

27. An 850-g (1.87-lb) baby boy, prematurely born at 27 weeks' gestational age, was intubated immediately and placed on positive pressure assisted ventilation. On the third day of life, his nurse noticed that he had tachycardia and a widened pulse pressure. Color Doppler echocardiography showed reverse pulmonary artery flow in diastole. A treatment with intravenous indomethacin was started. Which of the following best explains the reason for that therapy?

A. To speed up the maturation of the lungs
B. To increase lung surfactant formation
C. To decrease atrial contractility
D. To prevent thrombi on cardiac valves
E. To close the patent ductus arteriosus

Difficulty level: Medium

28. A 51-year-old woman complained to her physician of fatigue and shortness of breath. The woman, who was vegetarian, realized she had recently developed an unexplained desire to eat ice and also noted that her stools had become dark. She had been receiving piroxicam for 6 months to treat her rheumatoid arthritis. Physical examination was unremarkable. Which of the following disorders most likely caused the patient's symptoms?

A. Iron deficiency anemia
B. Respiratory alkalosis
C. Reye syndrome
D. Analgesic nephropathy
E. Aspirin hypersensitivity

Difficulty level: Easy

29. A 63-year-old woman recently diagnosed with osteoarthritis started treatment with ibuprofen. The biosynthesis of which of the following pairs of endogenous compounds was most likely inhibited by the drug?

A. Thromboxanes and leukotrienes
B. Prostaglandins and leukotrienes
C. Prostacyclin and thromboxanes
D. Prostaglandins and bradykinin
E. Thromboxanes and bradykinin
F. Prostacyclin and leukotrienes

Difficulty level: Easy

30. A 62-year-old man complained to his physician of epigastric pain. The man had been taking several ibuprofen tablets each day for the past 2 weeks because of arthritic pain. Endoscopy disclosed two superficial ulcers near the stomach antrum. Increased gastric secretion of which of the following compounds most likely contributed to the patient's disorder?

A. Gastrin
B. Hydrochloric acid
B. Bicarbonate secretion
D. Gastric mucus
E. Cholecystokinin

Questions: VII-4 Immunomodulating Drugs

Directions for questions **1–4**

Match each immunomodulating drug with the appropriate description (each lettered option can be selected once, more than once, or not at all).

A. Aldesleukin
B. Azathioprine
C. Basiliximab
D. Cyclosporine
E. Leflunomide
F. Mycophenolate mofetil
G. Muromonab-CD3
H. Sirolimus
I. Tacrolimus
J. Ustekinumab

Difficulty level: Easy

1. A recombinant form of a natural cytokine

Difficulty level: Easy

2. This drug binds to the CD25 α chain of the interleukin-2 receptor on activated T lymphocytes.

Difficulty level: Easy

3. A specific inhibitor of inosine monophosphate dehydrogenase

Difficulty level: Easy

4. A prodrug that is converted into mercaptopurine in the body

Difficulty level: Easy

5. A 56-year-old man with end-stage renal disease underwent a kidney transplant. He received immunosuppressive therapy that included a drug that suppresses cellular immunity, inhibits both prostaglandin and leukotriene synthesis, and increases the catabolism of immunoglobulin G (IgG) antibodies. Which of the following drugs has all of these actions?

A. Prednisone
B. Azathioprine
C. Tacrolimus
D. Muromonab-CD3
E. Cyclophosphamide

Difficulty level: Medium

6. A 27-year-old woman was admitted to the hospital with fever, malar butterfly erythema, arthralgia, intermittent pleuritic pain, and oral ulcers. Her lab tests revealed the following: serum creatinine 3.2 mg/dL, blood urea nitrogen (BUN) 35 mg/dL, and a high serum level of antinuclear antibodies. A diagnosis was made, and an appropriate therapy was started. Which of the following drugs most likely should be included in the therapeutic management of this patient?

A. Ustekinumab
B. Prednisone
C. BCG (bacilli Calmette-Guérin) vaccine
D. Interferon beta-1b
E. Aldesleukin

Difficulty level: Medium

7. A 39-year-old woman who has been suffering from myasthenia gravis for 4 years developed progressive dyspnea several days after an upper respiratory tract infection. Physical examination disclosed bilateral ptosis, bilateral facial weakness, and diminished upper and lower motor strength. An intravenous edrophonium injection improved muscle strength. A serum assay for antiacetylcholine receptor antibody was 4.8 (normal < 0.5). A promptly instituted treatment included a parenteral injection of prednisone. Which of the following statements best explains the most likely mechanism of action of the drug in this case?

A. Inhibition of plasma cholinesterase
B. Activation of cholinergic Nm receptors
C. Stimulation of synthesis of interleukin-2
D. Inhibition of T-cell activation and proliferation
E. Stimulation of synthesis of interleukin-1

Difficulty level: Easy

8. A 53-year-old man with a heart transplant underwent immunosuppressive treatment that included oral cyclosporine. Which of the following cells represent the main site of action of this drug?

    A. Macrophages
    B. Dendritic cells
    C. T-helper cells
    D. Plasma cells
    E. Natural killer cells

Difficulty level: Medium

9. A 54-year-old woman who underwent a kidney transplant developed nausea, vomiting, and diarrhea a few days after the surgery. The patient had received posttransplant therapy with cyclosporine and prednisone. A decision was made to substitute sirolimus for the cyclosporine. Which of the following actions most likely mediated the immunosuppressive effect of sirolimus?

    A. Stimulation of the synthesis of tumor necrosis factor
    B. Stimulation of B-cell proliferation
    C. Inhibition of histamine release
    D. Inhibition of T-cell proliferation
    E. Inhibition of calcineurin

Difficulty level: Medium

10. A 57-year-old man complained of a tingling sensation in his hands and peripheral edema. The man, who had received a heart transplant 1 month earlier, was in the hospital and scheduled for endomyocardial biopsy. Significant blood test results were potassium 6.1 mEq/L (normal 3.5–5.0 mEq/L), creatinine 3.8 mg/dL (normal 0.6–1.2 mg/dL), blood urea nitrogen (BUN) 42 mg/dL (normal 7–18 mg/dL). Current medications were cyclosporine, prednisone, and azathioprine to prevent rejection, omeprazole for heartburn, and diltiazem for arrhythmia. Biopsy results indicated no acute rejection. If the laboratory results were drug-related, which of the following was the most likely causative agent?

    A. Prednisone
    B. Cyclosporine
    C. Azathioprine
    D. Omeprazole
    E. Diltiazem

Difficulty level: Easy

11. A 66-year-old woman suffering from metastatic renal cancer started a pharmacotherapy that included aldesleukin. Which of the following classes of receptors most likely mediated the therapeutic effect of the drug in the patient's disease?

    A. Janus-kinase linked
    B. Metabotropic
    C. Ionotropic
    D. Intracellular
    E. Tyrosine-kinase linked

Difficulty level: Easy

12. A 44-year-old woman was in the coronary unit after a heart transplant performed 2 weeks earlier. Pertinent blood test results were white blood cell count $1.2 \times 10^3/mm^3$ (normal $4.5–11.0 \times 10^3/mm^3$), platelets $40,000/mm^{3.}$ (normal $150,000–400,000/mm^3$). Which of the following drugs most likely caused these findings?

    A. Cyclosporine
    B. Dobutamine
    C. Dopamine
    D. Azathioprine
    E. Fluorouracil

Difficulty level: Medium

13. A 41-year-old man came to the clinic complaining of an extensive rash, white plaquelike lesions in his mouth, dry eyes, hyperpigmentation of the tissues surrounding the eyes, and diarrhea. Three months earlier, the man, who was suffering from chronic myelogenous leukemia, underwent an allogeneic bone marrow transplant from his sister. He was successfully treated for his acute graft-versus-host disease and had no major health problems after that disease. Which of the following two-drug combinations would represent an appropriate immunosuppressive pharmacotherapy for the patient at this time?

    A. Prednisone and cyclosporine
    B. Cyclosporine and erythromycin
    C. Cyclophosphamide and doxorubicin
    D. Vinblastine and prednisone
    E. Doxorubicin and vinblastine

Difficulty level: Medium

14. A 43-year-old man who underwent a kidney transplant had been receiving an immunosuppressive treatment that included a macrolide antibiotic. The drug binds to a FK-binding proteins located in T cells, thus blocking gene expression for production of several cytokines. Which of the following drugs most likely works with this mechanism of action?

    A. Azithromycin
    B. Azathioprine
    C. Tacrolimus
    D. Cyclosporine
    E. Tobramycin

Difficulty level: Easy

15. A 42-year-old woman who underwent a liver transplant complained of nausea and vomiting, severe abdominal pain, and diarrhea 1 week after the surgery. The patient had been receiving a multidrug immunosuppressive therapy. If the patient's symptoms were drug-related, which of the following drugs most likely caused the reported adverse effects?

A. Etanercept
B. Mycophenolate mofetil
C. Doxorubicin
D. Leflunomide
E. Paclitaxel
F. Fluorouracil

Difficulty level: Easy

16. A 35-year-old woman who received a cadaveric liver transplant was treated with intravenous infusion of basiliximab immediately postoperatively. A few minutes later, she began to show wheezing, cyanosis, diaphoresis, pruritus, and a diffuse skin rash. Vital signs were pulse 128 bpm, blood pressure 98/50 mm Hg, respirations 22/min. Which of the following pathologic events most likely caused the patient's signs and symptoms?

A. Metabolic acidosis
B. Acute cardiac failure
C. Acute renal failure
D. Acute encephalopathy
E. Anaphylactoid reaction

Difficulty level: Easy

17. A 35-year-old man who underwent renal transplant showed signs of acute allograft rejection that was resistant to corticosteroid treatment. He was treated with muromonab-CD3 that was able to reverse the rejection. Which of the following actions most likely mediated the therapeutic effect of the drug in the patient's disease?

A. Inhibition of antibody formation by plasma cells
B. Inhibition of several enzymes involved in purine metabolism
C. Inhibition of calcineurin enzyme in T-cell cytoplasm
D. Stimulation of interleukin-1 synthesis in T cells
E. Neutralization of a surface protein receptor complex in T cells

Difficulty level: Easy

18. A 42-year-old man with end-stage renal disease underwent a kidney transplant. Therapeutic management of the patient included an intravenous injection of azathioprine just before surgery. Which of the following molecular actions most likely mediated the immunosuppressive effect of the drug in this patient?

A. Blockade of tumor necrosis factor-α (TNF-α) receptors
B. Inhibition of clonal expansion of T and B lymphocytes
C. Inhibition of antigen presentation by dendritic cells
D. Stimulation of genetic expression of interleukin-2
E. Stimulation of macrophage phagocytic activity

Difficulty level: Medium

19. A 42-year-old woman undergoing heart transplant received mycophenolate mofetil, cyclosporine, and prednisone before surgery. Which of the following statements best explains why mycophenolate mofetil is currently used instead of azathioprine to prevent rejection in solid organ transplantation?

A. Its immunosuppressive activity is definitely superior to that of azathioprine.
B. It has significantly fewer adverse effects than azathioprine.
C. It has drastically reduced the risk of graft-versus-host disease.
D. It selectively inhibits macrophage-mediated production of several interleukins.
E. It selectively inhibits antigen recognition by antigen-presenting cells.

Difficulty level: Medium

20. A 30-year-old man recently diagnosed with Crohn disease experienced substantial improvement after 1 month of prednisone therapy. Which of the following drugs would be appropriate to maintain remission of symptoms in this patient?

A. Sirolimus
B. Fluorouracil
C. Tacrolimus
D. Thalidomide
E. Azathioprine

Difficulty level: Medium

21. A 42-year-old woman who had been undergoing hemodialysis for 3 years was admitted to the hospital for a kidney transplant. Before and after surgery, she received cyclosporine, azathioprine, and prednisone. Four days after surgery, she developed acute allograft rejection. High-dose prednisone failed to resolve the rejection. Which of the following drugs could be used to treat this case of steroid-resistant rejection?

A. Dexamethasone
B. Muromonab-CD3
C. Aldesleukin
D. Methotrexate
E. Cyclophosphamide

Difficulty level: Easy

22. A 37-year-old man who was scheduled for a heart transplant received a triple immunosuppressive therapy just before surgery that included azathioprine and prednisone. Which of the following drugs was most likely the third agent of that combination drug regimen?

    A. Aldesleukin
    B. Cyclosporine
    C. Triamcinolone
    D. Infliximab
    E. Etanercept

Difficulty level: Easy

23. A 48-year-old woman who underwent a liver transplant had been receiving immunosuppression treatment with prednisone and cyclosporine. Despite the therapy, a liver biopsy still showed rejection 12 days after surgery, and the therapeutic team decided to substitute tacrolimus for cyclosporine. Which of the following cells represent the main site of action of tacrolimus?

    A. Macrophages
    B. Dendritic cells
    C. T-helper cells
    D. Plasma cells
    E. Natural killer cells

Difficulty level: Easy

24. A 53-year-old man who underwent liver transplantation for advanced biliary cirrhosis had been receiving immunosuppression treatment with prednisone and cyclosporine. Despite the therapy, a liver biopsy still showed rejection 14 days after surgery. Which of the following drugs could be substituted for cyclosporine to treat this case of cyclosporine-resistant rejection?

    A. Aldesleukin
    B. Vinblastine
    C. Tacrolimus
    D. Fluorouracil
    E. Paclitaxel

Difficulty level: Easy

25. A 65-year-old woman recently diagnosed with polymyositis had not improved after 2 weeks of treatment with prednisone. A decision was made to replace prednisone with an immunosuppressive drug that acts by inhibiting enzymes essential for purine biosynthesis. Which of the following drugs was most likely prescribed?

    A. Etanercept
    B. Cyclosporine
    C. Tacrolimus
    D. Sirolimus
    E. Azathioprine
    F. Infliximab

Difficulty level: Easy

26. A 45-year-old woman who underwent a liver transplant started an immunosuppressive therapy that included tacrolimus. The risk of which of the following drug-related disorders was most likely increased in this patient?

    A. Hypotension
    B. Hypokalemia
    C. Hypoglycemia
    D. Hemolytic anemia
    E. Neurotoxicity

Difficulty level: Medium

27. A 51-year-old man presented to the clinic with complaints of an enlarged, painful lymph node in his groin. One year earlier, he had undergone surgical resection of stage 2 malignant melanoma. A lymph node biopsy confirmed the recurrence of malignant melanoma. The patient started a course of chemotherapy that included the intravenous administration of aldesleukin. Which of the following molecular actions most likely mediated the therapeutic effect of the drug in the patient's disorder?

    A. Proliferation and differentiation of B and T lymphocytes
    B. Inhibition of macrophage phagocytic activity
    C. Inhibition of antigen presentation by dendritic cells
    D. Decreased synthesis of calcineurin
    E. Inhibition of activity of natural killer cells

Difficulty level: Easy

28. A 48-year-old woman presented to her ophthalmologist because of loss of central vision and pain on movement of her left eye. She reported that in the past she had had recurrent episodes of weakness and abnormal sensations in her arms and legs. The patient was referred to the neurologic clinic, where laboratory exams and brain magnetic resonance imaging confirmed the diagnosis of multiple sclerosis. The patient was prescribed a supportive therapy that included a recombinant cytokine endowed with immunostimulant properties. Which of the following drugs was most likely administered?

    A. Trastuzumab
    B. Infliximab
    C. Interferon beta-1b
    D. Prednisone
    E. Tacrolimus

Difficulty: Medium

29. A 27-year-old primipara woman delivered a baby boy at term. The woman was Rho(D) negative, and her husband was Rho(D) positive. The woman received an intravenous injection of Rho(D) immune globulin just after the delivery. The reason for this treatment was most likely to prevent which of the following events?

A. Placental crossing of fetal erythrocytes in subsequent pregnancies
B. Production of antibodies against fetal Rho(D)-positive erythrocytes
C. The mother's hemolytic disease in subsequent pregnancies
D. Production of fetal Rho(D)-positive erythrocytes in subsequent pregnancies
E. Placental crossing of fetal Rho(D) antibodies in subsequent pregnancies

Difficulty level: Easy

30. A 45-year-old woman received a deceased-donor kidney transplant. Within 12 hours of the transplantation, she started immunosuppressive pharmacotherapy that included cyclosporine. Which of the following actions most likely mediated the therapeutic effect of the drug in the patient's disease?

A. Stimulation of synthesis of tumor necrosis factor
B. Stimulation of B-cell differentiation into memory B cells
C. Inhibition of the apoptosis pathway in target cells
D. Stimulation of gene expression for interleukin-2 production
E. Inhibition of calcineurin enzyme

Questions: VII-5 Drugs for Arthritis and Gout

Directions for questions 1–4

Match each drug with the appropriate description (each lettered option can be selected once, more than once, or not at all).

A. Allopurinol
B. Azathioprine
C. Colchicine
D. Cyclosporine
E. Etanercept
F. Infliximab
G. Hydroxychloroquine
H. Leflunomide
I. Methotrexate
J. Rituximab

Difficulty level: Easy

1. An antimalarial drug used in rheumatoid arthritis

Difficulty level: Easy

2. A monoclonal antibody that binds to CD20 B lymphocytes

Difficulty level: Easy

3. A monoclonal antibody that binds to tumor necrosis factor-α

Difficulty level: Easy

4. This drug can inhibit the synthesis of inosinic acid.

Difficulty level: Easy

5. A 52-year-old woman recently diagnosed with mild rheumatoid arthritis started a therapy with nonsteroidal antiinflammatory drugs (NSAIDs), but 2 months later, the physician decided to add a disease-modifying antirheumatic drug (DMARD) to the therapeutic regimen. Which of the following is most likely the main advantage of DMARDs over NSAIDs in the treatment of rheumatoid arthritis?

A. To cause fewer adverse effects
B. To slow down the progression of bone and cartilage destruction
C. To improve symptoms after one week of therapy
D. To completely cure the disease, after 2 to 4 months of therapy
E. To completely abolish acute joint pain

Difficulty level: Easy

6. A 33-year-old man complained to his physician of low back pain and stiffness that were greatest on awakening in the morning and gradually improved throughout the day. The intermittent use of ibuprofen had been able to improve the symptoms in the past, but recently he had no relief. Magnetic resonance imaging confirmed the diagnosis of ankylosing spondylitis. Which of the following drugs would be appropriate for the patient at this time?

A. Hydroxychloroquine
B. Trastuzumab
C. Etanercept
D. Naproxen
E. Colchicine
F. Aldesleukin

Difficulty level: Easy

7. A 50-year-old woman with rheumatoid arthritis was recently diagnosed with refractory disease, and infliximab was added to her ongoing treatment. Which of the following endogenous compounds was most likely the molecular target of the drug?

   A. Interleukin-1
   B. Vascular endothelial growth factor
   C. Interleukin-10
   D. Epidermal growth factor
   E. Tumor necrosis factor-α

Difficulty level: Medium

8. A 48-year-old man was admitted to the emergency department with the chief complaint of an excruciating pain in his left ankle. The pain had started the previous night and increased over several hours. The patient reported that he sprained his ankle 1 week ago. On physical examination, the ankle appeared warm and tender, and the entire area was red and swollen. A synovial fluid analysis showed crystals engulfed by phagocytes. A diagnosis was made, and a pharmacotherapy was prescribed. Which of the following drugs would be most appropriate to treat the patient's pain?

   A. Codeine
   B. Indomethacin
   C. Methotrexate
   D. Aspirin
   E. Etanercept
   F. Allopurinol

Difficulty level: Easy

9. A 57-year-old man recently diagnosed with mild rheumatoid arthritis complained to his physician of joint pain despite ongoing therapy with ibuprofen. The man was a heavy smoker and had a history of chronic bronchitis with frequent acute exacerbations usually treated with antibiotics. The physician decided to add a disease-modifying antirheumatic drug (DMARD) to the treatment. Which of the following drugs would be most appropriate for the patient at this time?

   A. Leflunomide
   B. Hydroxychloroquine
   C. Rituximab
   D. Etanercept
   E. Azathioprine

Difficulty level: Easy

10. A 44-year-old woman suffering from rheumatoid arthritis recently had leflunomide added to her methotrexate therapy. Inhibition of which of the following enzymes most likely mediated the therapeutic effect of the drug in the patient's disease?

   A. Cyclooxygenase-1
   B. Type II topoisomerase
   C. Dihydrofolate reductase
   D. Dihydroorotate dehydrogenase
   E. Reverse transcriptase
   F. Peptidyl transferase

Difficulty level: Easy

11. A 55-year-old man complained to his physician that a rash had appeared the previous day on his thorax and legs. The patient was recently diagnosed with hyperuricemia and had been receiving allopurinol for 2 weeks. The physician suspected the rash was due to the ongoing pharmacotherapy and decided to discontinue allopurinol and to start a treatment with probenecid. The physician should advise the patient not to concurrently use which of the following drugs?

   A. Acetaminophen
   B. Ibuprofen
   C. Phenylephrine
   D. Aspirin
   E. Loratadine
   F. Diphenhydramine

Difficulty level: Easy

12. A 53-year-old woman recently diagnosed with gouty arthritis started a treatment with a drug that inhibits leukocyte migration and phagocytosis secondary to inhibition of tubulin polymerization. Which of the following drugs did the patient most likely take?

   A. Indomethacin
   B. Prednisone
   C. Colchicine
   D. Allopurinol
   E. Probenecid
   F. Piroxicam

Difficulty level: Medium

13. A 54-year-old Black woman was admitted to the hospital because of joint pain and a rash flare of erythematous maculopapular lesions on her neck, upper chest, and elbows. The patient was diagnosed with systemic lupus erythematosus 5 months earlier and had been receiving piroxicam since then. After further exams, another drug was added to her current pharmacotherapy. Which of the following drugs would be appropriate to administer at this time?

   A. Aspirin
   B. Indomethacin
   C. Ampicillin
   D. Hydroxychloroquine
   E. Clarithromycin
   F. Ciprofloxacin

Difficulty level: Hard

14. A 39-year-old woman complained to her physician of joint pain that had worsened over the past month. The pain was worst in the morning and prevented her from performing her household tasks for at least an hour after waking. She tried ibuprofen three times daily for 2 weeks, but relief was poor, and she stopped the medication because of epigastric pain. The woman was also suffering from chronic active hepatitis B, currently treated with lamivudine. On physical examination, the patient appeared uncomfortable with any movement. Her wrists, metacarpophalangeal joints, and knees showed bilaterally symmetrical swelling, tenderness, and warmth. Further exams confirmed the diagnosis, and a pharmacotherapy was prescribed. Which of the following drugs would be appropriate for the patient at this time?

- **A.** Methotrexate
- **B.** Aspirin
- **C.** Etanercept
- **D.** Piperacillin
- **E.** Ciprofloxacin
- **F.** Erythromycin

Difficulty level: Easy

15. A 32-year-old man diagnosed with rheumatoid arthritis had been taking methotrexate for 4 months. The disease was controlled initially, but the pain returned, and his rheumatologist decided to add a drug to the treatment regimen. The second drug is a recombinant fusion protein consisting of the extracellular portion of two tumor necrosis factor (TNF) receptor moieties. Which of the following drugs was most likely prescribed?

- **A.** Infliximab
- **B.** Etanercept
- **C.** Leflunomide
- **D.** Triamcinolone
- **E.** Cyclosporine
- **F.** Piroxicam

Difficulty level: Medium

16. A 15-year-old girl was admitted to the emergency department because of a sudden attack of severe abdominal pain accompanied by fever (103.5°F, 39.7°C). The patient had had two similar attacks 3 and 2 weeks ago that subsided spontaneously over the course of 48 hours. Multiple other family members had similar complaints. Physical examination showed a patient in moderate distress with evidence of pleural effusion in the right lung. Genetic testing showed a mutation in a gene of chromosome 16. Which of the following drugs would most likely prevent the recurrence of the attacks in this patient?

- **A.** Indomethacin
- **B.** Etanercept
- **C.** Methotrexate
- **D.** Prednisone
- **E.** Colchicine

Difficulty level: Easy

17. A 55-year-old man recently diagnosed with hyperuricemia started a treatment with allopurinol. Plasma levels of which of the following pairs of endogenous compounds most likely increased after a few days of therapy?

- **A.** Guanine and xanthine
- **B.** Xanthine and hypoxanthine
- **C.** Inosine and guanine
- **D.** Adenine and inosine
- **E.** Adenine and hypoxanthine

Difficulty level: Easy

18. A 44-year-old woman at a routine check-up was found to have a serum urate level of 18 mg/dL and a urine urate level of 800 mg/24 h. She started an appropriate treatment, and 3 weeks later her serum urate level was 7.2 mg/dL and urinary urate level was 530 mg/24 h. Which of the following drugs did the patient most likely take?

- **A.** Probenecid
- **B.** Aspirin
- **C.** Furosemide
- **D.** Allopurinol
- **E.** Indomethacin
- **F.** Naproxen

Difficulty level: Easy

19. A 43-year-old man suffering from rheumatoid arthritis complained to his physician that his joint pain had increased recently despite current naproxen and hydroxychloroquine therapy. The patient was otherwise healthy, and his past medical history was unremarkable. Which of the following drugs would be appropriate to add to the patient's therapy at this time?

- **A.** Diclofenac
- **B.** Acetaminophen
- **C.** Methotrexate
- **D.** Fentanyl
- **E.** Amitriptyline
- **F.** Carbamazepine

Difficulty level: Medium

20. A 55-year-old man complained to his physician of blurred vision, night blindness, light flashes, and photophobia. The man was diagnosed with mild rheumatoid arthritis 6 months ago and was taking a combination therapy that included a disease-modifying antirheumatic drug (DMARD). Ophthalmoscopy disclosed a macular area of hyperpigmentation surrounded by a zone of hypopigmentation on the left retina. Which of the following drugs most likely caused the patient's signs and symptoms?

A. Hydroxychloroquine
B. Etanercept
C. Methotrexate
D. Infliximab
E. Ibuprofen
F. Celecoxib

Answers and Explanations: VII-1 Histamine and Serotonin: Agonists and Antagonists

Questions 1–3

1. **E**
2. **A**
3. **B**

Learning objective: Outline the use of antihistamines to treat systemic itching.

4. **D** Itching is sometimes caused by exposure to sunlight, especially in the elderly. Because histamine is most often involved in itching, histamine H_1 antagonists are effective antipruritics. In this case, a second-generation antihistamine is the appropriate choice, as the patient has prostatic hypertrophy, which contraindicates first-generation antihistamines because of their antimuscarinic properties.

    A, B See correct answer explanation.

    C, E, F These drugs lack antipruritic properties.

Learning objective: Explain the mechanism of antimigraine action of ergot alkaloids.

5. **A** The effectiveness of ergot alkaloids in migraine seems to be primarily related to their cerebral vasoconstricting effects, which are apparently due to activation of both α adrenoceptors and serotonin (5-HT) receptors. The pathophysiology of migraine seems to include a vasomotor component, because the onset of headache is sometimes associated with increased amplitude of temporal artery pulsations; ergotamine can diminish these pulsations. Other mechanisms are probably also operative. For example, ergotamine blocks inflammation of the trigeminal neurovascular system. This action, possibly mediated by activation of 5-HT receptors, may be responsible for both the pain-relieving and the vasoconstricting effects of ergot alkaloids.

    B–E Ergotamine does not cause these effects. Moreover, these effects would increase, not decrease, the risk of a migraine attack.

Learning objective: Explain the mechanism of the antimigraine action of 5-$HT_{1B/1D}$ serotonin agonists.

6. **D** Triptans (e.g., sumatriptan and zolmitriptan) are specific 5-$HT_{1B/1D}$ agonists that are equally as or more effective than

ergot alkaloids in the acute treatment of migraine attack. There are two major proposed mechanisms for effectiveness of triptans in acute migraine headache:

- Vasoconstriction of cerebral vessels via the activation of vascular 5-HT_{1B} receptors
- Inhibition of release of neuropeptides with inflammatory properties via the activation of presynaptic 5-HT_{1D} receptors

Triptans are not intended for use in the prophylaxis of migraine.

    A Beta-blockers are effective for the prophylaxis of migraine in some patients, but they are of no value in the treatment of an ongoing migraine attack.

    B, C, E, F Drugs acting on these receptors cannot cure a migraine attack.

Learning objective: Outline the clinical uses of antihistamines.

7. **D** Drugs usually given to prevent an acute allergic reaction in patients at risk are glucocorticoids and histamine H_1 antagonists. First-generation H_1 antagonists are generally preferred when drug-induced sedation may be useful to reduce fear related to the procedure, as in this case.

    A–C, E, F These drugs are devoid of antiallergic properties.

Learning objective: Explain the reason for ergonovine use in postpartum bleeding.

8. **E** Uterine atony (absence of uterine contracture following the delivery of the placenta) is the most common cause of postpartum hemorrhage. When the hemorrhage does not respond to oxytocin administration, ergot alkaloids may be used to decrease bleeding. The uterus at term is extremely sensitive to the stimulant action of ergot alkaloids, and even an intermediate dose produces a prolonged and powerful spasm of the muscle that squeezes the uterine vessels, thus controlling bleeding.

    A Ergotamine can constrict uterine arteries, but this is not the main reason why the drug can stop postpartum bleeding.

    B–D Ergotamine does not have these effects.

Learning objective: Explain the mechanism of action of histamine H_1-receptor antagonists.

9. **D** Diphenhydramine is a first-generation histamine H_1-receptor antagonist. Most drugs of this class can also block muscarinic receptors. The drug easily crosses the blood–brain barrier and can block H_1 receptors and muscarinic receptors located in vestibular nuclei and in the nucleus of the tractus solitarius, thus decreasing the firing from these nuclei to the vomiting center.

    A–C, E All of these options have at least one receptor that is not involved in the mechanism of nausea and vomiting.

Learning objective: Describe the adverse effects of ergot alkaloids.

10. **C** Ergot alkaloids constrict most human blood vessels and can cause prolonged vasospasm when high doses are given. The vasospasm mainly affects the arms and legs and may result in gangrene. The vasospasm is refractory to most vasodilators, but nitroprusside or nitroglycerin infusion may be successful, as in this case.

    A, B, D–F All of these drugs can be used to relieve headache, but they do not cause peripheral vasospasm.

Learning objective: Describe the adverse effects of sumatriptan.

11. **C** Symptoms of chest pressure or tightness have been reported in up to 40% of patients treated with subcutaneous sumatriptan. These symptoms, most likely due to the serotonin $5\text{-}HT_{1B}$-mediated vasoconstricting action of the drug, are rarely serious, but in some cases the drug can cause coronary vasospasm and myocardial infarction.

    A, B, D, F These drugs are used for the treatment or prophylaxis of migraine, but they do not cause the symptoms reported by the patient.

    E Antihistamines are not used for migraine prophylaxis, and they do not cause the symptoms reported by the patient.

Learning objective: Describe the mechanism of action of antihistamines.

12. **E** Drugs effective against hay fever are histamine H_1-receptor competitive antagonists. Competitive means that the binding to the receptor is reversible; that is, the antagonism is pharmacological and surmountable.

    A–D, F H_1 antagonists have negligible blocking activity against H_2 and H_3 receptors.

Learning objective: Explain the mechanism of action of cyproheptadine.

13. **E** Cyproheptadine is a first-generation H_1 antagonist. Like other drugs of this class, it can also block muscarinic and serotonergic receptors (mainly $5\text{-}HT_2$). The blockade of M_3 receptors explains the dry mouth, constipation, and dysuria, while the increase in appetite was likely due to blockade of

$5\text{-}HT_2$ receptors in the hypothalamus. In fact, cyproheptadine has been used to treat anorexia, with mixed results.

    A–D, F See correct answer explanation.

Learning objective: Describe the contraindications of triptans.

14. **C** Triptans are contraindicated in patients with known or suspected coronary artery disease, because rare but serious adverse cardiac effects, including heart attacks, life-threatening disturbances of cardiac rhythm, and death, have been reported within a few hours of receiving one of these drugs. The mechanism of this adverse effect is likely related to the vasoconstricting actions of these drugs.

    A, B, D, E All of these drugs are used in the acute therapy and/or in prevention of migraine headache.

Learning objective: Describe the most common adverse effects of ergotamine.

15. **E** Ergot alkaloids cause nausea and vomiting in about 10% of patients. The effect is most likely due to activation of dopamine D_2 and serotonin $5\text{-}HT_3$ receptors in the chemoreceptor trigger zone.

    A Hallucinations occur only after administration of toxic doses of ergot alkaloids.

    B, C Ergotamine has powerful vasoconstricting actions. Therefore, these effects are unlikely.

    D Adynamic ileus is unlikely because ergotamine has stimulant effects on smooth muscle.

Learning objective: Describe the postreceptor mechanism of histamine H_1-receptor antagonists.

16. **C** Loratadine is a histamine H_1-receptor antagonist. Activation of H_1 receptors increases the synthesis of inositoltriphosphate and diacylglycerol, which in turn increases the cytoplasmic Ca^{2+} concentration in target cells. Most histamine effects due to activation of H_1 receptors are mediated by this increased availability of cytoplasmic Ca^{2+}. By blocking H_1 receptors, loratadine decreases the synthesis of inositoltriphosphate and diacylglycerol, thus antagonizing all histamine effects mediated by activation of H_1 receptors.

    A, B, D, E See correct answer explanation.

Learning objective: Explain the mechanism of action of loratadine.

17. **E** Histamine H_1 antagonists such as loratadine are used in allergic disorders because they block H_1 receptors in most peripheral organs and tissues. In this way, they prevent most histamine-induced effects.

    A Although some second-generation antihistamines can block histamine release, this is not the main mechanism of the antiallergic action of these drugs.

    B–D Loratadine does not cause these effects.

Learning objective: Describe the adverse effects of ergot alkaloids.

18. **C** Ergot alkaloids can cause peripheral vasospasm that can lead to pain, numbness, and tingling of the fingers and toes. The vasospasm, likely due to activation of α adrenoceptors and serotonin receptors, is often refractory to most vasodilators.

    A, B, D, E These drugs do not cause peripheral vasospasm.

Learning objective: Describe the main contraindications of ergot alkaloids.

19. **C** Ergot alkaloids such as ergotamine are contraindicated in patients with coronary artery disease and peripheral vascular disease because of the vasoconstricting properties of these drugs. It is even recommended that ergotamine not be given to patients in whom unrecognized coronary artery disease can be predicted by the presence of risk factors (hypertension, hypercholesterolemia, smoking, obesity, etc.), as in this case.

    A, B, D–F These drugs are used for the treatment of migraine, and they are not contraindicated in this patient.

Learning objective: Identify the endogenous compound that has its histamine-induced release blocked by H_1-receptor antagonists.

20. **D** Loratadine is a histamine H_1-receptor antagonist. Activation of H_1 receptors on vascular endothelium causes the release of nitric oxide, which is involved in the vasodilation, vascular permeability, and edema associated with acute inflammation. By blocking H_1 receptors, loratadine inhibits nitric oxide release, thus exerting a useful antiinflammatory response.

    A–C Histamine can induce the release of these endogenous compounds, but this release is mediated by the activation of H_2 receptors and therefore cannot be antagonized by H_1-receptor antagonists.

    E Histamine does not cause the release of bradykinin.

Learning objective: Outline the use of antihistamines in benign positional vertigo.

21. **A** The symptoms of the patient and the provocative test indicate that he was most likely affected by benign positional vertigo, a violent vertigo lasting less than 30 seconds and induced by certain head positions. The disorder is most likely due to formation of granular masses in the cupula of the semicircular canals. First-generation antihistamines such as diphenhydramine are often used to treat vestibular disturbances such as positional vertigo and Meniere syndrome. The beneficial effect is most likely due to blockade of histamine H_1 receptors in the nucleus of the tractus solitarius (vestibular pathways include histaminergic afferents to the nucleus of the tractus solitarius and to vestibular nuclei).

    B, C Ondansetron and dronabinol are antiemetic drugs, but they are not effective when nausea and vomiting are due to vestibular disturbances.

    D, F Ergotamine and propranolol have no effect on vestibular disturbances.

    E Loratadine is a second-generation H_1 receptor antagonist that does not cross the blood–brain barrier effectively and so cannot reach the nucleus of the tractus solitarius.

Learning objective: Describe the adverse effects of diphenhydramine.

22. **C** First-generation histamine H_1 antagonists such as diphenhydramine can cause pronounced sedation because they are able to cross the blood–brain barrier. This effect is more likely if the patient is already receiving another sedative drug, as in this case.

    A Second-generation H_1 antagonists are devoid of central depressive effects.

    B Glucocorticoid-induced central depressant effects are very rare.

    D–F All of these drugs can cause sedation, but they are not used to treat allergic disorders.

Learning objective: Outline the pharmacotherapy of systemic mastocytosis.

23. **C** Systemic mastocytosis is a disease of unknown origin characterized by an excessive accumulation of mast cells in various body tissues. Most symptoms of the disease are due to the extremely high plasma levels of histamine. Treatment with H_1 and H_2 antagonists represents a rational therapy.

    A, B, D, E See correct answer explanation.

Learning objective: Identify the drug used for migraine prophylaxis in a pregnant woman.

24. **B** Propranolol is the drug of choice for migraine headache prophylaxis because of its efficacy and favorable adverse effect profile. Beta-blockers are approved by the U.S. Food and Drug Administration for prevention of migraine headache, but their mechanism of action in this disease remains uncertain.

    A, C Ergot alkaloids are absolutely contraindicated in pregnant women because they could cause abortion due to the induction of powerful uterine contracture.

    D Valproic acid is an antiepileptic drug approved for prevention of migraine headache. However, it is contraindicated in pregnant women because of its substantial teratogenic risk.

    E Triptans are used to treat an impending migraine attack, not for chronic prophylaxis.

Learning objective: Describe the pharmacological effects of histamine H_1-receptor antagonists.

25. **A** First-generation histamine H_1 antagonists such as diphenhydramine have significant blocking activity on muscarinic receptors. This action relaxes the bladder detrusor, an effect that is without clinical consequences in normally healthy people, but that can further impair the voiding of the bladder in men with prostatic hypertrophy, as in this case.

    B The bladder external sphincter includes striated muscle and is not under the control of the autonomic nervous system.

    C The prostate capsule is constricted via α_1 receptors. Most antihistamines have negligible effects on these receptors.

    D The bladder internal sphincter has mainly α_1 receptors. Most antihistamines have negligible effects on these receptors.

    E Antihistamines have negligible effects on diuresis.

Learning objective: Describe the adverse effects due to selective serotonin reuptake inhibitor–triptan interaction.

26. **B** The patient's history and symptoms indicate the she was most likely suffering from serotonin syndrome, a rare but potentially fatal disorder that is related to an inappropriate increase of serotonergic transmission in the central nervous system (CNS). The syndrome can be caused by several drugs either alone or in combination, especially when given in high doses. The combination of two drugs that enhance serotonin transmission can be particularly dangerous. In this case, the patient was taking paroxetine, a selective serotonin reuptake inhibitor (SSRI). The addition of sumatriptan, a serotonin agonist, most likely triggered the syndrome. The U.S. Food and Drug Administration has issued a warning against the concomitant use of SSRIs and triptans.

    A, C–F None of these drugs cause an increase in serotonergic transmission in the CNS.

Learning objective: Identify the central site of action of sumatriptan.

27. **B** Sumatriptan and its congeners are currently first-line agents for the abortive therapy of acute, severe migraine attacks. The pathophysiology of migraine remains unknown, but the current view is that a complex series of neural and vascular events initiates migraine (the so-called neurovascular theory). The theory states that activation of the nucleus caudalis of the trigeminal nerve leads to the release of several potent vasodilating neuropeptides, which in turn causes dilation of cerebral blood vessels. This vasodilation seems to be a major cause of the throbbing headache of the migraine attack. By activating presynaptic serotonin 5-HT_{1D} receptors on trigeminal nerve endings, triptans can prevent the release of vasodilating neuropeptides.

    A, C–F See correct answer explanation.

Learning objective: Identify the drug that likely caused anticholinergic symptoms of drug overdose poisoning.

28. **B** The patient's syndrome indicated that he was poisoned by an anticholinergic drug. First-generation antihistamines such as diphenhydramine have significant antimuscarinic effects, and acute poisoning by these drugs is remarkably similar to that of atropine poisoning.

    A, C, D These drugs do not have antimuscarinic effects.

    E This drug is a second-generation antihistamine. Unlike first-generation, second-generation drugs are devoid of blocking activity on muscarinic receptors.

    F As stated above, the patient was poisoned by an antimuscarinic drug. However, atropine is unlikely, as the drug is not used to treat allergic symptoms.

Learning objective: Identify a drug that can aggravate open-angle glaucoma.

29. **D** Diphenhydramine is a first-generation histamine H_1 antagonist with pronounced sedative properties. Because of this, the drug is a component of over-the-counter preparations for insomnia. First-generation H_1 antagonists have prominent antimuscarinic actions. By blocking M_3 receptors in the ciliary muscle, these drugs can narrow the spaces of the trabecular meshwork and the lumen of Schlemm canal, thus hindering the outflow of the aqueous humor.

    A–C, E See correct answer explanation.

Learning objective: Explain why second-generation histamine H_1 antagonists are preferred over first-generation for the local treatment of allergic conjunctivitis.

30. **A** Unlike first-generation H_1 antagonists, second-generation H_1 antagonists are devoid of blocking activity on muscarinic receptors. Therefore, they do not have effects on pupil size and accommodation when applied into the conjunctival sac. This explains why only second-generation H_1 antagonists are used locally in allergic conjunctivitis.

    B Second-generation H_1 antagonists do not appreciably cross the blood–brain barrier and are therefore free of central nervous system properties. However, at most, this is a minor advantage when they are used locally in the eye because the systemic absorption of these drugs from the eye is negligible.

    C By blocking H_1 receptors, both first- and second-generation H_1 antagonists antagonize histamine-induced vasodilation.

    D Antihistamines are devoid of antibacterial activity.

    E Unlike first-generation, second-generation H_1 antagonists do not affect secretion of lacrimal glands because they are devoid of muscarinic M_3-receptor blocking activity.

Learning objective: Explain the mechanism of action of cromolyn sodium.

31. **B** The available therapeutic options for management of allergic conjunctivitis include ocular administration of antihistamines, decongestants, nonsteroidal antiinflammatory drugs (NSAIDs), and mast cell stabilizers. Chromone derivatives such as cromolyn sodium are drugs that can stabilize mast cells (but not basophils), thus inhibiting the release of chemical mediators from these cells.

    A This is the mechanism of action of antihistamines.

    C This is the mechanism of action of NSAIDs.

    D This is the mechanism of action of zafirlukast.

    E This is the mechanism of action of decongestants.

HISTAMINE AND SEROTONIN: AGONISTS AND ANTAGONISTS Answer key		
1. E	6. D	11. C
2. A	7. D	12. E
3. B	8. E	13. E
4. D	9. D	14. C
5. A	10. C	15. E
16. C	21. A	26. B
17. E	22. C	27. B
18. C	23. C	28. B
19. C	24. B	29. D
20. D	25. A	30. A
		31. B

Answers and Explanations: VII-2 Eicosanoids: Agonists, Antagonists, and Inhibitors

Directions: questions 1–6

1. **F**
2. **E**
3. **D**
4. **C**
5. **B**

Learning objective: Explain the mechanism of the antiglaucoma action of latanoprost.

6. **C** Latanoprost is a prostaglandin $F_{2\alpha}$ analogue that lowers the intraocular pressure by increasing the outflow of aqueous humor through the uveoscleral route. The effectiveness of the drug is similar to that of timolol. Moreover, latanoprost has additive effects when administered with β-blockers or α_2-adrenergic agonists.

    A, E These are mechanisms of action of cholinergic drugs.

    B This is the mechanism of action of β-blockers or α_2 agonists.

    D This is the mechanism of action of α agonists such as epinephrine and phenylephrine.

Learning objective: Explain the molecular mechanism of action of alprostadil in erection disorders.

7. **A** Alprostadil is synthetic prostaglandin E_1. When given by intraurethral administration, alprostadil acts by activating prostaglandin E_1 G protein–coupled receptors in penile vessels. This activation stimulates adenylyl cyclase, thus increasing the production of cyclic adenosine monophosphate (cAMP). An increased cAMP level increases Ca^{2+} efflux and decreases phosphorylation of myosin light chain both in vascular and nonvascular smooth muscle, thus leading to muscle relaxation. This relaxation allows increased inflow of blood into corpora cavernosa, thus causing penile erection.

    B–F See correct answer explanation.

Learning objective: Outline the therapeutic uses of dinoprostone.

8. **B** Prostaglandins E and F are able to terminate pregnancy at any stage by promoting uterine contractions. They are also able to ripen the cervix (i.e., to make it softer) by increasing proteoglycan content and changing the biophysical properties of collagen.

    Dinoprostone, a synthetic prostaglandin E_2, is administered intravaginally for ripening of the cervix in pregnant women at or near term whose cervix is not yet soft enough for oxytocin induction of labor.

    A Thromboxanes are not used as drugs.

    C Ergonovine can cause uterine contractions but has no cervical ripening properties.

    D–F Beta-2 agonists and nonsteroidal antiinflammatory drugs have uterine relaxant properties, and they are devoid of cervical ripening properties.

Learning objective: Outline the therapeutic uses of dinoprostone.

9. **E** In case of intrauterine fetal death, prostaglandins alone or with oxytocin can cause delivery effectively. Dinoprostone (prostaglandin E_2) is the prostaglandin currently used for this purpose.

    A–C These drugs do not have oxytocic properties.

    D Ergot alkaloids such as ergonovine can evoke rhythmic contraction and relaxation of the uterus when given in very small doses. At higher concentrations, however, these drugs elicit potentially dangerous powerful and prolonged contracture and therefore are not used to cause delivery.

Learning objective: Explain the molecular mechanism of action of zileuton.

10. **B** Zileuton is an inhibitor of 5-lipoxygenase, preventing leukotriene synthesis. It improves asthma control and reduces the frequency of asthma exacerbation, although its effects are less marked than those of inhaled glucocorticoids. The main advantage of the drug is that it can be taken orally.

    A, C–E See correct answer explanation.

Learning objective: Identify the drug used to induce medical abortion.

11. **E** The prescribed treatment most likely included mifepristone and misoprostol, the most common first-trimester medical abortion regimen. In the presence of progesterone, mifepristone acts as an antagonist at progesterone receptors. The inhibition of progesterone actions on the uterus in the early stage of pregnancy causes decidual breakdown, which leads to detachment of the blastocyst. Misoprostol, taken 24 to 48 hours later causes uterine contractions that expel the uterine contents. This medical abortion regimen terminates pregnancy in over 95% of women treated during the first 7 weeks after conception.

    A, B Large doses of these drugs can cause abortion and were used in the past to induce street abortions, but they are not used for medically induced abortion.

    C, D These drugs do not cause abortion.

Learning objective: Outline the therapeutic uses of alprostadil.

12. **B** When a baby is born with a congenital heart disease (transposition of the great arteries, pulmonary artery stenosis, etc.), it is important to maintain the patency of the ductus arteriosus before corrective surgery. Patency of the fetal ductus arteriosus depends primarily on prostaglandin E_2 and to a lesser extent on prostaglandin E_1. At birth, prostaglandin E_1 and E_2 levels are reduced because the increased blood oxygen speeds up prostaglandin metabolism, so the ductus arteriosus closes in 1 or 2 days. Alprostadil is a synthetic prostaglandin E_1 that can maintain the patency of the ductus arteriosus when given after birth. Because it is metabolized quickly (the half-life is about 10 minutes), it must be given by continuous infusion.

    A Cyclooxygenase inhibitors such as indomethacin inhibit the synthesis of prostaglandin E_2 and therefore are used to speed up the closure of the ductus arteriosus in case of delayed closure, which is common in premature infants.

    C, E Dinoprostone, a synthetic prostaglandin E_2, and misoprostol, a prostaglandin E_1 analogue, have activity on the ductus arteriosus, but they are not available for parenteral use.

    D Latanoprost is devoid of actions on the ductus arteriosus.

Learning objective: Explain the molecular mechanism of action of epoprostenol.

13. **E** Epoprostenol is a synthetic prostacyclin (prostaglandin I_2) that has powerful vasodilating activity. The drug has been approved for the treatment of primary pulmonary hypertension, a disease of unknown cause involving obliteration of medium and small pulmonary arteries and resulting in right ventricular failure or fatal syncope 2 to 5 years after detection. Epoprostenol activates specific prostaglandin I_2 receptors, causing relaxation of pulmonary arteries. Long-term therapy with this drug has been found to be highly effective in improving symptoms and prolonging survival.

    A–D See correct answer explanation.

Learning objective: Identify the eicosanoid that is increased during bleeding episodes.

14. **F** Activation of the thromboxane pathway is one of the body's defenses against bleeding. When bleeding occurs, thromboxanes (mainly A_2) are synthesized and released from cells in the bleeding area. Thromboxanes are powerful vasoconstricting agents that promote platelet aggregation and amplify the effect of other platelet-aggregating substances, such as thrombin. Both vasoconstriction and platelet aggregation help to block bleeding.

    A–E All of these endogenous substances are vasodilators, so their release following bleeding is unlikely.

Learning objective: Describe the ocular effects of latanoprost.

15. **D** Latanoprost is a synthetic prostaglandin $F_{2\alpha}$ that lowers the intraocular pressure without affecting the lens curvature or pupillary diameter. This is because it increases the outflow of the aqueous humor through the uveoscleral route, which is different from the Schlemm canal route. Drugs that increase outflow of the aqueous humor through the Schlemm canal cause increased lens curvature and miosis.

    A–C, E See correct answer explanation.

Learning objective: Identify the enzyme that catalyzes prostaglandin biosynthesis during inflammation.

16. **B** Cyclooxygenases are the enzymes that catalyze prostaglandin and thromboxane biosynthesis. Two different isoforms of cyclooxygenase have been found: cyclooxygenase-1 (COX-1) and cyclooxygenase-2 (COX-2). Whereas COX-1 is expressed in most tissues of the body and tends to be homeostatic in function, inflammatory mediators such as cytokines upregulate COX-2 expression, leading to high levels of COX-2 in inflamed tissues. COX-2, in turn, catalyzes the synthesis of prostaglandin E_2 and prostaglandin I_2, the predominant prostaglandins associated with inflammation. Both markedly enhance edema formation and leukocyte infiltration in the inflamed area.

A This enzyme is involved in tissue necrosis.

D This enzyme is involved in liver disease.

C, E, F See correct answer explanation.

Learning objective: Describe the adverse effects of prostaglandin E_2.

17. **C** Dysmenorrhea is a common disorder that usually starts during adolescence and tends to decrease with age and after pregnancy. Prostaglandin E_2, produced by the secretory endometrium, has a powerful contracting effect on uterine smooth muscle and is most likely the primary factor responsible for dysmenorrhea. Ibuprofen is a nonsteroidal antiinflammatory drug from the propionic acid class. By blocking prostaglandin biosynthesis, these drugs can relieve dysmenorrhea.

A, B, D, E All of these compounds are uterine relaxants, not stimulators of contraction.

Learning objective: Describe the adverse effects of misoprostol.

18. **D** Misoprostol is a prostaglandin E_1 analogue approved for prevention of nonsteroidal antiinflammatory drug-induced peptic ulcers. Diarrhea is the most common adverse effect of the drug (up to 30% of patients) and is the main reason for its infrequent clinical use.

A–C, E See correct answer explanation.

Learning objective: Explain the algesic effect of prostaglandins.

19. **D** When alprostadil, a synthetic prostaglandin E_1, is used intraurethrally to improve erectile dysfunction, penile pain is the most frequent adverse effect. The mechanism of this effect is most likely related to the algesic action of prostaglandins. These agents can lower the threshold of nociceptive afferent neurons, facilitating pain transmission to the spinal cord.

A–C, E All of these are actions in the central nervous system (CNS). Prostaglandins have very short half-lives and do not reach the CNS when administered peripherally.

Learning objective: Describe the action that mediates the therapeutic use of misoprostol.

20. **D** The patient's history and symptoms suggest that she was at risk of nonsteroidal antiinflammatory drug (NSAID)–induced ulcer. The prevalence of endoscopically confirmed peptic ulcer in NSAID users is 15 to 30% in the United States. When peptic ulcers develop in patients taking NSAIDs, the preferred approach is to stop the NSAID and to give an antiulcer drug, usually a proton pump inhibitor or a histamine H_2 antagonist. Prophylactic therapy should be considered for patients who are unable to discontinue NSAID therapy, as in this case. Misoprostol, a synthetic analogue of prostaglandin E_1, is the drug most often prescribed, as it is able to prevent (but not to treat) NSAID-induced ulcers. This preventive effect is most likely due to the following mechanisms:

- At low doses, misoprostol activates prostaglandin receptors on superficial epithelial cells of the stomach, increasing bicarbonate and mucus secretion (the so-called cytoprotective effect).
- At higher doses, it activates prostaglandin receptors on parietal cells of the stomach, decreasing gastric acid secretion (most likely the main mechanism).

A These are the mechanisms of action of sucralfate or of bismuth compounds. These drugs are much less effective than misoprostol when the ulcer is secondary to chronic ingestion of NSAIDs.

B This is the mechanism of action of antimuscarinic drugs. These drugs are no longer used as antiulcer agents.

C Gastrin receptor blockers are not yet available.

E Antibiotic drugs are not used in NSAID-induced peptic ulcer unless there is evidence of *Helicobacter pylori* infection.

EICOSANOIDS: AGONISTS, ANTAGOINISTS, AND INHIBITORS Answer key			
1. F	6. C	11. E	16. B
2. E	7. A	12. B	17. C
3. D	8. B	13. E	18. D
4. C	9. E	14. F	19. D
5. B	10. B	15. D	20. D

Answers and Explanations: VII-3 Nonsteroidal Antiinflammatory Drugs

Questions 1–7

1. **B**

2. **G**

3. **C**

4. **J**

5. **E**

6. **A**

7. **I**

Learning objective: Explain the mechanism of antipyretic action of nonsteroidal antiinflammatory drugs (NSAIDs).

8. **D** Ibuprofen is an NSAID of the propionic acid derivative class that is approved for children younger than 2 years. All NSAIDs inhibit prostaglandin biosynthesis by blocking cyclooxygenase both in the peripheral tissues and in the central nervous system. The release of prostaglandins (PGE_1, PGE_2) in the hypothalamus seems to be the ultimate factor that adjusts the hypothalamic thermoregulatory mechanism to maintain body temperature at a higher than normal level. By inhibiting prostaglandin synthesis, NSAIDs promote the return of the hypothalamic thermostat to the normal set point. Once the normal set point is restored, the temperature-regulating mechanisms operate (by dilation of superficial blood vessels, sweating, etc.) to reduce temperature.

    A–C All of these actions can lead to an antipyretic effect, but NSAIDs do not have these actions.

    E The inhibition of cyclooxygenase in peripheral tissues can lead to an antiinflammatory effect that can reduce fever. However, the main mechanism of the antipyretic effect of NSAIDs is central rather than peripheral.

    F Blockade of oxidative phosphorylation in skeletal muscle leads to hyperthermia, not to an antipyretic effect.

Learning objective: Identify the cause of ibuprofen-induced oliguria.

9. **A** Normal glomerular filtration rate (GFR) is maintained by a fine balance between prostaglandin-mediated dilation of afferent arterioles and angiotensin II–mediated vasoconstriction of efferent arterioles. Drugs that interrupt this homeostatic mechanism can cause renal failure. Because of the therapy with captopril, the angiotensin II–mediated vasoconstriction of the efferent arterioles was already lost. When a nonsteroidal antiinflammatory drug (NSAID) was added to the patient's regimen, his kidneys no longer had control of the afferent or efferent arteriolar tone, and renal failure ensued. In addition, it has been shown that NSAIDs can inhibit the diuretic effect of most diuretic agents, which can explain why in this patient even an increase in furosemide dosage had no effect.

    B Worsening of cardiac failure may be associated with oliguria, but this is unlikely in this case because the patient did show improvement with therapy.

    C Furosemide can increase, not decrease, renin secretion secondary to inhibition of Na^+ and Cl^- transport into the macula densa.

    D In patients with cardiac failure, digoxin usually increases, not decreases, GFR secondary to the increased cardiac output.

    E Severe hypokalemia impairs the concentrating ability of the kidney and therefore tends to cause polyuria, not oliguria.

Learning objective: Describe the poisoning due to salicylate overdose.

10. **E** The patient's symptoms, the marked hyperthermia, and the respiratory depression suggest severe poisoning by salicylates. This is supported by the lab results indicating mixed respiratory and metabolic acidosis (low pH, increased P_aCO_2, and decreased plasma bicarbonate content). This acid–base disturbance is typical of a high salicylate content in blood. In salicylate poisoning, the initial event (when salicylate concentration in blood is not yet high) is respiratory alkalosis caused by salicylate-induced stimulation of the respiratory center. Partial compensation is achieved, as usual, by increased renal excretion of bicarbonate. Therefore, the initial phase of poisoning (or when the poisoning is mild) is characterized by respiratory alkalosis (high pH, decreased levels of P_aCO_2 and bicarbonate). In a later phase, when salicylate blood levels become quite high, the respiratory center becomes depressed, and respiratory acidosis supervenes. This acidosis is uncompensated because a significant amount of bicarbonate has already been eliminated. Moreover, salicylates cause uncoupling of mitochondrial oxidative phosphorylation (which leads to hyperthermia) and inhibits the enzymes of the Krebs cycle, resulting in increased pyruvic and lactic acids. Lipolysis, gluconeogenesis, and glycolysis are also stimulated, leading to hyperglycemia and production of keto acids. Therefore, the final picture is mixed respiratory and metabolic acidosis, as in this case.

    A Acute alcohol poisoning can cause combative behavior, but hypothermia and hypoglycemia are typical signs of alcohol poisoning, and tinnitus is usually absent.

    B, C Poisoning by nonsteroidal antiinflammatory drugs other than salicylates does not usually cause profound impairment of the acid–base balance.

    D, F Poisoning by these drugs does not cause the set of symptoms showed by the patient.

Learning objective: Identify the drug that can cause nonsteroidal antiinflammatory drug (NSAID) hypersensitivity.

11. **C** The patient's history and symptoms suggest that the culprit drug was aspirin and that she was affected by aspirin hypersensitivity, a syndrome that can occur in 20 to 25% of middle-aged patients with asthma, chronic urticaria, or nasal polyps, as in this case. The reaction does not appear to be immunologic in nature, but instead seems to be a pseudoallergic reaction. The mechanism is not known, but it is likely related to the formation of increased amounts of leukotrienes and other products of the lipoxygenase pathway due to inhibition of the cyclooxygenase pathway. Patients with this syndrome experience a high degree of cross-sensitivity to other NSAIDs, which supports the conclusion that this reaction represents an abnormal response to a common pharmacological action.

A, D Bronchospasm induced by these drugs is exceedingly rare.

B, E These drugs do no not cause bronchospasm.

Learning objective: Outline the therapeutic use of acetaminophen in a patient with hemophilia.

12. **B** Because the patient is suffering from hemophilia, all nonsteroidal antiinflammatory drugs (NSAIDs) are contraindicated because they can decrease platelet aggregation and can provoke gastrointestinal bleeding. Acetaminophen is free from the above-mentioned effects and can be used as an analgesic in this patient.

A, C–F See correct answer explanation.

Learning objective: Describe disturbances of acid–base metabolism caused by high therapeutic doses of salicylates.

13. **B** The lab values indicate that the acid–base disturbance was respiratory alkalosis, which is an effect of high therapeutic doses of salicylates. These drugs stimulate respiration both directly (by a direct effect on the respiratory center in the medulla) and indirectly (by increased production of carbon dioxide due to increased oxygen consumption). Compensation is achieved by increased renal excretion of bicarbonate. Unless toxic doses are given, this stage seldom proceeds further.

A, C–E See correct answer explanation.

Learning objective: Explain the reason for hyperthermia due to salicylate overdose.

14. **D** The patient's signs and symptoms indicate he was suffering from salicylate overdose toxicity. Although salicylates have an antipyretic action, they can cause hyperthermia when given in too-high doses. This seems to be primarily due to the uncoupling of oxidative phosphorylation in skeletal muscle; that is, oxidation proceeds without phosphorylation, thus producing heat. This action is similar to that produced by dinitrophenol.

A–C, E See correct answer explanation.

Learning objective: Explain the mechanism of analgesic action of nonsteroidal antiinflammatory drugs (NSAIDs) in surgical pain.

15. **B** Prostaglandins are endogenous compounds that are released from damaged tissues and can sensitize nociceptors, causing pain. By inhibiting prostaglandin biosynthesis in the damaged area, NSAIDs cause an analgesic effect. Ketorolac is an effective analgesic but only a moderately effective antiinflammatory drug. Its analgesic efficacy seems greater than that of most other NSAIDs.

A NSAIDs do not act on prostaglandin receptors.

C, E NSAIDs do not cause these effects.

D Inhibition of prostaglandin biosynthesis in the central nervous system can occur and could contribute to the analgesic effect, but the effect is mainly a peripheral one.

Learning objective: Describe the main contraindications of nonsteroidal antiinflammatory drugs (NSAIDs).

16. **E** The history of the patient indicated aspirin hypersensitivity. This syndrome occurs in 0.3% of patients, but it can occur in 20 to 25% of middle-aged patients with asthma, nasal polyps, or chronic urticaria. The syndrome is not dose-related (it can occur with small amounts of aspirin) and does not appear to be immunologic in nature. Because there is a high degree of cross-sensitivity between aspirin and other NSAIDs, severe aspirin hypersensitivity is a contraindication to the use of any NSAIDs.

A–D See correct answer explanation.

Learning objective: Identify the antipyretic drug causing poisoning associated with extremely high transaminase levels.

17. **C** The patient's history and symptoms suggest that he was most likely suffering from acetaminophen poisoning. This poisoning is due to toxic metabolites (mainly *N*-acetyl-*p*-benzoquinone) that accumulate when glutathione is not available for conjugation. Usually these metabolites are rapidly conjugated with glutathione, but in the absence of glutathione, they react with cellular proteins, resulting in hepatotoxicity. This occurs after the ingestion of toxic doses or when alcohol is taken together with acetaminophen, as in both cases glutathione is depleted faster than it can be generated. The alcohol–acetaminophen syndrome occurs in a clinical setting in which acute, sometimes fulminant, hepatic necrosis develops after large doses of acetaminophen are taken during an alcoholic binge or a period of chronic, excessive alcohol intake. Peculiar to the alcohol–acetaminophen syndrome are the extremely high serum transaminase levels, as in this case. Early treatment consists of the administration of *N*-acetylcysteine, although at 48 hours or more after the ingestion, its use remains controversial.

A, B, D, E Overdose of all of the other listed drugs does not cause a significant increase in serum transaminase levels.

Learning objective: Outline the therapeutic uses of celecoxib in a patient with a relevant past medical history.

18. **E** Celecoxib is a selective inhibitor of cyclooxygenase-2. Drugs of this class (sometimes called coxibs) have analgesic, antipyretic, and antiinflammatory actions. However, they lack action on platelet aggregation and have lower adverse effects on the gastric mucosa than nonselective inhibitors of cyclooxygenases. These drugs are therefore preferred in patients at risk of peptic ulcer disease, as in this case.

A–D, F See correct answer explanation.

Learning objective: Describe the contraindications to the use of celecoxib.

19. **B** Celecoxib is a selective cyclooxygenase-2 (COX-2) inhibitor with antipyretic, analgesic, and antiinflammatory effects similar to those of other nonsteroidal antiinflammatory drugs (NSAIDs). It is a sulfa derivative and therefore is relatively contraindicated in this patient because of his previous serious allergic reaction to sulfonamides, even though the risk of an allergic reaction after administration of a sulfa derivative in a patient with sulfonamide hypersensitivity appears to be very low.

A, C–E See correct answer explanation.

Learning objective: Describe the nephropathy due to long-term use of nonsteroidal antiinflammatory drugs (NSAIDs).

20. **C** The culprit drug was most likely an NSAID such as diclofenac. Chronic use (6 to 8 months or more) of antipyretic analgesics can cause a nephropathy that is characterized by renal papillary necrosis (the primary lesion) and chronic interstitial nephritis. The cause of the disease is still uncertain, but it seems to be related, at least in part, to the chronic inhibition of prostaglandin biosynthesis, as prostaglandins play important roles in regulating renal function. The risk increases with the use of analgesic combinations, as in this case.

A, B The risk of nephropathy with chronic use of these analgesics is negligible.

D–F See correct answer explanation.

Learning objective: Explain the use of nonsteroidal antiinflammatory drugs (NSAIDs) in dysmenorrhea.

21. **B** The pain occurring during menses (dysmenorrhea) is thought to result from uterine contractions and ischemia, likely mediated by prostaglandins produced by the secretory endometrium. Contributing factors may include an extremely tight cervical os because of thermocautery or conization, as in this case. Pain occurs when the uterus attempts to expel tissue through the os. The analgesic effects of NSAIDs such as ibuprofen in the treatment of dysmenorrhea are mainly due to the inhibition of prostaglandin biosynthesis in the endometrium.

A NSAIDs do not act on prostaglandin receptors.

C Even if a central action (inhibition of prostaglandin biosynthesis in the central nervous system [CNS]) may contribute to the analgesic effect of NSAIDs, the effect is mainly peripheral. Acetaminophen is the only analgesic-antipyretic drug whose analgesic effect is thought to be primarily mediated by the inhibition of pain transmission in the CNS.

D Pelvic inflammatory disease may cause diffuse, continuous, low abdominal pain. In this case, however, the pain is present only during menses, so it is unlikely that it is due to pelvic inflammatory disease.

E Leukotrienes can increase nociceptive nerve ending sensitivity, but NSAIDs do not affect leukotriene synthesis.

Learning objective: Describe salicylate-induced Reye syndrome.

22. **F** The results of the autopsy and the history of the patient suggest that the cause of death was Reye syndrome. The syndrome consists of acute encephalopathy with fatty degeneration of the viscera. It is exceedingly rare and occurs almost exclusively in children younger than 18 years. Lethality is estimated to be about 20%. The cause of the syndrome is unknown, but risk factors involve use of salicylates in viral infections, as in this case.

A–E These drugs do not cause Reye syndrome.

Learning objective: Describe the contraindications to the use of celecoxib.

23. **C** Pain from osteoarthritis is usually treated initially with nonsteroidal antiinflammatory drugs. However, clinical data suggest that cyclooxygenase-2 (COX-2) inhibitors such as celecoxib are more likely to cause arterial thrombotic events, probably because they do not inhibit platelet aggregation that is mediated by thromboxane produced by the COX-1 enzyme. Therefore, COX-2-selective analgesics are contraindicated in patients with a history of previous thromboembolic disease, as in this case.

A, B, D, E See correct answer explanation.

Learning objective: Outline the uses of nonsteroidal antiinflammatory drugs (NSAIDs) in dysmenorrhea.

24. **D** Primary dysmenorrhea is cyclic pain associated with menses during ovulatory cycles but without demonstrable lesions affecting the reproductive cycle. The pain is thought to result from uterine contraction and ischemia, most likely mediated by the actions of prostaglandins produced by the secretory endometrium. NSAIDs taken 2 days before menses and continued for 2 or 3 days or as needed represents the first-line pharmacotherapy. Propionic acid derivatives are very effective in dysmenorrhea for many patients; in a variety of clinical trials, good to complete pain relief was reported for 40 to 100% of women using ibuprofen.

A Although acetaminophen is advertised as an analgesic for dysmenorrhea, it is much less effective than NSAIDs because it is a very poor inhibitor of cyclooxygenase in peripheral tissues.

B Beta-2 agonists can relax the uterus, but their action is much less effective than that of NSAIDs in dysmenorrhea, where prostaglandins play the main role.

C, E, F These drugs would increase, not decrease, uterine contractions.

Learning objective: Outline the use of ibuprofen in a patient with a relevant past medical history.

25. **D** Ibuprofen has been approved for use as an antipyretic in children and is currently available over the counter. Because most nonsteroidal antiinflammatory drugs have antipyretic activity, the initial choice is often based on specific patient-related contraindications.

    In this patient:

    A Aspirin is contraindicated because of the risk of Reye syndrome. This serious disorder mainly affects children or young adults, and predisposing factors include viral infection and salicylate therapy.

    B Indomethacin is not indicated for general use as an analgesic or antipyretic because of its toxicity.

    C Acetaminophen is contraindicated in this patient because of his congenital deficiency of red blood cell glutathione synthase. Acetaminophen is partially metabolized to N-acetyl-p-benzoquinoneimine, which is rapidly conjugated with glutathione. If glutathione stores are deficient, the metabolite reacts with hepatocyte macromolecules, resulting in hepatotoxicity. Patients with congenital deficiency of glutathione synthase are therefore at increased risk of acetaminophen toxicity.

    E, F These drugs are not used as antipyretics.

Learning objective: Outline the analgesic uses of piroxicam in a patient with a relevant past medical history.

26. **C** The symptoms and the history of the patient suggest the pain was caused by bone metastases, which are the most frequent metastases in prostatic carcinoma. Osseous metastases induce an inflammatory reaction with the production of prostaglandins that may cause osteolysis and sensitize free nerve endings, augmenting pain perception. Nonsteroidal antiinflammatory drugs (NSAIDs) effectively decrease prostaglandin and endoperoxide production and therefore can be useful for an initial treatment of metastatic bone pain. Piroxicam is a long-acting, nonselective, competitive inhibitor of cyclooxygenase that also inhibits polymorphonuclear cell migration and decreases oxygen radical production. All NSAIDs could be useful as analgesics, and the superiority of any particular drug for a particular patient cannot be predicted. Therefore, the initial choice is often based on specific patient-related contraindications.

    In this patient:

    A Aspirin is contraindicated because of his congenital glucose-6-phosphate dehydrogenase (G6PD) deficiency (salicylates can cause hemolytic anemia in patients with this deficiency).

    B Acetaminophen is a very weak inhibitor of cyclooxygenase in the presence of high concentrations of peroxide that are found in inflammatory lesions.

    D All propionic acid derivatives are contraindicated because of the serious allergic reaction to naproxen.

    E Tricyclic antidepressants such as amitriptyline are sometimes useful analgesics in neoplastic disorders when the pain is neuropathic (i.e., due to the damage of neuronal structures) but not when the pain is nociceptive (i.e., pain transmitted over intact neural pathways), as in this case.

Learning objective: Describe the use of indomethacin in a newborn baby with patent ductus arteriosus.

27. **E** The patient's symptoms and the echocardiography results suggest he had a patent ductus arteriosus, which can occur in up to 80% of premature infants with a birth weight less than 1200 g (2.65 lb). Patency of the ductus arteriosus is maintained in utero by the low partial pressure of oxygen and high concentration of prostaglandins, mainly PGE_1 and PGE_2, which have vasodilatory actions. Because of this, nonsteroidal antiinflammatory drugs have been found to speed up the closure of the ductus arteriosus in newborn babies. Indomethacin given intravenously is the treatment of choice and can achieve closure in more than 70% of neonates.

    A–D See correct answer explanation.

Learning objective: Describe nonsteroidal antiinflammatory drug (NSAID)–induced iron deficiency anemia.

28. **A** The patient's history and symptoms suggest that she was affected by iron deficiency anemia. Dark stools (due to gastric bleeding) and pica (craving to eat nonedible substances) are symptoms of iron deficiency anemia. Chronic occult bleeding is the most common cause of iron deficiency anemias in adults. It is present in up to 30% of patients chronically treated with NSAIDs. Iron deficiency from an inadequate diet can also contribute to the anemia, as may be relevant in this case (see the vegetarian habit of the patient).

    B–E See correct answer explanation.

Learning objective: Describe the mechanism of action of nonsteroidal antiinflammatory drugs (NSAIDs).

29. **C** Ibuprofen is an NSAID of the propionic acid derivative class. By inhibiting cyclooxygenases, these drugs impair the biosynthesis of both prostacyclin (prostaglandin I_2) and thromboxanes.

    A, B, D–F All of these options have at least one endogenous compound whose biosynthesis is not inhibited by NSAIDs.

Learning objective: Explain the mechanism of peptic ulcer formation by nonsteroidal antiinflammatory drugs (NSAIDs).

30. **B** Erosive gastritis, bleeding, and peptic ulcer are well recognized adverse effects of NSAIDs. The effects are the consequence of both systemic and local actions.

Systemic actions are related to inhibition of prostaglandin biosynthesis, which in turn leads to

- Increased gastric acid secretion (prostaglandins decrease this secretion by inhibiting cyclic adenosine monophosphate (cAMP)–mediated activation of the proton pump)
- Decreased bicarbonate and mucus secretion by gastric mucosa (which is increased by prostaglandins)

Local actions occur via an ion-trapping mechanism. Most NSAIDs are weak acids with an acid dissociation constant (pK_a) less than 5. Therefore, they are mainly nonionized (i.e., lipid soluble) in the stomach lumen and can cross the cell membrane by lipid diffusion. In the neutral environment of the cytoplasm, they become ionized (i.e., water soluble) and are trapped inside the cell, causing cell damage.

A, E Gastrin and cholecystokinin secretions are not affected by NSAIDs.

C, D See correct answer explanation.

NONSTEROIDAL ANTIINFLAMMATORY DRUGS Answer key		
1. B	6. A	11. C
2. G	7. I	12. B
3. C	8. D	13. B
4. J	9. A	14. D
5. E	10. E	15. B
16. E	21. B	26. C
17. C	22. F	27. E
18. E	23. C	28. A
19. B	24. D	29. C
20. C	25. D	30. B

Answers and Explanations: VII-4 Immunomodulating Drugs

Questions 1–4

1. **A**
2. **C**
3. **F**
4. **B**

Learning objective: Identify the immunosuppressive mechanisms of prednisone.

5. **A** An immunosuppressive drug therapy must be given to all patients undergoing organ transplant. No consensus exists on the best induction and maintenance immunosuppressive regimen, but most regimens rely on three or four agents, and one of these is almost always a glucocorticoid, such as prednisone. Glucocorticoids suppress primarily cellular immunity because of their ability to modify cellular function. In addition, they can inhibit phospholipase A_2, blocking both prostaglandin and leukotriene synthesis, and they increase the fractional catabolic rate of immunoglobulin G (IgG), the major class of antibody immunoglobulins, thus lowering the concentration of specific antibodies.

B–E All of these immunosuppressive drugs can suppress cellular immunity, but they do not affect eicosanoid synthesis or the catabolism of IgG antibodies.

Learning objective: Identify the drug used for the therapy of lupus erythematosus.

6. **B** The signs and symptoms of the patient indicate that she was most likely affected by lupus erythematosus. In fact, the patient showed 5 of the 11 signs and symptoms most often associated with this disease: malar (butterfly) erythema, arthritis, oral ulcers, renal disorder, and nuclear antibodies). According to the American College of Rheumatology, the diagnosis of lupus erythematosus is made when the patient has 4 or more of these 11 signs and symptoms. The cause of lupus erythematosus is unknown but is thought to involve autoimmune mechanisms. The therapy almost always includes corticosteroids, which are especially valuable for the more severe and life-threatening manifestations of the disease. Because in this case there are signs of renal insufficiency (see creatinine and blood urea nitrogen [BUN] values), steroid therapy is clearly indicated.

A Ustekinumab is approved for the treatment of plaque psoriasis only.

C–E These are immunostimulant drugs and therefore are contraindicated in autoimmune disease.

Learning objective: Describe the mechanism of glucocorticoids in autoimmune diseases.

7. **D** Myasthenia gravis is an acquired autoimmune disease characterized by exercise-induced muscle fatigue that resolves after rest. The pathogenesis is due to antibody-mediated destruction of cholinergic Nm receptor sites. The initiating event leading to antibody production is unknown. This patient most likely developed a myasthenic crisis (edrophonium improved muscle strength), which may be precipitated by infection but also can occur without apparent cause. Myasthenic crisis requires intensive management that includes selected anticholinesterase drugs such as neostigmine and immunosuppressive treatment with glucocorticoids and cyclosporine. The immunosuppressive effect of glucocorticoids is likely due to multiple

mechanisms of action. Especially important in this regard is the inhibition of T-cell activation (due to inhibition of synthesis of interleukin-1) and T-cell proliferation (due to inhibition of synthesis of interleukin-2).

A, B Glucocorticoids have no effect on plasma cholinesterase or nicotinic receptors.

C, E Glucocorticoids actually decrease the synthesis of these interleukins (see correct answer explanation).

Learning objective: Identify the cell type representing the site of action of cyclosporine.

8. **C** Cyclosporine is a selective inhibitor of T-helper cells, suppressing the early cellular response to antigenic stimuli. Its site of action is within the cytoplasm of T-helper cells, where it binds to an immunophilin called cyclophilin.

A, B, D, E These cells are not direct targets for cyclosporine.

Learning objective: Explain the mechanism of action of sirolimus.

9. **D** Sirolimus (formerly called rapamycin) resembles tacrolimus and binds to the same intracellular FK-binding proteins. However, whereas tacrolimus and cyclosporine block gene transcription, sirolimus acts later to block interleukin-2-dependent lymphocyte proliferation. This blockade is likely due to the inhibition of mammalian kinase (called mammalian target of rapamycin), an enzyme that is essential for cell-cycle progression. Therefore, the drug substantially inhibits T- and B-cell proliferation.

A–C, E See correct answer explanation.

Learning objective: Describe the adverse effects of cyclosporine.

10. **B** The lab tests suggest that the patient is suffering from renal insufficiency. Nephrotoxicity is the most common adverse effect of cyclosporine, occurring in up to 80% of treated patients. The pathophysiology of this adverse effect is still uncertain.

A, C–E These drugs have a negligible risk of nephrotoxicity.

Learning objective: Identify the receptor class activated by cytokines.

11. **A** Aldesleukin is a cytokine (recombinant interleukin-2). Most cytokines activate receptors that belong to the Janus-kinase family. These receptors are polypeptides consisting of an extracellular cytokine-binding domain and a cytoplasmic enzyme domain. When a cytokine binds to the extracellular domain, the intracellular domain binds to and phosphorylates a separate intracellular tyrosine kinase termed Janus kinase. This tyrosine kinase in turn phosphorylates other proteins called STAT (signal transduction and activation of transcription) that translocate to the nucleus and regulate transcription of specific genes.

B–E See correct answer explanation.

Learning objective: Describe the adverse effects of azathioprine.

12. **D** The profound leukopenia and thrombocytopenia exhibited by the patient suggest bone marrow suppression. Transplant patients always receive immunosuppressive therapy to prevent organ allograft rejection. Cyclosporine, azathioprine, and a glucocorticoid are the drugs most frequently used for this purpose. Azathioprine is a prodrug that is converted in the body to mercaptopurine, an antimetabolite anticancer drug. It is therefore a cytotoxic agent that can cause significant myelosuppression.

A Cyclosporine is the drug most frequently given for immunosuppression in transplant patients, but it does not cause myelosuppression.

B, C Dobutamine and dopamine are often given to heart transplant patients to increase cardiac output and renal blood flow, but they do not cause myelosuppression.

E Fluorouracil is an anticancer drug that is not used for immunosuppression.

Learning objective: Describe the immunosuppressive therapy used to treat chronic graft-versus-host disease (GVHD).

13. **A** The patient most likely suffered from chronic GVHD, which occurs in up to 70% of allogeneic bone marrow transplant patients. The most important risk factor for developing chronic GVHD is a prior diagnosis of acute GVHD. The mainstay of therapy of GVHD is long-term immunosuppressive therapy. Prednisone and cyclosporine are among the most commonly used agents for this purpose. The combination of cyclosporine and prednisone has resulted in higher survival when compared with prednisone or cyclosporine alone.

B–E Erythromycin, doxorubicin, and vinblastine are not immunosuppressive drugs.

Learning objective: Explain the molecular mechanism of action of tacrolimus.

14. **C** Antibiotics endowed with immunosuppressant properties include cyclosporine, tacrolimus, and sirolimus. They interfere with T-cell function by binding to immunophilins, small intracellular proteins that play a key role in T-cell response to cytokines. Cyclosporine binds to cyclophilin; tacrolimus and sirolimus bind to FK-binding proteins. The tacrolimus–protein complex binds to calcineurin, a cytoplasmic phosphatase, thus inhibiting calcineurin-mediated expression for production of several cytokines.

A Azithromycin is a macrolide antibiotic with antibacterial activity. It is devoid of immunosuppressive properties.

B Azathioprine is a cytotoxic drug with immunosuppressive properties, but it does not bind to an FK-binding protein.

D Cyclosporine also inhibits calcineurin actions, but it binds to cyclophilin, not to an FK-binding protein.

E Tobramycin is an aminoglycoside antibiotic devoid of immunosuppressive properties.

Learning objective: Identify the immunosuppressant drug used to prevent allograft rejection that frequently causes gastrointestinal adverse effects.

15. **B** Mycophenolate mofetil is currently used with prednisone and cyclosporine to prevent rejection in transplanted patients. Gastrointestinal effects are the most common adverse reactions associated with this drug and include severe abdominal pain (up to 60%) nausea and vomiting (up to 30%), diarrhea (up to 50%), and constipation (up to 40%).

A, C–F These drugs are not used to prevent allograft rejection.

Learning objective: Explain the anaphylactoid reaction to monoclonal antibodies.

16. **E** The patient was most likely experiencing an infusion-related reaction, which is a major adverse effect of most monoclonal antibodies. This reaction can be due to a cytokine release syndrome or an anaphylactoid reaction. The symptoms and signs of this patients point out that the syndrome was most likely an anaphylactoid reaction.

A–D These are not adverse effects of basiliximab.

Learning objective: Explain the molecular mechanism of action of muromonab-CD3.

17. **E** Muromonab-CD3 is a monoclonal antibody against CD3 molecules present on the surface of human thymocytes and mature T cells. CD3 molecules are necessary for a signal to be transduced to the cytoplasm after the T-cell receptor binds to the antigen. The drug binds and neutralizes the CD3 protein receptor complex, causing the death of T cells.

A Muromonab-CD3 has negligible effects on B cells.

B This is the mechanism of action of azathioprine.

C This is the mechanism of action of cyclosporine and tacrolimus.

D Stimulation of the synthesis of interleukin-1 would cause an immunostimulant, not an immunosuppressive, effect.

Learning objective: Explain the mechanism of the immunosuppressive action of azathioprine.

18. **B** Azathioprine is an immunosuppressive agent used in organ transplantation to prevent rejection. It is a prodrug that is converted in the body to mercaptopurine, an antimetabolite anticancer drug that blocks purine biosynthesis. This leads to cytotoxicity mainly toward cells with a high turnover rate, which includes T and B lymphocytes. Because the proliferation of these lymphocytes is inhibited, both cell- and antibody-mediated immune responses are inhibited. This also explains why most antimetabolite anticancer drugs have immunosuppressive actions. Azathioprine, however, appears to be a more effective immunosuppressive than mercaptopurine itself. The basis for this superiority is unknown.

Because azathioprine inhibits the early stages of cell differentiation and proliferation, the drug is useful for preventing rejection but is ineffective for the treatment of acute rejection.

A Azathioprine has no blocking activity on receptors of tumor necrosis factor-α (TNF-α).

C Antigen presentation by different antigen-presenting cells is an early step in the adaptive immune response. This step is not inhibited by azathioprine.

D, E These two actions would actually increase, not decrease, the immunologic response of the body.

Learning objective: Explain why mycophenolate mofetil currently replaces azathioprine to prevent rejection in a solid organ transplant.

19. **B** Mycophenolate mofetil is a prodrug that is biotransformed into mycophenolic acid. This active metabolite inhibits inosine monophosphate dehydrogenase, an enzyme involved in the de novo pathway of purine biosynthesis. However, unlike azathioprine, it does not inhibit enzymes involved in the salvage pathway of purine or pyrimidine biosynthesis. Thus, it selectively inhibits the proliferation of lymphocytes (including B and T lymphocytes), as these cells lack the enzymes of the alternative salvage pathway. Because of this, mycophenolate mofetil is cytotoxic only for lymphocytes, whereas azathioprine is cytotoxic for all rapidly growing cells. This explains why mycophenolate mofetil has significantly fewer adverse effects than azathioprine.

A The immunosuppressive activity of mycophenolate and azathioprine is roughly the same because both drugs are able to kill B and T lymphocytes.

C Graft-versus-host disease occurs after stem cell transplantation, not after solid organ transplantation.

D Mycophenolate mofetil has negligible effects on macrophages because these cells can utilize the salvage pathway for purine biosynthesis.

E Mycophenolate mofetil has no effect on antigen-presenting cells.

Learning objective: Identify the drug used to maintain remission in Crohn disease.

20. **E** Several studies have shown that glucocorticoids are ineffective in maintaining remission in Crohn disease, although a subset of patients require chronic administration of glucocorticoids to prevent recurrence of symptoms (termed steroid-dependent Crohn disease). Given the poor long-term efficacy of glucocorticoids, many experts attempt treatment with other immunosuppressive drugs. Azathioprine, methotrexate, and infliximab are effective in maintaining remission and are also used as a steroid-sparing strategy in patients with steroid-dependent Crohn disease.

A–D See correct answer explanation.

Learning objective: Describe the use of muromonab-CD3 to treat steroid-resistant organ allograft rejection.

21. **B** A high-dose glucocorticoid (usually intravenous methylprednisolone) is considered first-line therapy for acute rejection because it works very quickly in decreasing lymphocyte responsiveness and can reverse at least 75% of acute rejection episodes. Muromonab-CD3 is usually reserved for steroid-resistant rejection.

A Because prednisone failed to resolve the rejection, administration of another steroid would be irrational.

C Aldesleukin is an immunostimulant, not an immunosuppressive drug.

D, E Because a cytotoxic drug (azathioprine) failed to prevent rejection, the choice of other cytotoxic drugs is not appropriate.

Learning objective: Identify the immunosuppressive drug therapy given prior to heart transplant.

22. **B** Immunosuppressive therapy is given aggressively during the early transplant period because the risk of organ rejection is greater at this time. Azathioprine with prednisone was associated with a 50% organ survival rate. When cyclosporine was added, more than an 80% rate of organ survival was obtained.

A Aldesleukin is an immunostimulant drug, so its use would be irrational in this setting.

C Triamcinolone is a synthetic glucocorticoid. The combined use of prednisone and triamcinolone (two different glucocorticoids with equivalent effects) is superfluous.

D, E Infliximab and etanercept are immunosuppressive drugs that neutralize tumor necrosis factor-α (TNF-α). They are used only in Crohn disease and rheumatoid arthritis, both autoimmune diseases.

Learning objective: Identify the cell type representing the site of action of tacrolimus.

23. **C** Tacrolimus is not chemically related to cyclosporine but has a similar site and mechanism of action. Both drugs bind to immunophilins located in the cytoplasm of T-helper cells, suppressing the early cellular response to antigenic stimuli.

A, B, D, E These cells are not direct targets for tacrolimus.

Learning objective: Describe the therapeutic uses of tacrolimus.

24. **C** Patients who receive an initial immunosuppressant therapy with cyclosporine are sometimes converted to tacrolimus, either because of persistent drug reactions or of a poor response, as in this case. Tacrolimus has a mechanism of action very close to that of cyclosporine. Nevertheless, patient survival rates exceeding 80% have been reported in liver transplant patients who were converted from cyclosporine to tacrolimus because of failure of cyclosporine therapy.

A, B, D, E These drugs are not immunosuppressants.

Learning objective: Identify the immunosuppressive drug that can inhibit enzymes of de novo purine nucleotide biosynthesis.

25. **E** Azathioprine It is a prodrug that is biotransformed into mercaptopurine and then into the corresponding false nucleotide. The false nucleotide inhibits enzymes critical for the synthesis of phosphoribosylamine, which is an essential step in purine biosynthesis, as well as in the salvage pathway for purine conservation. The false nucleotide also causes DNA damage upon intercalation.

A–D, F These immunosuppressive drugs do not affect purine biosynthesis.

Learning objective: Describe the adverse effects of tacrolimus.

26. **E** Neurotoxicity and nephrotoxicity are the two major adverse effects of tacrolimus, occurring in more than 50% of patients receiving this drug. Neurotoxicity includes headache, insomnia, tremor, paresthesias, and seizures.

A–C Tacrolimus actually can cause hypertension, hyperkalemia, and hyperglycemia.

D Hemolytic anemia has been reported very rarely during tacrolimus treatment.

Learning objective: Explain the molecular mechanism of action of aldesleukin.

27. **A** Aldesleukin is recombinant interleukin-2 (IL-2) with a mechanism of action essentially identical to that of IL-2. Aldesleukin activates IL-2 receptors expressed on T-helper cells and stimulates a cytokine cascade involving various interferons, interleukins, and tumor necrosis factors. In this way, it induces proliferation of B and T cells (including cytotoxic T cells) and activation of natural killer cells and lymphokine-activated killer cells. The drug is approved for the adjunctive treatment of renal cell carcinoma and malignant melanoma. The mechanism of antitumor activity is unknown but is probably related to the activation of cytotoxic T cells. Aldesleukin is associated with serious cardiovascular, renal, and central nervous system toxicity, so extensive monitoring is required during therapy.

B–E All of these actions would lead to immunosuppressive, not immunostimulant, effects.

Learning objective: Identify the immunostimulant cytokine used in the therapy of multiple sclerosis.

28. **C** Interferon beta-1b is a cytokine produced by various cells, including fibroblasts and macrophages. Like other interferons, it has antiviral, immunomodulating, and antiproliferative activities. Interferon beta-1b was the first agent shown to have an effect on the course of multiple sclerosis (MS). The exact mechanism of its action is still unknown, but it is likely related to its immunomodulating properties, including the downregulation of the expression of class II major histocompatibility complex and of interferon-γ (gamma). It is thought that interferon-γ is a major factor responsible for triggering the autoimmune reaction leading to MS. It stimulates cytotoxic T cells and induces macrophages to produce proteinases that degrade the myelin sheath around the spinal cord.

A, B, D, E These drugs are not recombinant cytokines.

Learning objective: Explain the mechanism of action of Rho(D) immune globulin.

29. **B** Because the woman was Rho(D) negative, and her husband was Rho(D) positive, the baby had a 100% chance (if the father was homozygous) or a 50% chance (if the father was heterozygous) of being Rho(D) positive. When a Rho(D)-negative mother carries a Rho(D)-positive fetus, she will produce antibodies against Rho(D)-positive erythrocytes if these erythrocytes leak into the maternal circulation. This can occur during pregnancy, and the risk of this fetomaternal transfer increases as the pregnancy progresses. The risk is the highest during delivery. In subsequent pregnancies, these maternal antibodies are transferred to the fetus, leading to the development of hemolytic disease in the newborn (called erythroblastosis fetalis).

If Rho(D) immune globulin is administered just after delivery, it destroys the Rho(D)-positive fetal cells in the maternal bloodstream before she has an opportunity to make her own antibodies, thus preventing erythroblastosis fetalis in subsequent pregnancies. This is an example of passive immunization.

A Placental crossing of Rho(D)-positive erythrocytes in subsequent pregnancies is not prevented, so the mother must receive the Rho(D) immune globulin after each delivery to prevent sensitization. It should be remembered that passive immunization lasts for the lifetime of the administered antibodies. The half-life of Rho(D) immune globulin is 20 to 25 days.

C The drug actually prevents the hemolytic disease of the newborn, not of the mother.

D The production of Rho(D)-positive fetal erythrocytes is genetically determined.

E Rho(D) antibodies are produced by the mother, not by the fetus.

Learning objective: Explain the molecular mechanism of action of cyclosporine.

30. **E** The activity of cyclosporine is mediated through reversible inhibition of T-cell function, particularly T-helper cells. The drug binds to a T-helper cell cytoplasmic cyclophilin, then the complex binds to calcineurin (a phosphatase) and inhibits its action. This inhibition is thought to prevent activation of nuclear factors involved in the gene transcription of interleukin-2 and other cytokines. Because interleukin-2 is needed for T-cell activation and proliferation, these T-cell functions are suppressed.

A–D All of these actions would activate, not inhibit, immunity processes.

IMMUNOMODULATING DRUGS Answer key		
1. A	6. B	11. A
2. C	7. D	12. D
3. F	8. C	13. A
4. B	9. D	14. C
5. A	10. B	15. B
16. E	21. B	26. E
17. E	22. B	27. A
18. B	23. C	28. C
19. B	24. C	29. B
20. E	25. E	30. E

Answers and Explanations: VII-5 Drugs for Arthritis and Gout

Questions 1–4

1. **G**
2. **J**
3. **F**
4. **B**

Learning objective: Identify the advantage of disease-modifying antirheumatic drugs (DMARDs) over nonsteroidal antiinflammatory drugs (NSAIDs) in the treatment of rheumatoid arthritis.

5. **B** NSAIDs were once considered the first-line treatment of rheumatoid arthritis, but today they are used only as needed to control pain because it has been shown that they have little effect on bone and cartilage destruction. On the contrary,

DMARDs can arrest, or at least slow down, the progression of the disease. They are slow-acting drugs, and their effect may take 6 weeks to 6 months to become evident. Therefore, DMARD treatment should not be delayed beyond 3 months of arthritis diagnosis for the majority of patients.

A Most DMARDs can have frequent, and sometimes very serious, adverse effects.

C See correct answer explanation.

D There is no complete cure for rheumatoid arthritis. The progression of the disease can be arrested, but therapy must be continued indefinitely.

E Acute joint pain is not quickly abolished by DMARDs. NSAIDs remain an effective treatment for acute pain.

Learning objective: Outline the pharmacotherapy of ankylosing spondylitis.

6. **C** Ankylosing spondylitis is a systemic rheumatic disorder of unknown cause characterized by inflammation where ligaments attach to bone, mainly in the axial spine. The disorder is more frequent in men and usually begins between the ages of 20 and 40. In the past, the mainstay pharmacotherapy of ankylosing spondylitis was nonsteroidal antiinflammatory drugs (NSAIDs). More recently, it has been shown that anti–tumor necrosis factor agents such as etanercept are able to cause a rapid and sustained reduction in all clinical and laboratory measures of disease activity. NSAIDs and cyclooxygenase-2 selective inhibitors are still used in mild cases.

D Because ibuprofen was not effective, the efficacy of another propionic acid derivative would be unlikely.

A, B, E, F These drugs are of no value in ankylosing spondylitis.

Learning objective: Identify the molecular site of action of infliximab.

7. **E** Infliximab is a monoclonal antibody that binds with high affinity to soluble and possibly membrane-bound tumor necrosis factor-α (TNF-α). TNF-α is a proinflammatory cytokine that appears to be especially important in the inflammatory processes associated with autoimmune disorders, such as rheumatoid arthritis, ankylosing spondylitis, Crohn disease, and psoriasis. TNF-α-blocking agents such as infliximab are used in rheumatoid arthritis, especially when refractory disease is diagnosed, as in this case.

A–D Infliximab does not bind to these molecules.

Learning objective: Identify the appropriate drug to treat an attack of gout.

8. **B** The patient's signs and symptoms suggest that he is suffering from an acute gout attack. Although the metatarsophalangeal joint of the great toe is the most common joint affected by gout attack, other joints can be involved. The gout attack can be precipitated by overindulgence in purine-rich foods, alcohol, infection, or minor trauma, as in this case. Systemic treatment of acute gout attacks includes oral nonsteroidal antiinflammatory drugs (NSAIDs) or colchicine. NSAIDs such as indomethacin are often preferred because of the frequent and sometimes serious adverse effects of colchicine. Glucocorticoids administered intra-articularly after joint aspiration can be an effective and safe treatment for a gout attack.

A Codeine is a weak opioid analgesic devoid of antiinflammatory properties and is of no value in gout attack.

C, E Methotrexate and etanercept are effective in rheumatoid arthritis but are of no value in gouty arthritis.

D NSAIDs other than indomethacin have been proved effective in the treatment of acute gouty arthritis. When given in small doses, aspirin can inhibit the excretion of uric acid by the kidney, so it should not be used for analgesia in patients with gout.

F Allopurinol can decrease serum uric acid levels in patients with gout but cannot relieve the pain of a gouty attack.

Learning objective: Identify the appropriate disease-modifying antirheumatic drug (DMARD) in a patient with concomitant disease.

9. **B** The therapy of mild rheumatoid arthritis usually includes nonsteroidal antiinflammatory drugs (NSAIDs) that can control symptoms of pain and swelling, but DMARD treatment is almost always added within 3 months of the arthritis diagnosis. Hydroxychloroquine seems to be the least toxic among DMARDs and is usually the initial choice. Moreover, in this patient, immunosuppressant drugs are relatively contraindicated because of his frequent respiratory tract infections.

A, C–E See correct answer explanation.

Learning objective: Explain the mechanism of action of leflunomide.

10. **D** Leflunomide is a disease-modifying antirheumatic drug (DMARD) immunosuppressant approved for the treatment of rheumatoid and psoriatic arthritis. Its mechanism of action involves the inhibition of dihydroorotate dehydrogenase, an enzyme involved in pyrimidine synthesis. As a consequence, there is a reduction in uridine triphosphate levels and pyrimidine synthesis in leucocytes and other rapidly dividing cells. Leflunomide is about as effective as methotrexate in rheumatoid arthritis and enhances methotrexate activity when given concomitantly. Therefore, it is often added to methotrexate therapy, as in this case.

A–C, E, F See correct answer explanation.

Learning objective: Identify the drug that is contraindicated in patients taking probenecid.

11. **D** In humans, uric acid elimination is handled by the kidney through the following four active transport mechanisms located in subsequent segments of the proximal tubule:

- Glomerular filtration: all uric acid is freely filtered.
- Tubular reabsorption: 98% is reabsorbed.
- Tubular secretion: 50% is secreted.
- Postsecretory tubular reabsorption: 40% is reabsorbed.

Therefore, about 10% of the filtered uric acid load is finally eliminated by the kidney.

Uricosuric drugs such as salicylates and probenecid compete with uric acid for these transport mechanisms. They have a paradoxical effect because, depending on dosage, they may either decrease or increase the elimination of uric acid. It seems that the secretory mechanism is more sensitive to the blocking action of uricosuric drugs, so low doses block uric acid secretion only. Higher doses are able to block both mechanisms; therefore, as most uric acid is reabsorbed, the net result is increased elimination. Salicylates such as aspirin can completely antagonize the uricosuric action of probenecid. This interaction probably involves several mechanisms, including competition for renal tubular transport.

A–C, E, F These drugs are not contraindicated in a patient receiving probenecid.

Learning objective: Explain the mechanism of action of colchicine.

12. **C** Colchicine can be used to stop an acute gout attack or, most often, for the prevention of further attacks, as in this case. The drug binds to the intracellular protein, tubulin, thereby preventing its polymerization into microtubules and thus blocking mitosis in metaphase. Cells with the highest rate of division are affected early. Granulocyte migration into the inflamed area and phagocytosis of urate crystals by macrophages are inhibited, thus relieving the pain and inflammation of gouty arthritis. These actions are specific, and the drug is devoid of general analgesic or antiinflammatory effects.

A, B, F These drugs are effective in gouty arthritis but have different mechanisms of actions.

D, E These drugs can decrease the risk of gout attacks by decreasing the urate pool, not by inhibiting tubulin polymerization.

Learning objective: Outline the use of hydroxychloroquine in the treatment of systemic lupus erythematosus (SLE).

13. **D** The pharmacotherapy of SLE includes nonsteroidal antiinflammatory drugs (NSAIDs), antimalarials, immunosuppressants, and glucocorticoids. Antimalarials such as hydroxychloroquine are especially effective when the disease is mild and skin manifestations are prominent, as in this case. This drug has been shown to prevent relapses and to reduce morbidity and mortality. The mechanism of action of hydroxychloroquine is still unclear but is likely related to its antiinflammatory properties. A combination of an antimalarial and an NSAID is sometimes used in mild cases. However, a combination of glucocorticoids and immunosuppressive drugs is a first-line pharmacotherapy for treatment of severe SLE.

A, B Because the patient was already receiving an NSAID, adding another drug of the same class would be irrational.

C, E, F Antibiotics are of no value, unless an infection supervenes.

Learning objective: Outline the use of etanercept in rheumatoid arthritis.

14. **C** The patient's signs and symptoms indicate that she was most likely suffering from rheumatoid arthritis. When nonsteroidal antiinflammatory drugs (NSAIDs) are poorly effective and/or poorly tolerated, pharmacotherapy with disease-modifying antirheumatic drugs (DMARDs) is indicated. Methotrexate is the initial DMARD of choice for most patients because of its efficacy and relatively rapid onset of action. However, it can have dose-related hepatotoxicity and therefore is relatively contraindicated in this patient because of the presence of active hepatitis. Etanercept, a tumor necrosis factor-α antagonist approved for the treatment of rheumatoid arthritis, would be appropriate in this case.

A See correct answer explanation.

B Aspirin is associated with a higher incidence of gastrointestinal bleeding than other NSAIDs and is no longer commonly used for the treatment of rheumatoid arthritis. Moreover, in this patient, ibuprofen was not effective and poorly tolerated.

D–F Antibiotics are not currently used in the treatment of rheumatoid arthritis, but minocycline seems to be a useful adjunctive agent in some cases. The successful use of this drug supports the speculation that rheumatoid arthritis may have an infectious component.

Learning objective: Identify the drug that consists of the extracellular portion of two tumor necrosis factor (TNF) receptor moieties.

15. **B** Combination therapy with disease-modifying antirheumatic drugs (DMARDs) is currently a well-accepted approach because it has been shown that many DMARDS, when added to methotrexate, show improved efficacy. Etanercept is a recombinant fusion protein consisting of two portions of the extracellular domain of the TNF-α receptor linked to a portion of human immunoglobulin G$_1$. The drug binds with high affinity to TNF-α molecules.

A, C–E All of these drugs can be effective in rheumatoid arthritis, but they have different chemical structures.

Learning objective: Identify the drug used in the therapy of familial Mediterranean fever.

16. **E** The patient's history, symptoms, and lab tests suggest she was most likely suffering from familial Mediterranean fever, an inherited autosomal recessive disorder characterized by recurrent fever and serositis (mainly peritonitis but also pleuritis, arthritis, and pericarditis). Because of the chronic inflammatory process, these patients have a high incidence of amyloidosis and renal failure due to perivascular deposition of serum amyloid A protein. The use of colchicine has been associated with a dramatic reduction in the incidence of these complications. In fact, prophylactic colchicine provides complete remission or distinct improvement in about 85% of patients. The mechanism of this effect is still uncertain but is likely related to the antiinflammatory properties of the drug.

    A–D These drugs are not effective in familial Mediterranean fever.

Learning objective: Identify the two endogenous compounds that are increased after a few days of therapy with allopurinol.

17. **B** By inhibiting the enzyme xanthine oxidase, allopurinol inhibits the transformation of hypoxanthine into xanthine and of xanthine into uric acid. Therefore, the plasma level of uric acid will decrease with a small, concomitant rise of hypoxanthine and xanthine.

    A, C–E See correct answer explanation.

Learning objective: Identify the drug able to decrease uric acid in both serum and urine.

18. **D** Because the patient's urate levels are decreased after therapy both in serum and in urine, the drug must have decreased the formation of uric acid. Allopurinol inhibits the conversion of hypoxanthine to xanthine and xanthine to uric acid, thus decreasing uric acid formation.

    A Probenecid increases the renal excretion of uric acid and would have decreased uric acid in plasma but would have increased uric acid in the urine.

    B Aspirin would have decreased uric acid secretion at low/intermediate doses (causing hyperuricemia) and would have increased secretion at high doses (causing uricosuria).

    C Furosemide can cause hyperuricemia.

    E, F These drugs have negligible effects on uric acid secretion.

Learning objective: Outline the use of methotrexate in rheumatoid arthritis.

19. **C** Methotrexate is currently a first-line treatment for most patients with rheumatoid arthritis because of its high rate of response, relatively rapid onset of action (1 to 2 months), and long sustained efficacy. Moreover, it has been shown that the drug can enhance the action of some other disease-modifying antirheumatic drugs (DMARDs), including hydroxychloroquine, so it would be an appropriate drug to add to the ongoing therapy in this case.

    A, B The patient was already receiving a nonsteroidal antiinflammatory drug, so the addition of another drug of the same class would be of little value.

    D Fentanyl is a powerful opioid drug. Opioid analgesics are used in rheumatoid arthritis only exceptionally, on an as-needed basis, when the pain is excruciating.

    E, F Some antidepressants, such as amitriptyline, and some anticonvulsants, such as carbamazepine, are often effective in cases of neuropathic pain, but not for treatment of nociceptive pain such as occurs in rheumatoid arthritis.

Learning objective: Describe the adverse effects of hydroxychloroquine.

20. **A** The patient's signs and symptoms suggest he was most likely suffering from retinopathy, a rare adverse effect of hydroxychloroquine after long-term treatment. The drug is a disease-modifying antirheumatic drug (DMARD) used in rheumatoid arthritis, often in combination with other DMARD drugs. The drug has high affinity for pigmented (melanin-containing) structures and accumulates in the retina after long-term treatment.

    B–F All of these drugs can be used in rheumatoid arthritis, but they do not cause retinal damage.

DRUGS FOR ARTHRITIS AND GOUT (Answer key)							
1.	G	6.	C	11.	D	16.	E
2.	J	7.	E	12.	C	17.	B
3.	F	8.	B	13.	D	18.	D
4.	B	9.	B	14.	C	19.	C
5.	B	10.	D	15.	B	20.	A

VIII Chemotherapeutic Drugs

Questions: VIII-1 Bacterial Cell Wall Synthesis Inhibitors

Directions for questions **1–4**

Match each antibiotic drug with the appropriate description (each lettered option can be selected once, more than once, or not at all).

A. Ampicillin
B. Aztreonam
C. Cefepime
D. Cefotaxime
E. Cefotetan
F. Ceftazidime
G. Ceftriaxone
H. Cloxacillin
I. Ticarcillin
J. Piperacillin
K. Vancomycin

Difficulty level: Easy

1. A penicillinase-resistant penicillin

Difficulty level: Easy

2. A penicillin active against *Klebsiella* species

Difficulty level: Easy

3. A third-generation cephalosporin active against *Pseudomonas aeruginosa*

Difficulty level: Easy

4. This drug shows no cross-allergenicity with other β-lactam antibiotics.

Difficulty level: Easy

5. A 68-year-old man diagnosed with streptococcal pneumonia started treatment with a third-generation cephalosporin. Which of the following steps in the turnover of bacterial cell walls is specifically inhibited by this antibiotic?

A. Autolysin-mediated breaking of peptidoglycan chains
B. Elongation of linear amino sugar chains
C. Connection of two amino sugar chains by peptide bridges
D. Synthesis of *N*-acetylmuramic acid
E. Linking of two amino sugars by a glycosidic bond

Difficulty level: Easy

6. A 51-year-old woman recently diagnosed with acute bacterial cystitis started an appropriate antibiotic treatment. The administered drug achieves therapeutic concentration in the urine because it is primarily eliminated by the kidney through active secretion in the proximal tubule. Which of the following drugs did the patient most likely take?

A. Cephalexin
B. Azithromycin
C. Metronidazole
D. Tobramycin
E. Tetracycline

Difficulty level: Easy

7. A 23-year-old woman complained to her physician of urinary frequency, pain upon urination, and a mucopurulent vaginal discharge. One year earlier, the patient had undergone an anaphylactic reaction to penicillin. A Gram stain of the exudate revealed gram-negative cocci. Which of the following drugs would be contraindicated for this patient?

A. Doxycycline
B. Ciprofloxacin
C. Ceftriaxone
D. Erythromycin
E. Trimethoprim-sulfametoxazole

Difficulty level: Medium

8. A 32-year-old woman was seen at a clinic because of 2 days of headache with joint and muscle pain. Physical examination revealed nuchal rigidity and a petechial rash on the lower extremities. A Gram stain of her spinal fluid showed many neutrophils and many gram-negative, bean-shaped diplococci. Which of the following drugs would be most appropriate for the therapy of this patient?

A. Tetracycline
B. Penicillin G
C. Erythromycin
D. Aztreonam
E. Tobramycin
F. Metronidazole

Difficulty level: Medium

9. A 30-year-old woman was in labor with her second child. Her first baby had contracted neonatal meningitis due to contamination with *Streptococcus agalactiae* during delivery. To prevent recurrence of this infection in the second child, which of the following drugs would be most appropriate for treatment of both the mother and the baby?

A. Levofloxacin
B. Trimethoprim-sulfamethoxazole
C. Tetracycline
D. Gentamicin
E. Ampicillin

Difficulty level: Medium

10. A 24-year-old woman came to the clinic with a sore throat and low-grade fever. Physical examination showed tonsil exudates and tender cervical adenopathy. A Gram stain of the tonsil exudate demonstrated the presence of a high number of bacteria. A diagnosis was made, and penicillin G was prescribed, as the physician knew that the most likely offending pathogen was sensitive to the antibiotic. Which of the following bacteria did the physician most likely believe caused the patient's infection?

A. *Pseudomonas aeruginosa*
B. *Staphylococcus aureus*
C. *Clostridium difficile*
D. *Streptococcus pyogenes*
E. *Enterococcus faecalis*
F. *Haemophilus influenzae*
G. *Klebsiella pneumoniae*

Difficulty level: Medium

11. A 34-year-old man presented to the clinic with a painful ulcer on his penis. Regional lymph nodes were enlarged and painful. The man admitted to unprotected intercourse with a new partner while on a recent vacation. Darkfield microscopy and an FTA-ABS (fluorescent treponemal antibody absorption) test for syphilis were negative. A Gram stain of pus revealed short gram-negative bacilli in parallel chains. Which of the following would be the most appropriate pharmacotherapy for this patient?

A. Vancomycin
B. Nafcillin
C. Penicillin G
D. Ceftriaxone
E. Metronidazole

Difficulty level: Hard

12. A 41-year-old woman collapsed at home and was brought to the emergency department. Her husband stated she had complained recently of severe abdominal cramping, nausea,

vomiting, and diarrhea. Vital signs on admission were temperature 103°F (39.4°C), pulse 134 bpm, blood pressure 85/52 mm Hg, respirations 28/min. Physical examination showed a critically ill patient with an abdominal erythematous indurated area below the umbilicus and an 8-mm (0.31-inch) central ulcer. A fluorescent antibody test of a specimen from the ulcer identified group A streptococci. Which of the following pairs of drugs would be most appropriate for the emergency treatment of this patient?

A. Penicillin G and clindamycin
B. Tobramycin and metronidazole
C. Chloramphenicol and tetracycline
D. Erythromycin and amikacin
E. Piperacillin and aztreonam

Difficulty level: Medium

13. A 54-year-old man was admitted to the hospital with fever (100.6°F, 38.1°C), night sweats, arthralgias, and 15 lb (6.8 kg) of unintentional weight loss. Past history was significant for rheumatic fever at the age of 9 and for dental surgery 1 month ago. The symptoms started about 2 weeks after the dental procedure. Physical examination was significant for mitral regurgitation, subungual splinter hemorrhages, and hemorrhagic plaques on the soles of both feet. Three blood cultures were ordered, and an empiric therapy was started. Which of the following should be an appropriate treatment for the patient at this time?

A. Ampicillin and erythromycin
B. Piperacillin and chloramphenicol
C. Aztreonam and amikacin
D. Penicillin G and gentamicin
E. Dicloxacillin and ciprofloxacin

Difficulty level: Medium

14. A previously healthy 3-year-old child was admitted to the hospital with sore throat, fever, chills, painful swallowing, and dyspnea for the past 10 hours. Physical examination revealed a seriously ill patient with edematous erythema over the anterior neck, cervical lymph node enlargement, crackles in the left lung base, and diffuse wheezing best heard as stridor over the neck. Sputum Gram stain showed numerous gram-negative coccobacilli. A diagnosis of acute supraglottitis was made, and an emergency therapy was started. Which of the following drugs would be most appropriate for the patient's disease?

A. Dicloxacillin
B. Penicillin G
C. Ceftriaxone
D. Vancomycin
E. Cefazolin

Difficulty level: Medium

15. A 63-year-old homeless man was admitted to the hospital with fever, general malaise, and a swollen, painful leg. Physical examination showed a man in obvious distress with the following vital signs: blood pressure 88/50 mm Hg, heart rate 115 bpm, respirations 22/min, temperature 103.1°F (39.5°C). His right leg had a large wound and appeared swollen with a "bronze" discoloration and crepitation of the tissue. A presumptive diagnosis was made. An empiric therapy was started that included extensive debridement of the wound and administration of a drug that was able to cure the infection. The mechanism of action of the given drug most likely involved the inhibition of which of the following bacterial enzymes?

A. Acetyl transferase
B. Beta-lactamase
C. Transpeptidase
D. Autolytic enzymes
E. Transglycosylase

Difficulty level: Medium

16. A 56-year-old farmer presented to the clinic with a small, flat, hard swelling under the oral mucosa that formed a fistula discharging yellow granules. One month earlier, he had several teeth extracted because of paradental abscesses. Anaerobic cultures of the biopsy material showed small, spidery colonies containing gram-positive, non-acid-fast rods and branching filaments. A diagnosis was made, and an antibiotic therapy was prescribed. Which of the following drugs would be most appropriate for this patient?

A. Penicillin G
B. Aztreonam
C. Metronidazole
D. Gentamicin
E. Ciprofloxacin

Difficulty level: Easy

17. A 75-year-old man was admitted to the hospital for hip replacement. Which of the following antibiotics would be an appropriate prophylactic agent to be given before surgery?

A. Metronidazole
B. Tetracycline
C. Sulfamethoxazole
D. Aztreonam
E. Cefazolin
F. Erythromycin

Difficulty level: Medium

18. An 8-year-old girl was brought to the clinic because of fever (101.5°F, 38.6°C) and extensive skin abrasions on the right leg. Her mother explained that the girl had fallen off her bicycle a few days earlier and suffered several abrasions. Physical examination showed the skin of the right leg was hot, red, and edematous with a surface "peau d'orange" appearance. Regional lymphadenopathy was also present. A Gram stain from scrapings of the lesions showed the presence of a large number of gram-positive cocci. Which of the following drugs would be appropriate for the treatment of this patient?

A. Piperacillin
B. Aztreonam
C. Dicloxacillin
D. Tetracycline
E. Amikacin

Difficulty level: Easy

19. A 55-year-old woman recently diagnosed with bacterial pyelonephritis started a treatment with a β-lactam antibiotic that is resistant to most β-lactamases. Which of the following drugs was most likely administered?

A. Cephalexin
B. Ampicillin
C. Piperacillin
D. Ticarcillin
E. Cefepime
F. Cefazolin

Difficulty level: Medium

20. A 52-year-old man presented to his physician with an extensive skin rash on his trunk and limbs. The man had been suffering from non-Hodgkin lymphoma for 2 years. A few days earlier, he was diagnosed with acute bacterial pharyngitis and started on an antibiotic. The physician said the rash was most likely an allergic reaction to the antibiotic. Which of the following drugs most likely caused this reaction?

A. Amikacin
B. Amoxicillin
C. Doxycycline
D. Vancomycin
E. Sulfamethoxazole

Difficulty level: Easy

21. A 26-year-old man presented to the emergency department with sudden onset of fever (101.1°F, 38.5°C), oliguria, and a skin rash. The man had been receiving systemic pharmacotherapy for primary syphilis. Laboratory findings showed eosinophiluria and proteinuria. Further exams led to the

diagnosis of drug-induced tubulointerstitial nephritis. Which of the following antibiotics most likely caused the patient's disease?

A. Penicillin G
B. Cefepime
C. Rifampin
D. Nafcillin
E. Trimethoprim-sulfametoxazole

Difficulty level: Medium

22. A 73-year-old man diagnosed with pneumonia due to *Pseudomonas aeruginosa* was started on piperacillin, but 2 days later, the disease was not improved, and the physician suspected that the infective organism was resistant to the drug. Which of the following was most likely the mechanism of bacterial resistance to this antibiotic?

A. Increased affinity of penicillin-binding protein to the drug
B. Inhibition of drug binding to the 50S subunit
C. Decreased permeability of the bacterial cell membrane to the drug
D. Inhibition of the efflux pump of the bacteria cell membrane
E. Increased production of autolytic enzymes

Difficulty level: Medium

23. A 70-year-old female resident in a nursing facility was admitted to the hospital because of fever (101.4°F 38.6°C), diarrhea, and severe abdominal pain. Four days earlier, the patient had started antibiotic treatment because of acute tonsillitis due to β-hemolytic streptococci. Physical examination showed a critically ill patient with abdominal distention and absent bowel sounds. Colonoscopy revealed diffuse ulcerations and exudative plaques lining the colonic mucosa. Which of the following antibiotics most likely caused the patient's disease?

A. Gentamicin
B. Vancomycin
C. Rifampin
D. Aztreonam
E. Ampicillin

Difficulty level: Easy

24. A 34-year-old woman with no previous history of disease complained to her physician of burning on urination, bladder pain, and frequent urination of a small volume. A microorganism isolated from her urine grew on EMB (eosin methylene blue) agar, produced green colonies, was motile, and was urease-negative. A diagnosis of urinary tract infection was made, and antibiotic therapy was prescribed. Which of the following drugs would be appropriate for the patient's disease?

A. Erythromycin
B. Clindamycin
C. Vancomycin
D. Cephalexin
E. Penicillin G

Difficulty level: Hard

25. A 32-year-old male heroin addict was admitted to the hospital with a 2-day history of fever, shaking chills, rigors, and night sweats. His vital signs were blood pressure 100/60 mm Hg, pulse 120 bpm, respirations 24/min, temperature 102.2°F (39°C). Two-dimensional echocardiography revealed three small vegetations on the tricuspid valve. Three blood cultures were drawn, and empiric therapy was initiated. The cultures turned out to be positive for *Pseudomonas aeruginosa*, with the following antibiotic susceptibilities:

Drug	Minimum Inhibitory Concentration
Gentamicin	16 µg/mL
Tobramycin	2 µg/mL
Piperacillin	64 µg/mL
Ceftazidime	4 µg/mL
Imipenem	2 µg/mL

Surgical excision of the infected valve and a 6-week postoperative treatment were planned. Which of the following drug combinations would be most appropriate for the patient at this time?

A. Tobramycin and gentamicin
B. Ceftazidime and tobramycin
C. Imipenem and gentamicin
D. Ceftazidime and imipenem
E. Piperacillin and tobramycin

Difficulty level: Medium

26. A 22-year-old woman consulted her physician because of a postpartum breast infection. A Gram stain of the pus revealed gram-positive bacteria, and a susceptibility test showed resistance to all β-lactam antibiotics. Which of the following bacteria was most likely the offending pathogen?

A. *Listeria monocytogenes*
B. Methicillin-resistant *Staphylococcus aureus*
C. *Escherichia coli*
D. *Streptococcus pyogenes*
E. *Enterococcus faecalis*
F. *Clostridium tetani*
G. *Serratia marcescens*

Difficulty level: Easy

27. A 4-year-old boy was brought to the pediatrician by his mother because of respiratory difficulties. Medical history of the boy was significant for recurrent pulmonary infections. A Gram stain of the sputum revealed gram-positive cocci in grapelike clusters. Which of the following drugs would be an appropriate empiric treatment at this early stage?

A. Penicillin G
B. Ampicillin
C. Piperacillin
D. Dicloxacillin
E. Amoxicillin

Difficulty level: Medium

28. A 79-year-old female resident of a nursing facility complained of burning on urination and bladder pain. Microscopic examination of urine sediment revealed many gram-positive bacteria, and a urine culture indicated *Enterococcus faecalis* as the sole causative agent. Which of the following pairs of drugs would be most appropriate for the treatment of this patient?

A. Cefotetan and netilmicin
B. Cefepime and amikacin
C. Penicillin G and erythromycin
D. Ampicillin and tobramycin
E. Aztreonam and gentamicin

Difficulty level: Easy

29. A 54-year-old woman presented to her physician complaining of vaginal itching and a thick, white vaginal discharge. One week earlier, the woman had started treatment with amoxicillin because of a skin infection. Subsequent exams led to the diagnosis of candida vaginitis that the physician thought was a superinfection related to the amoxicillin treatment. Which of the following best explains why broad-spectrum penicillins can cause superinfections?

A. Impairment of host immunologic defense
B. Selection of viral-resistant mutants
C. Masking disease symptoms
D. Impairment of normal microflora of the host
E. Impairment of normal inflammatory reaction

Difficulty level: Easy

30. A 65-year-old woman was admitted to the emergency department with altered consciousness, fever, nausea, and vomiting. Vital signs on admission were blood pressure 90/50 mm Hg, pulse 115 bpm, respirations 20/min, temperature 103.6°F (39.8°C). Physical examination showed a patient in obvious distress with a stiff neck and positive Brudzinski

sign. Pupils were equal, poorly reactive to light, and papilledema was present. An empirical intravenous therapy was started with ampicillin, ceftriaxone, and vancomycin. Which of the following best explains the mechanism of action common to all of the given drugs?

A. Misreading of messenger RNA template code
B. Inhibition of tetrahydrofolate synthesis
C. Inhibition of RNA polymerization
D. Blockade of peptidyl-transfer RNA translocation
E. Inhibition of peptidoglycan synthesis

Difficulty level: Easy

31. A 61-year-old woman with poor dentition was scheduled to have all of her remaining teeth extracted for subsequent fitting of dentures. Past medical history was significant for numerous infections of the oral cavity. The woman had been suffering from mitral stenosis with mild cardiac insufficiency for 5 years. Which of the following drugs would be the most appropriate agent to prescribe to this woman before and after the extraction?

A. Amoxicillin
B. Gentamicin
C. Aztreonam
D. Piperacillin
E. Metronidazole

Difficulty level: Medium

32. A 5-year-old boy was brought to the clinic by his mother because of a localized, crusted lesion on his left leg. The mother reported that 3 days earlier, the boy had been bitten by his pet dog. A purulent discharge from the lesion was found to contain many small gram-negative coccobacilli. Which of the following correctly pairs the most likely offending pathogen with the appropriate treatment?

A. *Staphylococcus epidermidis:* oxacillin
B. *Clostridium difficile:* metronidazole
C. *Klebsiella pneumoniae:* vancomycin
D. *Serratia marcescens:* erythromycin
E. *Pasteurella multocida:* penicillin G

Difficulty level: Easy

33. A 6-year-old boy presented to his pediatrician with fever (101.3°F, 38.5°C) and sharp pain in his left ear. On physical examination, the left tympanic membrane was red, opaque, and bulging. Amoxicillin was prescribed, but 3 days later, the symptoms were not reduced. The pediatrician decided to modify the therapy and prescribed amoxicillin/potassium clavulanate. Which of the following best explains the advantage of adding potassium clavulanate to amoxicillin?

A. Inhibition of bacterial inactivation of amoxicillin
B. Extended antibacterial spectrum against *Pseudomonas aeruginosa*
C. Inhibition of renal secretion of amoxicillin
D. Increased amoxicillin entry into bacteria
E. Decreased amoxicillin allergenicity

A. Vancomycin
B. Ciprofloxacin
C. Penicillin G
D. Tobramycin
E. Metronidazole
F. Aztreonam

Difficulty level: Easy

34. A 34-year-old man was admitted to the emergency department because of flushing, itching, nausea, sneezing, and abdominal cramps. Five days earlier, the patient was diagnosed with syphilis and started on antibiotic treatment. Vital signs on admission were blood pressure 98/56 mm Hg, pulse 125 bpm, respirations 22/min. Physical examination showed a cyanotic patient with urticaria, angioedema, and wheezing. Which of the following antibiotics most likely caused the patient's signs and symptoms?

A. Azithromycin
B. Doxycycline
C. Metronidazole
D. Penicillin G
E. Amikacin
F. Clindamycin

Difficulty level: Medium

35. A 57-year-old woman consulted her physician because of fever (101°F, 38.3°C), chills, nausea and vomiting, and pain in the upper right quadrant. Subsequent exams led to the diagnosis of acute cholecystitis. An appropriate therapy was started, including a cephalosporin that is primarily eliminated in the bile. Which of the following drugs was most likely administered?

A. Ceftazidime
B. Cefoperazone
C. Cefotetan
D. Cefepime
E. Cephalothin

Difficulty level: Easy

36. A 33-year-old man presented to the clinic because he had noticed a red, painless nodule on the glans of his penis 1 week earlier. Three days after it appeared, the nodule became ulcerated, but only minimally painful. Physical examination showed an ulcer with an indurated base that exuded clear serum. Darkfield microscopy from the exudate showed numerous slender spiral microorganisms that were actively motile. A diagnosis was made, and a suitable therapy was prescribed. Which of the following drugs would be most appropriate for this patient?

Difficulty level: Medium

37. A 71-year-old diabetic man was admitted to the hospital with fever (101.2°F, 38.4°C) and a throbbing foot pain for the past 10 hours. Physical examination revealed a putrid smelling, pus-filled ulcer on the right foot. A metal probe inserted into the wound detected bone and a deep cavity. A Gram stain of the pus showed gram-positive cocci in chains, gram-negative diplococci, and gram-positive and -negative rods. Which of the following antibiotics would be most appropriate to give while blood and drainage cultures were processed?

A. Amoxicillin/clavulanate
B. Clindamycin
C. Linezolid
D. Metronidazole
E. Vancomycin

Difficulty level: Medium

38. A 53-year-old woman presented to the clinic complaining of 3 weeks of night sweats, cough productive of foul-smelling sputum, and about 10 lb (4.5 kg) of weight loss. Physical examination showed fever (101.3°F, 38.5°C), clear lung fields, and mild clubbing. Chest radiography showed a thick-walled abscess in the left lobe. Gram stain of the sputum revealed gram-negative rods, and aerobic cultures were negative. Which of the following correctly pairs the most likely causative pathogen with the appropriate treatment?

A. *Legionella pneumophila:* ampicillin
B. *Actinomyces israelii:* gentamicin
C. *Bacteroides fragilis:* imipenem
D. *Streptococcus pneumoniae:* aztreonam
E. *Listeria monocytogenes:* ceftazidime

Difficulty level: Easy

39. A 31-year-old woman recently diagnosed with acute tonsillitis started a treatment with amoxicillin. Which of the following molecular actions most likely contributed to the therapeutic effect of the drug in the patient's disease?

A. Activation of autolytic enzymes in the bacterial cell wall
B. Binding to the 30S bacterial ribosomal subunit
C. Activation of the efflux pump in bacterial cell membranes
D. Inhibition of transglycosylase in the bacterial cell wall
E. Inhibition of DNA-dependent RNA polymerase

Difficulty level: Medium

40. A 76-year-old man complained to his physician of a foul-smelling secretion from his left ear for the past 2 weeks. Further exams led to the diagnosis of chronic otitis media, and cultures from fluid secretions indicated *Bacteroides fragilis* as the main causative agent. An appropriate antibiotic treatment was started. Four days later, blood results indicated a prothrombin time of 25 seconds (normal 10–14 seconds). Which of the following drugs most likely caused this lab result?

A. Clindamycin

B. Chloramphenicol

C. Imipenem

D. Metronidazole

E. Ciprofloxacin

F. Cefotetan

Difficulty level: Easy

41. A 74-year-old man was recently diagnosed with pneumonia due to *Pseudomonas aeruginosa*. Past history of the patient was significant for a severe allergic reaction to ampicillin. A treatment was started with a β-lactam antibiotic that is highly resistant to β-lactamases and is active only against most gram-negative aerobic bacteria. Which of the following drugs was most likely given?

A. Imipenem

B. Ceftazidime

C. Amoxicillin

D. Aztreonam

E. Cefepime

Difficulty level: Easy

42. An 11-year-old girl was taken to the clinic because of fever (102°F, 38.8°C), shortness of breath, and cough productive of purulent sputum. A chest radiograph showed several areas of infiltration with possible abscess formation. Coagulase-positive bacteria were cultured from the blood, and a susceptibility test showed that they were methicillin-resistant. Treatment with vancomycin was started. Inhibition of which of the following molecular actions most likely mediated the therapeutic effect of the drug in the patient's disease?

A. Elongation of peptidoglycan

B. Relaxation of supercoiled DNA

C. Binding to ribosomal RNA

D. Translocation of peptidyl transfer RNA (tRNA)

E. Activation of autolytic enzymes

Difficulty level: Hard

43. A 7-year-old boy was admitted to the hospital with fever (102°F, 38.8°C) and joint pain in his knees and wrists. He had a history of a severe sore throat for 3 weeks. Vital signs on admission were blood pressure 122/80 mm Hg, heart rate 110 bpm, respirations 24/min. Physical examination showed red, hot, and painful knees and a nonpruritic rash with distinct disklike borders on his thighs and stomach. Subcutaneous, painless nodules were present over the bone surface of his elbows and knees. Heart auscultation revealed a mitral valve regurgitation murmur. Pertinent lab results on admission were erythrocyte sedimentation rate 80/h (normal < 10/h for children), antistreptolysin-O titer 410 IU (normal < 200 IU). A diagnosis was made, and a suitable therapy was prescribed. Which of the following pairs of drugs would be most appropriate for the initial treatment of this patient?

A. Penicillin G and naproxen

B. Amoxicillin and erythromycin

C. Ceftriaxone and acetaminophen

D. Tobramycin and aspirin

E. Penicillin G and acetaminophen

F. Amoxicillin and ceftriaxone

Difficulty level: Medium

44. A 7-year-old girl was admitted to the emergency department with fever (101.8°F, 38.8°C) and a productive cough of thick, greenish sputum. Her medical history was significant for cystic fibrosis and several episodes of pneumonia over the past 3 years. Gram stain of the sputum revealed gram-negative rods. Growth of bacteria on agar culture exhibited a blue-green pigment. Which of the following β-lactam drugs would be appropriate to include in the therapeutic regimen of this patient?

A. Piperacillin

B. Cephalothin

C. Amoxicillin

D. Clavulanic acid

E. Oxacillin

F. Penicillin G

Difficulty level: Medium

45. A 32-year-old man recently diagnosed with cellulitis caused by *Streptococcus pyogenes* started a treatment with ampicillin. The drug acts by binding to penicillin-binding proteins. Which of the following molecular actions is catalyzed by penicillin-binding proteins?

A. Transport of penicillins through porin channels

B. Transpeptidation reaction

C. Breakdown of the β-lactam ring

D. Inhibition of murein hydrolases

E. Binding of penicillins to the peptidoglycan layer

Difficulty level: Medium

46. A 64-year-old homeless man was taken to the emergency department because of chills, fever, nausea and vomiting, and a laceration in his left harm. Vital signs on admission were blood pressure 100/52 mm Hg, pulse 124 bpm, respirations 32/min, temperature (102.2°F, 39°C). Physical examination showed a critically ill patient with an infected wound, and microbiological tests from a wound specimen showed vancomycin-resistant *Staphylococcus aureus*. Emergency therapy was started. Which of the following drugs would be appropriate for this patient?

A. Cephalexin
B. Tobramycin
C. Aztreonam
D. Daptomycin
E. Imipenem
F. Gentamicin

Difficulty level: Medium

47. A 49-year-old man hospitalized for bacterial endocarditis had been receiving a treatment with two drugs given intravenously. One week into therapy, a routine urinalysis showed albuminuria, microscopic hematuria, and hyaline casts. Which of the following pairs of drugs most likely caused these findings?

A. Ampicillin and cephalexin
B. Amikacin and tobramycin
C. Erythromycin and tobramycin
D. Vancomycin and gentamicin
E. Aztreonam and erythromycin

Difficulty level: Easy

48. A 42-year-old man hospitalized for staphylococcal endocarditis developed hypotension, tachycardia, generalized pruritus, and facial flushing 15 minutes after receiving an intravenous injection of an antibiotic. Which of the following drugs most likely caused the patient's syndrome?

A. Imipenem
B. Vancomycin
C. Cefazolin
D. Oxacillin
E. Ampicillin
F. Cefepime

Difficulty level: Easy

49. A 49-year-old woman recently diagnosed with an uncomplicated urinary tract infection started a treatment with an antibiotic that impairs cell wall synthesis by inhibiting enolpyruvate transferase. Which of the following drugs has this mechanism of action?

A. Cephalothin
B. Vancomycin
C. Aztreonam
D. Fosfomycin
E. Imipenem

Difficulty level: Medium

50. A 53-year-old woman hospitalized for resection of breast carcinoma presented with fever (103.8°F, 39.4°C), cough, dyspnea, and viscid, currant jelly–like sputum 3 days after surgery. A Gram stain showed numerous gram-negative bacilli with large capsules. A chest radiograph showed dense right upper field infiltrates. A diagnosis of nosocomial pneumonia was made. Which of the following pairs of antibiotics would be most appropriate for the emergency therapy of this patient?

A. Vancomycin and oxacillin
B. Erythromycin and nafcillin
C. Cefoxitin and tobramycin
D. Penicillin G and gentamicin
E. Tetracycline and sulfametoxazole

Questions: VIII-2 Bacterial Protein Synthesis Inhibitors

Directions for questions **1–5**

Match each antibiotic drug with the appropriate description (each lettered option can be selected once, more than once, or not at all).

- **A.** Amikacin
- **B.** Azithromycin
- **C.** Chloramphenicol
- **D.** Clindamycin
- **E.** Demeclocycline
- **F.** Doxycycline
- **G.** Erythromycin
- **H.** Gentamicin
- **I.** Linezolid
- **J.** Neomycin
- **K.** Spectinomycin
- **L.** Streptomycin
- **M.** Paromomycin
- **N.** Tetracycline
- **O.** Tigecycline

Difficulty level: Easy

1. A glycylcycline antibiotic active against vancomycin-resistant staphylococci

Difficulty level: Easy

2. An aminoglycoside antibiotic active against amebiasis and giardiasis

Difficulty level: Easy

3. A macrolide antibiotic with a very long half-life (about 40 hours)

Difficulty level: Easy

4. A tetracycline antibiotic sometimes used in syndrome of inappropriate antidiuretic hormone secretion (SIADH)

Difficulty level: Easy

5. An aminoglycoside antibiotic sometimes used in hepatic encephalopathy

Difficulty level: Easy

6. A 45-year-old diabetic woman complained to her physician of pain in her right ear for the past 5 hours. Further exams led to the diagnosis of external otitis, and later the culture of ear exudate showed *Pseudomonas aeruginosa* as the main offending pathogen. The patient was given an antibiotic that causes misreading of the bacterial messenger RNA template leading to the production of aberrant bacterial proteins. Which of the following drugs was most likely administered?

- **A.** Piperacillin
- **B.** Ceftazidime
- **C.** Imipenem
- **D.** Aztreonam
- **E.** Gentamicin

Difficulty level: Easy

7. A 69-year-old man recently diagnosed with a *Proteus mirabilis* infection started treatment with a daily intramuscular injection of gentamicin. Which of the following pairs of properties best explains why the drug is usually administered once daily despite the short half-life of gentamicin (about 2 hours)?

- **A.** Time-dependent killing and bactericidal effect
- **B.** Extensive plasma protein binding and bactericidal effect
- **C.** Concentration-dependent killing and bacteriostatic effect
- **D.** Concentration-dependent killing and long postantibiotic effect
- **E.** Time-dependent killing and long postantibiotic effect

Difficulty level: Easy

8. A 3-year-old girl developed whooping cough. Parents and other close contacts of the patient should receive a 10-day course of which of the following drugs?

- **A.** Tetracycline
- **B.** Chloramphenicol
- **C.** Erythromycin
- **D.** Ciprofloxacin
- **E.** Ceftriaxone
- **F.** Ampicillin

Difficulty level: Easy

9. A 60-year-old man recently diagnosed with carcinoma of the colon was admitted to the hospital for colectomy. Which of the following drugs would be appropriate to be included in the oral prophylactic treatment of this patient to prevent surgical infection?

- **A.** Streptomycin
- **B.** Penicillin G
- **C.** Trimethoprim
- **D.** Neomycin
- **E.** Cephalothin
- **F.** Vancomycin

Difficulty level: Medium

10. A 45-year-old farmer presented to the clinic with fever (103.2°F, 39.5°C), chills, headache, and a dry cough. Chest x-ray showed extensive nodular infiltrates radiating from the hilum. History revealed that the man raised chickens and

that approximately 2 weeks ago he had lost a large number of them to an undiagnosed disease. The presumptive diagnosis of pneumonia was made, and an appropriate drug was prescribed. Which of the following correctly pairs the most likely offending pathogen with the appropriate treatment?

A. *Mycobacterium tuberculosis:* ceftazidime

B. *Chlamydia pneumoniae:* metronidazole

C. *Mycoplasma pneumoniae:* piperacillin

D. *Chlamydia trachomatis:* gentamicin

E. *Chlamydia psittaci:* doxycycline

Difficulty level: Easy

11. A 54-year-old man suffering from chronic renal insufficiency was about to receive gentamicin and piperacillin for sepsis, apparently due to gram-negative bacteria. The patient's creatinine clearance was about one half the normal value. The physician chose to change the dosage of gentamicin and maintain the normal dosing interval. Assuming that the usual gentamicin dose for sepsis is 100 mg every 8 hours, which of the following (in milligrams) would be an appropriate initial dose of gentamicin for this patient?

A. 110

B. 75

C. 200

D. 50

E. 150

F. 33

Difficulty level: Medium

12. A 51-year-old woman was admitted to the hospital with fever (102.7°F, 39.3°C), shaking chills, nausea and vomiting, flank pain, and hematuria. She had been suffering from chronic urinary tract infections for 1 year and from type II diabetes for 10 years. Further tests led to the diagnosis of acute pyelonephritis due to *Pseudomonas aeruginosa*. Which of the following pairs of drugs would be appropriate for this patient?

A. Piperacillin and tobramycin

B. Ampicillin and gentamicin

C. Imipenem and erythromycin

D. Cephalothin and amikacin

E. Ampicillin and doxycycline

Difficulty level: Easy

13. A 66-year-old woman complained to her physician of urinary urgency and burning pain during urination. A urine culture revealed that *Escherichia coli* was the offending organism, and a susceptibility test showed that the bacterium was resistant to aminoglycoside antibiotics. Which of the following mechanisms can account for the bacterial resistance to aminoglycosides?

A. Plasmid-mediated production of bacterial transferases

B. Decreased affinity of the drug for the 50S ribosomal subunit

C. Development of an active efflux pump

D. Mutation-induced change of bacterial peroxidase

E. Mutation-induced change of bacterial topoisomerases

Difficulty level: Medium

14. A 60-year-old man presented with fever (102°F, 38.9°C), general malaise, and tachypnea. The man had been hospitalized for the past 4 days for evaluation of stage C cardiac failure. Medical therapy on admission included furosemide, losartan, aspirin, and atenolol. Further tests led to the diagnosis of nosocomial pneumonia due to *Pseudomonas aeruginosa*, and a therapy with ceftazidime and amikacin was started. Because of his current cardiac therapy, the patient was at increased risk of which of the following adverse effects of amikacin?

A. Superinfections

B. Nephrotoxicity

C. Neuromuscular blockade

D. Ototoxicity

E. Peripheral neuritis

F. Optic nerve dysfunction

Difficulty level: Medium

15. A 62-year-old man complained to his physician of burning on urination and bladder pain. The man was wearing a permanent urinary catheter because of inoperable prostate hyperplasia. A urine culture was ordered, and a susceptibility test gave the following results:

Organism	Ticarcillin	Amikacin	Ceftazidime	Ciprofloxacin	TMP-SMX
Escherichia coli	S	S	I	S	S
Klebsiella pneumoniae	R	S	S	I	S
Pseudomonas aeruginosa	S	S	S	S	R
Proteus vulgaris	S	I	I	I	R

Abbreviations: I, intermediate; R, resistant; S, susceptible; TMP-SMX, trimethoprim-sulfametoxazole.

Which of the following drugs would be most appropriate for this patient?

A. Ticarcillin

B. Amikacin

C. Ceftazidime

D. Ciprofloxacin

E. Trimethoprim-sulfametoxazole

Difficulty level: Medium

16. A 72-year-old female resident of a nursing facility was admitted to the hospital because of steadily declining urine output over the past 3 days. The woman had been receiving an antibiotic for 2 weeks to treat a urinary tract infection apparently due to *Pseudomonas aeruginosa*. A urinalysis showed albuminuria, hematuria, and hyaline casts. Which of the following drugs most likely caused the patient's disorder?

   A. Piperacillin
   B. Tobramycin
   C. Aztreonam
   D. Vancomycin
   E. Rifampin

Difficulty level: Hard

17. A 35-year-old man presented with fever (101°F, 38.3°C), cough, and dyspnea. The man was hospitalized 1 week ago because he was found to be HIV positive, but no antiviral therapy had been initiated yet. Further exams led to the diagnosis of pneumonia, and 10 days of gentamicin therapy was able to cure the disease. Which of the following microorganisms was most likely the cause of the patient's acute illness?

   A. *Clostridium difficile*
   B. *Mycoplasma pneumoniae*
   C. *Bacteroides fragilis*
   D. *Borrelia recurrentis*
   E. *Enterobacter aerogenes*
   F. *Legionella pneumophila*

Difficulty level: Easy

18. A 45-year-old woman was diagnosed with a urinary tract infection due to gram-negative rods. The woman had been suffering from myasthenia gravis for 5 years. Which of the following antibiotics would be relatively contraindicated in this patient?

   A. Ceftriaxone
   B. Aztreonam
   C. Erythromycin
   D. Ciprofloxacin
   E. Tobramycin
   F. Cefepime

Difficulty level: Medium

19. A 15-year-old girl was admitted to the hospital because of fever (103.2°F, 39.5°C) and severe pain in her left leg. A bone scan showed inflammation in her left distal femur. Two blood cultures were positive for *Staphylococcus aureus*, and susceptibility testing showed that the bacterium was methicillin- and vancomycin-resistant. Therapy was started with an antibiotic that binds to the 23S portion of the 50S ribosomal subunit and inhibits the formation of the initiation complex. Which of the following drugs was most likely given?

   A. Tetracycline
   B. Erythromycin
   C. Imipenem
   D. Gentamicin
   E. Linezolid
   F. Tigecycline

Difficulty level: Easy

20. A 70-year-old woman complained to her physician of headache, nausea and vomiting, vertigo, tinnitus, and progressive loss of hearing. The woman had been receiving an antibiotic for 2 weeks to treat a urinary tract infection apparently due to *Serratia marcescens*. The drug used was most likely a member of which of the following antibiotic classes?

   A. Macrolides
   B. Tetracyclines
   C. Cephalosporins
   D. Sulfonamides
   E. Aminoglycosides

Difficulty level: Easy

21. A 14-year-old girl diagnosed with a respiratory tract infection started treatment with erythromycin. Which of the following molecular actions on bacterial cells most likely mediated the therapeutic effect of the drug in the patient's disease?

   A. Inhibition of DNA-dependent RNA polymerase
   B. Inhibition of DNA gyrase
   C. Production of aberrant bacterial proteins
   D. Blockade of translocation reaction
   E. Blockade of transfer RNA (tRNA) binding to the ribosome

Difficulty level: Easy

22. A 48-year-old-woman complained to her physician of fever (103.5°F, 39.7°C), nausea, vomiting, and bloody diarrhea for the past 3 days. Further exams identified the most likely offending pathogen, and a therapy with azithromycin was able to eliminate the diarrhea. Which of the following bacteria most likely caused the patient's disease?

A. *Escherichia coli*

B. *Campylobacter jejuni*

C. *Shigella dysenteriae*

D. *Salmonella enteritidis*

E. *Clostridium difficile*

F. *Entamoeba histolytica*

Difficulty level: Easy

23. A 17-year-old girl complained to her physician of watery diarrhea. Three days ago, she was diagnosed with streptococcal pharyngitis, and treatment with erythromycin was started. Which of the following best explains the most likely reason for this adverse effect of erythromycin?

A. Killing most bacteria of intestinal flora

B. Activation of motilin receptors in the gut

C. Inhibition of water reabsorption by colonic mucosa

D. Antibiotic-induced acute cholestatic hepatitis

E. Allergic reaction to erythromycin

Difficulty level: Medium

24. A 23-year-old woman complained to her physician of pain during urination and a mucoid-like vaginal discharge that started about 14 days after her last intercourse. A Gram stain of the exudate revealed gram-negative cocci. Treatment with ceftriaxone was prescribed. Which of the following drugs would be appropriate to add to the patient's regimen?

A. Ceftriaxone

B. Imipenem

C. Azithromycin

D. Aztreonam

E. Amikacin

F. Vancomycin

Difficulty level: Medium

25. A 68-year-old man hospitalized because of advanced renal insufficiency was found to have pneumonia due to *Pseudomonas aeruginosa*. An appropriate antibiotic treatment was planned, but the dose of the drug was reduced because its half-life can be 20 to 40 times longer in patients with kidney failure. Which of the following drugs was most likely prescribed?

A. Cefoperazone

B. Amikacin

C. Erythromycin

D. Clindamycin

E. Metronidazole

F. Vancomycin

Difficulty level: Medium

26. A 15-day-old baby boy was admitted to the pediatric ward with mucopurulent ocular discharge, edema of the eyelids, and peudomembrane formation. A Gram stain of the exudate revealed no microorganisms, but a Giemsa stain showed cells with cytoplasmic inclusions. Both topical and systemic treatments were prescribed. Which of the following drugs was most likely administered?

A. Tetracycline

B. Ampicillin

C. Ciprofloxacin

D. Trimethoprim-sulfamethoxazole

E. Erythromycin

F. Tobramycin

Difficulty level: Easy

27. A 65-year-old man complained to his physician of nervousness, insomnia, and palpitations. The man had been suffering from chronic obstructive pulmonary disease for several years and had been receiving therapy that included theophylline. A few days earlier, he had been diagnosed with streptococcal pharyngitis and started an appropriate treatment. The physician thought that the patient's symptoms were most likely due to an antibiotic–theophylline interaction. Which of the following antibiotics was most likely responsible for this interaction?

A. Penicillin G

B. Streptomycin

C. Doxycycline

D. Ceftriaxone

E. Erythromycin

F. Rifampin

Difficulty level: Medium

28. A 63-year-old alcoholic man presented to the emergency department with fever (102.2°F, 39°C), chest pain, and a cough producing mucoid sputum. Physical examination revealed a man in obvious distress with the following vital signs: blood pressure 140/85 mm Hg, pulse 55 bpm, respirations 22/min. Sputum culture showed gram-negative rods able to grow only on charcoal yeast extract agar. Which of the following antibiotics would be most appropriate for this patient?

A. Streptomycin

B. Penicillin G

C. Azithromycin

D. Vancomycin

E. Gentamicin

F. Metronidazole

Difficulty level: Easy

29. A 53-year-old man was admitted to the hospital with the admitting diagnosis of pneumonia. Further exams indicated that the pneumonia was due to *Mycoplasma pneumonia*, and treatment with an appropriate bacteriostatic antibiotic was started. The given drug most likely belonged to which of the following classes?

   A. Cephalosporins
   B. Aminoglycosides
   C. Macrolides
   D. Carbapenems
   E. Penicillins
   F. Fluoroquinolones

Difficulty level: Medium

30. A 48-year-old woman was hospitalized with the admitting diagnosis of polymorphic ventricular tachycardia. The woman had been suffering from depression and had been on amitriptyline for 3 months. Three days earlier, she complained of fever and sore throat and was started on antibiotics. Which of the following antibiotics most likely triggered the patient's tachycardia?

   A. Vancomycin
   B. Erythromycin
   C. Gentamicin
   D. Ceftriaxone
   E. Ampicillin
   F. Sulfametoxazole

Difficulty level: Medium

31. A 3-year-old boy was brought to the pediatrician's office by his mother because of a low-grade fever and a painful, enlarged inguinal lymph node. On questioning, the mother stated that the boy was scratched on his right leg by his pet cat 1 week earlier. A Gram stain of pus aspirated from the lymph node revealed many small, gram-negative rods. Which of the following correctly pairs the most likely offending pathogen with the appropriate treatment?

   A. *Enterococcus faecalis:* vancomycin
   B. *Clostridium difficile:* metronidazole
   C. *Bartonella enselae:* erythromycin
   D. *Bacteroides fragilis:* tobramycin
   E. *Actinomyces israelii:* penicillin G

Difficulty level: Medium

32. A 73-year-old man presented with fever (101.9°F, 38.8°C) and pain in the perineum and left buttock. Four days earlier, the man had undergone bowel surgery for colon cancer, which was complicated by escape of bowel contents into the peritoneal cavity. Medical history of the patient was significant for allergic reactions to several antibiotics, including penicillins and metronidazole. Further exams led to the diagnosis of acute peritonitis. The patient's illness responded to an empiric emergency treatment that included parenteral administration of clindamycin. Which of the following microorganisms was most likely the main cause of the patient's infection?

   A. *Legionella pneumophila*
   B. *Klebsiella pneumoniae*
   C. *Bacteroides fragilis*
   D. *Enterobacter aerogenes*
   E. *Proteus mirabilis*
   F. *Enterococcus faecalis*

Difficulty level: Medium

33. A 34-year-old pregnant woman developed severe pharyngitis that turned out to be due to *Streptococcus pyogenes*. Past history of the patient was significant for an anaphylactic reaction to ampicillin. Which of the following antibiotics would be most appropriate for this patient?

   A. Ceftriaxone
   B. Ceftazidime
   C. Imipenem
   D. Erythromycin
   E. Doxycycline
   F. Aztreonam

Difficulty level: Medium

34. A 58-year-old woman complained to her physician of bruising and nose bleeds. The woman, diagnosed with atrial fibrillation, had been taking warfarin for 1 year. One week earlier, she was diagnosed with mycoplasmal pneumonia and was started on antibiotic therapy. Which of the following drugs most likely mediated the patient's bleeding?

   A. Amoxicillin
   B. Erythromycin
   C. Amikacin
   D. Vancomycin
   E. Piperacillin
   F. Ceftriaxone

Difficulty level: Easy

35. A 23-year-old man complained to his physician of a severe sore throat and fever. Because the man was allergic to penicillin, erythromycin was prescribed, but 3 days later, the clinical picture was not improved. The physician changed the antibiotic because he suspected bacterial resistance to erythromycin. Which of the following mechanisms can account for resistance to macrolides?

A. Inhibition of the multidrug efflux pump

B. Production of drug-inactivating RNA polymerases

C. Alteration of the ribosomal binding site that prevents drug binding

D. Production of drug-inactivating glucuronosyl transferases

E. Inhibition of methylase enzymes that activate the drug

Difficulty level: Easy

36. A 49-year-old woman on vacation in the south of Italy presented with fever, headache, and a small, buttonlike skin ulcer, 5 mm (about 0.2 inch) in diameter, with a black center. The diagnosis of Mediterranean spotted fever was made, and the woman was prescribed doxycycline. Which of the following molecular actions most likely mediated the therapeutic effect of the drug in the patient's disease?

A. Inhibition of DNA-dependent RNA polymerase

B. Blockade of the formation of ribosomal initiation complex

C. Blockade of transpeptidation reaction

D. Blockade of binding of aminoacyl-transfer RNA (tRNA) to bacterial ribosomes

E. Inhibition of transpeptidase enzymes

Difficulty level: Medium

37. A 34-year-old woman presented to the clinic with mild fever (99.5°F, 37.5°C), fatigue, muscle and joint pain, and multiple red rashes with a clear center. She reported that 10 days ago she was bitten on the arm by a tiny tick. A circular skin lesion started at the bite site, expanded to 15 cm (about 6 inches) or so, and was followed by multiple, painless rashes. Physical examination confirmed the diagnosis of erythema migrans. Which of the following drugs would be appropriate for the patient at this stage?

A. Gentamicin

B. Metronidazole

C. Linezolid

D. Doxycycline

E. Vancomycin

Difficulty level: Medium

38. A 30-year-old man was admitted to the hospital with fever (103°F, 39.4°C), chills, tachycardia, vomiting, and muscle pain. He had the same symptoms 10 days earlier, just after a camping trip near the United States–Mexico border. The fever remained high for 3 days, then cleared abruptly. A thick blood smear with Giemsa stain revealed many threadlike bacteria with large, irregular coils. Which of the following correctly pairs the most likely disease with the appropriate treatment?

A. Syphilis: streptomycin

B. Brucellosis: streptomycin

C. Rocky Mountain spotted fever: doxycycline

D. Relapsing fever: doxycycline

E. Psittacosis: piperacillin

F. Histoplasmosis: ampicillin

Difficulty level: Easy

39. A 32-year-old woman on a vacation trip in East Asia was diagnosed with acute conjunctivitis. A topical treatment with chloramphenicol was able to completely heal the disease. Which of the following molecular actions most likely mediated the therapeutic efficacy of the drug in the patient's disease?

A. Inhibition of cross-linking of linear peptidoglycan chains

B. Blockade of the transpeptidation reaction of protein synthesis

C. Inhibition of relaxation of supercoiled bacterial DNA

D. Inhibition of ergosterol synthesis in the bacterial cell membrane

E. Misreading of the messenger RNA (mRNA) template in the ribosomal subunit

Difficulty level: Medium

40. An 1168-g (2.57-lb) preterm male born to a febrile mother presented with respiratory distress a few hours after the delivery. Physical examination and lab results suggested neonatal sepsis, and an empirical antibiotic therapy was instituted. Later, blood cultures indicated *Listeria monocytogenes* as the offending organism. Which of the following drugs would be most appropriate to administer in combination with ampicillin for the treatment of his infection?

A. Doxycycline

B. Gentamicin

C. Ceftriaxone

D. Erythromycin

E. Aztreonam

F. Metronidazole

Difficulty level: Easy

41. A 31-year-old pregnant woman who recently arrived from Uganda was diagnosed with lymphogranuloma venereum. The physician prescribed a treatment with erythromycin, as tetracyclines are contraindicated during pregnancy. Which of the following drug-induced adverse effects best describes the reason for this contraindication?

    A. Impairment of fetal growth
    B. Superinfections in the newborn
    C. Severe myelosuppression in the newborn
    D. Multiple fetal malformations
    E. Kernicterus in the newborn
    F. Early fetal death

Difficulty level: Medium

42. A 31-year-old man was hospitalized because of severe watery diarrhea, vomiting, and altered mental status. The man returned 1 day earlier from Latin America, where he visited with relatives, several of whom were recovering from an intestinal infection. Physical examination showed a critically ill patient with marked loss of tissue turgor, sunken eyes, and wrinkled skin. Lab tests on admission revealed hemoconcentration and severe metabolic acidosis. A diagnosis was made, and an emergency treatment was initiated that included the parenteral administration of doxycycline. Which of the following bacteria most likely caused the patient's disease?

    A. *Vibrio cholerae*
    B. *Bacteroides fragilis*
    C. *Enterobacter aerogenes*
    D. *Pseudomonas aeruginosa*
    E. *Clostridium difficile*

Difficulty level: Easy

43. A 24-year-old man was admitted to the hospital because of severe erythema that occurred a few minutes after exposure to sunlight. He reported that past and more prolonged exposures to sun had caused only a mild erythema. A few days earlier, the man had started on antibiotic treatment for nongonococcal urethritis. Which of the following antibiotics most likely caused the patient's erythema?

    A. Cefotetan
    B. Gentamicin
    C. Metronidazole
    D. Doxycycline
    E. Amoxicillin
    F. Linezolid

Difficulty level: Easy

44. A 33-year-old woman was hospitalized with fever (103.5°F, 39.7°C), chills, mental confusion, vomiting, and diarrhea. One week earlier, the woman had returned from a vacation in central Africa. A Giemsa stain confirmed the diagnosis of *Plasmodium falciparum* malaria. Because the patient came from a region with multidrug-resistant strains of *P. falciparum*, parenteral quinidine therapy was started. Which of the following would be a useful agent to add to her therapeutic regimen?

    A. Imipenem
    B. Azithromycin
    C. Doxycycline
    D. Gentamicin
    E. Piperacillin
    F. Cefepime

Difficulty level: Medium

45. A 76-year-old woman was admitted to the hospital because of fever (102.6°F, 39.2°C), shortness of breath, and cough productive of purulent sputum. X-ray of the chest showed several areas of infiltration with possible abscess formation. A blood culture indicated the infection was due to staphylococci, and a susceptibility test showed that they were resistant to methicillin and vancomycin. Which of the following antibiotic therapies would be most appropriate for this patient?

    A. Nafcillin
    B. Tetracycline
    C. Amikacin
    D. Cefoperazone
    E. Erythromycin
    F. Quinupristin/dalfopristin

Difficulty level: Easy

46. A 42-year-old farmer presented to his physician because he had fever that usually rose in the afternoon, subsided during the night, and was followed by drenching sweats. Further exams led to the diagnosis of brucellosis, and a suitable pharmacotherapy was prescribed. Which of the following pairs of drugs would be appropriate for the patient at this time?

    A. Rifampin and metronidazole
    B. Streptomycin and doxycycline
    C. Vancomycin and ampicillin
    D. Erythromycin and cephalothin
    E. Penicillin G and tobramycin

Difficulty level: Easy

47. A 38-year-old man presented to the hospital with fever (102.7°F, 39.2°C), severe retrobulbar headache, chills,

photophobia, muscular pains, and prostration. He reported he found a tick attached to his scalp 7 days earlier while camping in the mountains of Colorado. Physical examination revealed a rash of pink macules 2 to 5 mm (0.08–0.2 inch) spread all over his body. A presumptive diagnosis was made, and an empiric therapy was started. Which of the following antibiotics would be appropriate for this patient?

A. Imipenem
B. Doxycycline
C. Piperacillin
D. Gentamicin
E. Ceftazidime
F. Trimethoprim-sulfamethoxazole

Difficulty level: Easy

48. A 50-year-old woman recently diagnosed with gastric ulcer started a triple treatment for *Helicobacter pylori* infection that included tetracycline. Two weeks later, the *H. pylori* test was still positive, and the physician suspected the development of resistance to tetracycline. Which of the following mechanisms could account for the bacterial resistance to tetracyclines?

A. Increased access to the ribosomal binding site
B. Production of acetyltransferase enzymes
C. Increased permeability of the outer bacterial membrane
D. Production of RNA polymerase enzymes
E. Increased activity of the multidrug efflux pump

Difficulty level: Easy

49. A 25-year-old woman presented to the clinic because of vulvar itching and burning and a thick, cheesy vaginal discharge for the past 5 days. The woman had been taking an oral antibiotic for 2 months to treat moderate acne. Gram stain of a vaginal smear indicated *Candida albicans* as the offending pathogen. Which of the following drugs most likely contributed to the appearance of the patient's infection?

A. Cefazolin
B. Amikacin
C. Aztreonam
D. Fluconazole
E. Tetracycline
F. Metronidazole

Difficulty level: Medium

50. A 25-year-old man recently diagnosed with severe acne involving the face, back, and chest started a treatment that included tetracycline. The physician instructed the patient to avoid milk or dairy products within 2 hours of taking the medication, because dairy products can interact with tetracycline. Which of the following best explains the outcome of the interaction between tetracycline and dairy products?

A. Decreased drug binding to bacterial ribosome
B. Increased drug toxicity
C. Increased drug elimination
D. Decreased bacterial permeability to the drug
E. Decreased drug oral bioavailability

Questions: VIII-3 Inhibitors of Bacterial Nucleic Acid Synthesis or Function

Directions for questions **1–3**

Match each antibiotic drug with the appropriate description (each lettered option can be selected once, more than once, or not at all).

A. Ciprofloxacin
B. Metronidazole
C. Sulfadiazine
D. Sulfamethoxazole
E. Trimethoprim

Difficulty level: Easy

1. A prodrug that requires bacterial activation

Difficulty level: Easy

2. This drug blocks the last two steps in bacterial tetrahydrofolate biosynthesis

Difficulty level: Easy

3. Resistance to this drug may be due to a change in DNA gyrase

Difficulty level: Easy

4. An 83-year-old female resident in a nursing facility presented with fever (100.5°F, 38°C), dry cough, and general malaise. Further exams led to the diagnosis of hospital-acquired pneumonia due to *Pseudomonas aeruginosa*. Treatment was started with a drug that is effective against most gram-negative bacteria, as well as against some mycobacteria, mycoplasmas, chlamydiae, and rickettsiae. Which of the following drugs was most likely given?

A. Piperacillin
B. Ceftazidime
C. Ciprofloxacin
D. Erythromycin
E. Vancomycin

Difficulty level: Medium

5. A 53-year-old woman suffering from a urinary tract infection started a treatment with trimethoprim-sulfamethoxazole. One week later, burning upon urination was still pronounced, and the physician suspected that resistance to sulfamethoxazole had occurred. This resistance was most likely due to which of the following mechanisms?

   A. Increased permeability of bacterial cell membrane
   B. Decreased sulfonamide binding to bacterial ribosomes
   C. Increased production of para-aminobenzoic acid
   D. Decreased sulfonamides binding to dihydrofolate reductase
   E. Decreased activity of the multidrug efflux pump

Difficulty level: Medium

6. A 59-year-old man complained to his physician that his skin itched all over his body. Two weeks earlier, he had begun oral antibiotic therapy for acute pharyngitis. Physical examination showed a diffuse maculopapular rash. Which of the following drugs most likely caused the patient's dermatitis?

   A. Aztreonam
   B. Piperacillin
   C. Trimethoprim-sulfamethoxazole
   D. Vancomycin
   E. Gentamicin

Difficulty level: Easy

7. A 50-year-old obese man complained to his physician of a sharp pain in his left calf. Medical history indicated that 1 week ago he had started an antibiotic treatment for acute prostatitis. Further exams led to the diagnosis of Achilles tendon rupture. Which of the following drugs most likely led to the patient's leg pain?

   A. Ampicillin
   B. Doxycycline
   C. Ceftriaxone
   D. Erythromycin
   E. Ciprofloxacin

Difficulty level: Easy

8. A 46-year-old woman with a long history of recurrent urinary tract infection complained to her physician of burning on urination and bladder pain. The woman used antacids from time to time to treat annoying heartburn. The physician prescribed ciprofloxacin for 1 week and instructed the patient to avoid the use of antacids during the therapy. Which of the following statements best explains why antacids are contraindicated in patients taking fluoroquinolones?

   A. They decrease quinolone oral bioavailability.
   B. They increase the risk of quinolone-induced cartilage erosion.
   C. They decrease quinolone urinary excretion.
   D. They narrow the antibacterial activity spectrum of quinolones.
   E. They increase the risk of quinolone-induced torsades de pointes.

Difficulty level: Easy

9. A 22-year-old man who was on vacation in Mexico was seen at a local clinic because of malaise, fever (103.2°F, 39.5°C), tachycardia, nausea and vomiting, abdominal cramps and six loose, unformed, and bloody stools. The symptoms started 24 hours after a dinner at a local restaurant. A presumptive diagnosis was made, and pharmacotherapy was started. Which of the following drugs would be appropriate for this patient?

   A. Fluconazole
   B. Ciprofloxacin
   C. Cephalexin
   D. Vancomycin
   E. Dicloxacillin
   F. Linezolid

Difficulty level: Easy

10. A 49-year-old woman recently diagnosed with urinary tract infection started treatment with combined trimethoprim-sulfamethoxazole. Which of the following best explains the main reason for combining these two drugs?

   A. To retard the biotransformation of both drugs
   B. To decrease the risk of allergic reactions
   C. To increase patient compliance by administering a single preparation
   D. To obtain a bactericidal effect that is unlikely with either drug given alone
   E. To achieve longer duration of action of sulfamethoxazole

Difficulty level: Medium

11. A 64-year-old man was admitted to the hospital because of a 3-day history of fever, chest pain, cough, nausea, vomiting, and diarrhea. His past medical history was relevant for heavy cigarette smoking, surgery for prostatic hyperplasia, and intolerance to macrolide antibiotics. Vital signs were blood pressure 135/80 mm Hg, pulse 50 bpm, respirations 16/min, body temperature 102°F (38.8°C). A chest x-ray revealed a patchy infiltrate in the lower left lobe, and urinalysis showed microhematuria. Which of the following drugs would be appropriate for the therapy of the patient's disease?

A. Vancomycin
B. Gentamicin
C. Piperacillin
D. Ciprofloxacin
E. Erythromycin
F. Ceftriaxone

Difficulty level: Medium

12. A 30-year-old man recently diagnosed with otitis media started treatment with ciprofloxacin. A 7-day course was able to completely heal the disease. Which of the following bacteria most likely caused the patient's infection?

A. *Leptospira interrogans*
B. *Clostridium difficile*
C. *Nocardia asteroides*
D. *Borrelia burgdorferi*
E. *Haemophilus influenzae*

Difficulty level: Medium

13. A 47-year-old man was admitted to the hospital because of fever (103.1°F, 39.5°C), severe headache, weakness in his right arm and leg, and increasing drowsiness. The patient had a history of chronic sinusitis treated with a variety of oral antibiotics. His last episode of sinusitis occurred 1 month ago and apparently resolved with clindamycin therapy. A computed tomography scan revealed a left frontal lesion with a small amount of surrounding cerebral edema. A diagnosis of brain abscess was made, and the patient underwent stereotactic aspiration of the abscess under local anesthesia. Which of the following antibiotics would have been most appropriately included in the initial postsurgical therapy of this patient?

A. Amikacin
B. Metronidazole
C. Erythromycin
D. Aztreonam
E. Vancomycin

Difficulty level: Easy

14. A 42-year-old man recently diagnosed with mycoplasma pneumonia started a treatment with ciprofloxacin. Which of the following molecular actions most likely mediated the therapeutic effect of the drug in the patient's disease?

A. Inhibition of bacterial cell wall synthesis
B. Inhibition of relaxation of supercoiled bacterial DNA
C. Stimulation of synthesis of abnormal bacterial proteins
D. Inhibition of ergosterol synthesis in bacterial cell membrane
E. Stimulation of bacterial DNA helicase
F. Stimulation of bacterial DNA–dependent RNA polymerase

Difficulty level: Easy

15. A 50-year-old woman recently diagnosed with a urinary tract infection started treatment with trimethoprim-sulfamethoxazole. All symptoms disappeared after 1 week. Which of the following bacteria was most likely the cause of the patient's infection?

A. *Pseudomonas aeruginosa*
B. *Enterococcus fecium*
C. *Chlamydia trachomatis*
D. *Bacteroides fragilis*
E. *Escherichia coli*

Difficulty level: Easy

16. A 46-year-old woman complained of burning on urination and bladder pain. Her medical history was significant for recurrent urinary tract infections and for a congenital long QT syndrome detected during a routine visit 1 year ago. A clean catch midstream urine sample showed many gram-negative rods. Which of the following antibiotics would be contraindicated for this patient?

A. Ceftazidime
B. Aztreonam
C. Imipenem
D. Amoxicillin-clavulanate
E. Piperacillin
F. Ciprofloxacin

Difficulty level: Medium

17. A 37-year-old woman with AIDS was admitted to the hospital because of fever (100.4°F, 38°C), drenching night sweats, poor appetite, and an 18-lb (about 8-kg) weight loss over the past 3 months. She had a past medical history of intestinal candidiasis and cryptococcal meningitis. Physical examination revealed a cachectic woman with hepatospenomegaly. Chest radiography was unremarkable, and lab results showed a CD4+ lymphocyte count of 50 cells/mm^3. A presumptive diagnosis of *Mycobacterium avium* complex infection was made and later confirmed by a DNA probe test. Which of the following drugs should be included in the initial therapy of this patient?

A. Piperacillin
B. Acyclovir
C. Ciprofloxacin
D. Ceftazidime
E. Trimethoprim-sulfamethoxazole
F. Metronidazole

Difficulty level: Medium

18. A 44-year-old woman presented to the clinic with fever (101°F, 38.3°C) and cough productive of a small amount of greenish, thick sputum. The woman, suffering from pemphigus, had been receiving high-dose prednisone for 6 months. Physical examination revealed coarse breath sounds in the right lower lung, and a chest x-ray showed a 4-cm (1.6-inch) nodule with central cavitation. Examination of the sputum showed long branching filaments of gram-positive, acid-fast rods. Which of the following drugs would be appropriate to treat the patient's infection?

A. Ketoconazole
B. Rifampin
C. Erythromycin
D. Sulfadiazine
E. Amphotericin B

Difficulty level: Medium

19. A 47-year-old woman suffering from ulcerative colitis was admitted to the hospital with fever (103.5°F, 39.7°C) and severe abdominal pain. Physical examination showed an extremely ill patient with diffuse abdominal tenderness, profound dehydration, and bloody diarrhea. Further exams led to the diagnosis of fulminant colitis, and an emergency therapy was started. Which of the following antibiotics should be included in the treatment of this patient?

A. Metronidazole
B. Vancomycin
C. Ampicillin
D. Amikacin
E. Erythromycin
F. Trimethorpim-sulfamethoxazole

Difficulty level: Medium

20. A 36-year-old man presented to the clinic with fever (100.4°F, 38.6°C), nonproductive cough, mild dyspnea, and facial seborrheic dermatitis. The man was HIV seropositive, and his CD4 lymphocyte count was 100/mm³. A silver-stained preparation from bronchial lavage revealed a large number of cysts containing sporozoites. A diagnosis of pneumonia was made, and a treatment with trimethoprim-sulfamethoxazole for 14 days was able to cure the infection. Which of the following bacteria was most likely the cause of the patient's infection?

A. *Pseudomonas aeruginosa*
B. *Clostridium difficile*
C. *Mycoplasma pneumoniae*
D. *Rickettsia rickettsii*
E. *Treponema pallidum*
F. *Pneumocystis jiroveci*
G. *Enterococcus faecalis*

Difficulty level: Easy

21. A 52-year-old woman complained to her physician of recurrent epigastric pain. Endoscopy revealed a gastric ulcer, and biopsy results were positive for *Helicobacter pylori*. To eradicate *H. pylori,* the physician prescribed a therapy that included omeprazole and two antibiotics. Which of the following pairs of antibiotics would be appropriate for this patient?

A. Amoxicillin and gentamicin
B. Metronidazole and tetracycline
C. Erythromycin and vancomycin
D. Amoxicillin and rifampin
E. Metronidazole and vancomycin

Difficulty level: Easy

22. A 44-year-old man recently diagnosed with nocardiosis started a treatment with a high dose of sulfadiazine. Inhibition of which of the following bacterial enzymes most likely mediated the therapeutic effect of the drug in the patient's disease?

A. Purine phosphoribosyl transferase
B. Transpeptidase
C. Topoisomerase II
D. Dihydropteroate synthetase
E. Dihydrofolate reductase
F. RNA polymerase

Difficulty level: Medium

23. A 56-year-old man was admitted to the hospital with fever (101.7°F, 38.7°C), severe abdominal pain, and loose, bloody stools. Further exams led to the diagnosis of *Clostridium difficile*–associated colitis. Therapy with oral vancomycin was started, but 2 days later, the diarrhea was not improved. Which of the following changes in the therapy would be appropriate at this time?

A. Start on oral metronidazole.
B. Increase the dose of vancomycin.
C. Start on intravenous (IV) vancomycin.
D. Start on oral ceftazidime.
E. Start on IV amikacin.

Difficulty level: Medium

24. A 54-year-old alcoholic woman complained to her physician of weakness, drowsiness, and dyspnea on exertion. Medical history indicated she was diagnosed with acute cystitis 10 days earlier and started an antibacterial therapy. Pertinent results of blood tests were red blood cell count 3.2 × 10⁶/ mm³ (normal, female 3.5–5.5 × 10⁶/mm³), mean corpuscular volume 115 fL (normal 80–100 fL). Which of the following drugs most likely caused these lab results?

A. Ciprofloxacin
B. Vancomycin
C. Metronidazole
D. Trimethoprim
E. Doxycycline
F. Ceftazidime
G. Piperacillin

Difficulty level: Easy

25. A 75-year-old woman was admitted to the hospital with fever (102.6°F, 39.2°C), abdominal cramping, and foul-smelling, watery stools. A colonoscopy revealed exudative plaques attached to the surface of the inflamed colonic mucosa. The woman had been receiving high doses of ampicillin for 2 weeks to treat a urinary tract infection. Which of the following drugs would be most appropriate for this patient?

A. Piperacillin
B. Gentamicin
C. Doxycycline
D. Erythromycin
E. Metronidazole
F. Ciprofloxacin

Difficulty level: Easy

26. A 36-year-old woman complained to her physician that she became dizzy and suffered flushing and vomiting after drinking a double scotch. The woman, recently diagnosed with bacterial vaginosis, started an oral antibiotic therapy 1 week ago. Which of the following drugs most likely caused this interaction with alcohol?

A. Imipenem
B. Levofloxacin
C. Clindamycin
D. Piperacillin
E. Ceftriaxone
F. Metronidazole

Difficulty level: Medium

27. A 56-year-old Black woman complained to her physician of tiredness and fatigue. She also noticed that her urine had become dark. Medical history was significant for glucose-6-phosphate dehydrogenase deficiency and recurrent urinary tract infection. Five days earlier, the patient complained of burning sensation upon urination and started the prescribed antibiotic therapy. Urinalysis revealed bilirubin and urobilinogen. Which of the following drugs could have caused the patient's signs and symptoms?

A. Piperacillin
B. Gentamicin
C. Trimethoprim
D. Ceftriaxone
E. Ciprofloxacin
F. Sulfamethoxazole

Difficulty level: Medium

28. A 55-year-old woman complained to her physician of burning on urination, frequent urination, and bladder pain. A urine culture and susceptibility test showed that *Escherichia coli* was the main infecting organism and that it was resistant to ampicillin, cefotaxime, ciprofloxacin, and amikacin. Which of the following antibiotics would be most appropriate to treat the patient's infection?

A. Amoxicillin
B. Moxifloxacin
C. Vancomycin
D. Linezolid
E. Trimethoprim-sulfamethoxazole
F. Clindamycin

Difficulty level: Easy

29. A 34-year-old woman recently diagnosed with salpingitis due to *Bacteroides fragilis* started a treatment with a drug that is reduced by anaerobes to a highly reactive nitro radical anion able to damage bacterial DNA. Which of the following drugs did the patient most likely take?

A. Cefoxitin
B. Clindamycin
C. Imipenem
D. Metronidazole
E. Cefotetan

Difficulty level: Easy

30. A 28-year-old woman late in her third trimester of pregnancy complained to her physician of persistent burning upon urination. The patient's medical history was significant for recurrent urinary tract infections. An antibiotic treatment was prescribed. Which of the following drugs would be contraindicated in this patient because of a risk of kernicterus in the newborn?

A. Piperacillin
B. Sulfamethoxazole
C. Ceftriaxone
D. Imipenem
E. Gentamicin
F. Ciprofloxacin

Questions: VIII-4 Antimycobacterial Drugs

Directions for questions **1 and 2**

Match each antimycobacterial drug with the appropriate description (each lettered option can be selected once, more than once, or not at all).

- **A.** Amikacin
- **B.** Ciprofloxacin
- **C.** Clarithromycin
- **D.** Ethambutol
- **E.** Ethionamide
- **F.** Isoniazid
- **G.** Pyrazinamide
- **H.** Rifampin
- **I.** Streptomycin

Difficulty level: Easy

1. This drug imparts a harmless orange color to urine, sweat, and tears.

Difficulty level: Easy

2. This drug is effective against some atypical mycobacteria but not against *Mycobacterium tuberculosis.*

Difficulty level: Easy

3. A 31-year-old homosexual man was found to be HIV positive. Currently, he did not have symptoms of tuberculosis, but his tuberculin skin test was positive. A treatment with isoniazid was prescribed. The inhibition of synthesis of which of the following endogenous compounds most likely mediated the therapeutic effect of the drug in this patient?

- **A.** Mycolic acids
- **B.** Peptidoglycan
- **C.** Arabinosyl transferase
- **D.** Topoisomerase II
- **E.** DNA-dependent RNA polymerase

Difficulty level: Medium

4. A 56-year-old Hispanic man diagnosed with bone tuberculosis started a multidrug treatment, but 4 months later, the disease was minimally improved, and susceptibility testing showed a complete resistance to isoniazid. A high level of resistance of tubercle bacilli to isoniazid involves a decrease in the activity of which of the following enzymes?

- **A.** Catalase-peroxidase
- **B.** DNA-dependent RNA polymerase
- **C.** Topoisomerase II
- **D.** Acetyltransferase
- **E.** Transpeptidase

Difficulty level: Easy

5. A 49-year-old Asian woman recently diagnosed with tuberculosis started an appropriate multidrug therapy. Which of the drugs she was taking is inactivated by hepatic acetylation, the rate of which depends on genetic background?

- **A.** Streptomycin
- **B.** Ethambutol
- **C.** Rifampin
- **D.** Isoniazid
- **E.** Pyrazinamide

Difficulty level: Easy

6. A 36-year-old Black man recently diagnosed with pulmonary tuberculosis started a drug treatment that included rifampin. Inhibition of which of the following enzymes most likely mediated the therapeutic efficacy of rifampin in the patient's disease?

- **A.** DNA-dependent RNA polymerase
- **B.** Arabinosyl transferase
- **C.** Transpeptidase
- **D.** Topoisomerase II
- **E.** RNA-dependent DNA polymerase

Difficulty level: Easy

7. A 63-year-old man recently diagnosed with pulmonary tuberculosis started a multidrug treatment that included ethambutol. Inhibition of which of the following enzymes most likely mediated the therapeutic efficacy of the drug in the patient's disease?

- **A.** Dihydrofolate reductase
- **B.** Peptidyl transferase
- **C.** Arabinosyl transferase
- **D.** Enolpyruvate transpherase
- **E.** Dihydropteroate synthetase
- **F.** Transglycosylase

Difficulty level: Medium

8. A 34-year-old woman who was HIV positive presented with fever (100.8°F, 38.2°C), profuse night sweats, poor appetite, and a 20-lb (4.5-kg) weight loss over the past 5 months. Physical examination revealed a cachectic female with prominent oral thrush and mild splenomegaly. Her CD4+ lymphocyte count was 45 cells/mm^3 (normal > 500 cells/mm^3), and a DNA probe test confirmed the diagnosis of *Mycobacterium avium* complex infection. An appropriate multidrug regimen was started. Which of the following drugs was most likely included in the patient's pharmacotherapy?

A. Ceftriaxone
B. Linezolid
C. Metronidazole
D. Clarithromycin
E. Vancomycin

A. Piperacillin and tobramycin
B. Trimethoprim-sulfamethoxazole
C. Ciprofloxacin and azithromycin
D. Isoniazid and rifampin
E. Streptomycin and erythromycin

Difficulty level: Easy

9. A 28-year-old man underwent a tuberculin skin test (Mantoux method) that turned out to be positive. The man was the husband of a woman who had uncomplicated pulmonary tuberculosis treated at home with a multiple-drug regimen. The man was prescribed a drug to be taken daily for 6 months. Which of the following drugs was most likely given?

A. Amikacin
B. Ethambutol
C. Isoniazid
D. Ciprofloxacin
E. Pyrazinamide

Difficulty level: Easy

10. A 44-year-old woman complained of blurred vision and inability to distinguish green objects from red objects. The woman, recently diagnosed with cavitary pulmonary tuberculosis, had been receiving a three-drug combination regimen for 2 months. An eye examination indicated a narrowing of her visual field. Which of the following drugs most likely caused these adverse effects?

A. Isoniazid
B. Pyrazinamide
C. Streptomycin
D. Ethambutol
E. Ciprofloxacin

Difficulty level: Hard

11. A 34-year-old HIV-positive woman was admitted to the hospital because of a 4-week history of fatigue, increasing abdominal girth, exertional dyspnea, nocturnal dyspnea, and peripheral edema. Vital signs were pulse 80, blood pressure 90/70 mm Hg. Physical examination revealed prominent external jugular veins that became more distended during inspiration. The heart was slightly enlarged, and a third sound was noted in early diastole. A computed tomography scan showed a large pericardial effusion, and pericardiocentesis removed 500 mL of bloody fluid with a high protein content. A diagnosis of hemorrhagic pericarditis was made, and an appropriate therapy was prescribed. Which of the following pairs of drugs would be most appropriately included in the patient's regimen?

Difficulty level: Easy

12. A 10-year-old girl was brought to the emergency department by her mother, who said that her daughter had high fever (103.3°F, 39.6°C) and was irritable and lethargic. Physical examination showed nuchal rigidity and a positive Brudzinski sign. Subsequent exams led to the diagnosis of meningococcal meningitis. Which of the following drugs would have been appropriate prophylaxis for the health personnel assisting this girl?

A. Amikacin
B. Piperacillin
C. Isoniazid
D. Doxycycline
E. Rifampin

Difficulty level: Easy

13. A 47-year-old Hispanic man recently diagnosed with pulmonary tuberculosis started a multidrug treatment. One of the drugs he was given is active against most mycobacteria, many gram-positive and -negative bacteria, chlamydiae, rickettsiae, and poxviruses. Which of the following drugs has such a broad antibacterial spectrum?

A. Isoniazid
B. Rifampin
C. Streptomycin
D. Ethambutol
E. Pyrazinamide

Difficulty level: Medium

14. A 66-year-old man recently diagnosed with pulmonary tuberculosis started a three-drug treatment with isoniazid, rifampin, and ethambutol. The man, who had been suffering from atrial fibrillation for 4 years, was currently being treated with propranolol and warfarin. At this point, which of the following changes in the patient's therapeutic regimen would be appropriate?

A. Increase the dose of warfarin.
B. Decrease the dose of propranolol.
C. Add pyrazinamide to the current therapy.
D. Substitute isoniazid with streptomycin.
E. Substitute propranolol with digoxin.

Difficulty level: Medium

15. A 64-year-old alcoholic woman suffering from pulmonary tuberculosis complained of anorexia, nausea, and abdominal discomfort. She had been receiving isoniazid, ethambutol, and rifampin for 2 months. Lab results revealed an aspartate aminotransferase level of 330 U/L (normal 8–20 U/L). Which of the following best explains the reason for the patient's signs and symptoms?

    A. Rifampin-induced hemolytic anemia
    B. Rifampin-induced induction of the P-450 system
    C. Isoniazid-induced neuropathy
    D. Isoniazid-induced hepatitis
    E. Ethambutol-induced peripheral neuritis
    F. Ethambutol-induced hepatitis

Difficulty level: Easy

16. A 30-year-old man with AIDS was recently diagnosed with pulmonary tuberculosis and started a multidrug treatment with isoniazid, rifampin, pyrazinamide, and ethambutol. Which of the following best explains why ethambutol was added to the therapeutic regimen?

    A. To enhance the antibacterial activity of pyrazinamide
    B. To provide antibacterial activity against atypical mycobacteria
    C. To prevent the neurotoxic effects of isoniazid
    D. To prevent *Pneumocystis jiroveci* pneumonia
    E. To delay the emergence of drug resistance

Difficulty level: Medium

17. A 62-year-old man presented to the hospital complaining of anorexia, nausea and vomiting, and abdominal discomfort. He also had pain on motion and stiffness in several joints. The man, recently diagnosed with renal tuberculosis, started a four-drug combination regimen 1 month ago. Lab results showed serum aspartate aminotransferase of 280 U/L (normal 8–20 U/L) and serum uric acid of 25 mg /dL (normal 3.0–8.2 mg/dL). Which of the following drugs most likely caused the patient symptoms and signs?

    A. Rifampin
    B. Pyrazinamide
    C. Isoniazid
    D. Streptomycin
    E. Azithromycin

Difficulty level: Medium

18. A 35-year-old man recently diagnosed with pulmonary tuberculosis started a treatment with isoniazid, rifampin, pyrazinamide, and ethambutol, but 2 months later, susceptibility testing revealed a *Mycobacterium tuberculosis* resistant to isoniazid and pyrazinamide. These drugs were discontinued, and two other drugs were prescribed. Which of the following

pairs of drugs would be most appropriate for the patient at this time?

    A. Amikacin and vancomycin
    B. Ethionamide and azithromycin
    C. Imipemen and doxycycline
    D. Ceftriaxone and linezolid
    E. Streptomycin and moxifloxacin

Difficulty level: Easy

19. A 57-year-old man complained of a tingling sensation in his limbs and that his arms sometimes felt heavy. The man, who had been suffering from type II diabetes for 10 years, had been recently diagnosed with pulmonary tuberculosis and had been receiving isoniazid and rifampin for 1 month. The concomitant use of which of the following drugs would have most likely prevented the patient's neurologic symptoms?

    A. Folic acid
    B. Pyridoxine
    C. Cyanocobalamin
    D. Vitamin B_2
    E. Folinic acid

Difficulty level: Easy

20. A 13-year-old boy had been receiving a multidrug treatment for bone tuberculosis. After 4 months of therapy, susceptibility testing showed that the mycobacterium was resistant to isoniazid and rifampin. Which of the following was most likely the mechanism of mycobacterial resistance to rifampin in this patient?

    A. Blockade of mycolic acid synthesis
    B. Gene-induced changes in bacterial topoisomerase II
    C. Gene-induced changes in bacterial RNA polymerase
    D. Gene-induced changes in bacterial peptidyl transferase
    E. Increased bacterial acetylation of the drug

Difficulty level: Easy

21. A 44-year-old man who recently moved from Mexico to Los Angeles presented to the hospital because of a diffuse skin disease. Skin examination showed macules, nodules, and plaques over his face and thorax. Further exams led to the diagnosis of lepromatous leprosy, and an appropriate therapy was started. Which of the following drugs should be included in the therapeutic regimen of this patient?

    A. Ampicillin
    B. Ceftriaxone
    C. Metronidazole
    D. Dapsone
    E. Fluconazole
    F. Ivermectin

Difficulty level: Easy

22. A 33-year-old man had been receiving a multidrug treatment for pulmonary tuberculosis. After 3 months of therapy, susceptibility testing showed that the mycobacterium was resistant to isoniazid and ethambutol. Which of the following was most likely the mechanism of mycobacterial resistance to ethambutol in this patient?

A. Gene-induced changes in bacterial topoisomerase II
B. Increased bacterial metabolism of the drug
C. Gene-induced changes in bacterial arabinosyl transferase
D. Decrease activity of the bacterial multiefflux pump
E. Gene-induced changes in bacterial RNA polymerase
F. Decreased bacterial permeability to the drug

Questions: VIII-5 Antifungal Drugs

Directions for questions **1–3**

Match each antifungal drug with the appropriate description (each lettered option can be selected once, more than once, or not at all).

A. Amphotericin B
B. Caspofungin
C. Fluconazole
D. Flucytosine
E. Griseofulvin
F. Itraconazole
G. Nystatin
H. Terbinafine

Difficulty level: Easy

1. The antifungal spectrum of this drug is limited to *Candida* and *Aspergillus* species.

Difficulty level: Easy

2. This drug has the broadest antifungal spectrum but is used only in case of severe mycoses because of its toxicity.

Difficulty level: Easy

3. The mechanism of action of this drug involves the inhibition of the synthesis of β-glucan, an essential constituent of a fungal cell wall.

Difficulty level: Easy

4. A 42-year-old HIV-positive woman was recently diagnosed with invasive histoplasmosis and started a therapy with amphotericin B. Which of the following molecular actions most likely mediated the therapeutic effect of the drug in the patient's disease?

A. Activation of fungal cytochrome P-450 enzymes
B. Pore formation in fungal cell membrane
C. Inhibition of fungal cytochrome P-450 enzymes
D. Inhibition of fungal mitosis
E. Pore formation in the fungal cell wall

Difficulty level: Easy

5. A 39-year-old man living in New Mexico was recently diagnosed with pulmonary coccidioidomycosis. A treatment was started with a drug that acts by inhibiting the fungal P-450 system. Which of the following drugs was most likely administered?

A. Amphotericin B
B. Nystatin
C. Fluconazole
D. Flucytosine
E. Griseofulvin
F. Terbinafine

Difficulty level: Easy

6. A 42-year-old man with AIDS was admitted to the hospital because of a recent onset of tonic-clonic seizures. Physical examination suggested acute meningitis, and lab tests indicated cryptococcal infection. A treatment with amphotericin B and flucytosine was initiated but had to be suspended due to the appearance of severe adverse effects. An alternative treatment was initiated. Which of the following drugs would be most appropriate for the patient at this time?

A. Terbinafine
B. Griseofulvin
C. Nystatin
D. Caspofungin
E. Fluconazole

Difficulty level: Hard

7. A 53-year-old man presented to the clinic because of painful, erosive, markedly pruritic lesions on the glans penis, scrotum, and inguinal region for the past week. The man had a 10-year history of poorly controlled diabetes mellitus. Physical examination showed irregular, shallow, erythematous ulcerations. A wet preparation of ulcer secretions showed budding cells with pseudohyphae. A diagnosis was made, and an oral therapy was prescribed. Which of the following drugs would be appropriate for this patient?

A. Nystatin
B. Metronidazole
C. Fluconazole
D. Acyclovir
E. Mebendazole
F. Griseofulvin

Difficulty level: Easy

8. A 40-year-old woman with AIDS was admitted to the hospital because of fever (103.2°F, 39.5°C), cough, and chest pain over the past 12 hours. Physical examination revealed verrucose and vesicular skin lesions on her arms and face, and a chest x-ray showed scattered pulmonary lesions compatible with a granulomatous process. A blood culture displayed typical yeasts with chlamydospores. Which of the following correctly pairs the most likely offending pathogen with the appropriate treatment?

A. *Cryptococcus neoformans:* amphotericin B
B. *Trichophyton tonsurans:* griseofulvin
C. *Histoplasma capsulatum:* fluconazole
D. *Aspergillus fumigatus:* fluconazole
E. *Candida albicans:* amphotericin B

Difficulty level: Easy

9. A 43-year-old woman recently diagnosed with chromoblastomycosis started a treatment that included a drug that acts by inhibiting fungal DNA synthesis. Which of the following drugs was most likely given?

A. Fluorouracil
B. Cytarabine
C. Flucytosine
D. Griseofulvin
E. Fluconazole
F. Terbinafine

Difficulty level: Medium

10. A 30-year-old Mexican man who was a lifelong resident of the San Joaquin Valley, California, was admitted to the hospital because of a 4-day history of low-grade fever (99.9°F, 37.7°C), severe headache, irritability, and fatigue. Physical

examination showed stiff neck and Kerning sign. Microscopic analysis of the spinal fluid revealed spherules filled with endospores. Which of the following drugs was most likely administered to this patient for an appropriate therapy?

A. Itraconazole
B. Nystatin
C. Terbinafine
D. Fluconazole
E. Flucytosine
F. Zidovudine

Difficulty level: Hard

11. A 31-year-old man with AIDS was admitted to the emergency department with fever (102.4°F, 39.1°C), headache, confusion, muddled thinking, and vomiting. Physical examination revealed nuchal rigidity, diplopia, and loss of vision. An agglutination test of the spinal fluid for capsular polysaccharide antigen turned out to be positive. Which of the following treatments would be most appropriate for this patient?

A. Ampicillin and erythromycin
B. Saquinavir and foscarnet
C. Pyrimethamine and sulfadiazine
D. Amphotericin B and flucytosine
E. Tolnaftate and nystatin
F. Terbinafine and griseofulvin

Difficulty level: Medium

12. A 68-year-old man hospitalized because of prostate cancer developed fever (103.8°F, 39.9°C) 4 days after prostatectomy despite empirical antibacterial therapy. He had a urinary catheter and was treated with a combination of broad-spectrum antibiotics. The patient had been suffering from chronic renal insufficiency for the past year. Urinalysis showed many budding yeasts and cultures that were positive for *Candida albicans*. Which of the following drugs would be appropriate for systemic antifungal treatment of this patient?

A. Amphotericin B
B. Caspofungin
C. Piperacillin
D. Metronidazole
E. Griseofulvin
F. Nystatin

Difficulty level: Easy

13. A 37-year-old woman suffering from AIDS was recently diagnosed with systemic candidiasis, and an intravenous antifungal treatment was prescribed. One week later, the following lab results were obtained: serum creatinine 5.9 mg/dL (normal: 0.6–1.2 mg/dL), blood urea nitrogen (BUN)

53 mg/dL (normal 7–18 mg/dL), plasma potassium 2.3 mmol/L (normal 3.5–5.0 mmol/L). Which of the following drugs most likely caused these abnormal lab results?

A. Amphotericin B
B. Fluconazole
C. Griseofulvin
D. Flucytosine
E. Cyclosporine
F. Tobramycin

Difficulty level: Easy

14. A 29-year-old man presented to his physician with an annular lesion with raised borders on his left hand. Microscopic examination of skin scrapings revealed branching hyphae. The diagnosis of tinea manus was made, and the patient was prescribed terbinafine. Which of the following skin structures was most likely the site of action of the prescribed drug?

A. Stratum basale
B. Stratum spinosum
C. Stratum corneum
D. Pigment layer
E. Hair follicle
F. Hair shaft

Difficulty level: Medium

15. A 9-year-old girl was brought to the pediatrician by her mother because the girl had several small hairless patches on her scalp. Upon close physical examination, patches looking like black dots were seen on the skin surface. Microscopic examination revealed a dense sheath of spores around the hair. Which of the following drugs given orally would be appropriate for this patient?

A. Acyclovir
B. Metronidazole
C. Terbinafine
D. Vancomycin
E. Amphotericin B
F. Flucytosine

Difficulty level: Easy

16. A 34-year-old man with AIDS was admitted to the hospital because of fever (103.7°F, 39.8°C), severe headache, and mental confusion. Further exams led to the diagnosis of cryptococcal meningitis. An intravenous (IV) dose of hydrocortisone was administered, then an antibiotic therapy was started that included an IV infusion of amphotericin B. Hydrocortisone was most likely given to decrease which of the following drug-related adverse effects?

A. Red man syndrome
B. Nephrotoxicity
C. Hepatotoxicity
D. Infusion reaction
E. Hemolytic anemia
F. Exfoliative dermatitis

Difficulty level: Easy

17. A 33-year-old woman presented to her gynecologist with a 4-day history of perineal pruritus and a nonmalodorous, thick, cheesy vaginal discharge. The only medication the woman was taking was an oral contraceptive. A wet preparation of vaginal secretion showed budding yeast cells and pseudohyphae. A diagnosis was made, and a local therapy was prescribed. Which of the following correctly pairs the most likely offending pathogen with the appropriate treatment?

A. *Candida albicans:* griseofulvin
B. *C. albicans:* terbinafine
C. *C. albicans:* nystatin
D. *Blastomyces dermatitidis:* caspofungin
E. *B. dermatitidis:* terbinafine
F. *B. dermatitidis:* nystatin

Difficulty level: Medium

18. A 34-year-old man presented with fever (103.5°F, 39.6°C), cough, increasing dyspnea, and bloody sputum. The man, suffering from a non-Hodgkin lymphoma, was in the hospital for the second cycle of chemotherapy. A chest x-ray disclosed diffuse alveolar infiltrates on the right lobe and multiple small cavitary lesions on the left lobe. Bronchoalveolar lavage revealed fungal forms typical of the *Aspergillus* genus. Which of the following drugs would be appropriate for this patient?

A. Flucytosine
B. Terbinafine
C. Griseofulvin
D. Voriconazole
E. Nystatin

Difficulty level: Easy

19. A 63-year-old woman recently diagnosed with onychomycosis started a treatment with terbinafine. Inhibition of which of the following enzymes most likely mediated the therapeutic effect of the drug in the patient's disease?

A. Thymidylate synthase
B. Lanosterol synthetase
C. Squalene epoxidase
D. Transpeptidase
E. 7α-hydroxylase

Difficulty level: Medium

20. A 36-year-old HIV-positive man living near the Mississippi River was admitted to the hospital with a 3-week history of cough, productive yellow sputum, and progressive dyspnea of exertion, as well as a 14-lb (6.4-kg) weight loss. Physical examination disclosed prominent hepatospenomegaly and diffuse lymphadenopathy. Pertinent lab results on admission were CD4+ lymphocyte count 320 cells/mm^3 (normal > 500 cells/mm^3), lactate dehydrogenase 5000 IU/L (normal < 600 IU/L). A blood stain showed neutrophils containing small uninucleated, encapsulated microorganisms. A diagnosis was made, and an appropriate pharmacotherapy was started. Which of the following drugs would be most appropriate for this patient?

A. Amphotericin B
B. Isoniazid
C. Terbinafine
D. Streptomycin
E. Nystatin

Difficulty level: Easy

21. A 45-year-old farmer complained to his physician of a red itchy rash over his thorax and arms. One week earlier, the man had been diagnosed with a fungal infection on his face and started an appropriate drug treatment. After physical examination, the physician told the patient that the rash was most likely a photosensitivity reaction to the drug. Which of the following drugs most likely caused the adverse effect in this patient?

A. Flucytosine
B. Amphotericin B
C. Caspofungin
D. Griseofulvin
E. Doxycycline
F. Ciprofloxacin

Difficulty level: Medium

22. A 42-year-old HIV-positive woman was admitted to the emergency department with the admitting diagnosis of pneumonia. Further exams led to the diagnosis of cryptococcal pneumonia, and a treatment with liposomal amphotericin B was started. Which of the following best explains the primary advantage of liposomal preparations over the regular colloidal suspension of amphotericin B?

A. Decreased interactions with other drugs
B. Increased antifungal activity spectrum
C. Decreased systemic toxicity
D. Decreased drug clearance
E. Increased oral bioavailability

Difficulty level: Medium

23. A 34-year-old man with AIDS was admitted to the emergency department and diagnosed with severe invasive candidiasis. He was initially treated with an antifungal drug to rapidly reduce fungal burden, and the drug was then replaced with another agent for chronic therapy. Which of the following pairs of drugs were most likely given?

A. Amphotericin B and terbinafine
B. Caspofungin and griseofulvin
C. Caspofungin and metronidazole
D. Amphotericin B and fluconazole
E. Amphotericin B and mebendazole
F. Caspofungin and terbinafine

Difficulty level: Easy

24. A 45-year-old woman with AIDS had been receiving fluconazole for an esophageal *Candida* infection. The therapy was initially effective, but over time its efficacy decreased, and the physician thought that development of resistance had occurred. Which of the following was most likely the mechanism of fungal resistance to fluconazole in this patient?

A. Gene-induced changes in fungal topoisomerase II
B. Increased fungal metabolism of the drug
C. Gene-induced changes in fungal cytochrome P-450 enzymes
D. Decreased activity of fungal multiefflux pump
E. Gene-induced changes in fungal RNA polymerase
F. Decreased fungal permeability to the drug

Questions: VIII-6 Antiviral Drugs

Directions for questions **1–3**

Match each antiviral drug with the appropriate description (each lettered option can be selected once, more than once, or not at all).

A. Abacavir
B. Didanosine
C. Efavirenz
D. Enfuvirtide
E. Fomivirsen
F. Lamivudine
G. Maraviroc
H. Oseltamivir
I. Raltegravir
J. Ritonavir
K. Stavudine
L. Trifluridine
M. Zalcitabine

Difficulty level: Easy

1. A nucleoside reverse transcriptase inhibitor used to treat both HIV and hepatitis B viral infections

Difficulty level: Easy

2. This drug is active against HIV-1 but not against HIV-2 or other retroviruses.

Difficulty level: Easy

3. This drug is administered by intravitreal injection to treat cytomegalovirus retinitis.

Difficulty level: Easy

4. At a routine clinic visit, a 40-year-old man with a long history of AIDS was found to have a CD4+ lymphocyte count of 122 cells/mm³ (normal > 500 cells/mm³) despite his current highly active antiretroviral therapy. The physician decided to change the therapy and to include a drug that blocks the integration of reverse-transcribed HIV DNA into the chromosomes of host cells. Which of the following drugs was most likely given?

A. Zidovudine
B. Atazanavir
C. Lopinavir
D. Ritonavir
E. Raltegravir

Difficulty level: Medium

5. A 35-year-old man with AIDS started a therapy that included a combination of lopinavir–ritonavir. Which of the following statements best explains the main reason for this combination regimen?

A. Lopinavir prevents ritonavir resistance.
B. Lopinavir inhibits ritonavir metabolism.
C. Lopinavir enhances ritonavir intestinal absorption.
D. Ritonavir prevents lopinavir resistance.
E. Ritonavir inhibits lopinavir metabolism.
F. Ritonavir enhances lopinavir intestinal absorption.

Difficulty level: Easy

6. A 30-year-old man with AIDS presented to the clinic complaining of recent weight gain. The man had been using a highly active antiretroviral therapy for 6 months. Physical examination showed a patient with truncal obesity and cushingoid appearance. Lab tests revealed hyperglycemia and hyperlipidemia. A drug from which of the following antiretroviral drug classes most likely caused these adverse effects?

A. Entry inhibitors
B. Nucleoside reverse transcriptase inhibitors
C. Nonnucleoside reverse transcriptase inhibitors
D. Integrase inhibitors
E. Protease inhibitors

Difficulty level: Medium

7. A 34-year-old woman reported to her physician that she had experienced genital burning pain for the past 2 days. The pain and burning were worse during urination and accompanied by fever and malaise. Physical examination revealed multiple blisters and ulcerative lesions in the vaginal area. A presumptive diagnosis of herpes genitalis was made, and an oral drug was prescribed. Which of the following steps of the viral growth cycle was most likely primarily inhibited by the prescribed drug?

A. Entry
B. Uncoating
C. Transcription
D. Translation
E. Proteolytic cleavage
F. Assembly

Difficulty level: Medium

8. A 33-year-old woman with AIDS was recently diagnosed with cytomegalovirus retinitis. The ophthalmologist prescribed a drug that must be phosphorylated first by virus-specific enzymes, then by host cell enzymes to become active. Which of the following drugs was most likely given?

A. Foscarnet
B. Ribavirin
C. Ganciclovir
D. Acyclovir
E. Vidarabine
F. Zidovudine

Difficulty level: Easy

9. An 80-year-old man was brought from a nursing home to the emergency department with chief complaints of fever (102.8°F, 39.3°C), cough, headache, malaise, anorexia, and photophobia. Conventional antibiotic therapy was ineffective, and 3 days later, influenza virus was detected from sputum. Over the next week, three other nursing home patients developed similar symptoms. Vaccination and chemoprophylaxis were planned for all nursing home residents and staff. Which of the following drugs would be appropriate to administer as a prophylactic measure?

A. Acyclovir
B. Foscarnet
C. Ribavirin
D. Ganciclovir
E. Oseltamivir
F. Zidovudine

Difficulty level: Medium

10. A 72-year-old man was admitted to the hospital with a 1-week history of malaise, night sweats, and increasing shortness of breath. Blood tests on admission were notable for hemoglobin 10 mg/dL (normal > 13.5 mg/dL) and creatinine 3.2 mg/dL (normal 0.6–1.2 mg/dL). On admission, physical examination showed a cyanotic and dyspneic patient in obvious distress. Auscultation revealed decreased lung sounds bilaterally. A viral culture from bronchoalveolar lavage was positive for herpes simplex virus. Parenteral therapy with acyclovir was started. The patient was at increased risk of developing which of the following adverse effects as a result of this therapy?

A. Hepatic cirrhosis
B. Renal failure
C. Hemolytic anemia
D. Neutropenia
E. Agranulocytosis
F. Pancreatitis

Difficulty level: Easy

11. A 74-year-old diabetic woman was brought to the emergency department with fever (102.7°F, 39.3°C), shaking chills, cough, headache, and malaise. Physical examination showed profound dyspnea, and rales were audible on auscultation of both lungs. Chest x-ray showed bilateral infiltrates, and blood gas analysis revealed significant hypoxia. A Gram stain of the sputum showed no bacteria. Fluorescent antibodies identified influenza A virus on cells of nasal aspirates. An appropriate therapy was started that included a drug that acts by inhibiting viral uncoating. Which of the following drugs was most likely given?

A. Foscarnet
B. Ganciclovir
C. Zidovudine
D. Amantadine
E. Cidofovir
F. Indinavir

Difficulty level: Easy

12. A 34-year-old man presented to the clinic with jaundice and complaints of incapacitating fatigue and vague intermittent abdominal pain for the past month. The patient had a history of intravenous drug abuse and alcohol abuse. Hepatitis serologic tests were positive for hepatitis B surface antigen. Which of the following drugs would be appropriate for this patient?

A. Enfuvirtide
B. Atazanavir
C. Amantadine
D. Interferon alfa-2a
E. Ganciclovir
F. Foscarnet

Difficulty level: Easy

13. A 30-year-old man with AIDS was recently diagnosed with cytomegalovirus retinitis, and a therapy with ganciclovir was started. Two weeks later, the disease was not much improved, and the ophthalmologist decided to add a drug that, unlike ganciclovir, can directly inhibit DNA polymerase without requiring activation by phosphorylation. Which of the following drugs was most likely prescribed?

A. Acyclovir
B. Lopinavir
C. Ribavirin
D. Foscarnet
E. Trifluridine
F. Nevirapine

Difficulty: Easy

14. A 23-year-old man had recurrent genital herpes that was effectively treated each time by acyclovir. The patient asked his physician why the treatment was not able to prevent recurrence. Which of the following would be the most appropriate answer for the physician to give?

   A. Acyclovir has a very short duration of action.
   B. Recurrence is due to a new contact with infected partners.
   C. Antiviral drugs have no effect on the latent state of viral disease.
   D. Recurrence is due to a hypersensitivity reaction to viral proteins.
   E. Resistance to acyclovir is the rule after one cycle of therapy.

Difficulty level: Medium

15. A 56-year-old man suffering from viral hepatitis B had started a treatment with interferon alfa-2a, but 9 months later, he was still positive for hepatitis B early antigen. The gastroenterologist decided to stop interferon and start another drug. Which of the following drugs would be appropriate for the patient at this time?

   A. Ganciclovir
   B. Lopinavir
   C. Raltegravir
   D. Nevirapine
   E. Didanosine
   F. Lamivudine

Difficulty level: Easy

16. A 34-year-old woman with AIDS was found to have a CD4+ lymphocyte count of 45 cells/mm³ (normal > 500 cells/mm³) at her last clinic visit. The patient had an extensive history of treatment with a variety of antiretroviral drugs and had been taking zidovudine, lamivudine, and ritonavir. A tropism test showed that her HIV used the CCR5 receptor to enter the host cells. Therapy was started with a drug that prevents entry. Which of the following drugs was most likely given?

   A. Ribavirin
   B. Enfuvirtide
   C. Didanosine
   D. Maraviroc
   E. Indinavir
   F. Atazanavir

Difficulty level: Easy

17. A 35-year-old man with AIDS was found to have a CD4+ lymphocyte count of 190 cells/mm³ (normal > 500 cells/mm³) at his last follow-up visit. The patient had an extensive history of treatment with a variety of drug regimens. He was currently taking, lopinavir, ritonavir, lamivudine, maraviroc, and raltegravir. Which of these drugs acts by inhibiting the viral enzyme that uses viral RNA to make a complementary DNA copy?

   A. Lopinavir
   B. Ritonavir
   C. Maraviroc
   D. Raltegravir
   E. Lamivudine

Difficulty level: Easy

18. A 43-year-old man with AIDS complained to his physician of multiple painful ulcers on his tongue and palate. Exfoliative cytology led to the diagnosis of herpes simplex infection, and therapy with oral acyclovir was initiated. Two weeks later, no improvement was seen, and the dose of the drug was increased, but without success. Which of the following was most likely the cause of failure of acyclovir therapy?

   A. Mutation of aspartate protease
   B. Viral transpeptidase deficiency
   C. Viral thymidine kinase deficiency
   D. Viral neuraminidase deficiency
   E. Mutation of reverse transcriptase

Difficulty level: Easy

19. A 5-month-old baby girl born prematurely at 31 weeks' gestation was found to have bronchopulmonary dysplasia and required oxygen administration. A respiratory syncytial virus (RSV) outbreak was ongoing in the community, and the pediatrician decided to prescribe a drug to prevent RSV infection. Which of the following drugs would be appropriate for this baby?

   A. Raltegravir
   B. Lopinavir
   C. Amantadine
   D. Lamivudine
   E. Palivizumab
   F. Trastuzumab

Difficulty level: Easy

20. A 61-year-old woman suffering from the hepatitis B virus (HBV) underwent a follow-up examination. She was found to have more than 10^5 HBV DNA copies/mL and alanine transaminase of 210 U/L (normal 8–20 U/L). Therapy with entecavir was started. Inhibition of which of the following viral enzymes most likely mediated the therapeutic effect of the drug in the patient's disease?

A. DNA polymerase
B. Phosphotransferase
C. RNA polymerase
D. HIV protease
E. Thymidine kinase
F. Neuraminidase

Difficulty level: Easy

21. A 47-year-old man with AIDS was found to have a CD4+ lymphocyte count of 170 cells/mm³ (normal > 500 cells/mm³) at his last clinic visit. The patient had an extensive history of treatment with a variety of antiretroviral drugs and had been currently taking abacavir, lamivudine, and atazanavir. The physician decided to add enfuvirtide to the current therapy. Which of the following steps of the viral growth cycle was most likely inhibited by the prescribed drug?

A. Entry
B. Uncoating
C. Transcription
D. Translation
E. Proteolytic cleavage
F. Assembly

Difficulty level: Medium

22. A 40-year-old man was recently found to be HIV positive, and he started a highly active antiretroviral therapy (HAART) with lamivudine, stavudine, and atazanavir. Which of the following two steps in the HIV growth cycle were specifically affected by this drug regimen?

A. Entry and proteolytic cleavage
B. Entry and uncoating
C. Transcription and attachment
D. Attachment and uncoating
E. Transcription and proteolytic cleavage

Difficulty level: Easy

23. A 32-year-old woman visited her physician complaining of very painful blisters on her abdomen. Physical examination showed localized blisters on her left abdomen consistent with a cutaneous zoster infection. Therapy with acyclovir was started. Which of the following enzymes was most likely inhibited by the administered drug?

A. Transpeptidase
B. DNA polymerase
C. Aspartate protease
D. Reverse transcriptase
E. Neuraminidase
F. Integrase

Difficulty level: Easy

24. A 71-year-old man was brought to the emergency department because of fever (103.2°F, 39.6°C), chills, dyspnea, and generalized aches in his back and legs. Social history of the patient was significant for an outbreak of flu in the community. A clinical diagnosis of influenza was made, and treatment with a neuraminidase inhibitor was started. Which of the following actions most likely mediated the therapeutic effect of the drug in the patient's disease?

A. Prevention of virus release from infected cells
B. Blockade of fusion of the virus with the host cell
C. Inhibition of viral transcription
D. Inhibition of viral proteolytic cleavage
E. Inhibition of viral protein synthesis

Difficulty level: Medium

25. A 31-year-old man with AIDS was recently diagnosed with cytomegalovirus pneumonia. The patient's current medications included zidovudine, didanosine, and atazanavir. Intravenous therapy with ganciclovir was started. Which of the following adverse effects would be predicted to be most likely to occur due to the concurrent administration of ganciclovir and the antiretroviral drugs?

A. Anemia and neutropenia
B. Retinal detachment
C. Cataract
D. Sexual dysfunction
E. Hyperglycemia
F. Lactic acidosis

Difficulty level: Medium

26. A 34-year-old woman with AIDS had been taking an antiretroviral therapy that included zalcitabine and stavudine. Which of the following adverse effects would be predicted to be most likely, as it is shared by both drugs?

A. Nephrolithiasis
B. Myelosuppression
C. Hallucinations
D. Peripheral neuropathy
E. Altered body fat distribution

Difficulty level: Easy

27. A 35-year-old man recently diagnosed with herpes simplex keratitis started a topical therapy with eye drops. Which of the following drugs would be appropriate for this patient?

A. Adefovir
B. Lopinavir
C. Nevirapine
D. Zidovudine
E. Trifluridine
F. Zanamivir

Difficulty level: Medium

28. A 35-year-old HIV-positive man presented for a follow-up visit. His CD4+ lymphocyte count was 350 cells/mm^3 (normal > 500 cells/mm^3). A highly active antiretroviral therapy (HAART) was initiated. Which of the following triple-drug regimens was most likely used?

A. Flucytosine + acyclovir + atazanavir
B. Didanosine + ganciclovir + zidovudine
C. Vidarabine + foscarnet + didanosine
D. Ribavirin + atazanavir + zidovudine
E. Zidovudine + didanosine + atazanavir

Difficulty level: Easy

29. A 34-year-old pregnant woman was admitted to the hospital at term for delivery. Two weeks earlier, the woman was diagnosed with asymptomatic HIV. An oral dose of nevirapine was given to the woman at the onset of labor. Which of the following best explains the reason for this administration?

A. To start a highly effective antiretroviral therapy
B. To reduce AIDS symptoms in the near future
C. To prevent bleeding after delivery
D. To prevent HIV transmission in the newborn
E. To prevent respiratory distress syndrome in the newborn

Difficulty level: Medium

30. A 31-year-old HIV-positive man at a routine clinic visit was found to have a CD4+ lymphocyte count of 122 cells/mm^3 (normal > 500 cells/mm^3). A highly active antiretroviral therapy was started that included a drug that does not require phosphorylation to become active. Which of the following is an antiretroviral drug with this property?

A. Efavirenz
B. Foscarnet
C. Stavudine
D. Lamivudine
E. Abacavir
F. Didanosine

Difficulty level: Easy

31. A 34-year-old man with AIDS presented to the clinic because of fever (103.4°F, 39.7°C), malaise, myalgias, nausea, and diarrhea. Three weeks earlier, the patient had started a highly active antiretroviral therapy. He stated that the symptoms were most prominent several hours after each dose and that they seemed to be getting progressively worse with each dose. Physical examination disclosed a fine maculopapular rash over his face, trunk, and arms. Which of the following drugs most likely caused the patient's syndrome?

A. Zidovudine
B. Ribavirin
C. Foscarnet
D. Abacavir
E. Lamivudine
F. Zanamivir

Difficulty level: Medium

32. A 12-day-old premature baby boy developed a poor feeding pattern, irritability, and respiratory distress. His mother, who had suffered several episodes of genital herpes, had presented to the hospital in labor with premature rupture of the membranes. Physical examination of the baby revealed several small vesicular skin lesions located on the scalp, and dendritic keratitis was present in both eyes. Which of the following drugs would be appropriate to include in the therapeutic treatment of this baby?

A. Atazanavir
B. Acyclovir
C. Zidovudine
D. Pentamidine
E. Fluconazole
F. Metronidazole

Difficulty level: Easy

33. A 25-year-old man recently diagnosed with AIDS started an antiretroviral therapy that included atazanavir. Which of the following steps of the viral growth cycle was primarily inhibited by this drug?

A. Entry
B. Uncoating
C. Transcription
D. Translation
E. Proteolytic cleavage
F. Assembly

Difficulty level: Easy

34. A 39-year-old man with AIDS was taking an antiretroviral therapy that included a drug with a pronounced inhibitory effect on CYP3A4. Which of the following drugs most likely has this inhibitory action?

A. Atazanavir
B. Zidovudine
C. Lamivudine
D. Ritonavir
E. Enfuvirtide

Difficulty level: Hard

35. A 71-year-old woman was admitted to the hospital with a 2-day history of progressive dyspnea, fever, cough, and wheezing. A chest radiograph was normal, but a bronchoscopy showed marked erythema of the trachea and bronchi, with multiple ulcerations. A bronchial biopsy confirmed the diagnosis of herpetic tracheobronchitis. The patient received intravenous acyclovir for 3 days, but no improvement was seen. Resistance to acyclovir was suspected, and an alternative drug was given intravenously. Which of the following drugs would be most appropriate for the patient at this time?

A. Foscarnet
B. Atazanavir
C. Amantadine
D. Zidovudine
E. Trifluridine

Difficulty level: Easy

36. A 43-year-old woman with AIDS started a highly active antiretroviral therapy with zidovudine, lamivudine, and atazanavir. Which of the following reasons best explains an important rationale for triple therapy in AIDS patients?

A. To destroy both the replicating and nonreplicating viral genome
B. To increase the half-life of any one of the agents
C. To delay the appearance of drug resistance
D. To inhibit each other's drug metabolism
E. To expand the antimicrobial efficacy to opportunistic infections

Difficulty level: Hard

37. A 43-year-old HIV-positive woman was admitted to the hospital with a 2-day history of nausea, vomiting, and severe epigastric pain radiating through to the back. The woman had been taking an antiretroviral therapy for 3 months. Vital signs on admission were: blood pressure 100/50 mm Hg, heart rate 130 bpm, respirations 32/min and shallow. Physical examination showed an acutely ill and sweaty patient with abdominal distention, tenderness in the epigastric area, and absent bowel sounds. Lab results on admission revealed serum amylase of 520 IU/L (normal < 115 IU/L). A preliminary diagnosis was made. Which of the following antiviral drugs most likely caused the patient's disorder?

A. Zidovudine
B. Lamivudine
C. Didanosine
D. Abacavir
E. Ribavirin
F. Acyclovir

Difficulty level: Medium

38. A 5-year-old girl was admitted to the emergency department because of fever (102°F, 38.8°C) and disorientation in time and space. Soon after admission, the patient had a seizure. Ceftriaxone and dexamethasone were initiated, but the next day, the patient became lethargic and lapsed into a coma. Examination of the cerebrospinal fluid revealed no bacteria. A computed tomography scan of the head showed decreased density in a small area of the right parietal lobe of the brain. Intravenous acyclovir was started, and 5 days later, the child was alert, responsive, and actively moving. Which of the following diseases most likely caused the patient's signs and symptoms?

A. *Neisseria* meningitis
B. Toxoplasmic encephalitis
C. Cryptococcal meningitis
D. Cytomegalovirus encephalitis
E. Herpes encephalitis

Difficulty level: Medium

39. A 41-year-old woman with AIDS started a highly active antiretroviral therapy that included abacavir and efavirenz. Which of the following adverse effects would most likely be predicted because it was shared by both drugs?

A. Erythematous skin rash
B. Hallucinations
C. Liver cirrhosis
D. Pancreatitis
E. Macrocytic anemia
F. Lactic acidosis

Difficulty level: Medium

40. A 23-year-old woman with AIDS came to the clinic complaining of floating spots in her vision and difficulty in reading. Funduscopic examination revealed the presence of alternating areas of hemorrhagic tissue and fluffy white patches in the proximity of the retinas of both eyes, consistent with hemorrhagic retinitis. Which of the following drugs would be appropriate for the treatment of the patient's ocular disorder?

A. Amantadine
B. Ribavirin
C. Ganciclovir
D. Lopinavir
E. Gentamicin
F. Doxycycline

Questions: VIII-7 Antiprotozoal Drugs

Directions for questions **1–5**

Match each antiprotozoal drug with the appropriate description (each lettered option can be selected once, more than once, or not at all).

A. Chloroquine
B. Clindamycin
C. Doxycycline
D. Iodoquinol
E. Mefloquine
F. Metronidazole
G. Paromomycin
H. Primaquine
I. Pyrimethamine
J. Quinine
K. Sodium stibogluconate
L. Sulfadoxine
M. Nifurtimox

Difficulty level: Easy

1. An effective blood schizonticide also used in the treatment of rheumatoid arthritis

Difficulty level: Easy

2. This drug can kill most anaerobic bacteria and anaerobic protozoa.

Difficulty level: Easy

3. An antimalarial drug with a very long half-life (about 20 days)

Difficulty level: Easy

4. This antimalarial drug can kill the late tissue schizonts of *Plasmodium vivax* and *Plasmodium ovale.*

Difficulty level: Easy

5. The first-line agent to treat acute American trypanosomiasis (Chagas disease)

Difficulty level: Easy

6. A 45-year-old male reporter who was about to leave for Honduras started a prophylactic antimalarial treatment with chloroquine. Which of the following molecular actions most likely mediated the prophylactic effect of the drug in this man?

A. Inhibition of dihydropteroate synthase
B. Blockade of translocation of peptidyl transfer RNA (tRNA)
C. Incorrect amino acid incorporation into the polypeptide chain
D. Inhibition of DNA-dependent RNA polymerase
E. Prevention of polymerization of free heme into hemozoin

Difficulty level: Easy

7. A 55-year-old man who was about to leave for a vacation trip to Central Africa started a prophylactic treatment with mefloquine. Which of the following plasmodia can be effectively killed by the drug?

A. *Plasmodium vivax* hypnozoites
B. *P. falciparum* gametocytes
C. *P. vivax* tissue schizonts
D. *P. falciparum* tissue schizonts
E. *P. malariae* blood schizonts
F. *P. malariae* tissue schizonts

Difficulty level: Easy

8. A 43-year-old man who was about to leave for a vacation in the Amazon basin was advised by his physician to take malarone (atovaquone and proguanil) as a prophylactic measure, as chloroquine resistance was widespread in those regions. Which of the following reasons best explains the likely mechanism of plasmodial resistance to chloroquine?

A. Increased inactivation of the drug
B. Increased activity of the DNA repair mechanism
C. Increased drug transport out of plasmodia cells
D. Decreased chloroquine-binding sites on plasmodia cells
E. Decreased conversion of free heme into hemozoin

Difficulty level: Easy

9. A 45-year-old Black man reported to his physician that a few days earlier he had noticed a persistent yellow color in his eyes. One week ago, coming back from a trip to Central America, the man had started a treatment that included primaquine. Blood tests disclosed the following:

- Red blood cell count: 3.8×10^6/mm³ (normal, male 4.3–5.9×10^6/mm³)
- Hemoglobin: 9 g/dL (normal, male 13.5–17.5 g/dL)
- Reticulocytes: 3.7% of red cells (normal 0.5–1.5%)
- White blood cell count: 15,000/mm³ (normal 4500–11,000/ mm³)

The physician told the patient that he probably had a genetically induced enzyme defect that could explain his blood test results. Which of the following enzymes was most likely abnormal in this patient?

A. Thymidylate synthase
B. Uroporphyrinogen decarboxylase
C. Pyruvate kinase
D. Dihydrofolate reductase
E. Glucose-6-phosphate-dehydrogenase

Difficulty level: Medium

10. A 41-year-old woman who had recently returned from a trip to Kenya was admitted to the hospital because of malaise, myalgia, abdominal pain, and fever (104°F, 40°C). Recent history was significant for two paroxysmal attacks of chills, fever, and vomiting. The first attack lasted a day and was followed by a second, 36 hours later. Physical examination revealed an acutely ill patient complaining of severe abdominal pain. Palpation showed a tender, soft, and enlarged spleen. Examination of a stained blood specimen revealed ringlike and crescentlike forms within the red blood cells. Which of the following pairs of drugs would be appropriate for this patient?

A. Artesunate and doxycycline
B. Primaquine and clindamycin
C. Pyrimethamine and metronidazole
D. Chloroquine and paromomycin
E. Mefloquine and ciprofloxacin

Difficulty level: Easy

11. A 38-year-old man was planning a vacation to sub-Saharan Africa, where chloroquine-resistant strains of *Plasmodium falciparum* are present. Which of the following drug combinations would be appropriate to prevent malaria infection in this man?

A. Primaquine–quinine
B. Mefloquine–metronidazole
C. Atovaquone–proguanil
D. Doxycycline–iodoquinol
E. Chloroquine–paromomycin

Difficulty level: Medium

12. A 30-year-old epileptic woman presented to the clinic with a 5-day history of loose stools containing bloody mucus. Upon physical examination, her abdomen was soft but nontender. Laboratory examination of fresh stool showed *Entamoeba histolytica* trophozoites. A computed tomography scan was negative for gut wall or liver amebiasis. Which of the following drugs would be appropriate for this patient?

A. Metronidazole
B. Chloroquine
C. Clindamycin
D. Paromomycin
E. Pyrimethamine
F. Sulfadoxine

Difficulty level: Medium

13. A 30-year-old man with AIDS was admitted to the hospital with the preliminary diagnosis of pneumonia. Further tests led to the diagnosis of toxoplasmosis, and an appropriate combination therapy was started. Inhibition of which of the following protozoal enzymes most likely mediated the therapeutic effect of the therapy in this patient?

A. Purine phosphoribosyl transferase
B. Ornithine decarboxylase
C. Ferredoxin oxidoreductase
D. Glucose-6-phosphate dehydrogenase
E. Dihydrofolate reductase

Difficulty level: Easy

14. A 31-year-old man returning from a trip to Malaysia was admitted to the hospital with a 2-day history of fever, chills, and bouts of diarrhea. A Giemsa blood smear demonstrated *Plasmodium vivax* trophozoites. The patient was placed on chloroquine for 5 days and was then instructed to take another drug for 14 days. Which of the following drugs would be appropriate for the 14 days of therapy?

A. Primaquine
B. Mefloquine
C. Quinidine
D. Pyrimethamine
E. Doxycycline
F. Sulfadoxine

Difficulty level: Medium

15. A 29-year-old married woman complained to her physician of soreness of her vulva and pain during intercourse. Further tests led to a definitive diagnosis, and an appropriate therapy was started. The prescribed antibiotic acts by damaging microbial DNA through a highly reactive nitro radical anion. Which of the following drugs was most likely administered to the patient and to her husband?

A. Ampicillin
B. Gentamicin
C. Erythromycin
D. Metronidazole
E. Cefoperazone

Difficulty level: Medium

16. A 38-year-old woman who had recently returned from a vacation in Greece developed a red papule on her right arm that enlarged slowly and began to ulcerate but caused no pain. A few days later, multiple skin lesions developed. A smear taken from the skin lesions demonstrated the presence of amastigotes. Which of the following drugs would be most appropriate for this patient?

A. Metronidazole
B. Sodium stibogluconate
C. Doxycycline
D. Ceftriaxone
E. Chloroquine
F. Clindamycin

Difficulty level: Medium

17. A 31-year-old homosexual man presented to the clinic with a 10-day history of abdominal pain and multiple brown, watery stools. Physical examination revealed a tall man with abdominal distress. Vital signs were blood pressure 125/75 mm Hg, pulse 78 bpm, temperature 103.5°F (39.7°C). His abdomen was slightly distended with a tender mass palpable in the lower right quadrant, which an ultrasound examination revealed to be an abdominal abscess. A serologic test was positive for *Entamoeba histolytica*. Which of the following pairs of drugs would be appropriate for this patient?

A. Metronidazole and iodoquinol
B. Chloroquine and clindamycin
C. Metronidazole and pyrimethamine
D. Doxycycline and iodoquinol
E. Chloroquine and ciprofloxacin
F. Pyrimethamine and ciprofloxacin

Difficulty level: Medium

18. A 1700-g (3.8-lb) preterm female newborn presented with hydrocephalus and seizures. Further tests led to the diagnosis of congenital toxoplasmosis, and an appropriate therapy was started. Which of the following drug combinations would be most appropriate for this baby?

A. Gentamicin and piperacillin
B. Sulfadiazine and pyrimethamine
C. Vancomycin and ceftazidime
D. Isoniazid and rifampin
E. Streptomycin and tetracycline

Difficulty level: Medium

19. A 51-year-old alcoholic woman complained to her physician of abdominal discomfort and occasional foul-smelling diarrhea alternating with constipation for the past 3 weeks. The symptoms started after her return from a vacation trip to Guatemala. Heart-shaped trophozoites with four pairs of flagella and round cysts were observed in her stool specimen. Which of the following drugs would be most appropriate to prescribe to this patient?

A. Paromomycin
B. Metronidazole
C. Primaquine
D. Ciprofloxacin
E. Pyrimethamine
F. Fluconazole

Difficulty level: Easy

20. A 34-year-old black man living in the United States was planning to visit his seriously ill father who lives in Uganda. He was going to be accompanied by his wife and son. Knowing that chloroquine-resistant strains of malaria are present in Uganda, which of the following drugs used alone would be the most appropriate prophylaxis for the man, his wife, and their son before entering Uganda?

A. Primaquine
B. Metronidazole
C. Pyrimethamine
D. Mefloquine
E. Chloroquine
F. Quinine

Difficulty level: Medium

21. A 32-year-old woman complained to the nurse of a sudden increase in her heart rate. Four days earlier, the woman, who had recently returned from a trip to Uganda, was hospitalized with the presumptive diagnosis of malaria. The woman had been suffering from anorexia nervosa for 1 year. The *Plasmodium vivax* infection was confirmed, and the patient started an appropriate therapy. An electrocardiogram led to the diagnosis of torsades de pointes. Which of the following drugs most likely caused the patient's arrhythmia?

   A. Quinine
   B. Chloroquine
   C. Metronidazole
   D. Iodoquinol
   E. Artesunate
   F. Pyrimethamine

Difficulty level: Easy

22. A 44-year-old woman complained to her physician that the drug she was taking caused an oral thrush. One week earlier, the woman was diagnosed with amebiasis and started an appropriate treatment. Examination of the oral cavity showed white patches of a cheesy substance on a friable oral mucosa. Which of the following drugs most likely caused the adverse effect in this patient?

   A. Paromomycin
   B. Iodoquinol
   C. Tobramycin
   D. Metronidazole
   E. Mebendazole
   F. Fluconazole

Questions: VIII-8 Anthelmintic Drugs

Directions for questions **1–5**

Match each anthelmintic drug with the appropriate description (each lettered option can be selected once, more than once, or not at all).

   A. Albendazole
   B. Diethylcarbamazine
   C. Ivermectin
   D. Mebendazole
   E. Praziquantel
   F. Pyrantel pamoate

Difficulty level: Easy

1. The agent of choice for echinococcosis

Difficulty level: Easy

2. A drug active against most trematodes and cestodes

Difficulty level: Easy

3. A benzimidazole derivative with less than 10% oral bioavailability

Difficulty level: Easy

4. The agent of choice for onchocerciasis

Difficulty level: Easy

5. This drug most likely acts by increasing worm cell permeability to Ca^{2+}.

Difficulty level: Easy

6. A 14-year-old boy living in a rural area of the southern United States was diagnosed with strongyloidiasis. Treatment with ivermectin was started. Which of the following molecular actions on the worm cells most likely mediated the therapeutic effect of the drug in this patient?

   A. Inhibition of DNA polymerase
   B. Blockade of nicotinic receptors
   C. Inhibition of protein synthesis
   D. Activation Cl^- channels
   E. Increased membrane Ca^{2+} permeability

Difficulty level: Easy

7. A 56-year-old homeless man living in a poor area of southern California was seen at a local clinic because of abdominal pain, nausea, and vomiting over the past 12 hours. Physical examination revealed a malnourished man with diffuse abdominal tenderness. Stool exam showed numerous eggs of *Ascaris lumbricoides* and *Trichuris trichiura,* as well as rhabditiform larvae of *Strongyloides stercoralis.* An appropriate treatment was ordered. Which of the following drugs would be most appropriate to treat the patient's mixed worm infection?

   A. Metronidazole
   B. Diethylcarbamazine
   C. Ivermectin
   D. Praziquantel
   E. Mebendazole

Difficulty level: Medium

8. A 10-year-old boy who recently moved from India to the United States was admitted to the hospital with fever (103.4°F, 39.6°C) and acute lymphedema of the scrotum. Further exams led to the diagnosis of bancroftian filariasis, and pharmacotherapy was prescribed. Which of the following drugs would be most appropriate for this boy?

A. Mebendazole
B. Praziquantel
C. Metronidazole
D. Chloroquine
E. Diethylcarbamazine

Difficulty level: Medium

9. A 5-year-old boy was seen in his pediatrician's office. His mother said the boy had been very irritable and complained of abdominal discomfort and perianal pruritus on two occasions the previous week. The mother also noticed some very small motile worms in the boy's stools. Exam of a cellophane tape swab placed over the perianal skin demonstrated translucent eggs. Which of the following drugs would be appropriate for this child?

A. Ivermectin
B. Praziquantel
C. Pyrimethamine
D. Metronidazole
E. Mebendazole
F. Diethylcarbamazine

Difficulty level: Medium

10. A 31-year-old man was seen at a clinic with fever (103.2°F, 39.5°C), chills, nausea, abdominal pain, myalgia, and urticaria rashes. The man had taken a vacation trip to the Amazon River 4 weeks earlier. Stool exams upon admission disclosed eggs with a lateral spine and miracidium larvae inside. A diagnosis was made, and a pharmacotherapy was started. Which of the following pairs correctly matches the most likely offending pathogen with the appropriate treatment?

A. *Schistosoma mansoni:* praziquantel
B. *Taenia solium:* metronidazole
C. *Echinococcus granulosus:* ivermectin
D. *Enterobius vermicularis:* praziquantel
E. *Necator americanus:* metronidazole
F. *Diphyllobothrium latum:* ivermectin

Difficulty level: Easy

11. A 24-year-old man living in the US Great Lakes region was recently diagnosed with diphyllobothriasis. The physician prescribed a single tablet of praziquantel. Which of the following molecular actions on the worm cells most likely mediated the therapeutic effect of the drug in this patient?

A. Activation of topoisomerase II
B. Blockade of muscarinic receptors
C. Inhibition of gamma-aminobutyric acid (GABA)–mediated neurotransmission
D. Increased membrane permeability to calcium
E. Activation of GABA-mediated neurotransmission

Difficulty level: Easy

12. A 6-year-old girl who was living in a rural area of Texas was recently diagnosed with trichuriasis. Tablets of mebendazole were prescribed for 3 days. Which of the following molecular actions on the worm cells most likely mediated the therapeutic effect of the drug in this patient?

A. Stimulation of nicotinic receptors at the neuromuscular junction
B. Inhibition of dihydrofolate reductase
C. Enhancement of gamma-aminobutyric acid (GABA)–mediated neurotransmission
D. Inhibition of heme polymerase
E. Increased membrane permeability to calcium
F. Inhibition of microtubule polymerization and assembly

Difficulty level: Medium

13. A 53-year-old woman who had spent most of her adult life as a missionary in Senegal was referred to an ophthalmologist for evaluation of diminished visual acuity. An eye exam showed sclerosing keratitis and chorioretinal lesions. Physical examination disclosed firm, nontender subcutaneous nodules on her elbows, iliac bones, and knees. A skin biopsy showed microfilariae. Which of the following drugs would be appropriate for this patient?

A. Diethylcarbamazine
B. Praziquantel
C. Ivermectin
D. Fluconazole
E. Metronidazole

Difficulty level: Medium

14. A 32-year-old woman who recently moved to the United States from Japan was seen at the clinic because of dyspnea, chest pain, and blood in her sputum. Chest x-rays showed a diffuse infiltrate with pleural effusion. Lab exam of sputum was negative for pathogen bacteria but disclosed numerous large operculated eggs. A presumptive diagnosis was made, and pharmacotherapy was started. Which of the following drugs would be appropriate for this patient?

A. Metronidazole

B. Mebendazole

C. Diethylcarbamazine

D. Ivermectin

E. Praziquantel

Difficulty level: Medium

15. A 7-year-old girl who was living in a poor sanitation area of Mexico was brought by her mother to the family physician's office. The mother reported that the previous day, the girl had complained of abdominal cramps and was frightened by seeing some large, motile worms in her stools. Which of the following drugs would be appropriate for this girl?

A. Primaquine

B. Mebendazole

C. Fluconazole

D. Metronidazole

E. Praziquantel

F. Mefloquine

Difficulty level: Easy

16. A 41-year-old man was admitted to the hospital with fever (103.5°F, 39.7°C), dizziness, prostration, skin rashes, tachycardia, hypotension, and pain in the muscles, joints, and lymph glands. The man, who had lived in Guatemala for several years, was recently diagnosed with onchocerciasis and had started an appropriate medical therapy the day before. Which of the following drugs most likely caused the patient's syndrome?

A. Ivermectin

B. Praziquantel

C. Mebendazole

D. Ketoconazole

E. Amphotericin B

F. Mefloquine

Difficulty level: Medium

17. A 45-year-old man who raised sheep in California complained to his physician of abdominal pain over the past 3 days. Physical examination disclosed an abdominal mass, and a subsequent computed tomography scan showed a large liver

cyst. Aspiration of the cyst revealed hydatid sand. Pharmacotherapy was started, and the patient was scheduled for surgical removal of the cyst. Which of the following drugs would be appropriate for the patient at this time?

A. Metronidazole

B. Chloroquine

C. Ivermectin

D. Diethylcarbamazine

E. Albendazole

F. Ketoconazole

Difficulty level: Medium

18. A 13-year-old boy who had recently moved from Costa Rica to Los Angeles complained to the school nurse of vague abdominal pain and that he kept seeing "white noodle-like" objects in his stools. Examination of a cellophane tape swab placed over the perianal area and stool samples demonstrated proglottids and numerous free eggs. Which of the following drugs would be appropriate for this boy?

A. Ivermectin

B. Artemisin

C. Praziquantel

D. Metronidazole

E. Amphotericin B

F. Fluconazole

Difficulty level: Medium

19. A 10-year-old boy who was living in a poor rural area of the southeastern United States was seen at a clinic because of weakness, tachycardia, abdominal cramps, and diarrhea over the past 2 days. Physical examination disclosed a pale boy with evident signs of growth retardation. Blood tests revealed hypochromic-microcytic anemia, eosinophilia, and thrombocytopenia. A stool analysis showed occult blood and numerous thin-shelled oval eggs in the four-cell stage of segmentation. A diagnosis was made, and a medical therapy was prescribed. Which of the following pairs correctly matches the most likely offending pathogen with the appropriate treatment?

A. *Schistosoma mansoni:* ivermectin

B. *Onchocerca volvulus:* metronidazole

C. *Ascaris lumbricoides:* metronidazole

D. *Enterobius vermicularis:* ivermectin

E. *Necator americanus:* mebendazole

F. *Diphyllobothrium latum:* mebendazole

Difficulty level: Easy

20. A 6-year-old girl recently diagnosed with enterobiasis started a treatment with mebendazole, but after two cycles of therapy, many worms were still found in her stools. The physician decided to prescribe an alternative treatment. Which of the following drugs would be appropriate for the patient at this time?

A. Pyrantel pamoate
B. Praziquantel
C. Diethylcarbamazine
D. Metronidazole
E. Fluconazole

Difficulty level: Medium

21. A 46-year-old woman was admitted to the emergency department with fever (102.2°F, 39°C), diarrhea, poor appetite, and fatigue over the past 48 hours. History revealed that 2 weeks earlier, the woman had been diagnosed with ascariasis and started an appropriate treatment for 3 days. The treatment was repeated 4 days before admission. Physical examination showed a febrile patient with an erythematous rash over the chest and trunk. Pertinent blood exam results on admission were alanine aminotransferase 350 U/L (normal > 40 U/L), eosinophils 18% (normal > 3%). Tests for hepatitis A, B, and C were negative. Ultrasound of the abdomen was negative. Stools were negative for ova and parasites. A liver biopsy showed multiple granulomas with multinucleate

cells and active inflammation. Which of the following drugs most likely caused the patient's syndrome?

A. Mebendazole
B. Praziquantel
C. Diethylcarbamazine
D. Metronidazole
E. Fluconazole

Difficulty level: Medium

22. A 34-year-old man complained to his physician that the drug he was taking caused nausea, abdominal pain, loose stools, and itching. Three days earlier, the man had been diagnosed with *Taenia solium* infection and had started an appropriate therapy. The physician told the patient that his symptoms were common adverse effects of the drug and should subside in 1 or 2 days. Which of the following drugs most likely caused the patient's symptoms?

A. Diethylcarbamazine
B. Ivermectin
C. Pyrantel pamoate
D. Praziquantel
E. Metronidazole
F. Miconazole

Questions: VIII-9 Antineoplastic Drugs

Directions for questions 1–4

Match each anticancer drug with the appropriate molecular mechanism of action (each lettered option can be selected once, more than once, or not at all).

A. Asparaginase
B. Carmustine
C. Etoposide
D. Fluorouracil
E. Hydroxyurea
F. Imatinib
G. Methotrexate
H. Paclitaxel
I. Trastuzumab
J. Vincristine

Difficulty level: Easy

1. Covalent binding with nucleophilic groups on DNA bases

Difficulty level: Easy

2. Inhibition of ribonucleotide reductase

Difficulty level: Easy

3. Inhibition of thymidylate synthetase

Difficulty level: Easy

4. Inhibition of a mutated tyrosine kinase present in certain cancer cells

Difficulty level: Easy

5. A 63-year-old woman complained to her physician of intermittent back pain that was worse at night. History revealed that the woman had undergone a modified radical mastectomy 2 years earlier for infiltrating ductal carcinoma of the breast that turned out to be HER-2 (human epidermal growth factor receptor 2) positive. A computed tomography scan revealed bone metastases, and she was scheduled for high-dose combination chemotherapy. Which of the following drugs was most likely included in her treatment regimen?

A. Clomiphene
B. Leuprolide
C. Trastuzumab
D. Flutamide
E. Asparaginase
F. Finasteride

6. A 15-year-old boy suffering from acute lymphoblastic leukemia received a consolidation anticancer therapy that included high-dose methotrexate. Leucovorin was also given after methotrexate. Which of the following concepts specifically underlies this therapeutic strategy?

   A. log kill
   B. Recruitment
   C. Pulsing
   D. Combined modality strategy
   E. Rescue therapy

7. A 52-year-old woman recently diagnosed with malignant glioblastoma received radiation therapy followed by a cycle of combination therapy that included carmustine. Which of the following statements best explains why carmustine is most often used to treat central nervous system neoplasms?

   A. It inhibits only neuronal tumor cells.
   B. It can easily enter the brain.
   C. It has negligible neurologic adverse effects.
   D. It is taken up into neurons by the amine pump.
   E. It has a very long half-life (10 days).

8. A 61-year-old woman with advanced Hodgkin lymphoma began chemotherapy with the ABVD (doxorubicin, bleomycin, vinblastine, and dacarbazine) regimen. Which of the following molecular actions most likely mediated the therapeutic effect of doxorubicin in the patient's disease?

   A. It intercalates between DNA strands and inhibits topoisomerase II.
   B. It prevents microtubule disassembly into tubulin monomers.
   C. It prevents assembly of tubulin dimers into microtubules.
   D. It alkylates nucleophilic groups on DNA bases.
   E. It blocks the synthesis of both ribonucleotides and deoxynucleotides.

9. A 47-year-old man with non-Hodgkin lymphoma was admitted to the hospital to receive his fourth cycle of CHOP (cyclophosphamide, doxorubicin, vincristine, and prednisone) regimen plus rituximab. Physical examination revealed tachycardia, shortness of breath that worsened soon after lying flat, neck vein distention, pulmonary rales, and ankle edema. Which of the following drugs most likely caused these adverse effects?

   A. Cyclophosphamide
   B. Doxorubicin
   C. Prednisone
   D. Vincristine
   E. Rituximab

10. A 13-year-old boy was admitted to the hospital with a 10-day history of fever, general malaise, dizziness, and nosebleed. He had a 1-week history of an upper respiratory tract infection. A blood test revealed normochromic, normocytic anemia, and a differential white blood cell count showed 11% lymphoblasts. A bone marrow biopsy showed 95% lymphoblasts. Which of the following pairs of drugs would be most appropriate for the patient at this time?

    A. Cisplatin and etoposide
    B. Flutamide and goserelin
    C. Vincristine and prednisone
    D. Tamoxifen and anastrozole
    E. Fluorouracil and cisplatin

11. A 61-year-old man was found to have recurrent colon cancer. The primary tumor was removed 8 months previously, at which time adjuvant chemotherapy with fluorouracil and carboplatin was begun. The oncologist suspected that the cancer recurrence was related to resistance to fluorouracil. Which of the following mechanisms best explains the resistance to this drug?

    A. Decreased ability to phosphorylate pyrimidines
    B. Decreased activity of the cell efflux pump
    C. Increased intracellular concentration of a reduced folate
    D. Decreased activity of topoisomerase
    E. Decreased activity of thymidylate synthase

12. A 24-year-old man was admitted to the hospital because of abdominal discomfort and shortness of breath. The man was diagnosed with testicular cancer 16 month earlier, for which he underwent a radical inguinal orchiectomy. An abdominal computed tomography revealed a 10-cm mass, and a chest radiograph showed multiple nodules in the lung. The first course of a three-drug combination chemotherapy was started. Which of the following drugs was most likely included in the patient's combination chemotherapy?

    A. Carmustine
    B. Methotrexate
    C. Cytarabine
    D. Cisplatin
    E. Mercaptopurine
    F. Asparaginase

Difficulty level: Easy

13. A 26-year-old man complained of numbness in his fingers and the soles of his feet. Three weeks previously, he had started chemotherapy for acute lymphoblastic leukemia. Physical examination showed loss of ankle jerk and depression of deep tendon reflexes. Which of the following drugs most likely caused the patient's signs and symptoms?

    A. Vincristine
    B. Prednisone
    C. Methotrexate
    D. Mercaptopurine
    E. Doxorubicin

Difficulty level: Easy

14. A 44-year-old man recently diagnosed with Hodgkin lymphoma was about to receive his first MOPP (mechlorethamine, vincristine, procarbazine and prednisone) regimen. Which of the following components of this regimen is given intravenously and has vesicant activity that may cause tissue necrosis and sloughing in case of extravasation?

    A. Prednisone
    B. Vincristine
    C. Procarbazine
    D. Mechlorethamine

Difficulty level: Easy

15. A 47-year-old woman recently diagnosed with acute myelogenous leukemia started remission chemotherapy with daunorubicin and cytarabine. Which of the following molecular actions most likely mediated the therapeutic effect of cytarabine in the patient's disease?

    A. Inhibition of topoisomerase II
    B. Inhibition of DNA chain elongation
    C. Inhibition of adenosine deaminase
    D. Inhibition of microtubule assembly
    E. Inhibition of microtubule disassembly

Difficulty level: Easy

16. A 4-year-old boy diagnosed with Wilms tumor underwent surgery, followed by 18 weeks of vincristine and dactinomycin therapy. Which of the following molecular actions most likely mediated the therapeutic effect of dactinomycin in the patient's disease?

    A. Alkylation of nucleophilic groups on RNA bases
    B. Inhibition of dihydrofolate reductase
    C. Inhibition of pyrimidine biosynthesis
    D. Binding to double-stranded DNA
    E. Inhibition of free radical formation
    F. Inhibition of tyrosine kinases

Difficulty level: Easy

17. A 55-year-old man presented to his physician with complaints of swollen lymph nodes, occasional fevers, and night sweats. The biopsy of a supraclavicular lymph node led to the diagnosis of diffuse B-cell lymphoma. A standard therapeutic regimen was implemented with cyclophosphamide, doxorubicin, vincristine, and prednisone. Which of the following molecular actions most likely mediated the therapeutic effect of cyclophosphamide in the patient's disease?

    A. Formation of covalent bonds with DNA bases
    B. Prevention of DNA chain elongation
    C. Inhibition of thymidylate synthase
    D. Prevention of DNA resealing
    E. Inhibition of microtubule assembly

Difficulty level: Easy

18. A 59-year-old woman recently diagnosed with stage IV adenocarcinoma of the lung started the first cycle of anticancer chemotherapy. The regimen included a drug that binds to tubulin and prevents microtubule disassembly. Which of the following drugs has this mechanism of action?

    A. Asparaginase
    B. Trastuzumab
    C. Paclitaxel
    D. Methotrexate
    E. Cytarabine
    F. Hydroxyurea

Difficulty level: Easy

19. A 53-year-old man recently diagnosed with small cell lung cancer started chemotherapy with cisplatin and etoposide. Which of the following molecular actions most likely mediated the therapeutic effect of etoposide in the patient's disease?

    A. Inhibition of dihydrofolate reductase
    B. Inhibition of thymidylate synthase
    C. Prevention of resealing of nicked strands of DNA
    D. Alkylation of nucleophilic groups on RNA bases
    E. Inhibition of microtubule disassembly

Difficulty level: Easy

20. A 60-year-old man was admitted to the hospital with fever (100.1°F, 38.4°C), dyspnea, and nonproductive cough. Two weeks earlier, the patient had completed five courses of chemotherapy with cyclophosphamide, doxorubicin, vincristine, prednisone, and bleomycin for large-cell lymphoma. Chest x-ray showed diffuse bilateral infiltrates, and a lung biopsy revealed inflammation and fibrosis with no evidence of lymphoma. Bacterial, fungal, and viral cultures were negative. Which of the drugs administered to the patient most likely caused his pulmonary disorder?

   A. Cyclophosphamide
   B. Doxorubicin
   C. Vincristine
   D. Prednisone
   E. Bleomycin

Difficulty level: Easy

21. A 59-year-old woman with inoperable lung cancer had been receiving combination chemotherapy. Lab tests revealed the following plasma levels: creatinine 5.5 mg/dL (normal 0.6–1.2 mg/dL), blood urea nitrogen (BUN) 45 mg/dL (normal 7–18 mg/dL), Mg^{2+} 0.2 mmol/L (normal 1.5–2.0 mmol/L). Which of the following drugs most likely caused these lab results?

   A. Fluorouracil
   B. Doxorubicin
   C. Vincristine
   D. Cisplatin
   E. Paclitaxel

Difficulty level: Easy

22. A 6-year-old boy suffering from acute lymphoblastic leukemia started combination maintenance therapy. One of the administered drugs is inactive in its parent form and must be metabolized by the enzyme hypoxanthine-guanine phosphoribosyl transferase into a monophosphate nucleotide. Which of the following drugs undergoes this activation?

   A. Methotrexate
   B. Fluorouracil
   C. Cytarabine
   D. Asparaginase
   E. Doxorubicin
   F. Mercaptopurine

Difficulty level: Easy

23. A 60-year-old man underwent surgery to remove an adenocarcinoma of the colon. Because the regional lymph nodes showed evidence of tumor involvement, adjuvant therapy was initiated after surgery. Which of the following drugs would be most appropriately included in the therapeutic regimen of this patient?

   A. Cytarabine
   B. Fludarabine
   C. Asparaginase
   D. Hydroxyurea
   E. Fluorouracil

Difficulty level: Medium

24. A 45-year-old man recently diagnosed with small cell lung cancer started his first course of combination chemotherapy with cisplatin, topotecan, and etoposide. Which of the following peripheral blood cells most likely decreased first in this patient?

   A. Lymphocytes
   B. Platelets
   C. Monocytes
   D. Granulocytes
   E. Erythrocytes

Difficulty level: Easy

25. A 50-year-old woman underwent surgery to remove an ovarian carcinoma. Following surgery, she started her first course of combination chemotherapy in order to eradicate the remaining tumor cells. Which of the following pairs of drugs were most likely included in her combination regimen?

   A. Mercaptopurine and asparaginase
   B. Methotrexate and hydroxyurea
   C. Cytarabine and prednisone
   D. Methotrexate and tamoxifen
   E. Cisplatin and paclitaxel

Difficulty level: Easy

26. A 10-year-old boy suffering from acute lymphoblastic leukemia started maintenance therapy that included high dose methotrexate. Two weeks later, a blood test with differential showed a white blood cell count of 1800/mm³ (normal 4500–11,000/mm³). The oncologist believed the result was related to an excessive dose of methotrexate and ordered an antidote agent. Which of the following drugs would be appropriate for the patient at this time?

   A. Vitamin B_{12}
   B. Pyridoxine
   C. Folic acid
   D. Vitamin B_3
   E. Leucovorin

Difficulty level: Medium

27. A 49-year-old man presented to the clinic with increasing fatigue, anorexia, weight loss and widespread ecchymoses. A blood test revealed a white blood cell count of 70,000/mm³ with 90% myeloblasts, and a bone marrow biopsy showed blast cells that made up about 40% of the nucleated cells in the marrow (normal < 5%). A diagnosis was made and a pharmacotherapy was prescribed. Which of the following drugs should be included in the initial treatment of this patient?

A. Cisplatin
B. Paclitaxel
C. Bleomycin
D. Cytarabine
E. Fluorouracil

Difficulty level: Medium

28. A 32-year-old man recently diagnosed with acute myelogenous leukemia received standard remission chemotherapy with daunorubicin and cytarabine. Drug dosage was maximized to a toxicity limit of a 2-log decrease in blood platelets. Which of the following represents the percentage of platelets killed by the drug regimen?

A. 99.9%
B. 99%
C. 90%
D. 80%
E. 70%

Difficulty level: Easy

29. A 10-year-old hospitalized boy complained of tinnitus and hearing loss. The boy had been diagnosed with neuroblastoma and was receiving his first course of combination chemotherapy. Which of the following drugs most likely caused the patient's symptoms?

A. Cyclophosphamide
B. Vincristine
C. Doxorubicin
D. Dactinomycin
E. Cisplatin

Difficulty level: Medium

30. A 42-year-old man with stage III Hodgkin lymphoma received six courses of chemotherapy with the ABVD (doxorubicin, bleomycin, vinblastine, and dacarbazine) regimen. Which of the drugs in this regimen acts mainly in the G_2 phase of the tumor cell cycle?

A. Doxorubicin
B. Bleomycin
C. Vinblastine
D. Dacarbazine

Difficulty level: Medium

31. A 6-year-old hospitalized child complained of pain when urinating. A urine sample was cloudy and red. The child, diagnosed with neuroblastoma, had begun a chemotherapy program 5 days earlier. Which of the following drugs most likely caused the patient's symptoms?

A. Paclitaxel
B. Vincristine
C. Topotecan
D. Cisplatin
E. Doxorubicin
F. Cyclophosphamide

Difficulty level: Medium

32. A 7-year-old girl was seen by her pediatrician because of a 1-week history of upper respiratory tract infection, increasing weakness, and bleeding gums. Physical examination revealed hepatosplenomegaly. A blood test with differential showed a white blood cell count of 65,000/mm³ (normal 4500–11,000/mm³) with 43% lymphoblasts. A bone marrow biopsy revealed 92% lymphoblasts. A diagnosis was made, and the girl received a therapy that included the intrathecal administration of a drug. Which of the following drugs was most likely injected intrathecally?

A. Methotrexate
B. Paclitaxel
C. Etoposide
D. Bleomycin
E. Cisplatin
F. Chlorambucil

Difficulty level: Easy

33. A 36-year-old woman recently diagnosed with Hodgkin lymphoma started her first cycle of ABVD (doxorubicin, bleomycin, vinblastine, and dacarbazine) chemotherapy. Which of the following molecular actions most likely mediated the therapeutic effect of bleomycin in the patient's disease?

A. Formation of free radicals that cause DNA fragmentation
B. Inhibition of tubulin polymerization
C. Inhibition of thymidylate biosynthesis
D. DNA alkylation that blocks DNA strand scission
E. Inhibition of tetrahydrofolate biosynthesis

Difficulty level: Easy

34. A 40-year-old woman recently diagnosed with lymphoblastic T-cell lymphoma received her first combination chemotherapeutic regimen that included cyclophosphamide, vincristine, doxorubicin, and prednisone. From which of the following adverse effects was the patient most likely to suffer during the first day of treatment?

A. Neuropathy
B. Hemorrhagic cystitis
C. Pulmonary fibrosis
D. Congestive heart failure
E. Nausea and vomiting

Difficulty level: Easy

35. A 46-year-old woman who had undergone a radical mastectomy for infiltrating ductal carcinoma started adjuvant combination therapy with the CMF (cyclophosphamide, methotrexate, and fluorouracil) regimen. Which of the following was the initial molecular action that most likely mediated the therapeutic effect of methotrexate in the patient's disease?

A. Inhibition of purine biosynthesis
B. Inhibition of DNA chain elongation
C. Inhibition of single-stranded DNA resealing
D. DNA fragmentation through free radical formation
E. Inhibition of microtubule assembly

Difficulty level: Medium

36. A 47-year-old man presented to the clinic because of a 1-week history of low-grade fever, anorexia, increasing weakness, and weight loss. A blood test showed a white blood cell count of 90,000/mm³ (normal 4500–11,000/mm³) with 90% neutrophils and a platelet count of 500,000/mm³ (normal 150,000–400,000/mm³). Chromosomal studies on a bone marrow aspirate found the presence of the Philadelphia chromosome. A diagnosis was made, and a therapy was started. Which of the following drugs would be most appropriate to include in the patient's therapeutic regimen?

A. Hydroxyurea
B. Erythropoietin
C. Oprelvekin
D. Etoposide
E. Asparaginase
F. Fluorouracil

Difficulty level: Easy

37. An 8-year-old girl recently diagnosed with acute lymphoblastic leukemia started her first cycle of remission chemotherapy. The antineoplastic regimen included a drug that acts by depleting the body of an amino acid that can be synthesized by normal cells but not by neoplastic cells. Which of the following drugs has this mechanism of action?

A. Vincristine
B. Asparaginase
C. Daunorubicin
D. Prednisone
E. Methotrexate
F. Cytarabine

Difficulty level: Medium

38. A 69-year-old woman diagnosed with colon cancer started adjuvant chemotherapy with intravenous fluorouracil following surgery to remove the primary tumor. Which of the following drugs was most likely given concomitantly with the fluorouracil to increase its cytotoxic activity?

A. Folic acid
B. Asparaginase
C. Leucovorin
D. Trastuzumab
E. Sargramostim
F. Tamoxifen

Difficulty level: Easy

39. A 62-year-old man with testicular cancer was undergoing his first cycle of combination chemotherapy (cisplatin, vinblastine, and neomycin). Two years earlier, the patient had suffered from myocardial infarction. Which of the following procedures should be implemented to counteract the most common organ toxicity of cisplatin?

A. Administration of leucovorin
B. Vigorous hydration and furosemide
C. Administration of sargramostim
D. Short therapy cycles
E. Administration of prednisone

Difficulty level: Easy

40. A 5 year-old girl was found to have a lung nodule during a scheduled follow-up visit. The girl had undergone surgery for stage III Wilms tumor and then had been receiving a triple therapy with vincristine, doxorubicin, and dactinomycin for 10 weeks. The oncologist concluded that the tumor had become multidrug resistant. Which of the following mechanisms most likely mediated the simultaneous resistance to doxorubicin, vincristine, and dactinomycin in this patient?

A. Decreased activity of DNA repairing pathways
B. Decreased sensitivity of a target enzyme
C. Decreased cellular uptake of the drug
D. Loss of enzymes needed for drug activation
E. Enhanced activity of an outward transport system

Difficulty level: Medium

41. A 53-year-old woman recently diagnosed with ovarian cancer started her first cycle of combination chemotherapy with paclitaxel, cisplatin, and cyclophosphamide. Which of the following drugs should also be administered to counteract a specific adverse effect of cyclophosphamide?

A. Erythropoietin
B. Leucovorin
C. Mercaptoethane sulfonate
D. Acetylcysteine
E. Vitamin K

Difficulty level: Hard

42. A 65-year-old man presented to his family physician with a persistent cough. A routine complete blood count showed the following: hemoglobin 9 g/dL (normal, male 13.5–17.5 g/dL), white blood cell count 40,000/mm³ (normal 4500–10,500/mm³) with 85% lymphocytes (normal 25–33%), platelet count 90,000/mm³ (normal 150,000–400,000/mm³). Bone marrow examination revealed normal cellularity with 45% of nucleated cells lymphocytes. A diagnosis of leukemia was confirmed. Which of the following anticancer drug regimens would be most appropriate for this patient?

A. Etoposide and asparaginase
B. Vincristine and cisplatin
C. Hydroxyurea and topotecan
D. Methotrexate and paclitaxel
E. Chlorambucil and prednisone

Difficulty level: Easy

43. A 54-year-old man recently diagnosed with inoperable lung cancer started induction chemotherapy that included a drug that acts by forming both inter- and intrastrand cross-links in the DNA molecule. Which of the following drugs was most likely given?

A. Paclitaxel
B. Etoposide
C. Vincristine
D. Cisplatin
E. Fluorouracil

Difficulty level: Medium

44. A 35-year-old man diagnosed with malignant testicular teratoma was hospitalized to receive his fourth cycle of the BEP (bleomycin, etoposide, and cisplatin) regimen. The patient was most likely at increased risk of which of the following adverse effects as a result of his therapy?

A. Chronic myelogenous leukemia
B. Syndrome of inappropriate antidiuretic hormone (SIADH) secretion
C. Polymorphic ventricular tachycardia
D. Pulmonary embolism
E. Pneumonitis leading to lung fibrosis

Difficulty level: Easy

45. An 8-year-old girl suffering from acute lymphoblastic leukemia completed her remission chemotherapy with a multidrug regimen and started maintenance therapy with a regimen that included a cell cycle–specific anticancer drug administered daily, for 7 days every 4 weeks. Which of the following drugs did the patient most likely take for maintenance therapy?

A. Daunorubicin
B. Doxorubicin
C. Mercaptopurine
D. Cisplatin
E. Carmustine

Difficulty level: Easy

46. A 7-year-old boy recently diagnosed with Wilms tumor started a combination anticancer therapy that included vincristine. Inhibition of which of the following functions in cancer cells most likely mediated the therapeutic effect of the drug in the patient's disease?

A. Tubulin polymerization
B. Resealing of single-stranded DNA
C. Resealing of double-stranded DNA
D. Purine biosynthesis
E. RNA biosynthesis

Difficulty level: Medium

47. A 53-year-old woman recently diagnosed with ovarian cancer started a treatment that included paclitaxel. The patient was most likely at increased risk of which of the following adverse effects as a result of her therapy?

A. Kidney failure
B. Liver failure
C. Peripheral neuropathy
D. Urinary tract infection
E. Tuberculosis

Difficulty level: Medium

48. A 56-year-old woman with a long history of heavy smoking presented with cough, fever, chest pain, and bloody sputum. A chest x-ray revealed a 3.5-cm (1.4-in.) hilar mass, and a transbronchial biopsy showed infiltrating groups of anaplastic small cells with hyperchromatic nuclei and no nucleoli. Which of the following drugs was most likely appropriately included in the therapeutic regimen of this patient?

A. Isoniazid
B. Ceftazidime
C. Streptomycin
D. Asparaginase
E. Cytarabine
F. Etoposide

Difficulty level: Medium

49. A 56-year-old man recently had a routine blood test during his annual checkup. The test showed a white blood cell count of 42,000/mm³ (normal 4500–11,000/mm³). The only pertinent physical finding was splenomegaly. A bone marrow aspirate revealed hypercellular marrow with 15% blasts, and cytogenetic analysis found the presence of the Philadelphia chromosome. A diagnosis was made, and a therapy was started. Which of the following drugs would be most appropriate to include in the patient's therapeutic regimen?

A. Methotrexate
B. Trastuzumab
C. Bleomycin
D. Etoposide
E. Asparaginase
F. Imatinib

Difficulty level: Easy

50. A 10-year-old girl recently diagnosed with acute lymphoblastic leukemia received her first cycle of induction chemotherapy, which included asparaginase. Risk of which of the following adverse effects was most likely increased because of the administration of this drug?

A. Myelosuppression
B. Renal failure
C. Hypoglycemia
D. Heart failure
E. Hypersensitivity reactions

Answers and Explanations: VIII-1 Bacterial Cell Wall Synthesis Inhibitors

Questions 1–4

1. **H**
2. **J**
3. **F**
4. **B**

Learning objective: Explain the mechanism of action of β-lactam antibiotics.

5. **C** Cephalosporins are β-lactam antibiotics. The mechanism of action of all β-lactam antibiotics involves the inhibition of transpeptidase, the enzyme that catalyzes the final connection (cross-link) of two amino sugar chains by peptide bridges. In this way, the synthesis of peptidoglycans is inhibited.

   A, B, D, E See correct answer explanation.

Learning objective: Describe the renal elimination of cephalosporins.

6. **A** Most community-acquired urinary tract infections are due to *Escherichia coli*. First-, second-, and third-generation cephalosporin, fluoroquinolones, and trimethoprim-sulfametoxazole are first-line agents for these infections. Most cephalosporins are eliminated by the kidney, mainly by active secretion in the proximal tubule (two notable exceptions are ceftriaxone and cefoperazone, which are excreted mainly through the biliary tract). In most cases, concentrations in urine are higher than those in plasma.

   B Macrolides are mainly eliminated by biliary excretion.

   C Metronidazole is mainly eliminated by liver metabolism.

   D Aminoglycosides are excreted almost entirely by glomerular filtration only.

   E Renal excretion of tetracyclines occurs by glomerular filtration and tubular reabsorption.

Learning objective: Identify the drug contraindicated in a patient with previous allergic reaction to β-lactam drugs.

7. **C** The signs of the patient and the lab results strongly suggest the diagnosis of gonorrhea. Ceftriaxone would be the first-line agent for gonorrhea, but a previous anaphylactic reaction to penicillin contraindicates the use of most β-lactam drugs.

   A, B, D, E All of these antibiotics are effective against *Neisseria gonorrhoeae*; they are not first-line agents, but none of them are contraindicated in this case.

Learning objective: Identify the drug used to treat *Neisseria meningitidis*.

8. **B** The patient's symptoms and lab results indicate that she was most likely suffering from meningitis due to *N. meningitidis*. In this disease, the preferred treatments are penicillin G (4 million units intravenously every 4 hours) and a third-generation cephalosporin (mainly ceftriaxone).

   A, C Although *N. meningitidis* is sensitive to these antibiotics, a bactericidal drug must be given in serious infectious diseases.

   D, E These antibiotics are mainly active against gram-negative bacilli.

   F *N. meningitidis* is not sensitive to metronidazole.

Learning objective: Identify the antibiotic given to prevent infections due to *Streptococcus agalactiae.*

9. **E** Beta-lactam antibiotics are drugs of choice for streptococcal infections. *S. agalactiae* is a group B streptococcus sensitive to penicillins. Penicillin G or ampicillin is used with excellent results for antimicrobial prophylaxis against group B streptococci.

   A–C Streptococci may be sensitive to quinolones, sulfonamides, and tetracyclines, but these antibiotics are not recommended in children and newborns because of several potential adverse effects.

   D When given alone, aminoglycoside antibiotics are not effective against streptococci.

Learning objective: Identify the bacterium still sensitive to penicillin G.

10. **D** The patient was most likely suffering from streptococcal pharyngitis, the most common disease caused by *Streptococcus pyogenes*, a group A β-hemolytic streptococcus. Group A streptococci are still exquisitely sensitive to penicillin G. Penicillin therapy of streptococcal pharyngitis reduces the risk of subsequent acute rheumatic fever. However, current evidence suggests that the incidence of glomerulonephritis that follows streptococcal infections is not reduced to a significant degree by treatment with penicillin.

    A–C, E–G All of these bacteria are now resistant to penicillin G.

Learning objective: Identify the drug used to treat chancroid.

11. **D** The history of the patient and the site of the ulcer suggest a sexually transmitted disease. Among these diseases, those characterized by ulcer on the penis include chancroid (caused by *Haemophilus ducreyi*), lymphogranuloma venereum (caused by *Chlamydia trachomatis*), granuloma inguinale (caused by *Donovania granulomatis*), syphilis (caused by *Treponema pallidum*), and genital herpes (caused by herpes simplex virus). The presence of gram-negative bacilli excludes viral infections such as genital herpes, as well as chlamydia and donovania infections (chlamydia and donovania are intracellular bacteria). Syphilis is unlikely because of the negative darkfield microscopy and FTA-ABS (fluorescent treponemal antibody absorption) test. Therefore, the patient's disease is most likely caused by *H. ducreyi*, a gram-negative bacterium that is sensitive to second- and third-generation cephalosporins, trimethoprim-sulfametoxazole, quinolones, and tetracyclines. Ceftriaxone is most often used because it has a long half-life (about 7 hours) and therefore can provide a long minimum bactericidal concentration (most β-lactam antibiotics exhibit time-dependent killing).

    A–C These antibiotics are not effective against gram-negative bacteria.

    E Metronidazole is not effective against *H. ducreyi.*

Learning objective: Identify the two antibiotics used to treat streptococcal septic shock syndrome.

12. **A** In addition to being among the most common of all human pathogens, group A streptococci have emerged in recent years as important causes of life-threatening invasive and suppurative infections. This patient likely had streptococcal septic shock syndrome, which is an especially lethal streptococcal disease. In 60% of patients with this syndrome, the organism is contracted through the skin or the genital mucosa. Patients are usually otherwise healthy children or adults. Pyrogenic exotoxins are thought to play a crucial role in the pathogenesis. Streptococcal septic shock syndrome follows a fulminant clinical course with a mortality rate of 50%. The principles of management include aggressive resuscitation, prompt surgical exploration and débridement of soft tissue infections, and antibiotic therapy. Penicillin-resistant isolates have yet to be observed for group A streptococci, so penicillin G remains an agent of choice. Patients may fail to achieve optimal response to penicillin G because large concentrations of bacteria in the lesion reach a stationary growth phase (in the absence of cell division, penicillin cannot have a bactericidal effect). Clindamycin has multiple effects against group A streptococcal infections. Its efficacy is not affected by inoculum size or growth stage; it is a potent suppressor of bacterial toxin synthesis, facilitates phagocytosis of *Streptococcus pyogenes* by inhibiting protein synthesis, and suppresses the synthesis of penicillin-binding proteins, which are enzymes involved in cell wall synthesis. Therefore, most clinicians recommend combined therapy with penicillin and clindamycin.

    B Tobramycin and metronidazole are not effective against gram-positive bacteria.

    C Chloramphenicol and tetracycline are bacteriostatic agents, and most strains of streptococci are now resistant to these drugs.

    D Erythromycin is effective against streptococci but is a bacteriostatic drug, and amikacin is effective mainly against gram-negative bacteria.

    E Piperacillin and aztreonam are β-lactam antibiotics mainly effective against gram-negative bacteria.

Learning objective: Outline the therapy for infective endocarditis most likely due to viridans streptococci.

13. **D** The patient's history and clinical presentation suggest that the man is suffering from infective endocarditis. He appears chronically ill and represents the typical patient with subacute disease. He has mitral valve prolapse, which is the predominant defect in infective endocarditis, and he also exhibits several peripheral manifestation of infective endocarditis, including hemorrhages in the hands and feet. The gram-positive bacteria most commonly involved in infective endocarditis are streptococci and staphylococci. Streptococci of the viridans group are the principal cause of endocarditis in an abnormal heart valve (which is present in this case), and they reach the bloodstream typically after dental trauma. The temporal relationship between the dental procedure and the onset of symptoms makes it the most obvious cause of the disease. Most viridans streptococci are sensitive to penicillins and cephalosporins. Single-drug regimens include high-dose penicillin G or ceftriaxone for 2 to 4 weeks. When empirical therapy is needed, the guidelines suggest high-dose penicillin G plus an aminoglycoside, as in this case. This is a synergistic combination that can achieve bactericidal activity against resistant streptococcal species.

A, B These are combinations of a bactericidal plus a bacteriostatic antibiotic. In general, these combinations should be avoided (with few exceptions), as an antagonistic interaction can occur in many cases.

C These antibiotics are mainly effective against gram-negative bacteria.

E Dicloxacillin is effective against mutant streptococci, but many strains of streptococci are now resistant to fluoroquinolones, and there is no synergism between penicillins and fluoroquinolones.

Learning objective: Identify the antibiotic used to treat acute supraglottitis.

14. **C** Acute supraglottitis can occur at any time in life, but its incidence is highest in children ages 2 to 5 years. Most patients are febrile, many have cervical lymph node enlargement, and occasionally cellulitis appears over the anterior neck. Acute supraglottitis can be fulminant in onset and, if suspected clinically, must always be considered an emergency, as sudden, complete airway obstruction is impending. The disease is almost always due to *Haemophilus influenzae* type b. A third-generation cephalosporin (ceftriaxone) and ampicillin-sulbactam are the antibiotics of choice.

A, B, D, E *H. influenzae* is not sensitive to any of the other listed antibiotics.

Learning objective: Explain the mechanism of action of β-lactam antibiotics.

15. **C** The appearance of the lesion (crepitation, bronze discoloration) indicates that the patient was most likely suffering from gas gangrene (myonecrosis). The disease can be caused by many bacteria, including bacteroides, enterobacteriaceae, streptococci, and staphylococci, but the most frequent pathogen is *Clostridium perfrigens*. Penicillin G, in high doses, is still the drug of choice for *C. perfrigens* infection. The mechanism of action of β-lactam antibiotics involves the inhibition of transpeptidase, the enzyme that catalyzes the final cross-link step in the synthesis of peptidoglycan.

A, B, D, E These enzymes are not inhibited by penicillins.

Learning objective: Identify the drug used to treat actinomycosis.

16. **A** The patient's history (a lesion after a local trauma), the site and type of lesion, and the appearance of the biopsy material suggest that the patient was suffering from actinomycosis. The disease is a chronic, suppurative, and granulomatous infection caused most often by *Actinomyces israelii*. The bacterium is sensitive to penicillins, cephalosporins, macrolides, tetracyclines, and sulfonamide-trimethoprim. Penicillin G remains the treatment of choice.

B–E None of the other listed drugs are effective in actinomycosis.

Learning objective: Identify the antibiotic used for surgical prophylaxis in high-risk patients.

17. **E** Because surgical wound infections are major nosocomial infections, antimicrobial prophylaxis is advisable in open heart surgery, surgery for placement of prosthetic materials, any surgeries performed on an immunocompromised host, high-risk patients in preparation for contaminated and clean-contaminated surgical procedures, and orthopedic surgery, as in this case. The goal of antimicrobial prophylaxis is to decrease bacterial counts below the critical level necessary to cause infection. Cefazolin is the drug most frequently used for surgical prophylaxis when skin flora is the source of contamination because of its excellent activity against staphylococci.

A Metronidazole is not used for surgical prophylaxis, as it is active only against anaerobic microorganisms.

B, C, F Bacteriostatic agents are not used for microbial prophylaxis because bacteremia can reoccur when the drug is no longer present.

D Aztreonam is active only against gram-negative bacteria and therefore is not suitable to prevent infection due to staphylococci.

Learning objective: Identify the drug used to treat cellulitis.

18. **C** The patient was most likely suffering from cellulitis. Acute bacterial infection of the skin and subcutaneous tissue is most often caused by streptococci or staphylococci. For most patients, empiric treatment effective against both bacteria is adequate. Because most staphylococcal isolates produce penicillinase, the best initial treatment is a β-lactamase-resistant penicillin, such as dicloxacillin, or a third-generation cephalosporin, or a carbapenem.

    A, B, E These drugs are mainly effective against gram-negative bacteria.

    D Most gram-positive cocci are now resistant to tetracyclines.

Learning objective: identify the β-lactam antibiotic that is resistant to most β-lactamases.

19. **E** Cefepime is a fourth-generation cephalosporin. The drugs of this class are resistant to most plasmid- and chromosomally mediated β-lactamases. In general, resistance to β-lactamases increases from first- to fourth-generation cephalosporins.

    A, F These drugs are first-generation cephalosporins with a limited resistance to β-lactamases.

    B–D These penicillins are β-lactamase sensitive.

Learning objective: Describe the adverse effects to β-lactam drugs.

20. **B** Acute pharyngitis is predominantly a viral infection but is also often caused by group A β-hemolytic streptococci. Because the patient was diagnosed with bacterial pharyngitis, he was most likely treated with a penicillin. Allergic reactions are the most frequent adverse effects of penicillins. They occur in up to 10% of patients previously exposed to the drug. Patients suffering from infectious mononucleosis, fungus infection, leukemia, and lymphoma are especially at risk, as in this case. Although allergic reactions can be caused by the intact drug molecule, most antigenic determinants of penicillin hypersensitivity are breakdown products. Both the intact molecule and the breakdown products act as haptens after their covalent reaction with proteins. The major antigenic determinant is the penicilloyl moiety, which is formed when the β-lactam ring is opened. When an allergic reaction occurs during the course of the therapy, the drug should be discontinued (if a valid alternative drug is available), because there is a chance, although small, that the reaction could worsen.

    A, C–E All of these antibiotics can cause allergic reactions, but they are not currently used to treat acute pharyngitis.

Learning objective: Identify the antibiotic most likely responsible for tubulointerstitial nephritis in a patient treated for syphilis.

21. **A** The signs and symptoms of the patient (the skin rash and eosinophiluria) suggest that the tubulointerstitial nephritis is due to drug allergy. Penicillin is the drug of choice for primary syphilis, so it is the most likely offending drug.

    B–E Allergic tubulointerstitial nephritis can occur with all of the drugs listed, but these drugs are not currently used to treat primary syphilis.

Learning objective: Describe the mechanisms of bacterial resistance to β-lactam drugs.

22. **C** Resistance to β-lactam antibiotics is due to four main mechanisms:

    • Production of β-lactamase enzymes (by far the most important mechanism). Beta-lactamases hydrolyze the β-lactam ring, thus producing penicilloic acids that are devoid of antibacterial activity.
    • Development of penicillin-binding proteins that have decreased affinity for the antibiotic (the mechanism for penicillin resistance in pneumococci)
    • Decreased permeability of the cell membrane to the drug (the mechanism for resistance in many gram-negative bacteria)
    • Development of an active efflux pump (the mechanism for resistance in some gram-negative bacteria)

    A, D, E These mechanisms would increase, not decrease, the sensitivity of bacteria to β-lactam antibiotics.

    B This is a mechanism of resistance to antibiotics that inhibit protein synthesis.

Learning objective: Identify the drug that poses the highest risk of antibiotic-associated colitis.

23. **E** The patient most likely developed antibiotic-associated pseudomembranous colitis (AAPC) due to *Clostridium difficile*. The disease has emerged as a major threat to elderly patients. Ampicillin, clindamycin, cephalosporins, and fluoroquinolones are the most common antibiotics associated with the condition. Other causative agents are penicillins, erythromycin, trimethoprim-sulfamethoxazole, and tetracyclines. Ampicillin was most likely given to the patient to cure tonsillitis and therefore was the most plausible offending agent.

    A–D All of these antibiotics very rarely cause AAPC, and they are not used to treat streptococcal tonsillitis.

Learning objective: Identify the antibiotic used to treat urinary tract infection due to *Escherichia coli.*

24. **D** The lab tests suggest that the patient's urinary tract infection was most likely due to *E. coli*, a gram-negative rod that accounts for about 80% of urinary tract infections. *E. coli* is sensitive to cephalosporins, broad-spectrum penicillins, aminoglycosides, trimethoprim-sulfametoxazole, tetracyclines, and fluoroquinolones. However, several strains are now resistant to broad-spectrum penicillins, tetracyclines, and trimethoprim-sulfametoxazole. Cephalosporins and fluoroquinolones remain first-line agents.

    A–C, E All of these drugs are effective mainly against gram-positive bacteria.

Learning objective: Identify the two antibiotics used to treat valve endocarditis after susceptibility testing.

25. **B** The clinical picture suggests that the patient had a valve endocarditis. Endocarditis occurring in injection drug users, especially when infection involves the tricuspid valve, is commonly caused by *Staphylococcus aureus* strains, many of which are methicillin-resistant, but the results of susceptibility testing indicated that *Pseudomonas aeruginosa* was the cause of valve endocarditis in this patient. There is substantial evidence that a β-lactam and an aminoglycoside antibiotic exert a synergistic effect in serious infections caused by a number of bacteria, including *P. aeruginosa*. It appears that β-lactam drugs that are cell wall active increase the active transport of aminoglycosides into many bacteria, including staphylococci, enterococci, and *P. aeruginosa*. In choosing the right antibiotic combination, the results of susceptibility testing must be taken into account. Theoretically, all of the tested drugs can be effective against *P. aeruginosa*. Nevertheless, the combination of ceftazidime and tobramycin or imipenem and tobramycin (not listed) appears to be the best in this case (see below).

    A Although both tobramycin and gentamicin are active against *P. aeruginosa*, a β-lactam plus an aminoglycoside must be given to provide in vivo synergy and prevent resistant subpopulations from emerging during therapy.

    C Because both imipenem and gentamicin are effective against *P. aeruginosa,* the combination could seem appropriate. Although the sensitivity of gentamicin is less than that of tobramycin, this could be overcome by increasing the gentamicin dose. However, aminoglycoside antibiotics have significant dose-dependent toxicity, and a minimum inhibitory concentration (MIC) higher than 3 to 4 µg/mL is predictive of toxicity.

    D *P. aeruginosa* is very sensitive to both imipenem and ceftazidime. However, the combination of these two drugs would be additive, not synergistic, as both share the same mechanism of action.

E The very high MIC of piperacillin indicates that the *Pseudomonas* strain of this patient is resistant to the drug.

Learning objective: Describe the staphylococcal resistance to β-lactam antibiotics.

26. **B** *Staphylococcus aureus* is the most common causative pathogen of mastitis. Methicillin-resistant staphylococci are resistant through acquisition (via transposon) of penicillin-binding proteins with a very low affinity for all β-lactam antibiotics.

    A, D, F These bacteria are sensitive to most penicillins.

    C, E, G These bacteria are sensitive to broad-spectrum penicillins, imipenem, and aztreonam, as well as to some third- and fourth-generation cephalosporins.

Learning objective: Identify the antibiotic used to treat staphylococcal infections.

27. **D** The appearance of gram-positive cocci arranged in clusters suggests that the causative agent is staphylococcal. *Staphylococcus aureus* is the most common pathogen of staphylococcal respiratory tract disease. Because about 90% of *S. aureus* isolates produce penicillinase, the best initial treatment is a β-lactamase-resistant penicillin.

    A–C, E All of these penicillins are β-lactamase-sensitive.

Learning objective: Outline the therapeutic uses of ampicillin plus tobramycin in urinary tract infection due to *Enterococcus faecalis*.

28. **D** The woman most likely had a urinary tract infection. *Escherichia coli* is still the predominant pathogen in nosocomial acquired urinary tract infections, but other pathogens are increasingly involved, including *Enterococcus faecalis*. Broad-spectrum penicillins, as well as vancomycin and teicoplanin, are active against this bacterium. However, monotherapy inhibits but does not kill the enterococci. Therefore, an aminoglycoside is always given together with the first drug.

    A, B No cephalosporins are active against enterococci.

    C Most enterococcal strains are now resistant to penicillin. Macrolides are not active against enterococci.

    E Aztreonam is active only against gram-negative bacteria.

Learning objective: Explain the main reason for antibiotic-induced superinfections.

29. **D** Superinfections are new infections that occur during antibacterial therapy of a primary infection. Superinfection is due to removal of the inhibitory influence of the microflora that normally inhabits certain parts of the body (oropharynx, intestine, vagina, etc.). In fact, many members of the normal microflora appear to produce antibacterial substances, and they also presumably compete for essential nutrients. The broader the spectrum of an antibiotic, the greater the alteration of the normal microflora. When the normal microflora

is altered, a single microorganism can become predominant, invade the host, and cause infection.

A–C, E Antibiotics do not cause these actions.

Learning objective: Explain the mechanism of action common to ampicillin, ceftriaxone, and vancomycin.

30. **E** The signs and symptoms of the patient strongly suggest a diagnosis of meningitis. When the patient is very ill and the offending organism is unknown, an empiric triple antibiotic therapy is usually given pending cerebrospinal fluid test results. Third-generation cephalosporins such as ceftriaxone are active against most gram-positive and -negative bacteria. Because many methicillin-resistant cocci are increasingly prevalent, vancomycin is usually added. Ampicillin is added to cover *Listeria* species. All of these antibiotics act by inhibiting the synthesis of peptidoglycan. Ampicillin and ceftriaxone inhibit the transpeptidation reaction, blocking cross-link formation. Vancomycin inhibits transglycosylase, blocking further elongation of peptidoglycan chains.

A This is the mechanism of action of aminoglycosides.

B This is the mechanism of action of trimethoprim-sulfametoxazole.

C This is the mechanism of action of rifampin.

D This is the mechanism of action of macrolides.

None of the above-mentioned drugs are used alone to treat gram-negative bacillary meningitis, either because they do not cross the blood–brain barrier (aminoglycosides) or because they are not effective against some gram-negative bacteria (i.e., *Pseudomonas aeruginosa*).

Learning objective: Identify the antibiotic used prophylactically in at-risk patients undergoing dental surgery.

31. **A** Antibiotic prophylaxis is generally recommended for patients at risk who are undergoing procedures associated with significant bacteremia. These include any dental procedure that is likely to cause bacteremia secondary to bleeding from tissues. Because this patient is at risk of infective endocarditis as a result of the ongoing heart disease, antibiotic prophylaxis is advisable. Antimicrobial prophylaxis should be addressed to viridans streptococci, as they are the most common cause of endocarditis following dental procedures. Amoxicillin is currently recommended for prophylaxis in susceptible individuals undergoing upper respiratory tract or dental surgery, as in this case.

B–D All of these antibiotics are mainly active against gram-negative bacteria and therefore not suitable to prevent streptococcal infections.

E Metronidazole is not active against streptococci.

Learning objective: Identify the antibiotic used to treat *Pasteurella multocida* infection.

32. **E** *P. multocida* is part of the normal oral flora of dogs and cats and therefore is the most common microorganism in human wounds inflicted by bites from these animals. It is sensitive to penicillin G, which is still the drug of first choice.

A, B *Staphylococcus epidermidis* and *Clostridium difficile* are gram-positive bacteria.

C, D *Klebsiella pneumoniae* and *Serratia marcescens* are enterobacteriaceae that only exceptionally infect superficial wounds. Moreover, they are not sensitive to erythromycin and vancomycin.

Learning objective: Explain the mechanism of action of potassium clavulanate.

33. **A** The patient's symptoms and physical examination suggest the diagnosis of acute otitis media, one of the most common infectious diseases afflicting infants and children. The main bacteria causing otitis media in children are *Streptococcus pneumoniae, Haemophilus influenzae,* and *Moraxella catarrhalis.* Most clinicians advocate a stepped approach to the antimicrobial therapy, which involves initial treatment with amoxicillin or trimethoprim-sulfamethoxazole. If this regimen does not reduce symptoms within 3 days, amoxicillin/clavulanate or cefuroxime or ceftriaxone should be substituted for the initial therapy, as was done in this case. Potassium clavulanate is a β-lactamase inhibitor that blocks many, but not all, β-lactamase enzymes, protecting amoxicillin from inactivation by β-lactamase-producing bacteria.

B Beta-lactamase inhibitors extend the antibacterial spectrum of amoxicillin, but *Pseudomonas aeruginosa* remains resistant.

C, D Beta-lactamase inhibitors do not significantly affect the kinetics of penicillins.

E Beta-lactamase inhibitors do not affect the allergenicity of β-lactam antibiotics.

Learning objective: Describe the acute anaphylactic reaction to penicillin G.

34. **D** The signs and symptoms of the patient indicate that he was most likely suffering from an acute anaphylactic reaction to penicillin G, which is the treatment of choice in all stages of syphilis.

A, B These drugs are sometimes used in the treatment of syphilis for penicillin-allergic patients, but they have a much lower risk of allergic reactions.

C, E, F These drugs are not used in the treatment of syphilis because *Treponema pallidum* is intrinsically resistant to these antibiotics.

Learning objective: Identify the cephalosporin that is mainly eliminated with the bile.

35. **B** The antibiotic therapy for acute cholecystitis is usually initiated to treat possible infection, but evidence of benefit is still modest. Empiric therapy is directed against gram-negative enteric organisms such as *Escherichia coli, Klebsiella,* and *Enterobacter* species. Cefoperazone and ceftriaxone are the two cephalosporins primarily eliminated with the bile. Both are active against the above-mentioned bacteria; therefore, cefoperazone can be appropriate for the empiric treatment of acute cholecystitis, as in this case.

    A, C–E These drugs are mainly eliminated by tubular secretion.

Learning objective: Describe the appropriate antimicrobial therapy for primary syphilis.

36. **C** The signs and symptoms of the patient, as well as the dark-field exam, suggest that he is suffering from primary syphilis. Penicillin G is the drug of choice for the treatment of all stages of syphilis. A single intramuscular injection of benzathine penicillin G is appropriate for the early stage, as in this patient. If penicillin G is contraindicated, doxycycline or ceftriaxone can be used.

    A, B, D–F These drugs are not effective against *Treponema pallidum.*

Learning objective: Identify the drug given to treat acute osteomyelitis.

37. **A** The signs and symptoms of the patient suggest that he was most likely suffering from acute osteomyelitis following a diabetic foot ulcer. The Gram stain was polymicrobial, and the putrid smell was specific for anaerobic microorganisms. Amoxicillin/clavulanate is a broad-spectrum antibiotic active against gram-positive cocci, gram-negative rods, and anaerobic bacteria. If the patient had a history of methicillin-resistant staphylococci, the addition of vancomycin or linezolid would be appropriate.

    B Clindamycin is active against gram-positive cocci and anaerobes but not against gram-negative rods.

    C, E Linezolid and vancomycin are active only against gram-positive cocci.

    D Metronidazole is active only against anaerobes.

Learning objective: Identify the antibiotic used to treat bacteroides abscess.

38. **C** The putrid sputum and the negative aerobic culture point out that the offending pathogen was most likely an anaerobic bacterium. *Bacteroides fragilis is* the most common pathogen associated with anaerobic infections. It is very sensitive to imipenem, clindamycin, and broad-spectrum penicillins plus β-lactamase inhibitors. Other effective antibiotics are metronidazole and some cephalosporins.

A *Legionella pneumophila* is an aerobic, gram-negative rod and is not sensitive to ampicillin.

B *Actinomyces israelii* is an anaerobic rod, but it is gram-positive and not sensitive to gentamicin.

D *Streptococcus pneumoniae* is an aerobic, gram-positive coccus and is not sensitive to aztreonam.

E *Listeria monocytogenes* is an aerobic, gram-positive rod and is not sensitive to cephalosporins.

Learning objective: Explain the mechanism of action of β-lactam antibiotics.

39. **A** The mechanism of action of β-lactam antibiotics includes the following two actions:

- They bind to specific β-lactam receptors called penicillin-binding proteins located on the cytoplasmic membrane. These proteins are enzymes endowed with various catalytic functions that are inhibited by binding to the antibiotic. The most important enzymes inhibited are transpeptidases, which catalyze the final cross-link step in the synthesis of murein (also called peptidoglycan). Because peptidoglycan layers are constituents of bacterial cell walls, the synthesis of the cell wall is blocked.
- Autolytic enzymes (called autolysins or murein hydrolases) are present in the cell wall and degrade the peptidoglycan. Beta-lactam antibiotics can activate these autolysins (apparently by blocking an autolysin inhibitor), thus promoting the lysis of bacteria.

    B This is the mechanism of action of tetracyclines.
    C This is a mechanism of resistance to antibiotics.
    D This is the mechanism of action of vancomycin.
    E This is the mechanism of action of rifampin.

Learning objective: Identify the antibiotic that can cause hypoprothrombinemia.

40. **F** *Bacteroides fragilis* has been isolated from up to 28% of patients with chronic otitis media. Antibiotics effective against bacteroides are metronidazole, clindamycin, and β-lactam drugs, including imipenem, broad-spectrum penicillins plus β-lactamase inhibitors, cefoxitin, and cefotetan. Hypoprothrombinemia has been associated with the use of certain cephalosporins, including cefoperazone, cefotetan, and cefamandole. The mechanism of hypoprothrombinemia is still uncertain but seems to be related to the methylthiotetrazole side chain of these cephalosporins, as this group can inhibit the carboxylation of glutamic acid, the vitamin K–dependent step in the synthesis of clotting factors. Because of this, the hypoprothrombinemia can be rapidly reversed by the administration of vitamin K.

    A–D These drugs are active against bacteroides, but hypoprothrombinemia is exceedingly rare.

    E Most quinolones have negligible activity against bacteroides.

Learning objective: Identify the antibiotic to be used in a patient allergic to β-lactam drugs.

41. **D** Aztreonam is a β-lactam antibiotic with excellent activity against only most gram-negative, aerobic bacteria, including *Pseudomonas aeruginosa*. It has negligible allergic cross-reactivity with other β-lactam antibiotics and is therefore useful for treating gram-negative infections in patients with a history of prior allergic reaction to β-lactam drugs, as in this case.

    A–C, E All of these antibiotics are contraindicated in this patient because of his hypersensitivity to β-lactam drugs.

Learning objective: Explain the mechanism of the antimicrobial action of vancomycin.

42. **A** The patient's signs, symptoms, and lab tests indicate that she was most likely suffering from pneumonia due to methicillin-resistant (MR) *Staphylococcus aureus*. The patient received vancomycin, a drug of choice for MR staphylococcal infections. Vancomycin binds to the terminus of nascent peptidoglycan pentapeptides. The binding inhibits transglycosylase, the enzyme that catalyzes the elongation of peptidoglycan chains, preventing formation of linear peptidoglycan chains. The binding also inhibits transpeptidase, but because transglycosylation precedes transpeptidation, inhibition of transglycosylase is the primary mechanism of action of the drug.

    B–E These actions are not inhibited by vancomycin.

Learning objective: Identify the two drugs used for the initial treatment of acute rheumatic fever.

43. **A** The patient's clinical picture suggests that he was affected by acute rheumatic fever. The disease is a nonsuppurative complication of an infection with group A streptococci. The diagnosis of acute rheumatic fever requires two of the following major manifestations of the illness: carditis, migratory polyarthritis, chorea, erythema marginatum, and subcutaneous nodules. The patient has four such features. In acute rheumatic fever, it is appropriate to administer a therapeutic course (at least 10 days) of parenteral penicillin. In severe cases, aggressive use of antiinflammatory drugs is required. Salicylates remain the drugs of choice, but other nonsteroidal antiinflammatory drugs (NSAIDs, e.g., naproxen) can also be used in children. If a therapeutic effect has not been achieved after the fourth day, NSAIDs should be abandoned in favor of a glucocorticoid.

    B, C, F Amoxicillin and ceftriaxone are less effective against streptococci than penicillin G. Moreover an antiinflammatory drug must be given in acute rheumatic fever.

D Aminoglycoside antibiotics are poorly effective against streptococci.

E Acetaminophen is an antipyretic but not an antiinflammatory drug. Therefore, it is not useful in acute rheumatic fever, for which NSAIDs are given mainly to counteract the acute inflammatory reaction.

Learning objective: Identify the antibiotic used to treat *Pseudomonas aeruginosa* infections.

44. **A** The patient's history and the lab results suggest that she is suffering from a pulmonary infection due to *Pseudomonas aeruginosa*. All patients with cystic fibrosis eventually develop endobronchial colonization and infection. Commonly offending respiratory pathogens are *Staphylococcus aureus*, *Haemophilus influenzae,* and *P. aeruginosa*. Of these, *P. aeruginosa* has become the most common pathogen isolated in chronically colonized patients. For infections due to *P. aeruginosa*, a combination of two bactericidal antibiotics is the rule, and an antipseudomonal penicillin, such as piperacillin (or an antipseudomonal cephalosporin), plus an aminoglycoside is the most commonly used treatment.

    B–F None of these antibiotics are active against *P. aeruginosa*.

Learning objective: Explain the action of penicillin-binding proteins.

45. **B** Penicillin-binding proteins are specific targets for β-lactam antibiotics. They are located in the bacterial cytoplasmic membrane, and some of them are transpeptidases that catalyze the cross-linking of the peptidoglycan amino sugar chain by peptide bridges. This gives the cell wall its structural rigidity. By binding to these transpeptidase enzymes, β-lactam antibiotics block the transpeptidation reaction and therefore the synthesis of peptidoglycan.

    A Porin channels are aqueous channels present on the outer membrane of gram-negative bacteria. Beta-lactam antibiotics enter the cell through these channels. Penicillin-binding proteins do not affect this process.

    C The breakdown of the β-lactam ring is catalyzed by β-lactamases, not by transpeptidases.

    D Beta-lactam antibiotics can activate, not inhibit, murein hydrolases, which are enzymes able to destroy the cell wall.

    E Beta-lactam antibiotics bind to penicillin-binding proteins, not to the peptidoglycan layer.

Learning objective: Outline the therapeutic uses of daptomycin.

46. **D** The patient's signs, symptoms, and lab tests indicate that he was most likely suffering from sepsis due to vancomycin-resistant *Staphylococcus aureus*. Currently available antibiotics for vancomycin-resistant staphylococci are daptomycin, quinupristin/dalfopristin, linezolid, and tigecycline. Daptomycin is a bactericidal antibiotic active against gram-positive bacteria, including vancomycin-resistant staphylococci and enterococci. Its mechanism of action is not fully understood, but it is known that the drug binds to bacterial cell membranes via calcium-dependent insertion of its lipid tail. This likely results in formation of a pore, causing a loss of cellular potassium and resulting in rapid cell death. Because of this unique mechanism of action, there is no cross-resistance with other antibiotics, and resistance mechanisms are not known. A rare but serious adverse effect of the drug is myopathy, and creatine phosphokinase levels should be monitored.

   A, C, E Vancomycin-resistant staphylococci are resistant to all β-lactam drugs.

   B, F Aminoglycoside antibiotics are not effective against most gram-positive bacteria.

Learning objective: Describe the nephrotoxicity due to concomitant treatment with vancomycin and gentamicin.

47. **D** Treatment of bacterial endocarditis requires the use of one or most often two bactericidal antibiotics. A cell wall synthesis inhibitor plus an aminoglycoside is the first-line treatment, as a synergistic effect can be obtained (the cell wall synthesis inhibitor enhances the bacterial uptake of the aminoglycoside). In this case, vancomycin plus gentamicin was the most likely treatment because the patient showed signs of nephrotoxicity. The incidence of nephrotoxicity associated with vancomycin alone is very low, but it increases substantially (up to 20%) in patients receiving vancomycin plus an aminoglycoside, as in this case.

   A, E These combinations are not used for bacterial endocarditis and are not nephrotoxic.

   B This combination can cause nephrotoxicity, but it is irrational to use together two antibiotics with the same mechanism of action.

   C This combination can cause nephrotoxicity (due to the aminoglycoside), but it is not used for bacterial endocarditis. In general, a combination of a bactericidal plus a bacteriostatic antibiotic should be avoided, as an antagonistic interaction would occur in many cases.

Learning objective: Describe the infusion reaction associated with vancomycin.

48. **B** The patient most likely received vancomycin, a first-line agent for methicillin-resistant staphylococci. A common reaction to vancomycin is the so-called red man syndrome, which can occur after intravenous infusion of the antibiotic

and includes hypotension, tachycardia, generalized pruritus, and facial flushing, as in this case. The syndrome is most likely caused by histamine release.

   A, C–F Although all of these antibiotics are effective against staphylococci, they do not cause histamine release.

Learning objective: Explain the mechanism of action of fosfomycin.

49. **D** Fosfomycin is an antibiotic mainly active against enterobacteriaceae, including *Escherichia coli*, enterococci, and *Klebsiella, Enterobacter, Proteus,* and *Serratia* species. The drug is approved for urinary tract infection due to susceptible bacteria because it is eliminated mainly by the kidney and attains high concentration in the urine. Fosfomycin acts by inhibiting enolpyruvate transferase, the enzyme that catalyzes the synthesis of *N*-acetylmuramic acid, an essential precursor for peptidoglycan synthesis. In this way, bacterial cell wall synthesis is inhibited.

   A–C, E All of these drugs can block bacterial cell wall synthesis, but they act with different mechanisms of action.

Learning objective: Identify the two antibiotics used to treat *Klebsiella* pneumonia.

50. **C** Nearly 1% of hospitalized patients develop pneumonia, which has a 20 to 50% mortality rate. The predominant organisms causing nosocomial pneumonia are aerobic gram-negative bacilli, including *Klebsiella pneumoniae, Escherichia coli, Proteus mirabilis, and Pseudomonas aeruginosa*. Less common causes are *Staphylococcus aureus, Streptococcus pneumoniae,* and anaerobes. The most frequent and best characterized pathogen is *Klebsiella pneumoniae*, which causes Friedlander pneumonia, a disease that can have a fulminant course and a mortality rate of about 50%, despite the availability of effective antibiotics. In this case, the typical appearance of the sputum (a homogeneous mixture of blood and mucus resembling currant jelly) and the results of lab tests and x-ray suggest Friedlander pneumonia. Cephalosporins are drugs of first choice against *Klebsiellae*. However, due to the seriousness of the disease, most authorities suggest the use of an aminoglycoside together with a cephalosporin.

   A, B, D, E All of the other listed options have at least one antibiotic that is not effective against *Klebsiellae*.

BACTERIAL CELL WALL SYNTHESIS INHIBITORS Answer key							
1.	H	6.	A	11.	D	16.	A	21.	A
2.	J	7.	C	12.	A	17.	E	22.	C
3.	F	8.	B	13.	D	18.	C	23.	E
4.	B	9.	E	14.	C	19.	E	24.	D
5.	C	10.	D	15.	C	20.	B	25.	B
26.	B	31.	A	36.	C	41.	D	46.	D
27.	D	32.	E	37.	A	42.	A	47.	D
28.	D	33.	A	38.	C	43.	A	48.	B
29.	D	34.	D	39.	A	44.	A	49.	D
30.	E	35.	B	40.	F	45.	B	50.	C

Answers and Explanations: VIII-2 Bacterial Protein Synthesis Inhibitors

Questions 1–5

1. **O**
2. **L**
3. **B**
4. **E**
5. **J**

Learning objective: Explain the mechanism of action of gentamicin.

6. **E** Gentamicin is an aminoglycoside antibiotic. These drugs bind irreversibly to specific 30S ribosomal subunits and inhibit bacterial protein synthesis in at least three ways:

   - Blockade of the "initiation complex," the complex formed for initiation of translation that consists of the 30S microsomal subunit, messenger RNA (mRNA), transfer RNA (tRNA), and some initiation factors. This blockade leads to an mRNA chain with only a single ribosome on it, the so-called monosome.
   - Misreading of mRNA templates, which leads to the production of aberrant proteins. These proteins may be inserted into cell membranes, altering permeability and further stimulating aminoglycoside transport (energy-dependent phase II transport).
   - Blockade of translocation (i.e., the ribosome advancement of three nucleotides is blocked)

   For external otitis, the drug would be given topically as ear drops. Gentamicin can be ototoxic, especially if given systemically.

   A–D All of these antibiotics are active against *Pseudomonas aeruginosa*, but they do not cause misreading of the bacterial mRNA template.

Learning objective: Explain concentration-dependent killing and the postantibiotic effect.

7. **D** The aminoglycoside bactericidal effect is concentration-dependent; that is, increasing concentrations kill an increasing proportion of bacteria and at a more rapid rate. They also have a long postantibiotic effect, that is, persistent suppression of bacterial growth for several hours beyond the time that measurable drug is present. Most antibiotics exhibit this effect against gram-positive cocci. Antibiotics that possess this effect against gram-negative bacilli are aminoglycosides, fluoroquinolones, and tetracyclines.

   Because of these two properties, a given total amount of aminoglycoside may have better efficacy and lower toxicity when administered as a higher single daily dose than when given as a lower dose two or three times daily.

   A, E The bactericidal effect of aminoglycosides is not time-dependent.

   B Protein binding is totally unrelated to the duration of the antibiotic effect.

   C Aminoglycosides are bactericidal, not bacteriostatic.

Learning objective: Identify the drug used for prophylaxis of whooping cough.

8. **C** Erythromycin and azithromycin are agents of choice for whooping cough. If they are given during the catarrhal stage, they can ameliorate the disease. After paroxysms are established, these drugs have no clinical effect, but they decrease the duration of infectiousness, thus preventing spread. Contacts of all ages, whether vaccinated or not, should receive a 10-day course of erythromycin.

   A, B, D These drug are active against *Bordetella pertussis* but are contraindicated in children.

   E, F These drugs are not active against *B. pertussis*.

Learning objective: Identify the antibiotic used for antimicrobial prophylaxis in colorectal surgery.

9. **D** Antibiotic prophylaxis is widely used for surgical procedures to decrease the degree of bacterial contamination during surgery. Prophylaxis is especially advisable for colorectal surgery, owing to the large number of bacteria comprising the intestinal flora. Oral nonadsorbable antibiotics function effectively as intestinal decontaminants because high intraluminal drug concentrations can be easily achieved. An oral antimicrobial regimen used for colorectal surgical prophylaxis is neomycin (for aerobic enterobacteriaceae) plus erythromycin (for anaerobes). Neomycin is preferred over other aminoglycosides because of its wider spectrum of antibacterial activity.

   A See correct answer explanation.

   B Penicillin G given orally is rapidly destroyed by gastric juices.

   C, E, F These antibiotics are not active against enterobacteriaceae or anaerobes.

Learning objective: Identify the antibiotic used to treat psittacosis.

10. **E** The patient's history suggests that he was affected by psittacosis, a pneumonia caused by *Chlamydia psittaci*. The organism is found mainly in psittacine birds, but other birds can also be affected. Human infection usually occurs by inhalation of dust from feathers of infected birds. Chlamydiae are sensitive to tetracyclines, macrolides, and quinolones. Doxycycline is often the preferred drug.

    A–D All of the listed bacteria can cause pneumonia, but none of them are sensitive to the paired drug.

Learning objective: Calculate the dose of gentamicin to be given to a patient with renal insufficiency, given sufficient data.

11. **D** Aminoglycosides are excreted almost entirely by the kidney, and their clearance is essentially equal to the glomerular filtration rate. Because these drugs have a narrow therapeutic index, dosing must be reduced in patients with impaired renal function.

    In general, the dose in a patient with renal impairment may be corrected by multiplying the average dose for a normally healthy person by the ratio of the patient's altered to normal creatinine clearance (about 100 mL/min). In other words, the dose must be reduced proportionally to the reduction of creatinine clearance. In this case, as the patient's creatinine clearance is about one half the normal value, the dose should be one half the normal dose.

    A–C, E, F See correct answer explanation.

Learning objective: Identify the pair of drugs used to treat acute pyelonephritis due to *Pseudomonas aeruginosa*.

12. **A** Acute pyelonephritis is a well-known complication of chronic lower urinary tract infections. Among patients ages 20 to 50 years, urinary tract infection is about 50-fold greater in women, and pyelonephritis occurs by the ascending route despite the dynamics of urine flow. In this patient, diabetes could predispose to renal infections, possibly because diabetics have altered antibacterial defense mechanisms. Because the patient is acutely ill, and *P. aeruginosa* is the causative agent of her disease, she should be treated with an anti-*Pseudomonas* penicillin (or cephalosporin) plus an aminoglycoside. Both drugs are bactericidal against *P. aeruginosa*, and penicillins are synergistic with aminoglycosides by increasing the uptake of these drugs by many gram-positive and -negative bacteria.

    B–D Only one of the two listed antibiotics is effective against *P. aeruginosa*.

    E Ampicillin and tetracyclines are not effective against *P. aeruginosa*.

Learning objective: Describe the bacterial resistance to aminoglycosides.

13. **A** Resistance to aminoglycosides is primarily due to plasmid-mediated production of bacterial transferases that phosphorylate, acetylate, and adenylate the drug. Less common mechanisms of resistance are decreased permeability of the bacterium to the drug and decreased affinity of the drug for the 30S ribosomal subunit. Resistance appears most frequently to gentamicin and least frequently to amikacin.

    B Resistance can be due to decrease in the affinity of the drug for the 30S (not for the 50S) ribosomal subunit.

    C This is a mechanism of resistance to penicillins.

    D This is the mechanism of resistance to isoniazid.

    E This is the mechanism of resistance to quinolones.

Learning objective: Identify the risk of drug reaction with an aminoglycoside in a patient taking furosemide.

14. **D** Aminoglycosides can cause ototoxicity, which is more likely in patients receiving other ototoxic drugs, including loop diuretics such as furosemide.

    A, C–F All of these are potential adverse effects of aminoglycosides, but their risk is not increased by the concomitant administration of the drugs used by the patient.

Learning objective: Identify the antibiotic most appropriate for a patient with urinary tract infection based on results of a susceptibility test.

15. **B** Approximately 20% of catheterized patients develop urinary tract infections. In this disease, the choice of the most suitable antibiotic is often dictated by antimicrobial susceptibility tests, as the disease does not require immediate empiric antimicrobial therapy. The results of susceptibility tests are reported qualitatively by indicating for each microorganism if it is susceptible, intermediate, or resistant to a given antibiotics. In this case, amikacin was the drug collectively most active against the tested bacteria.

    A, C–E On the whole, these drugs are less effective than amikacin against the bacteria isolated from the patient's urine.

Learning objective: Identify the antibiotic that caused nephrotoxicity in a patient suffering from infection.

16. **B** The patient's urinalysis indicates nephrotoxicity. Aminoglycoside antibiotics are active against *Pseudomonas aeruginosa and* can cause nephrotoxicity in 8 to 26% of patients receiving these drugs for more than 1 week. Risk factors include old age, as in this case.

    A, C Piperacillin and aztreonam are active against *P. aeruginosa*, but they do not cause nephrotoxicity.

    D, E Vancomycin and rifampin can cause nephrotoxicity, but they are not active against *P. aeruginosa*.

Learning objective: Identify the bacterium sensitive to aminoglycosides.

17. **E** The efficacy of gentamicin therapy indicated that an aerobic gram-negative rod was the most likely offending organism. Aminoglycosides are mainly active against aerobic gram-negative rods, including *Klebsiella pneumoniae, Pseudomonas aeruginosa, Haemophilus influenzae, Escherichia coli, Proteus mirabilis, Proteus vulgaris, Enterobacter aerogenes,* and *Serratia marcescens,* as well as against some mycobacteria (*Mycobacterium tuberculosis and Mycobacterium avium-intracellulare*). *Enterobacter* pneumonia is usually hospital-acquired and occurs mainly in immunocompromised patients, as in this case.

    A–D, F Aminoglycosides are not active against *Clostridia,* mycoplasma, bacteroides, *Borrelia,* and *Legionella* species.

Learning objective: Identify the antibiotic that is contraindicated in a patient suffering from myasthenia gravis.

18. **E** Tobramycin is an aminoglycoside antibiotic. These drugs are associated with neuromuscular blockade and may cause neuromuscular weakness lasting hours to days. Therefore, they are relatively contraindicated in patients receiving anesthetics or neuromuscular-blocking agents and in patients with neuromuscular diseases such as myasthenia gravis and parkinsonism. The U.S. Food and Drug Administration has a black box warning for use of tobramycin in patients with these diseases.

A–D These drugs are effective in urinary tract infections and do not enhance the neuromuscular blockade caused by diseases or drugs.

Learning objective: Explain the mechanism of action of linezolid.

19. **E** The patient's signs and symptoms indicate that she was most likely suffering from acute hematogenous osteomyelitis, which classically has been a disease of children. Linezolid is a relatively new antibiotic that inhibits protein synthesis by binding to the 23S portion of the 50S ribosomal subunit and preventing formation of the initiation complex. The ultimate effect is mainly bacteriostatic. The drug is active against methicillin-resistant (MR) and vancomycin-resistant (VR) staphylococci.

A–D All of these antibiotics have a different mechanism of action, and they are not active against MR and VR staphylococci

F Tigecycline is active against MR and VR staphylococci but has a different mechanism of action; it binds instead to the 30S ribosomal subunit and prevents binding of the aminoacyl-transfer RNA (tRNA) to the acceptor site.

Learning objective: Identify the class of antibiotics that can cause dose-dependent ototoxicity.

20. **E** Aminoglycosides cause dose-dependent ototoxicity that involves both cochlear and vestibular function. Nausea, vomiting, and vertigo indicate impairment of vestibular function, and tinnitus and decreased hearing capacity point out that cochlear function is affected.

A Macrolides can rarely cause ototoxicity, but they are not active against *Serratia marcescens*.

B Some tetracyclines (minocycline) can cause vestibular disturbances, but they are not active against *S. marcescens*.

C, D Cephalosporins and sulfonamides do not cause ototoxicity.

Learning objective: Explain the mechanism of action of macrolides.

21. **D** Macrolide antibiotics inhibit bacterial protein synthesis mainly by blocking translocation of the newly synthesized peptidyl-transfer RNA (tRNA) from the acceptor site to the donor site of the ribosome. They are mainly bacteriostatic, but they may be bactericidal at higher doses.

A This is the mechanism of action of rifampin.

B This is the mechanism of action of quinolones.

C This is the mechanism of action of aminoglycosides.

E This is the mechanism of action of tetracyclines.

Learning objective: Identify the bacterium sensitive to macrolides.

22. **B** *Campylobacter jejuni* accounts for most cases of diarrhea in the United States. The diarrhea is usually bloody, especially when fever is present, as in this case. Macrolides such as azithromycin are effective against *Campylobacter* species.

A, C, D, F These bacteria can cause diarrhea, but they are resistant to macrolides.

E Some *Clostridia* species are sensitive to macrolides, but *Clostridium difficile* is not.

Learning objective: Describe the mechanism of erythromycin-induced diarrhea.

23. **B** Nausea, vomiting, diarrhea, and abdominal pain may accompany the administration of macrolides. These effects are dose-related and occur more commonly in children and young adults. The mechanism that underlies these adverse reactions is still uncertain but is most likely related to macrolide-mediated activation of motilin receptors in the gut.

A Erythromycin is not active against most enterobacteriaceae. In fact, superinfections are exceedingly rare.

C Erythromycin does not affect water reabsorption by colonic mucosa.

D Macrolides (mainly erythromycin estolate) can rarely cause cholestatic hepatitis, but diarrhea is not a symptom of that disease.

E Allergic reactions to macrolide antibiotics are very rare and include mainly fever and skin eruptions.

Learning objective: Describe the use of macrolides in gonococcal urethritis.

24. **C** The patient's symptoms and lab results suggest the diagnosis of gonococcal urethritis. Because up to 50% of women with gonorrhea have coinfection with *Chlamydia trachomatis,* azithromycin is usually added to ceftriaxone treatment. Other offending pathogens sometimes responsible for coinfection are *Ureaplasma urealyticum* and *Mycoplasma genitalium;* both are also sensitive to macrolides. Azithromycin is often preferred because a single dose is usually effective.

A, B, D–F None of these antibiotics are effective against chlamydiae, mycoplasmas, or ureaplasmas.

Learning objective: Identify the antibiotic that should be used in a patient with renal insufficiency and an infection due to *Pseudomonas aeruginosa*.

25. **B** Amikacin is an aminoglycoside antibiotic. Because aminoglycosides are very polar drugs, they are water soluble, undergo little hepatic metabolism, and are excreted almost entirely by glomerular filtration. As a result, their half-lives can increase enormously in patients with kidney failure. Aminoglycosides have a narrow therapeutic window, so two dosing schedules are currently used to avoid toxicity: reduction of the dose or extension of dosing intervals. Both methods have advantages and disadvantages.

    A Cefoperazone is an anti-*Pseudomonas* cephalosporin but is excreted mainly in the bile, so its dosage does not need to be changed in the presence of kidney failure.

    C–F These antibiotics are not effective against *P. aeruginosa*.

Learning objective: Identify the drug used to treat inclusion conjunctivitis.

26. **E** The patient's symptoms and the lab results indicate that the baby most likely has inclusion conjunctivitis, an infection due to *Chlamydia trachomatis* that the newborn acquired during passage through an infected birth canal. Macrolides, tetracyclines, quinolones, and trimethoprim-sulfamethoxazole are effective against chlamydiae, but tetracyclines, quinolones, and sulfonamides are relatively contraindicated in children. Erythromycin remains the first-line agent for inclusion conjunctivitis in the newborn.

    A, C, D See correct answer explanation.

    B, F Beta-lactam antibiotics and aminoglycosides are not effective against chlamydiae.

Learning objective: Describe the main drug interactions involving macrolides.

27. **E** The patient's symptoms were most likely due to an increased plasma concentration of theophylline. Erythromycin metabolites inhibit the P-450 system, thus increasing plasma concentration of several drugs given concomitantly, including theophylline, carbamazepine, valproic acid, corticosteroids, digoxin, and warfarin.

    A–D, F These drugs do not interact with theophylline.

Learning objective: Identify the drug used to treat Legionnaires' disease.

28. **C** The patient's symptoms (high fever with bradycardia) and lab results indicate that he was most likely suffering from Legionnaires' disease, a pneumonia caused by *Legionella* species (mainly *Legionella pneumophila*). More than 60% of patients with Legionnaires' disease exhibit bradycardia, and positive cultures in charcoal yeast extract agar are diagnostic. *L. pneumophila* is sensitive to macrolides, fluoroquinolones, tetracyclines, trimethoprim-sulfamethoxazole, and rifampin. Azithromycin, alone or with rifampin, is a first-line agent.

    A, B, D–F None of these antibiotics are effective against *L. pneumophila*.

Learning objective: Identify a class of antibiotics that exhibits mainly bacteriostatic activity.

29. **C** Macrolides are mainly bacteriostatic antibiotics with excellent activity against mycoplasmas.

    A, B, D, E All of these antibiotics have bactericidal activity. Moreover, they are not active against mycoplasmas.

    F Fluoroquinolones are active against mycoplasmas, but they are bactericidal, not bacteriostatic.

Learning objective: Identify the antibiotic that can trigger polymorphic ventricular tachycardia in patients at risk.

30. **B** Macrolide antibiotics can cause prolongation of the electrocardiogram QT interval, a condition that increases the risk of polymorphic ventricular tachycardia. This primarily occurs when macrolides are given in high doses or are given together with other drugs that can prolong the QT interval. These include several antiarrhythmic drugs, H_1 antagonists, neuroleptics, tricyclic antidepressants, antimalarials, and quinolones. In this case, the patient was taking amitriptyline, a tricyclic antidepressant, so she was at increased risk of developing ventricular tachycardia when erythromycin was taken.

    A, C–F These drugs do not appear to prolong the QT interval.

Learning objective: Identify the antibiotic used to treat cat scratch disease.

31. **C** The boy most likely suffered from cat scratch disease, a benign illness caused by *Bartonella enselae*, a gram-negative rod that infects at least 30% of domestic cats. Cat scratch disease is usually self-limited and does not require treatment in normal adults. In very young children or in immunocompromised patients, a macrolide is the drug of choice.

    A, B, E *Enterococcus faecalis*, *Clostridium difficile*, and *Actinomyces israelii* are gram-positive bacteria.

    D *Bacteroides fragilis* is an anaerobic gram-negative rod that causes mainly intra-abdominal infections and is not sensitive to aminoglycosides.

Learning objective: Identify the microorganism sensitive to clindamycin.

32. **C** The fact that the patient's infection started after surgery with contamination of the peritoneum and that clindamycin was chosen for therapy points out that the main offending pathogen was most likely *Bacteroides fragilis*. Clindamycin is a lincosamide antibiotic with very good activity against

Bacteroides (including *B. fragilis*). The drug is not first choice in bacteroides infections because β-lactam antibiotics and metronidazole are usually preferred, but the patient was allergic to both.

A, B, D, E All of these microorganisms are resistant to clindamycin.

Learning objective: Identify the antibiotic used for streptococcal pharyngitis in a person allergic to penicillins.

33.   **D** Erythromycin is the drug of choice for streptococcal infections in a patient allergic to penicillins.

A–C A serious allergic reaction to penicillins contraindicates the use of all β-lactam antibiotics except aztreonam.

E Many streptococcal strains are now resistant to tetracyclines, and these antibiotics are contraindicated in pregnant women.

F Aztreonam is active only against gram-negative bacteria.

Learning objective: Describe the main erythromycin drug interactions.

34.   **B** Macrolides are first-line agents for infection due to *Mycoplasma pneumoniae*.

Erythromycin metabolites inhibit the P-450 system, so they can increase the plasma concentration of several drugs given concomitantly, including warfarin. Therefore, the patient's bleeding was most likely due to an increased plasma concentration of warfarin.

A, C–F These drugs do not affect plasma concentration of warfarin and are not active against mycoplasma species.

Learning objective: Describe the mechanisms of bacterial resistance to macrolides.

35.   **C** Resistance to macrolides is mainly plasmid-mediated. The two main mechanisms of this resistance are

• Modification of the binding site on the 50S ribosomal subunit. This modification is due to the production of a methylase enzyme that adds a methyl group to the ribosomal binding site, "protecting" the site from binding by macrolides.

• Increased activity of the multidrug efflux pump

A, E See correct answer explanation.

B, D RNA polymerases and glucuronosyl transferases are not drug-inactivating enzymes.

Learning objective: Explain the mechanism of action of tetracyclines.

36.   **D** Mediterranean spotted fever is a disease caused by *Rickettsia conorii*. Doxycycline is a tetracycline antibiotic that has become the drug of choice for most rickettsial diseases because of its efficacy, long half-life, and very good oral bioavailability. Tetracyclines bind reversibly to the 30S ribosomal

subunit and block the access of aminoacyl-transfer RNA (tRNA) to the acceptor side of the messenger RNA (mRNA) ribosome complex. This prevents the addition of amino acids to the growing peptide chain and therefore inhibits bacterial protein synthesis.

A This is the mechanism of action of rifampin.

B This is one of the mechanisms of action of aminoglycosides.

C This is the mechanism of action of chloramphenicol.

E This is the mechanism of action of β-lactam antibiotics.

Learning objective: Identify the drug used to treat Lyme disease.

37.   **D** The history and the symptoms of the patient indicate that she was most likely suffering from Lyme disease, a tick-borne borreliosis caused by *Borrelia burgdorferi*. The first stage of the disease begins as a red macule that expands (hence the name erythema migrans), often with a central clearing, to a diameter as large as 50 cm (about 20 inches). The second stage occurs within weeks to months of the onset of erythema and is characterized by arthritis (about 50% of patients) and/or neurologic and cardiac abnormalities (less than 20% of patients). *B. burgdorferi* is susceptible to the action of tetracyclines, macrolides, penicillins, and some second- and third-generation cephalosporins. Tetracyclines are still the drug of choice for the erythema migrans, whereas ceftriaxone is the preferred drug for the second stage of the disease.

A–C, E These antibiotics are not effective against *Borrelia*.

Learning objective: Identify the drug used to treat relapsing fever.

38.   **D** The lab results indicate that spirochetes are the offending pathogens, and the patient's symptoms are consistent with the diagnosis of relapsing fever. The disease is caused by several *Borrelia* species and transmitted by lice or ticks. In the United States, the disease is endemic in areas where there are ticks that harbor *Borrelia* (usually remote settings in the western mountains and semiarid plains). The disease is characterized by recurrent febrile paroxysms lasting 3 to 5 days and separated by intervals of apparent recovery, as in this case. *Borrelia* species are sensitive to tetracyclines, macrolides, penicillins, and some second- and third-generation cephalosporins. Doxycycline is often the preferred drug.

A Syphilis is caused by a spirochete, but the symptoms are quite different, and the disease cannot be cured by streptomycin.

B Brucellosis can be cured by streptomycin but is not caused by a spirochete.

C Rocky Mountain spotted fever can be cured by tetracyclines but is not caused by a spirochete.

E, F These diseases are not caused by spirochetes and cannot be cured by β-lactam antibiotics.

Learning objective: Explain the mechanism of action of chloramphenicol.

39. **B** Chloramphenicol enters the cell by facilitated diffusion and binds reversibly with the 50S ribosomal subunit. At this site, it prevents binding of the amino acid–containing end of the aminoacyl transfer RNA (tRNA) to the acceptor site of the 50S ribosomal subunit. Thus, the peptide at the donor site cannot be transferred to its amino acid acceptor, and the transpeptidation reaction cannot occur. The drug is used very rarely for systemic treatment because of its toxicity but is frequently used topically, as in this case, as it has a very broad activity spectrum.

    A This is the mechanism of action of β-lactam drugs.

    C This is the mechanism of action of fluoroquinolones.

    D This is the mechanism of action of antifungal azoles.

    E This is the mechanism of action of aminoglycosides.

Learning objective: Outline the therapy for neonatal listeriosis.

40. **B** Neonatal sepsis occurs in about 1 in 1000 live births. Preterm newborns are especially at risk. Mortality ranges from 10 to 50% and is higher in those with early-onset disease. The most common pathogens found in neonatal sepsis are streptococci and staphylococci, but another important and often overlooked pathogen is *Listeria monocytogenes.* A penicillin (ampicillin or penicillin G) with an aminoglycoside (mainly gentamicin) is the standard therapy against neonatal listeriosis. Ampicillin is very effective against *Listeria,* and the aminoglycoside may provide synergy.

    A, D Tetracyclines and macrolides are both active against *Listeria,* but bacteriostatic antibiotics are rarely first-choice agents in case of severe, life-threatening infections.

    C, E, F Cephalosporins, aztreonam, and metronidazole are not active against *Listeria.*

Learning objective: Explain the reason for contraindication of tetracyclines during pregnancy.

41. **A** Lymphogranuloma venereum is a chlamydial disease endemic in parts of Africa, characterized by a transitory primary skin lesion followed by suppurative lymphadenitis and lymphangitis. Doxycycline and erythromycin rapidly heal the disease. Tetracyclines are bound to calcium deposited in newly formed bone and teeth of young children and in fetal bones. Therefore, they may cause inhibition of fetal growth if given during pregnancy.

    B–E Tetracyclines have a negligible risk of these adverse effects.

Learning objective: Identify bacterium sensitive to tetracyclines.

42. **A** The patient's signs and symptoms and the fact that doxycycline was chosen for therapy indicate that the offending pathogen was most likely *Vibrio cholerae.* Cholera is endemic in portions of Asia, Africa, and South and Central America. The disease can be subclinical, mild, or fulminant and potentially lethal. Early treatment with an effective antibiotic can stop diarrhea in 48 hours (thus decreasing fluid loss) and shorten the duration of the carrier state. *V. cholerae* is sensitive to macrolides, tetracyclines, and fluoroquinolones. Doxycycline is often the preferred agent.

    B–E All of these bacteria are resistant to tetracyclines.

Learning objective: Describe the adverse effects of doxycycline.

43. **D** The patient's history and symptoms indicate that he was most likely suffering from a phototoxic reaction due to doxycycline. Tetracyclines can cause phototoxicity that usually has the clinical appearance of an exaggerated sunburn reaction. Other antibiotics that can cause phototoxicity are fluoroquinolones and sulfonamides.

    A–C, E, F The risk of a phototoxic reaction with these drugs is negligible. Moreover, these antibiotics are not active against nongonococcal urethritis, which is usually caused by *Chlamydia trachomatis* or *Ureaplasma urealyticum.*

Learning objective: Identify the drug used together with quinidine to treat *Plasmodium falciparum* malaria.

44. **C** Tetracyclines are effective against some protozoa, including *P. falciparum.* They are mainly used, together with quinine or quinidine, in cases of severe malarial attack, as in this case. Doxycycline is the preferred drug and should overlap quinidine for 2 or 3 days before the latter is discontinued.

    A, B, D–F These drugs are not effective against *Plasmodia.*

Learning objective: Identify the antibiotic used to treat infection due to vancomycin-resistant *Staphylococcus aureus.*

45. **F** In recent years, methicillin-resistant (MR) staphylococci have been associated with the emergence of resistance to vancomycin, too. Because vancomycin was considered the last-line therapy for MR staphylococci, these findings are worrisome. The combination of quinupristin plus dalfopristin, two antibiotics of the streptogramin family, has been shown to be effective against vancomycin-resistant (VR) staphylococci, as well as VR *Enterococcus faecium,* and currently represents a first-line treatment against these bacteria.

    A–E VR staphylococci are usually resistant to all the listed antibiotics.

Learning objective: Identify the pair of drugs used to treat brucellosis.

46. **B** Brucellosis is a zoonotic infectious disease characterized by an acute febrile stage and a chronic stage with relapses of fever, sweats, and vague pains. *Brucellae* are sensitive to several antibacterial drugs, including aminoglycosides, tetracyclines, chloramphenicol, imipenem, rifampin, fluoroquinolones, and trimethoprim-sulfamethoxazole. Because treatment with a single agent has been associated with a high incidence of relapse, combination therapy is used whenever possible. The combination of doxycycline and an aminoglycoside (streptomycin, gentamicin, or amikacin) for 4 weeks followed by the combination of doxycycline and rifampin for 4 to 8 weeks seems to be the most effective regimen.

A Rifampin is effective against brucellae, but metronidazole is not.

C–E Brucellae are not sensitive to vancomycin, macrolides, penicillins, and cephalosporins.

Learning objective: Identify the drug used to treat Rocky Mountain spotted fever.

47. **B** The classic triad of fever, rash, and history of tick exposure strongly suggests the diagnosis of Rocky Mountain spotted fever. The disease is caused by *Rickettsia rickettsii* and can be serious, with a mortality rate of about 5%, largely due to delay in initiating specific treatment. Rickettsiae are sensitive to tetracyclines, chloramphenicol, macrolides, and fluoroquinolones, but tetracyclines such as doxycycline remain the drugs of choice.

A, C–F These drugs are not effective against rickettsiae.

Learning objective: Describe the mechanisms of bacterial resistance to tetracyclines.

48. **E** Resistance to tetracyclines is mainly plasmid mediated. The major mechanisms are

- Increased activity of the multidrug efflux pump
- Decreased uptake of the drug
- Production of ribosome protection proteins that prevent the access of tetracyclines to the ribosome

Plasmids that include genes involved in the production of the tetracycline efflux pump commonly include resistance genes for several antibiotics.

A–D See correct answer explanation.

Learning objective: Identify the antibiotic causing candidiasis in a patient with acne.

49. **E** The patient's genital candidiasis was most likely a superinfection caused by antibiotic-mediated alteration of the normal genital microflora. Because the woman had acne, she most likely received tetracycline, the most common antibiotic used in moderate to severe acne. *Propionibacterium acnes* is an anaerobic corynebacterium that resides in normal skin and participates in the pathogenesis of acne. The bacterium is very sensitive to tetracyclines and macrolides. The risk of superinfection is higher with broad-spectrum antibiotics such as tetracyclines. Long-term treatment with these drugs, as in this case, further increases the risk.

A–D, F None of these drugs are used to treat acne, and they rarely cause superinfections.

Learning objective: Describe the outcome of interaction between tetracyclines and dairy products.

50. **E** Tetracycline absorption (except that of doxycycline and minocycline) is impaired by some cations (Ca^{2+}, Mg^{2+}, Fe^{2+}, Al^{3+}) because tetracyclines can chelate these cations, forming a complex that cannot permeate the intestinal wall. Therefore, products that contain a large amount of these cations (e.g., milk and dairy products, antacids, and iron and zinc supplements) must not be administered with tetracyclines. The decrease in drug oral bioavailability is pronounced (50–90%).

A–D See correct answer explanation.

BACTERIAL PROTEIN SYNTHESIS INHIBITORS Answer key				
1. O	6. E	11. D	16. B	21. D
2. L	7. D	12. A	17. E	22. B
3. B	8. C	13. A	18. E	23. B
4. E	9. D	14. D	19. E	24. C
5. J	10. E	15. B	20. E	25. B
26. E	31. C	36. D	41. A	46. B
27. E	32. C	37. D	42. A	47. B
28. C	33. D	38. D	43. D	48. E
29. C	34. B	39. B	44. C	49. E
30. B	35. C	40. B	45. F	50. E

Answers and Explanations: VIII-3 Inhibitors of Bacterial Nucleic Acid Synthesis or Function

Questions 1–3

1. **B**
2. **E**
3. **A**

Learning objective: Describe the antibacterial spectrum of fluoroquinolones.

4. **C** Ciprofloxacin is a fluoroquinolone antibiotic. These drugs have a broad antibacterial spectrum that includes some gram-positive bacteria, most gram-negative bacteria, and some mycobacteria, mycoplasmas, chlamydiae, and rickettsiae.

    A, B Piperacillin and ceftazidime are effective against *Pseudomonas aeruginosa* but not against mycobacteria, mycoplasmas, chlamydiae, and rickettsiae.

    D Erythromycin is effective against mycobacteria, mycoplasmas, chlamydiae, and rickettsiae but not against *P. aeruginosa* and mycobacteria.

    E Vancomycin is effective only against gram-positive bacteria.

Learning objective: Explain the mechanism of resistance to sulfonamides.

5. **C** Many bacteria originally sensitive to sulfonamides are now resistant. Resistance to trimethoprim-sulfamethoxazole is less frequent than resistance to either of the agents alone, but it still occurs in several cases. When resistance develops, it is usually persistent and irreversible. Mechanisms of resistance to sulfonamides are

   - Decreased affinity for sulfonamides by dihydropteroate synthetase
   - Decreased bacterial permeability to the drug
   - Increased production of para-aminobenzoic acid (PABA). For example, some resistant staphylococci may synthesize 70 times as much PABA as do the susceptible parental strains.

    A, E These mechanisms would increase, not decrease, the bacterial sensitivity to sulfonamides.

    B Sulfonamides do not act by binding to bacterial ribosomes.

    D Sulfonamides do not act by binding to dihydrofolate reductase.

Learning objective: Identify the drug that can cause dermatitis in a previously sensitized person.

6. **C** The patient's history and symptoms suggest that he had an allergic reaction to trimethoprim-sulfametoxazole. Rash is a common adverse effect associated with sulfonamide use and is most frequently due to hypersensitivity. Moreover, trimethoprim-sulfamethoxazole has been reported to cause up to three times as many dermatologic reactions as do sulfonamides alone.

    A, B, D, E These drugs are not currently used to treat acute pharyngitis, and they are not given orally.

Learning objective: Describe the adverse effects of fluoroquinolones.

7. **E** Fluoroquinolones have been associated with an increased risk of tendon rupture that can occur even after short-term use of these drugs. This adverse effect has been officially reported in literally hundreds of patients. The mechanism of this action seems related to a direct cytotoxic effect of the drug on the ligament tissue. In fact, in vitro exposure of tendon tissue to ciprofloxacin resulted in a decrease in fibroblast proliferation, a decrease in collagen synthesis, and a significant increase in matrix-degrading proteolytic activity.

    A–D These drugs do not cause tendon rupture.

Learning objective: Describe the main drug interactions with fluoroquinolones.

8. **A** Products containing divalent and trivalent cations (Mg^{2+}, Ca^{2+}, Zn^{2+}, Al^{3+}, Fe^{2+}), such as antacids, milk products, and Fe^{2+}-containing medications, invariably cause a significant decrease in intestinal absorption of fluoroquinolones (up to 70%) because fluoroquinolones can chelate the cations, forming insoluble compounds. This may result in therapeutic failures. It is therefore imperative that clinicians question patients regarding other medications, both prescription and nonprescription, that they may be taking and instruct them to avoid certain products, as in this case.

    B–E See correct answer explanation.

Learning objective: Outline the therapeutic uses of ciprofloxacin.

9. **B** The patient's history and symptoms indicate that he was most likely suffering from traveler's diarrhea, a disease defined as three or more loose stools per day plus at least one enteric symptom. The disease is due to enterobacteriaceae, with *Escherichia coli* being the causative agent in more than 50% of cases. Many antimicrobial agents have been shown to shorten the duration and severity of diarrhea, but because of the increasing resistance of enterobacteriaceae, currently fluoroquinolones, and to a lesser extent trimethoprim-sulfamethoxazole, are recommended for the empiric treatment of traveler's diarrhea.

    A, C–F These drugs are not active against most enterobacteriaceae.

Learning objective: Explain the rationale of the trimethoprim-sulfamethoxazole combination.

10. **D** The trimethoprim-sulfamethoxazole combination kills sensitive bacteria, whereas sulfonamides and trimethoprim are both bacteriostatic drugs. The synergistic effect of the combination is most likely due to the inhibition of two consecutive steps in the synthesis of tetrahydrofolic acid, which is essential for the synthesis of purines and then for the synthesis of DNA.

A, E The combination does not affect the pharmacokinetics of either drug.

B Because both drugs can cause allergic reactions, the risk of those reactions, if anything, should be increased, not decreased.

C It is well known that patient compliance is increased when fewer pills must be taken, but this is not the reason for the drug combination.

Learning objective: Outline the therapeutic uses of ciprofloxacin.

11. **D** The patient's signs and symptoms indicate that he was suffering from pneumonia. The associated relative bradycardia, gastrointestinal symptoms, and microhematuria suggest Legionnaires' disease, a pneumonia caused by *Legionella* species (mainly *Legionella pneumophila*), which accounts for 1 to 3% of all pneumonias. *L. pneumophila* is sensitive to macrolides, fluoroquinolones, tetracyclines, trimethoprim-sulfamethoxazole, and rifampin. Erythromycin, alone or with rifampin, is the treatment of choice. Fluoroquinolones such as ciprofloxacin may be useful in case of intolerance to macrolides, as in this case.

A, B, C, F *L. Pneumophila* is not sensitive to these antibiotics.

E See correct answer explanation.

Learning objective: Describe the antibacterial spectrum of fluoroquinolones.

12. **E** *Haemophilus influenzae* can cause otitis media in adults, although *Streptococcus pneumoniae* and *Staphylococcus aureus* are more common. *H. influenzae* is very sensitive to fluoroquinolones, such as ciprofloxacin.

A–D These bacteria do not cause otitis media and are resistant to fluoroquinolones.

Learning objective: Outline the therapeutic uses of metronidazole.

13. **B** Brain abscesses most commonly arise from a contiguous, suppurative source of infection (sinusitis, mastoiditis, and dental infection), as in this case. Streptococci are implicated in about 60% of cases and include both anaerobic and microaerophilic streptococci. Bacteroides are found in about 40% of cases. Antibiotic therapy for brain abscess needs to be sufficiently broad to cover the most likely pathogens. A combination of penicillin G and metronidazole is used in most cases. Metronidazole achieves abscess fluid concentration equal to or in excess of serum levels and is bactericidal against anaerobes. Moreover, in this case, the apparent good activity of clindamycin in the previous sinusitis points out that anaerobes are most likely the main bacteria of the patient's abscess.

A, C–E These antibiotics are not active against anaerobes.

Learning objective: Explain the mechanism of action of fluoroquinolones.

14. **B** Ciprofloxacin is a fluoroquinolone antibiotic. Fluoroquinolones inhibit bacterial DNA synthesis by blocking the following enzymes:

- Topoisomerase II (also called DNA gyrase). The blockade prevents the relaxation of supercoiled DNA, which is required for normal transcription (prevalent mechanism in gram-negative bacteria).
- Topoisomerase IV. The blockade interferes with separation of replicated chromosomal DNA during cell division (prevalent mechanism in gram-positive bacteria).

A This is the mechanism of action of β-lactam antibiotics.

C This is the mechanism of action of aminoglycosides.

D This is the mechanism of action of antifungal azoles.

E Helicases are enzymes involved in DNA strand separation during replication. Fluoroquinolones have no activity on these enzymes.

F This is the mechanism of action of rifampin.

Learning objective: Identify the bacterium that is sensitive to trimethoprim-sulfamethoxazole.

15. **E** The successful treatment indicates that the offending pathogen was sensitive to trimethoprim-sulfamethoxazole. *Escherichia coli* is the most common causative agent of urinary tract infection and is sensitive to trimethoprim-sulfamethoxazole, even though resistance has significantly increased in recent years.

A–D All of these bacteria are resistant to trimethoprim-sulfamethoxazole.

Learning objective: Describe the main contraindications of fluoroquinolones.

16. **F** Fluoroquinolones are largely used for urinary tract infections because of their excellent activity against most gram-negative bacteria, but they are contraindicated in people with long QT interval of any cause, as they can increase QT interval, predisposing to polymorphic ventricular tachycardia.

A–E All of these antibiotics are active against gram-negative rods and are not contraindicated in persons with long QT intervals.

Learning objective: Outline the therapeutic uses of ciprofloxacin.

17. **C** Disseminated *Mycobacterium avium* complex (MAC) infection is common in end-stage AIDS patients. The risk of developing the infection is strongly associated with a CD4+ lymphocyte count of less than 100 cells/mm³. Transient bacteremia is followed by invasion of tissues resulting in organ dysfunction. Any organ can be involved, and patients often present with nonspecific symptoms, as in this case.

    The current recommended regimen for MAC infection includes three drugs. Clarithromycin plus ethambutol are the preferred two, and the third agent may be ciprofloxacin, rifambutin, or imipenem.

    A, B, D−F None of these drugs are effective against MAC.

Learning objective: Outline the therapeutic uses of sulfonamides.

18. **D** The patient's signs (a cavitary lesion seen on a chest x-ray) and lab results suggest the diagnosis of nocardiosis. *Nocardia asteroides* is the most common pathogen in nocardiosis, an opportunistic infection associated with several risk factors, including immunosuppression, as in this case (see the prolonged corticosteroid treatment). In nocardiosis, sulfonamides are first-line agents. Alternative drugs include penicillins, aminoglycosides, and tetracyclines (doxycycline and minocycline).

    A−C, E These antibiotics are not effective against *Nocardia*.

Learning objective: Outline the therapeutic uses of metronidazole.

19. **A** Fulminant colitis is a rare but severe form of pancolitis, an inflammation affecting the entire colon. Patients with pancolitis are at risk of developing toxic megacolon, and an emergency treatment must include intravenous fluid and electrolyte therapy, high-dose corticosteroids, and antibiotics. Because *Bacteroides fragilis* is the most abundant bacterium in the human colon, metronidazole remains a first-line agent. Fluoroquinolones, clindamycin, cefoxitin, and cefotetan may be alternatives.

    B−F These antibiotics are not effective against *B. fragilis*.

Learning objective: Identify the bacterium that is sensitive to trimethoprim-sulfamethoxazole.

20. **F** The patient's history, the lab results, and the prescribed therapy suggest that the pneumonia was due to *Pneumocystis jiroveci*, a well-recognized opportunistic infection in AIDS patients. The pathogen grows extracellularly in the surfactant layer of the lung. The blockade of the oxygen exchange interface results in hypoxemia and cyanosis. The medication of choice for pneumocystis pneumonia is trimethoprim-sulfamethoxazole; pentamidine is also effective and may be given as an alternate drug.

    A−E, G *Pseudomonas aeruginosa*, *Clostridium difficile*, mycoplasmas, rickettsiae, spirochetes, and enterococci are resistant to trimethoprim-sulfamethoxazole.

Learning objective: Outline the therapeutic uses of metronidazole.

21. **B** A variety of regimens have been used to eradicate *Helicobacter pylori*, each with different dosing schedules, adverse effects, and cost. Combination therapy with two or three antibiotics plus an H_2 antagonist or a proton pump inhibitor is associated with the highest rate of eradication. Antibiotics effective against *H. pylori* are amoxicillin, clarithromycin, metronidazole, and tetracycline.

    A, C−E None of these pairs include two antibiotics effective against *H. pylori*.

Learning objective: Explain the mechanism of action of sulfonamides.

22. **D** Sulfonamides are competitive inhibitors of the bacterial enzyme dihydropteroate synthetase, which is responsible for the incorporation of para-aminobenzoic acid (PABA) into dihydropteroic acid, the immediate precursor of folic acid. Because bacterial cells use PABA to synthesize folic acid, the synthesis of folic acid is inhibited. This in turn inhibits the synthesis of bacterial purines that are needed for the synthesis of nucleic acids. In contrast, mammalian cells use preformed folic acid that is present in the diet and therefore are not sensitive to the action of sulfonamides.

    A−C, E These enzymes are not inhibited by sulfonamides.

Learning objective: Describe the use of metronidazole in *Clostridium difficile*-associated colitis.

23. **A** The oral agents most commonly used to treat pseudomembranous colitis due to *C. difficile* are vancomycin and metronidazole. The two drugs have comparable efficacy, but when vancomycin fails, a treatment with metronidazole is the most appropriate course of action.

    B, C Oral vancomycin produces fecal concentrations that are 100 times the concentration needed to inhibit *C. difficile*, so increasing the dose or using intravenous vancomycin are not useful options.

    D, E These antibiotics are not effective against *C. difficile* infections.

Learning objective: Identify the antibiotic that can cause megaloblastic anemia.

24. **D** The patient was most likely treated with trimethoprim-sulfamethoxazole, a first-line drug combination for urinary tract infection. The patient's symptoms and the lab results indicate that she was most likely suffering from megaloblastic anemia. Trimethoprim may cause the predictable adverse effects of an antifolate drug, including megaloblastic anemia. The anemia is rare in healthy individuals but can occur in patients who are already folate-deficient from different causes, such as poor diet, malabsorption syndromes, malignancy, or alcoholism, as in this case.

    A−C, E−G These drugs do not affect folate metabolism.

Learning objective: Outline the therapeutic uses of metronidazole.

25. **E** The patient's history and symptoms indicate that she was most likely affected by *Clostridium difficile*–associated pseudomembranous colitis. The disease has emerged as a major threat to elderly patients receiving certain antibiotics. Ampicillin, clindamycin, and cephalosporins are the antibiotics most commonly associated with the condition. Other drugs are penicillins, erythromycin, trimethoprim-sulfamethoxazole, fluoroquinolones, and tetracyclines. Ampicillin was most likely the causative antibiotic in this case. Metronidazole and vancomycin are the two first-line agents for *C. difficile*–associated colitis.

    A–D, F None of these antibiotics are effective against *C. difficile*.

Learning objective: Describe the main drug interactions with metronidazole.

26. **F** Bacterial vaginosis is due to a complex alteration of vaginal flora in which lactobacilli decrease and anaerobic pathogens overgrow. Topical or oral metronidazole is the agent of choice. The drug can inhibit aldehyde dehydrogenase and therefore can cause a disulfiram-like effect due to accumulation of acetaldehyde in people drinking alcohol concomitantly. The reaction may cause flushing, throbbing headache, nausea and vomiting, hypotension, and mental confusion.

    A–E None of these antibiotics interact with alcohol.

Learning objective: Identify the antibiotic that can cause acute hemolytic anemia in patients with congenital glucose-6-phosphate dehydrogenase deficiency.

27. **F** The patient most likely received trimethoprim-sulfamethoxazole, a drug combination frequently used to treat urinary tract infection. The patient's signs and symptoms (tiredness, dark urine) suggest that she was suffering from acute hemolytic anemia, a disease that can develop in persons with congenital deficiency of glucose-6-phosphate dehydrogenase when given oxidant chemicals. Glucose-6-phosphate dehydrogenase is a key enzyme in reduction reactions, and these reactions appear to be essential for maintenance of cellular integrity. A deficiency of this enzyme results in an exaggerated sensitivity to the hemolytic effect of certain oxidant drugs such as sulfonamides, antimalarials, and certain nonsteroidal antiinflammatory drugs.

    A–E These drugs do not have significant oxidant properties.

Learning objective: Outline the therapeutic use of trimethoprim-sulfamethoxazole.

28. **E** Trimethoprim-sulfamethoxazole is still a first-line agent against urinary tract infection due to *E. coli*, even though resistance has increased over the past several years. Moreover, the drug is effective against several enterobacteriaceae (with the exception of *P aeruginosa* and anaerobes) that are usually present in urinary tract infections.

    A, B Because the bacterium was resistant to ampicillin and ciprofloxacin, it would be illogical to use amoxicillin or moxifloxacin because cross-resistance would be likely.

    C, D, F These antibiotics are not effective against *E. coli*.

Learning objective: Explain the mechanism of action of metronidazole.

29. **D** Metronidazole is an antibiotic active against most microaerophile and anaerobic bacteria and anaerobic protozoa. These microorganisms, unlike their aerobic counterparts, contain electron transport components called ferredoxins that can donate electrons to metronidazole. This donation forms a highly reactive nitro radical anion that damages bacterial DNA. The ultimate effect is bactericidal.

    A–C, E All of these antibiotics are active against *Bacteroides fragilis,* but they have mechanisms of action different from that of metronidazole.

Learning objective: Explain the adverse fetal effects of trimethoprim-sulfamethoxazole in pregnant women.

30. **B** Trimethoprim-sulfamethoxazole combination is currently used for urinary tract infection, but sulfonamides have a definite risk of causing kernicterus in neonates if given to mothers during the third trimester of pregnancy. These drugs displace unconjugated bilirubin from plasma albumin, thereby allowing free bilirubin to enter the brain. The risk is high in neonates because bilirubin conjugation is already defective due to the low levels of glucuronosyl transferase.

    A, C, D These drugs are used in urinary tract infections and are not contraindicated in pregnancy.

    E, F Aminoglycosides and fluoroquinolones are relatively contraindicated in pregnancy, but not because they can cause kernicterus. Aminoglycosides can induce fetal ototoxicity, and fluoroquinolones can cause articular cartilage erosion.

INHIBITORS OF BACTERIAL NUCLEIC ACID SYNTHESIS OR FUNCTION Answer key					
1.	B	6.	C	11.	D
2.	E	7.	E	12.	E
3.	A	8.	A	13.	B
4.	C	9.	B	14.	B
5.	C	10.	D	15.	E
16.	F	21.	B	26.	F
17.	C	22.	D	27.	F
18.	D	23.	A	28.	E
19.	A	24.	D	29.	D
20.	F	25.	E	30.	B

Answers and Explanations: VIII-4 Antimycobacterial Drugs

Questions 1 and 2

1. **H**
2. **C**

Learning objective: Explain the mechanism of action of isoniazid.

3. **A** Isoniazid is used alone for the prophylaxis of tuberculosis in at-risk patients, including those who are HIV positive, as in this case. The drug inhibits the synthesis of mycolic acids, which are specific constituents of the mycobacterial cell wall. This can explain, at least in part, why isoniazid is effective only against mycobacteria.

    B The synthesis of peptidoglycan is inhibited by β-lactam antibiotics.

    C Arabinosyl transferase is inhibited by ethambutol.

    D Topoisomerase II is inhibited by fluoroquinolones.

    E DNA-dependent RNA polymerase is inhibited by rifamycins.

Learning objective: Identify the enzyme involved in mycobacterial resistance to isoniazid.

4. **A** Isoniazid is a prodrug that must be converted into the active compound by a mycobacterial catalase-peroxidase. Resistance is often associated with the deletion of the *katG* gene that codes for the synthesis of catalase peroxidase. In this way, activation of the prodrug cannot occur.

    B–E These enzymes are not involved in the mechanism of resistance of mycobacteria to isoniazid.

Learning objective: Describe the metabolism of isoniazid.

5. **D** Isoniazid is metabolized by hepatic acetylation, which is under genetic control. Patients may be fast acetylators (mainly among people of Asian origin) or slow acetylators (mainly among people of European and African origin). Fast acetylators require higher dosage than slow acetylators to obtain equivalent therapeutic effects.

    A–C, E These drugs are not metabolized by acetylation.

Learning objective: Explain the mechanism of action of rifampin.

6. **A** Rifampin inhibits DNA-dependent RNA polymerase in mycobacteria and other sensitive microorganisms by binding to the β subunit of the enzyme to form a stable drug–enzyme complex. This leads to suppression of initiation of chain formation in RNA synthesis. The ultimate effect is bactericidal.

    B This enzyme is inhibited by ethambutol.

    C This enzyme is inhibited by β-lactam antibiotics.

    D This enzyme is inhibited by fluoroquinolones.

    E This enzyme is inhibited by reverse transcriptase inhibitors.

Learning objective: Explain the mechanism of action of ethambutol.

7. **C** Ethambutol inhibits arabinosyl transferase, disrupting the synthesis of arabinogalactan, an essential component of the mycobacterial cell wall. The ultimate effect is bacteriostatic.

    A This enzyme is inhibited by trimethoprim.

    B This enzyme is inhibited by chloramphenicol.

    D This enzyme is inhibited by fosfomycin.

    E This enzyme is inhibited by sulfonamides.

    F This enzyme is inhibited by vancomycin.

Learning objective: Identify the antibiotic that is most likely included in the pharmacotherapy of *Mycobacterium avium* complex (MAC) infection.

8. **D** MAC infection is common in end-stage AIDS patients, and the risk of developing the infection is the highest when the CD4+ lymphocyte count is less than 50 cells/mm^3, as in this case. MAC is much less susceptible than *Mycobacterium tuberculosis* to most antimycobacterial drugs, and in most cases disseminated MAC is incurable and therapy is lifelong. Drug regimens for MAC should include at least three drugs, and one of these must be a macrolide, such as clarithromycin or azithromycin, as these are the only antibiotics for which a correlation between in vitro susceptibility tests for MAC and clinical response has been demonstrated. Other drugs active against MAC are rifampin, ethambutol, ethionamide, imipenem, and fluoroquinolones.

    A–C, E These drugs are not active against MAC.

Learning objective: Describe the prophylactic use of isoniazid in close contacts of people with active tuberculosis.

9. **C** Isoniazid is the drug of choice to prevent tuberculosis in skin test converters and in close contacts of patients with active disease, as in this case. The drug is given as the sole agent for at least 6 and up to 12 months. In people at high risk of infection with multidrug-resistant strains (i.e., HIV-positive patients), preventive therapy is usually performed with more than one drug.

    A, B, D, E These drugs are not used for prophylaxis of tuberculosis unless the patient is at high risk of infection.

Learning objective: Describe the adverse effects of ethambutol.

10. **D** The signs and symptoms of the patient are most likely due to ethambutol-induced optic neuritis, a serious adverse effect of the drug that is dose- and duration-related. Because of this, periodic visual acuity testing is desirable during ethambutol therapy. Recovery is usually, but not always, complete when the drug is discontinued.

    A–C, E These drugs do not cause optic neuritis.

Learning objective: Outline the pharmacotherapy for hemorrhagic mycobacterial pericarditis.

11. **D** This patient demonstrates many of the clinical features of constrictive pericarditis, including an inspiratory increase of systemic venous pressure (Kussmaul sign), third heart sound, and narrow pulse pressure. The slow development of symptoms and the large amount of bloody fluid removed by pericardiocentesis indicate subacute effusive-constrictive pericarditis. The two most common causes for hemorrhagic pericarditis are tuberculosis (TB) and metastatic carcinoma. Because the patient is HIV positive, TB is much more likely. In fact, TB is the leading cause of death in HIV-infected people worldwide. Antimycobacterial therapy should be carried out if a TB origin can be diagnosed, is suspected, or cannot be excluded in a patient with chronic constrictive pericarditis. Isoniazid and rifampin are the leading drugs for TB even if, as in this case, a four-drug regimen including pyrazinamide and ethambutol should be administered because TB pericarditis is a serious infection, and HIV patients are also at risk of developing TB meningitis.

    A–C, E These combinations contain at least one drug not active against *Mycobacterium tuberculosis*.

Learning objective: Identify the drug to be used prophylactically in close contacts of patients with meningococcal meningitis.

12. **E** Rifampin is the drug of first choice for chemoprophylaxis of close contacts of patients with meningococcal meningitis. The potential for a close contact to become infected with *Neisseria meningitidis* is 500 to 800 times greater than for the total population. The drug should be administered as soon as possible because the risk of secondary disease is greatest within 2 to 5 days after exposure to the index case. Other drugs used for chemoprophylaxis include ceftriaxone and ciprofloxacin.

    A–D These antibiotics are not active against *N. meningitidis*.

Learning objective: Describe the antibacterial spectrum of rifampin.

13. **B** The antimicrobial spectrum of rifampin is broad. The drug is active against most mycobacteria; most gram-positive bacteria, including methicillin-resistant staphylococci; and many gram-negative bacteria, including *Escherichia coli, Proteus, Klebsiella, Legionella, Brucella, Haemophilus, Chlamydia,* and *Rickettsia* species and poxviruses.

    A, D, E These drugs are active only against mycobacteria.

    C Aminoglycoside antibiotics are active mainly against gram-negative aerobic bacteria.

Learning objective: Describe the appropriate therapy for a patient treated with rifampin when another drug is given concomitantly.

14. **A** Rifampin is a strong inducer of the hepatic P-450 system and can increase the metabolism of many drugs, including glucocorticoids, oral contraceptives, methadone, β-blockers, and warfarin. Therefore, the dose of warfarin should be increased to maintain an appropriate anticoagulant effect.

    B The dose of propranolol should be raised, not reduced, because the metabolism of the drug is increased.

    C–E All of these options are irrational.

Learning objective: Describe the hepatotoxicity of isoniazid.

15. **D** The symptoms of the patient and the lab results indicate that she was most likely suffering from isoniazid-induced hepatitis, which is the most frequent major toxic effect of isoniazid. It occurs in about 1% of patients and can lead to potentially fatal multilobular necrosis. The risk increases with age and in alcoholics, as in this case.

    A–C, E These disorders cause neither the symptoms reported by the patient nor an increase in aminotransferase level.

    F Ethambutol-induced hepatitis is a very rare disorder.

Learning objective: Describe the main reason for the use of ethambutol in the pharmacotherapy of tuberculosis (TB).

16. **E** The main reason for the use of any drug combination in the therapy of TB is to delay the emergence of resistance. In the case of ethambutol, this is by far the primary reason, as the drug has only weak bacteriostatic activity against *Mycobacterium tuberculosis* and cannot add significant antibacterial effect to a given therapeutic regimen.

    A–D All of these options are irrational.

Learning objective: Describe the adverse effects of pyrazinamide.

17. **B** The gastrointestinal symptoms and the high aminotransferase levels (which suggest some liver dysfunction), together with the joint pain and hyperuricemia, strongly indicate that pyrazinamide is the drug that caused these adverse effects. Hepatotoxicity is the major limiting adverse effect of pyrazinamide, is dose-related, and is far less common today with current dosing regimens. Arthralgia is also common and dose-related. Hyperuricemia is seen in more than 50% of patients taking the drug and is likely due to inhibition of uric acid secretion.

    A Rifampin very rarely causes hepatitis but can substantially increase the risk of hepatotoxicity when given together with pyrazinamide. However, it does not cause hyperuricemia.

    C Isoniazid can cause hepatotoxicity, but hyperuricemia is very rarely reported.

    D, E These drugs do not cause hepatotoxicity or hyperuricemia.

Learning objective: Describe the therapeutic strategy for multi-drug-resistant tuberculosis (TB).

18. **E** The starting treatment of this patient is standard for active TB, but when resistance occurs, the treatment must be changed. There is no standard regimen for multidrug-resistant TB, but it is critical to avoid adding or substituting a single drug to a failing regimen. Adding one drug at a time leads to the sequential selection of drug resistance. Therefore, two or more previously unused drugs, chosen among the second-line agents, should be substituted. Second-line agents include some aminoglycoside antibiotics (mainly streptomycin; amikacin is also active), ethionamide, cycloserine, p-aminosalicylic acid, and fluoroquinolones. Most fluoroquinolones have excellent antimycobacterial activity in vitro; moxifloxacin seems the most active clinically.

    A–D All of these combinations contain at least one drug that is not active against *Mycobacterium tuberculosis*.

Learning objective: Describe the use of pyridoxine to prevent isoniazid-induced neurotoxicity.

19. **B** The patient is most likely suffering from isoniazid-induced peripheral neuropathy. Neurotoxicity is the most common adverse effect of isoniazid when the daily dose exceeds 6 mg/kg (unless pyridoxine is given concurrently), likely because the drug promotes the excretion of pyridoxine, a vitamin involved in several metabolic transformations, including the synthesis of some neurotransmitters (gamma-aminobutyric acid, norepinephrine, and serotonin). The risk of neurotoxicity is increased in slow acetylators, alcoholics, and diabetics, as in this case. Peripheral neuropathy is the main sign of isoniazid neurotoxicity (it can affect as many as 20% of patients at risk), but high doses can also provoke memory loss, confusion, hallucinations, and seizures. Most neurotoxic effects can be prevented or corrected by pyridoxine supplementation without losing the antibacterial effect.

    A, C–E These drug are useless in isoniazid-induced neurotoxicity.

Learning objective: Explain the most common mechanism of bacterial resistance to rifampin.

20. **C** Resistance to rifampin results primarily from mutation in the gene that codes for the β subunit of RNA polymerase. This mutation prevents binding of rifampin to the enzyme.

    A, B, D, E These enzymes are not involved in the bacterial resistance to rifampin.

Learning objective: Identify the first-line agent to treat leprosy.

21. **D** Leprosy is an exceedingly rare disease in the developed world, but about 5000 cases are reported each year in the United States, mainly in immigrants from Mexico and Central America, as in this case. Lepromatous leprosy is the most severe form of the disease because life-threatening complications (erythema nodosum leprosum and necrotizing skin reaction) can develop. Dapsone, a sulfone derivative, is the mainstay of therapy. The drug concentrates in the infected skin, which explains, at least in part, its undisputed efficacy. Other drugs active against *Mycobacterium leprae* are rifampin, clofazimine, macrolides, tetracyclines, and fluoroquinolones.

    A–C, E, F These antibiotics are not effective against *M. leprae*.

Learning objective: Explain the mechanism of bacterial resistance to ethambutol.

22. **C** A general mechanism of resistance to antimycobacterial drugs is related to mutation of genes that encode for the synthesis of enzymes that are inhibited by the drug. This mutation inhibits binding of the drug to the enzyme, preventing antibacterial activity. Ethambutol resistance is thought to result primarily from mutation in the gene that encodes for mycobacterial arabinosyl transferase, the enzyme specifically inhibited by the drug.

    A, B, D–F These actions are not involved in the mycobacterial resistance to ethambutol.

ANTIMYCOBACTERIAL DRUGS Answer key			
1. H	6. A	11. D	16. E
2. C	7. C	12. E	17. B
3. A	8. D	13. B	18. E
4. A	9. C	14. A	19. B
5. D	10. D	15. D	20. C
			21. D
			22. C

Answers and Explanations: VIII-5 Antifungal Drugs

Questions 1–3

1. **B**
2. **A**
3. **B**

Learning objective: Explain the mechanism of action of amphotericin B.

4. **B** Amphotericin B binds to fungal cell membranes and causes the formation of artificial pores through which ions and small molecules are lost. This causes the death of the fungal cell.

    A, C–E See correct answer explanation.

Learning objective: Identify the antifungal drug that acts by inhibiting the fungal P-450 system.

5. **C** *Coccidioides immitis* is sensitive to amphotericin B and antifungal azoles. Azole antifungals, primarily fluconazole and itraconazole, have replaced amphotericin B as initial therapy for most chronic pulmonary and disseminated infections. Amphotericin B is now usually reserved for patients with rapidly progressive coccidioidal infections. Azoles act by inhibiting the cytochrome P-450 system in fungal cells. The inhibition blocks the synthesis of ergosterol in the fungal cell membrane, leading to an antifungal effect. Relative selectivity occurs because the affinity for mammalian P-450 isozymes is less than that for the fungal isozymes. However, azoles can also block mammalian P-450 isozymes in the liver, which can explain the increased plasma concentration of many other drugs when coadministered with azoles.

    A, B, D–F These drugs do not block the fungal synthesis of ergosterol.

Learning objective: Identify the alternative drug to be used to treat cryptococcal meningitis when amphotericin B is not tolerated.

6. **E** Cryptococcal meningitis is common in patients with AIDS and is always fatal if untreated. Amphotericin B and flucytosine represents the standard therapy but is associated with frequent adverse reactions, including renal insufficiency and bone marrow suppression. Fluconazole is a useful alternative in patients who experience severe adverse effects. The antifungal spectrum of azoles includes *Cryptococcus neoformans*, but fluconazole is the preferred azole in case of meningitis

because it easily crosses the blood–brain barrier. AIDS patients with cryptococcal meningitis frequently are treated indefinitely with fluconazole to prevent recurrence of clinical disease.

   A, B Terbinafine and griseofulvin are effective only against superficial mycoses due to dermatophytes.

   C Nystatin is structurally similar to amphotericin B and has the same mechanism of action and the same antifungal spectrum in vitro, but it is too toxic to be used systemically.

   D Caspofungin is effective only against *Candida* and *Aspergillus* species.

Learning objective: Identify the drug used to treat genital candidiasis.

7. **C** The patient's symptoms and lab results suggest he was suffering from genital candidiasis, which can occur in people without underlying illnesses but is more common in those with diabetes mellitus or with the use of certain drugs (broad-spectrum antibiotics, corticosteroids, or immunosuppressants). Budding yeast cells and pseudohyphae of *Candida albicans*, the most common *Candida* species causing candidiasis, can be detected by microscopic examination of biologic specimens. *C. albicans* is sensitive to most antifungal drugs, but for genital candidiasis, a topical or oral azole derivative or topical nystatin is the first-line treatment. Oral and topical therapies are therapeutically equivalent.

   A Nystatin is effective against *Candida* species, but it is used only topically because of its toxicity.

   B, D, E These agents are not antifungal drugs.

   F Griseofulvin is not effective against *C. albicans*.

Learning objective: Outline the pharmacotherapy of systemic candidiasis.

8. **E** The patient's signs, symptoms, and x-ray suggest a systemic mycosis. Lab results confirm the diagnosis of systemic candidiasis, which accounts for about 80% of major systemic fungal infections. Amphotericin B, antifungal azoles, and echinocandins are first-line agents for systemic candidiasis.

   A–D All of these fungal infections are paired with the appropriate treatment, but they do not produce chlamydospores in blood cultures.

Learning objective: Explain the mechanism of action of flucytosine.

9. **C** Flucytosine is accumulated in fungal cells and is converted by a cytosine deaminase to 5-fluorouracil (selectivity occurs because mammalian cells do not accumulate and do not deaminate flucytosine). Fluorouracil is in turn metabolized to 5-deoxyfluorouridylic acid, a potent inhibitor of thymidylate synthetase, the enzyme responsible for converting deoxyuridine monophosphate to deoxythimidine monophosphate. This reduces the availability of thymidylic acid, impairing DNA synthesis. The drug is not used alone but is given together with itraconazole in chromoblastomycosis to avoid the development of resistance.

A, B Fluorouracil and cytarabine can inhibit DNA synthesis in mammalian cells but are not accumulated in fungal cells and therefore are devoid of antifungal activity.

D–F These antifungal drugs do not inhibit DNA synthesis.

Learning objective: Identify the drug used to treat meningeal coccidioidomycosis.

10. **D** The patient' signs and symptoms suggest the diagnosis of meningitis, and the lab results confirm that the man was suffering from meningeal coccidioidomycosis. The infection is caused by *Coccidioides immitis*, a soil mold that lives in semiarid regions of the globe, including the southwestern United States. Inhalation of the arthrospores leads to a primary infection that is asymptomatic in 60% of individuals. Others develop a flulike self-limited illness called valley fever or desert rheumatism. Following inhalation, the arthrospores form spherules that contain endospores. In biologic specimens, these spherules are diagnostic of *C. immitis* infection. In less than 1% of individuals, a secondary or disseminated infection evolves within a year after the primary one. This secondary infection is often life-threatening and can affect many parts of the body and tissues, but the most frequent are the bone, joints, and meninges. Untreated meningitis is always fatal.

C. immitis is sensitive to amphotericin B and antifungal azoles. Fluconazole is the first-line agent for meningeal coccidioidomycosis. It easily crosses the blood–brain barrier, and cerebrospinal fluid concentrations are 50 to 90% of plasma concentrations.

A Itraconazole is effective against *C. immitis,* but penetration into the brain is negligible.

B, C These antifungal drugs are not effective against *C. immitis.*

E, F These agents are not antifungal drugs.

Learning objective: Outline the pharmacotherapy of cryptococcal meningitis.

11. **D** The patient's history, signs and symptoms, and lab results suggest the diagnosis of cryptococcal meningitis. After toxoplasmosis, cryptococcosis is the most common central nervous system infection associated with AIDS. *Cryptococcus neoformans* is a yeast that is characterized by a thick polysaccharide capsule. During infection, the capsular polysaccharide is dissolved in spinal fluid and can be detected by an agglutination test that is diagnostic of cryptococcosis. *C. neoformans* is sensitive to amphotericin B, flucytosine, and antifungal azoles. The current treatment recommended for acute cryptococcal meningitis is amphotericin B plus flucytosine. Synergism between the two drugs has been demonstrated in vitro and in vivo. It may be related to enhanced penetration of flucytosine through the amphotericin-damaged fungal cell membrane.

A–C These agents are not antifungal drugs.

E, F These antifungal drugs are not effective against *C. neoformans.*

Learning objective: Identify the drug used to treat candiduria.

12. **B** The patient is suffering from candiduria, a condition often related to the placement of an indwelling urinary catheter, especially if the patient is taking broad-spectrum antibiotics, as in this case. Eradication of *Candida* in the urine includes the removal of the catheter and an antifungal treatment. Treatment options include amphotericin B, fluconazole, and an echinocandin such as caspofungin. However, in this patient, amphotericin B, which directly damages renal tubules, is contraindicated because of chronic renal dysfunction. Echinocandins are the newest class of antifungal drugs. They act by inhibiting the synthesis of β-glucan, an essential constituent of the fungal cell wall. Their antifungal spectrum is limited to *Candida* and *Aspergillus* species. Echinocandins are approved for treatment of mucocutaneous or disseminated candidiasis.

A See correct answer explanation.

C, D Piperacillin and metronidazole are not antifungal drugs.

E Though an antifungal drug, griseofulvin is not effective against *C. albicans.*

Learning objective: Recognize the adverse effects of amphotericin B.

13. **A** The lab results indicate that the patient was suffering from renal insufficiency. Amphotericin B is the drug of choice for many systemic mycoses, but it can cause serious, dose-dependent renal dysfunction due to direct damage of renal tubules. Azotemia, renal tubular acidosis, and K^+ wasting are the most prominent symptoms.

B–D These antifungal drugs do not cause renal toxicity.

E, F These agents are nephrotoxic but are not antifungal drugs.

Learning objective: Identify the site of action of terbinafine.

14. **C** Tinea manus is a cutaneous mycosis caused by dermatophytes that infect only the superficial, keratinized tissues. These fungi are probably restricted to the nonviable, keratinized tissues (stratum corneum, hairs, nails) because most are unable to grow at 37°C (98.6°F). Dermatophytoses can be treated locally with several antifungal drugs, but a first-line agent for systemic treatment is terbinafine. The drug has good oral bioavailability and is deposited in newly formed keratinized tissues, where it exerts its antifungal action.

A, B, D, E See correct answer explanation.

F Terbinafine can be deposited in the hair shaft, where it can cure tinea capitis, but in this case, the fungus is in the skin's stratum corneum, not in the hair.

Learning objective: Identify the drug used to treat mycoses due to *Trichophyton tonsurans*.

15. **C** The microscopic examination of the hair suggests the diagnosis of "black dots" tinea capitis, a skin mycosis caused by *T. tonsurans*. Cutaneous mycoses are caused by fungi (mainly dermatophytes) that infect only the superficial keratinized tissues. Dermatophytes are sensitive to terbinafine, antifungal azoles, griseofulvin, and amphotericin B, but the first two are agents of choice in cutaneous mycoses because they are deposited in newly forming skin, where they bind to keratin, protecting the skin from the infection. Griseofulvin is less frequently used today because of its toxicity.

A, B, D These agents are not antifungal drugs.

E Amphotericin B is only used topically for cutaneous mycoses.

F Flucytosine is a systemic antifungal drug but is not effective against dermatophytes.

Learning objective: Describe the use of glucocorticoids to prevent amphotericin B–related infusion reaction.

16. **D** The intravenous administration of amphotericin B can cause an infusion reaction with fever, chills, muscle spasms, headache, vomiting, and hypotension. Premedication with nonsteroidal antiinflammatory drugs, antihistamines, or glucocorticoids can alleviate the syndrome. The cause of this reaction is still uncertain, but histamine and prostaglandin release seems to be involved.

A–C, E, F See correct answer explanation.

Learning objective: Outline the pharmacological therapy of genital candidiasis.

17. **C** The patient's symptoms and lab results suggest that she was suffering from vulvovaginal candidiasis, the most common opportunistic mycosis of the genital tract in women taking oral contraceptives. Other predisposing factors are pregnancy, menstruation, diabetes mellitus, and use of broad-spectrum antibiotics, corticosteroids, or immunosuppressive drugs. Budding yeast cells and pseudohyphae of *Candida albicans*, the most common *Candida* species causing candidiasis, can be detected by microscopic examination of biologic specimens. Local therapy of vulvovaginal candidiasis includes azoles and nystatin. Cure rates for uncomplicated vulvovaginal candidiasis are 80 to 95% with topical or oral azoles and 70 to 90% with nystatin.

A, B, D–F All of these mycoses are incorrectly paired with the appropriate therapeutic agent.

Learning objective: Identify the drug used to treat invasive pulmonary aspergillosis.

18. **D** Fungi of the genus *Aspergillus* usually coexist with man in harmless symbiosis. In special circumstances, however, some species may play an opportunistic role in producing disease in humans. Patients with chemotherapy-induced neutropenia or impaired immune responses from any cause are at high risk for invasive pulmonary aspergillosis, as in this case. Recent studies indicate that the isolation of aspergilli in bronchoalveolar lavage fluid correlates strongly with histologic evidence of parenchymal invasion. The disease must be treated aggressively with amphotericin B or voriconazole, which most experts now consider a first-line agent. Despite treatment, the mortality rate remains high (30–90%).

A Flucytosine is effective in vitro against *Aspergillus* species but is not clinically effective in case of invasive aspergillosis.

B, C These antifungal drugs are not effective against *Aspergillus* species.

E Nystatin is too toxic for parenteral administration and is only used topically.

Learning objective: Explain the mechanism of antifungal action of terbinafine.

19. **C** Terbinafine is an antifungal drug that inhibits fungal squalene epoxidase, the enzyme that catalyzes the conversion of lanosterol into ergosterol. The inhibition leads to the accumulation of squalene, which is toxic to dermatophytes. The drug is deposited in keratinized tissue and is used in the treatment of dermatophytoses, mainly onychomycosis. The drug is fungicidal and is therefore more effective than griseofulvin, which is fungistatic.

A, B, D, E See correct answer explanation.

Learning objective: Identify the drug used to treat disseminated histoplasmosis.

20. **A** The fact that uninucleated, encapsulated microorganisms are found intracellularly suggests an infection with *Histoplasma capsulatum*. Other intracellular microorganisms are either multinucleate, such as blastomyces, or not encapsulated, such as the intracellular stage of several pathogenic protozoa. Infection with *H. capsulatum* is extremely common. In the vast majority of cases, it is subclinical, or it may manifest itself as a mild, self-limited pneumonia. Progressive disseminated histoplasmosis usually occurs in people with suppressed cell-mediated immunity, especially if they are from endemic areas (Mississippi River valleys and the Caribbean basin), as in this case. Most laboratory findings are nonspecific, but the lactate dehydrogenase level can reach 10 times above normal. Progressive disseminated histoplasmosis has a high fatality rate. Amphotericin B remains the first-line agent, but mild cases can be treated initially with parenteral azoles.

    B–E See correct answer explanation.

Learning objective: Describe griseofulvin-induced photosensitivity.

21. **D** The location of the fungal infection suggests that the patient was most likely suffering from tinea barbae, a dermatophytosis most often caused by fungi of the *Trichophyton* genus. Griseofulvin and terbinafine are the agents of choice. Griseofulvin can cause both a phototoxic and a photoallergic reaction in sun-exposed areas. Other antifungal drugs that can cause photosensitivity effects are antifungal azoles.

    A–C These antifungal drugs are not effective against dermatophytosis, and they do not cause photosensitivity.

    E, F These antibiotics can cause photosensitivity but are not effective against fungal infections.

Learning objective: Explain the main advantage of liposomal preparations of amphotericin B.

22. **C** In liposomal preparations of amphotericin B, the drug is contained inside lipid delivery vehicles. The drug binds to the lipids of these vehicles with an affinity that is lower than that for fungal ergosterol but higher than that for human cholesterol. Thus, the drug is more likely to be delivered to fungi than to human cells. Moreover, some fungi contain lipases that can liberate free amphotericin B directly at the site of infection. Therefore, the liposomal preparations allow a reduction of toxicity; that is, they improve the therapeutic index of the drug. However, although laboratory experiments found very large differences between the lethal dose of liposomal formulations and those of regular formulations, the clinical improvement obtained with the liposomal vehicles is, at best, moderate.

    A Decreased interactions with other drugs could occur, but this is not the main advantage of liposomal preparations.

    B Amphotericin B is the active molecule, and the antifungal activity spectrum is the same.

    D The clearance of liposomal preparations can be decreased or increased, but this is not the reason for their advantage over the regular preparation.

    E Intestinal absorption of all amphotericin B formulations is negligible.

Learning objective: Outline the therapy for severe invasive candidiasis.

23. **D** Because of its broad spectrum of fungicidal activity, amphotericin B remains the first-line agent for nearly all severe fungal infections. Due to toxicity, the drug is often used initially to rapidly reduce fungal load and then is replaced by another less toxic antifungal agent, as in this case.

    A–C, E, F All of these pairs include at least one drug that is not effective against systemic candidiasis.

Learning objective: Explain the mechanism of resistance to fluconazole.

24. **C** Fungal resistance to drugs in the azole class tends to occur gradually over the course of prolonged drug therapy. In *Candida* infections, resistance occurs by way of mutations in the gene that encodes for an enzyme of the P-450 system. These mutations prevent the azole drug from binding and inhibiting the enzyme. Development of resistance to one azole in this way confers resistance to all drugs in the class.

    A, B, D–F These actions are not involved in the mycobacterial resistance to fluconazole.

ANTIFUNGAL DRUGS Answer key			
1. B	6. E	11. D	16. D
2. A	7. C	12. B	17. C
3. B	8. E	13. A	18. D
4. B	9. C	14. C	19. C
5. C	10. D	15. C	20. A
			21. D
			22. C
			23. D
			24. C

Answers and Explanations: VIII-6 Antiviral Drugs

Questions 1–3

1. **F**
2. **C**
3. **E**

Learning objective: Describe the mechanism of action of raltegravir.

4. **E** Raltegravir is an integrase inhibitor. Drugs from this class block the transfer of reverse-transcribed HIV DNA into the chromosomes of host cells, thus preventing the final step of provirus integration. It is used mainly when standard antiretroviral therapy is not effective for a given patient, as in this case.

    A This drug is a reverse transcriptase inhibitor.

    B–D These drugs are protease inhibitors.

Learning objective: Explain the reason for a ritonavir–lopinavir combination.

5. **E** Ritonavir is a powerful inhibitor of the CYP3A4 enzymes. Even when given in subtherapeutic doses, the drug inhibits the metabolism of lopinavir with a resultant increase of lopinavir plasma levels. This permits lower or less frequent dosing with greater tolerability. Therefore, in this combination, ritonavir is mainly acting as a pharmacokinetic enhancer, and for this reason it is currently given mainly in association with another protease inhibitor.

    A–D, F See correct answer explanation.

Learning objective: Describe the adverse effects of protease inhibitors.

6. **E** Most protease inhibitors can cause a Cushing-like syndrome with central obesity, dorsocervical fat enlargement (buffalo hump), and peripheral wasting. The syndrome is related to an impairment of glucose and lipid metabolism (hyperlipidemia and hyperglycemia with insulin resistance are common) and may affect up to 50% of patients receiving protease inhibitors for several months.

    A–D These antiretroviral drugs do not cause a Cushing-like syndrome.

Learning objective: Identify which step of the viral growth cycle is inhibited by acyclovir.

7. **C** The prescribed drug was most likely acyclovir, a first-line agent for herpes genitalis. Oral therapy speeds up the healing and reduces the frequency of reactivation episodes. Acyclovir must be activated by phosphorylation, then the triphosphate compound competitively inhibits viral DNA polymerase, thus blocking DNA synthesis. Transcription is therefore inhibited.

    A, B, D–F See correct answer explanation.

Learning objective: Explain the mechanism of action of gancyclovir.

8. **C** Ganciclovir and acyclovir are nucleoside analogues that must be phosphorylated first by virus-specific enzymes. Both drugs are phosphorylated by a viral thymidine kinase in herpes simplex virus (HSV)–infected cells. Ganciclovir is also phosphorylated by a specific viral phosphotransferase in cytomegalovirus (CMV)–infected cells. This explains why both drugs are active against HSV, but only ganciclovir is effective against CMV.

    A Foscarnet is used in CMV retinitis, but it does not require activation by phosphorylation.

    B, D Ribavirin and acyclovir have no activity against CMV infections.

    E, F Vidarabine and zidovudine are nucleoside analogues that must be phosphorylated to become active. However, for these drugs, phosphorylation is carried out by host cell enzymes only, and these drugs are not effective against CMV.

Learning objective: Outline the prophylactic use of neuraminidase inhibitors.

9. **E** Vaccination plus chemoprophylaxis against influenza is advisable for residents of nursing homes or other chronic care facilities and personnel who have extensive contacts with high-risk patients, as in this case. Oseltamivir and zanamivir are inhibitors of neuraminidases produced by influenza A and B viruses. These enzymes cleave sialic acid residues from cell surfaces, thus promoting the release of newly formed virus from the surface of infected cells. Both drugs cause a significant reduction of the symptoms of influenza A and B and are therefore preferable to amantadine, which is effective only against influenza A. Resistance to neuraminidase inhibitors was uncommon until recently, but now rates of resistance to oseltamivir among H1N1 virus (a subtype of influenza A) have risen abruptly and dramatically.

    A–D, F These drugs are not effective against influenza viruses.

Learning objective: Describe the adverse effects of acyclovir.

10. **B** The patient was most likely suffering from herpes simplex virus (HSV) pneumonia, a disease that affects primarily immunocompromised and elderly people. Acyclovir is a first-line agent for HSV infection. More than 90% of acyclovir is eliminated unchanged by the kidneys, and nephrotoxic effects can occur with parenteral administration as a result of crystallization of the drug within the nephron. Acyclovir has low solubility in urine. Low urine volume associated with volume contraction may contribute to crystalluria, which in turn can lead to azotemia, renal tubular obstruction, renal failure, and death. Crystalluria is more likely to occur during administration of large parenteral doses, as in this case. Renal failure is more likely in this patient because of his renal insufficiency (see creatinine levels).

    A, C–F Acyclovir has no significant toxicity on the bone marrow, liver, or pancreas.

Learning objective: Explain the mechanism of action of amantadine.

11. **D** Amantadine and rimantadine are adamantane derivatives approved for both prophylaxis and therapy of influenza A. They act by preventing uncoating of the virus once it is fused into host cell membranes. These drugs can reduce the severity of symptoms and the duration of illness and are mainly used in elderly patients or in those with underlying diseases, as in the present case The drugs have no effect on influenza B and C viruses or parainfluenza viruses. Unfortunately, more than 90% of circulating influenza A viruses are now resistant to adamantane derivatives.

    A–C, E, F These antiviral drugs are not active against influenza viruses.

Learning objective: Outline the use of interferon alfa-2a in viral hepatitis B.

12. **D** The chronic occurrence of jaundice in a young patient is suggestive of hepatitis, and the presence of hepatitis B surface antigen (HBsAG) in serum is diagnostic for hepatitis B virus (HBV) infection. Approximately 5% of the world's population is infected with HBV. The most prominent risk factors associated with the disease are sexual contacts (> 50%) and injected drug use (15%). Subclinical infections are common, but 25% of carriers develop chronic active hepatitis. Worldwide, one million deaths a year are attributed to HBV-related diseases, including hepatocellular carcinoma. Drugs for the treatment of chronic hepatitis B include interferons, adefovir, entecavir, tenofovir, and lamivudine. These drugs are only moderately effective in treating the disease. Remission may be sustained, but in many patients, viral replication reappears following cessation of therapy. Interferons are cytokines that possess antiviral, immunomodulating, and antiproliferative actions. They induce over two dozen proteins in the host cells that contribute to viral resistance through different mechanisms, including inhibition of viral penetration and uncoating, synthesis of viral DNA and RNA, and viral assembly and release.

    A–C, E, F These antiviral drugs are not effective against HBV.

Learning objective: Explain the mechanism of action of foscarnet.

13. **D** Foscarnet is an inorganic pyrophosphate analogue that inhibits viral DNA polymerase, RNA polymerase, and HIV reverse transcriptase directly without requiring activation by phosphorylation. The drug, given only by intravenous injection, is effective in the treatment of cytomegalovirus (CMV) infections, including retinitis, colitis, and esophagitis. It is often given together with ganciclovir because it has been shown that the combination is superior to either agent alone in delaying the progression of retinitis. Adverse effects can be severe, and renal impairment may occur in up to 30% of patients.

    A–C, E, F None of these drugs are effective in CMV retinitis.

Learning objective: Explain why antiviral drugs cannot prevent recurrence of viral diseases.

14. **C** Herpes viruses replicate in the skin or mucous membranes at the initial site of infection, then migrate up the neuron and become latent in the sensory ganglion cells. The virus can be reactivated from the latent state by a variety of factors, including sunlight, hormonal changes, trauma, stress, and fever. Upon reactivation, the virus migrates down the neuron and replicates in the skin, causing lesions. No currently available antiviral drugs can attack viruses during latency; they act only on actively replicating viruses.

    A, B, D, E See correct answer explanation.

Learning objective: Outline the therapeutic uses of lamivudine.

15. **F** Lamivudine is the first nucleoside analogue approved by the U.S. Food and Drug Administration for use in patients with hepatitis B virus (HBV). It inhibits HBV DNA polymerase and HIV reverse transcriptase by competing with deoxycytidine triphosphate for incorporation into the viral DNA. Lamivudine is an effective agent for patients with chronic hepatitis B. It can suppress HBV DNA to undetectable levels in about 40% of patients and can normalize liver transaminase in up to 75% of patients. Unfortunately, resistance is a problem, developing in up to 70% of patients after 5 years of therapy.

    A–E These antiviral drugs are not effective against HBV.

Learning objective: Explain the mechanism of action of maraviroc.

16. **D** Maraviroc binds to the host protein CCR5 receptor, one of the two chemokine receptors necessary for entrance of HIV into CD4+ cells. This blocks the fusion of viral and cellular

membranes, preventing viral entry. It has been shown that about 50% of patients in whom at least two antiviral regimens had failed were infected with R5 HIV-1. Because maraviroc is active exclusively against HIV strains that use CCR5 but not against other HIV strains, tropism testing should be performed before starting a treatment with this drug, as in this case.

A Ribavirin is not an antiretroviral agent.

B Enfuvirtide is an entry inhibitor but targets a gp41 subunit of the viral envelope.

C Didanosine is a reverse transcriptase inhibitor.

E, F Indinavir and atazanavir are protease inhibitors.

Learning objective: Identify the drug that acts by inhibiting reverse transcriptase.

17. **E** Lamivudine is a reverse transcriptase inhibitor. Reverse transcriptase is an enzyme specific to retroviruses that uses viral RNA to make a complementary single-stranded DNA copy. The copy is then duplicated to form the double-stranded proviral DNA, which migrates into the nucleus and becomes integrated with the genetic material of the host cell. All reverse transcriptase inhibitors can block the initial phase of viral replication. In this way, they can prevent the infection of new cells, but they do not affect chronically infected cells in which the HIV genome is already integrated into the host genome.

A–D These drugs do not affect reverse transcriptase activity.

Learning objective: Explain the most common reason of failure of acyclovir therapy.

18. **C** Acyclovir resistance is the most common cause of failure of acyclovir therapy. Acyclovir-resistant strains of the herpes simplex and varicella zoster viruses arise chiefly from mutations in the thymidine kinase gene that result in little or no production of the enzyme. Because viral thymidine kinase is essential for conversion of acyclovir to active derivatives, resistance to the drug ensues. Resistant strains are most commonly reported in severely immunocompromised patients receiving an extended course of the drug, as in this case.

A, B, D, E None of these enzymes are involved in the mechanism of action of acyclovir.

Learning objective: Outline the prophylactic uses of palivizumab.

19. **E** Palivizumab is a humanized monoclonal antibody that binds to the A antigen site on the F surface protein of respiratory syncytial virus (RSV). It is approved for the prevention of RSV infection in high-risk infants and children, such as those with pulmonary dysplasia, as in this case.

A–D, F These drugs are not effective against RSV infection.

Learning objective: Explain the mechanism of action of entecavir.

20. **A** Entecavir is a guanosine derivative that inhibits hepatitis B virus (HBV) DNA polymerase. The drug is more effective than lamivudine against hepatitis B and is highly effective in lamivudine-resistant strains. Clinical resistance to entecavir is very rare (< 1% at 4 years).

B–F These enzymes are not inhibited by entecavir.

Learning objective: Explain the mechanism of action of enfuvirtide.

21. **A** Enfuvirtide inhibits HIV-1 entry into the host cell by binding to the gp41 subunit of the viral envelope glycoprotein, preventing the conformational changes required for the fusion of viral and cellular membranes. It has no activity against HIV-2.

B–F See correct answer explanation.

Learning objective: Identify the steps of the HIV growth cycle specifically affected by nucleoside reverse transcriptase inhibitors and protease inhibitors.

22. **E** Lamivudine and stavudine are nucleoside reverse transcriptase inhibitors (NRTIs). They block the reverse transcription of RNA into DNA. Atazanavir is a protease inhibitor that blocks the proteolytic cleavage of immature budding particles, thus preventing the assembly of structural proteins around genomic RNA to form a nucleocapsid.

A–D At least one of these two steps is not affected by NRTIs or protease inhibitors.

Learning objective: Explain the mechanism of action of acyclovir.

23. **B** Drugs for varicella zoster virus (VZV) infection include acyclovir, famciclovir, and penciclovir. These drugs are activated by phosphorylation, catalyzed by the virus-specific thymidine kinase in infected cells. The triphosphate derivatives are potent inhibitors of both viral DNA and mammalian DNA polymerase. However, viral DNA polymerase is more sensitive to inhibition than the DNA polymerase of the host cell.

A, C–F These enzymes are not inhibited by acyclovir.

Learning objective: Explain the mechanism of action of oseltamivir.

24. **A** Oseltamivir and zanamivir are inhibitors of neuraminidase, an enzyme produced by influenza A and B viruses. The enzyme cleaves sialic acid residues from cell surfaces, promoting the release of newly formed virus from the surface of infected cells. By blocking the enzyme, these drugs inhibit virus release from the infected cells.

B–E See correct answer explanation.

Learning objective: Describe the adverse effects of ganciclovir.

25. **A** Ganciclovir is a drug of choice for cytomegalovirus (CMV) infections. The dose-limiting toxicity of both zidovudine and ganciclovir is bone marrow suppression; therefore, anemia and neutropenia can be predicted from the concurrent administration of ganciclovir and zidovudine.

    B, C Retinal detachment and cataracts are adverse effects of ganciclovir that can occur following intravitreal administration of the drug for CMV retinitis. They do not occur when the drug is administered intravenously for systemic anti-CMV therapy.

    D Sexual dysfunction is not an adverse effect of the drugs the patient has been receiving.

    E Hyperglycemia can occur after prolonged administration of protease inhibitors such as atazanavir, but it does not occur with ganciclovir.

    F Lactic acidosis has been reported with the use of nucleoside reverse transcriptase inhibitors such as zidovudine and didanosine, but it is does not occur with ganciclovir.

Learning objective: Describe the adverse effects common to zalcitabine and stavudine.

26. **D** Peripheral neuropathy is a dose-limiting adverse effect of both zalcitabine and stavudine, which can occur in up to 30% of patients. It is slowly reversible upon the prompt discontinuation of the drug.

    A Nephrolithiasis is a potential adverse effect of indinavir, not of zalcitabine and stavudine.

    B Myelosuppression is a typical adverse effect of zidovudine. Zalcitabine and stavudine very rarely cause myelosuppression.

    C Zalcitabine and stavudine easily enter the central nervous system, but hallucinations are not reported.

    E Altered body fat distribution is a typical adverse effect of protease inhibitors. Zalcitabine and stavudine do not cause this effect.

Learning objective: Outline the therapeutic uses of trifluridine.

27. **E** Herpes simplex keratitis is a common ocular disorder and one of the most frequent causes of blindness in the United States. The illness is usually treated topically, and trifluridine eye drops 8 or 9 times daily are effective in most cases. The drug is phosphorylated intracellularly by host cell enzymes and then competes with thymidine triphosphate for incorporation by the viral DNA polymerase, thus inhibiting the enzyme. Incorporation into both viral and host DNA prevents its systemic use. The drug is not effective against herpes zoster keratitis. Another pharmacotherapy used occasionally for herpes simplex keratitis is oral acyclovir, especially for recurrent infection.

    A Adefovir is used for viral hepatitis.

    B–D Lopinavir, nevirapine, and zidovudine are used for HIV infection.

    F Zanamivir is used for influenza.

Learning objective: Outline the highly active antiretroviral therapy (HAART) for AIDS.

28. **E** HAARTs are prescribed to many HIV-positive patients even before they develop symptoms of AIDS. These therapies have dramatically altered the natural progression of infection and significantly improved the quality of life of many HIV-infected patients. HAART usually includes two nucleoside reverse transcriptase inhibitors (NRTIs; e.g., zidovudine and didanosine), plus a protease inhibitor (e.g., atazanavir) or a nonnucleoside reverse transcriptase inhibitor (NNRTI).

    A–D All of these drug combinations include at least one drug that is not an antiretroviral agent.

Learning objective: Outline the antiretroviral therapy to prevent mother-to-infant HIV transmission during pregnancy.

29. **D** It is known that HIV can be transmitted to the fetus or newborn during pregnancy, delivery, or breast feeding. It has been shown that certain antiretroviral drugs, when given to the mother and to the newborn during the perinatal period, can prevent the transmission of HIV. Zidovudine, given for 6 weeks before delivery, was used in the past, but recently it has been found that nevirapine is more convenient, as a single dose of the drug is effective when administered to women at the onset of labor and followed by an oral dose to the neonate within 3 days after the delivery.

    A A highly effective antiretroviral therapy (HAART) usually includes more than one drug.

    B A single dose of an antiretroviral drug cannot prevent AIDS.

    C Nevirapine is not an oxytocic drug. Moreover, oxytocic drugs are given after the delivery, not at the onset of labor.

    E Prevention of newborn respiratory distress syndrome is usually achieved with glucocorticoid antenatal therapy.

Learning objective: Identify the antiretroviral drug that does not need phosphorylation to become active.

30. **A** The highly active antiretroviral therapy (HAART) can be nonnucleoside based, that is, one nonnucleoside reverse transcriptase inhibitor (NNRTI) plus two nucleoside reverse transcriptase inhibitor (NRTIs). Efavirenz is an NNRTI. Unlike NRTIs, no NNRTIs require phosphorylation to be activated.

    B Foscarnet does not require phosphorylation to be activated, but it is not an antiretroviral drug.

    C–F Because these drugs are NRTIs, they required phosphorylation to become active.

Learning objective: Describe the main adverse effects of abacavir.

31. **D** The patient was most likely suffering from a hypersensitivity reaction to abacavir. This is a multiorgan systemic illness that occurs in up to 8% of HIV-infected patients who initiate therapy with abacavir. Abacavir hypersensitivity reaction can cause life-threatening complications if abacavir is continued despite progressive symptoms. In addition, among persons who have experienced the abacavir hypersensitivity reaction, subsequent rechallenge with abacavir following discontinuation can cause an immediate and potentially fatal reaction.

A, E These drugs very rarely cause hypersensitivity reactions.

B, C, F These drugs are not active against HIV.

Learning objective: Outline the therapeutic uses of acyclovir.

32. **B** The mother's history (several episodes of genital herpes) and the patient's signs (prematurity, respiratory distress, and cutaneous vesicles) suggest that the baby was suffering from congenital herpes, a disease that affects about 1 in 3000 live births and is acquired, in most cases, during passage through the birth canal. The diagnosis is confirmed by the finding of dendritic keratitis, which is pathognomonic of herpetic keratoconjunctivitis. Antiherpes drugs include acyclovir, several acyclovir congeners, foscarnet, ganciclovir, cidofovir, and trifluridine. Acyclovir is still the first-line agent for systemic treatment. Foscarnet and cidofovir can be used for acyclovir-resistant strains. Trifluridine can be used topically to manage keratitis.

A, C Atazanavir and zidovudine are antiretroviral drugs used only in HIV infection.

D–F These drugs are not antiviral agents.

Learning objective: Identify the step of viral growth cycle blocked by atazanavir.

33. **E** During the late stage of the HIV growth cycle, the gene products become immature budding particles. The immature core (noninfectious) is cleaved into smaller infectious particles by viral aspartate protease. Atazanavir is a protease inhibitor that blocks the proteolytic cleavage, preventing viral maturation. Unlike other protease inhibitors, it does not appear to be associated with the impairment of glucose and lipid metabolism.

A–D, F None of these steps are affected by protease inhibitors.

Learning objective: Identify the protease inhibitor with the most pronounced inhibitory effect on CYP3A4.

34. **D** All of the antiretroviral protease inhibitors are substrates and inhibitors of CYP3A4, with ritonavir having the most pronounced inhibitory effect and saquinavir the least. As a result, there is a huge potential for drug–drug interactions with other antiretroviral agents and other commonly used medications. This potential is also exploited therapeutically in the marketed ritonavir–lopinavir combination. Ritonavir acts as a pharmacokinetic enhancer by inhibiting lopinavir metabolism.

A–C, E These drugs have no clinically significant inhibitory effect on CYP3A4.

Learning objective: Outline the therapeutic uses of foscarnet.

35. **A** Herpetic tracheobronchitis has been documented in both immunocompromised and immunocompetent individuals. Normal hosts typically are elderly individuals. Early detection of herpetic tracheobronchitis appears critical so that acyclovir, which is a drug of first choice for herpes simplex virus (HSV) infections, can be given during the time of peak viral replication, which tends to coincide with symptomatic clinical illness. The most common cause of failure of acyclovir therapy is the presence of thymidine kinase–deficient strains of HSV. Because acyclovir must be phosphorylated by a viral thymidine kinase to become a nucleotide analogue that inhibits viral DNA polymerase, these strains are acyclovir-resistant. In this case, foscarnet, which directly inhibits viral DNA polymerase, represents a useful alternative.

B–D Atazanavir, amantadine, and zidovudine are not active against HSV.

E Trifluridine is effective against HSV, but it is very toxic and therefore is only used topically.

Learning objective: Explain the main reason for a triple therapy in HIV infection.

36. **C** The primary goal of highly active antiretroviral therapy is to delay the emergence of resistance, as mutations conferring resistance to one drug do not necessarily confer resistance to other drugs. An additional benefit of the combination therapy is to decrease the risk of toxicity associated with any one of the agents, as the drugs have different toxicity profiles.

A There are no drugs able to kill nonreplicating viruses.

B, D This can occur in rare cases but is not the purpose of the combination therapy.

E Antiviral drugs usually have no effect on opportunistic infections, which are primarily bacterial infections.

Learning objective: Describe the most serious adverse effect of didanosine.

37. **C** The patient's signs, symptoms, and lab tests indicate that she was most likely suffering from acute pancreatitis, the most serious adverse effect associated with didanosine therapy. The effect is dose-dependent and can occur in up to 7% of patients on antiretroviral therapy with this drug.

    A, B, D The risk of acute pancreatitis with these drugs is negligible.

    E, F These drugs are not antiretroviral agents.

Learning objective: Outline the therapeutic uses of acyclovir.

38. **E** The patient's signs and symptoms suggested the presumptive diagnosis of bacterial meningitis, but the lack of efficacy of antibiotic therapy and the negative cerebrospinal fluid result raised the suspicion of herpes simplex virus (HSV) encephalitis, the most common sporadic viral infection of the central nervous system. Acyclovir is the first-line agent for HSV infection, and the efficacy of therapy confirms that the patient was suffering from herpes encephalitis.

    A See correct answer explanation.

    B, C These diseases are rare in patients without HIV and cannot be cured with antiviral drugs.

    D Cytomegalovirus (CMV) infection occurs mainly in immunocompromised patients or is congenital, and acyclovir is not active against CMV.

Learning objective: Describe the most likely adverse effect of the concurrent administration of abacavir and efavirenz.

39. **A** Abacavir and efavirenz can frequently cause skin rashes. Abacavir can cause allergic reactions in up to 8% of patients,

and erythematous skin rash occurs in about one half of patients presenting such reactions. Efavirenz can cause skin rashes in up to 28% of patients. Because the patient was taking both drugs, there is a high probability that an erythematous skin rash might occur.

B Efavirenz can cause psychotic symptoms, but the frequency of such adverse effects is exceedingly low.

C–E The risk of these adverse effects is negligible.

Learning objective: Outline the therapeutic uses of ganciclovir.

40. **C** Hemorrhagic retinitis in an AIDS patient suggests the diagnosis of cytomegalovirus (CMV) retinitis, which accounts for more than 75% of CMV end-organ disease in HIV-positive patients. Treatment options for CMV retinitis include ganciclovir, foscarnet, and cidofovir. These drugs are administered intravenously or by intraocular injections. Fomivirsen is another drug used for CMV retinitis and is administered only by intraocular injection.

    A, B, D These antiviral drugs are not used for CMV retinitis.

    E, F These drugs are not antiviral agents.

ANTIVIRAL DRUGS Answer key							
1.	F	6.	E	11.	D	16.	D
2.	C	7.	C	12.	D	17.	E
3.	E	8.	C	13.	D	18.	C
4.	E	9.	E	14.	C	19.	E
5.	E	10.	B	15.	F	20.	A
21.	A	26.	D	31.	D	36.	C
22.	E	27.	E	32.	B	37.	C
23.	B	28.	E	33.	E	38.	E
24.	A	29.	D	34.	D	39.	A
25.	A	30.	A	35.	A	40.	C

Answers and Explanations: VIII-7 Antiprotozoal Drugs

Questions 1–5

1. A

2. **F**

3. **E**

4. **H**

5. **M**

Learning objective: Explain the mechanism of action of chloroquine.

6. **E** Malarial parasites grow in host erythrocytes by ingesting hemoglobin, a process that generates free radicals and heme as highly reactive by-products. Heme polymerizes into an unreactive malarial pigment called hemozoin. Chloroquine inhibits plasmodial heme polymerase, the enzyme that polymerizes heme into hemozoin, and the buildup of free heme causes the death of parasites.

    A–D See correct answer explanation.

Learning objective: Identify the species and stages of *Plasmodium* that can be killed by mefloquine.

7. **E** Mefloquine is a blood schizonticide that is moderately effective against gametocytes, except those of *Plasmodium falciparum*. It has no effect on primary tissue schizonts or hypnozoites. Mefloquine is especially useful as a chemoprophylactic agent for travelers in areas that are chloroquine-resistant, as in this case.

    A–D, F See correct answer explanation.

Learning objective: Explain the mechanism of plasmodial resistance to chloroquine.

8. **C** Chloroquine acts by being accumulated in the food vacuole, where it inhibits heme polymerase. Resistant strains are able to efflux the drug by an active pump mechanism and release

the drug at least 40 times faster than sensitive strains, thereby rendering the drug ineffective. Chloroquine resistance is maintained throughout the whole life cycle and is transferred to the progeny. Cross-resistance has been demonstrated with other 4-amino quinolines but not to quinine, mefloquine, or antifolates.

A, B, D, E See correct answer explanation.

Learning objective: Identify the enzyme defect that can cause hemolytic anemia in a patient receiving primaquine.

9. **E** The patient's history and lab tests indicate that he was suffering from hemolytic anemia. The disorder was most likely triggered by primaquine in a person with a genetically induced glucose-6-phosphate dehydrogenase deficiency (G6PD), an X-linked disorder. Over 100 mutant forms of the enzyme have been identified, but the most common one is the drug-sensitive variety. The enzyme defect occurs in about 10% of American Black males. Hemolysis affects the older red blood cells (RBCs) after exposure to drugs that produce peroxide and causes oxidation of RBC membranes. A vast array of drugs can induce hemolysis in people with G6PD deficiency, including primaquine and other antimalarial drugs (chloroquine, quinine). The degree of hemolytic anemia varies greatly. Jaundice, reticulocytosis, and leukocytosis are common, as in this case.

A–D See correct answer explanation.

Learning objective: Describe the emergency treatment for falciparum malaria.

10. **A** The history and the signs of the patient, together with the lab results, indicate that she was most likely affected by falciparum malaria. Because infections with *Plasmodium falciparum* in nonimmune patients can progress rapidly to a fatal outcome, therapy should be initiated promptly. Artemisin-based combination therapy is currently the standard treatment for severe falciparum malaria. Artesunate is given for 3 days, followed by a 7-day oral course of doxycycline or clindamycin. Artemisin derivatives are very rapidly acting blood schizonticides against all human malaria parasites. The mechanism of antimalarial activity of artemisins is still uncertain but likely results from the production of toxic free radicals.

B–E See correct answer explanation.

Learning objective: Identify the drugs used for antimalarial prophylaxis in people visiting areas with chloroquine-resistant *Plasmodium falciparum*.

11. **C** Atovaquone–proguanil combination (Malarone) is a standard prophylactic regimen for chloroquine-resistant *P. falciparum*. Resistance to atovaquone alone develops easily in *P. falciparum*, but the addition of proguanil markedly reduces this resistance.

A, B, D, E In these drug combinations, at least one drug is not active against *P. falciparum*.

Learning objective: Identify the appropriate antiamebic drug for a patient suffering from epilepsy.

12. **D** The patient's symptoms and lab tests indicate that she was suffering from amebic dysentery. Because the patient apparently had no extraintestinal amebiasis (see the negative computed tomography scan), a luminal amebicide is appropriate. Paromomycin is a second-line luminal amebicide. In this patient, however, metronidazole is relatively contraindicated because of epilepsy (the drug is relatively contraindicated in patients with any neurologic disorder).

A See correct answer explanation.

B Chloroquine is effective only against liver amebiasis.

C, E, F These drugs are not effective against *Entamoeba histolytica*.

Learning objective: Explain the molecular mechanism of action of pyrimethamine.

13. **E** The patient most likely received a sulfadiazine–pyrimethamine combination that represents the standard therapy for toxoplasmosis. Pyrimethamine selectively inhibits protozoal dihydrofolate reductase, a key enzyme for folate biosynthesis in the parasite. This in turn leads to failure in DNA synthesis and nuclear division.

A–D See correct answer explanation.

Learning objective: identify the drug active against the late exo-erythrocytic stage of *Plasmodium vivax* and *P. ovale*.

14. **A** Primaquine is the only agent able to prevent relapse of infection due to the late exoerythrocytic stage of *P. vivax* and *P. ovale*. It is therefore commonly given to achieve a radical cure of vivax or ovale malaria.

B–F See correct answer explanation.

Learning objective: Explain the mechanism of action of metronidazole.

15. **D** The woman was most likely suffering from trichomoniasis, a protozoal infection of the vagina that may be asymptomatic or may cause inflammatory disorders in the genital tract. Metronidazole is a first-line agent for trichomoniasis. Its mechanism of action most likely involves damage of protozoal DNA through the formation of a highly reactive nitro radical anion. Therapy must include sex partners in order to avoid reinfection.

A–C, E These antibiotics are not effective against *Trichomonas vaginalis*.

Learning objective: Outline the pharmacotherapy in the case of leishmaniasis.

16. **B** The patient's history, signs, and lab tests indicate that she was most likely suffering from cutaneous leishmaniasis. *Leishmania tropica* is the causative agent in southern Europe. Drugs of choice for leishmaniasis include antimony compounds (e.g., sodium stibogluconate), pentamidine, amphotericin B, and certain azoles (itraconazole). Sodium stibogluconate is the classic therapy for all species of *Leishmania*. Resistance to the drug has led to failure of this therapy in India but not in other parts of the world.

    A, C–F These drugs are not effective against leishmaniasis.

Learning objective: Outline the pharmacotherapy of extraintestinal amebiasis.

17. **A** The patient's symptoms and lab tests indicate that he was most likely suffering from an amebic abscess presumably located on the gut wall (ameboma). For extraintestinal amebiasis, metronidazole is the drug of choice. A luminal amebicide such as iodoquinol or paromomycin must be given concomitantly to eradicate the infection.

    B–F In these drug combinations, at least one of the drugs is not active against *Entamoeba histolytica*.

Learning objective: Outline the pharmacotherapy of congenital toxoplasmosis.

18. **B** *Toxoplasma gondii* is a small intracellular protozoan that can infect people worldwide. Asymptomatic infections are common in immunocompetent individuals, but the disease can be life-threatening in newborns. A combination of sulfadiazine and pyrimethamine represents the treatment of choice for toxoplasma infection. The treatment must be continued for 1 year. Treatment of infants without substantial neurologic disease at birth using pyrimethamine and sulfadiazine has resulted in normal cognitive, neurologic, and auditory outcomes for all patients. Treatment of infants who had moderate or severe neurologic disease at birth has resulted in normal neurologic and/or cognitive outcomes for more than 72% of patients. The best alternative therapy for patients intolerant to sulfonamides is clindamycin and pyrimethamine. Alternative therapies are trimethoprim–sulfamethoxazole, azithromycin, and doxycycline.

    A, C–E These drug combinations are not effective against *T. gondii*.

Learning objective: Identify the appropriate pharmacotherapy for an alcoholic person suffering from giardiasis.

19. **A** The patient's symptoms and lab test results (heart-shaped trophozoites with four pairs of flagella) indicate that she was suffering from giardiasis. Metronidazole would be the drug of choice for this disease but is contraindicated in this patient because she is an alcoholic. Concurrent alcohol consumption with metronidazole causes a disulfiram-like effect that can be dangerous (psychotic reactions have been reported in alcoholics receiving metronidazole). Paromomycin is active against *Giardia lamblia* and can be a useful option when metronidazole is contraindicated, as in this case.

    B See correct answer explanation.

    C–F These drugs are not effective against giardiasis.

Learning objective: Describe the prophylactic use of mefloquine in people visiting areas with chloroquine-resistant *Plasmodium falciparum*.

20. **D** Resistance to chloroquine is now very common in many areas of Africa. Mefloquine has strong schizonticidal activity and is effective against many chloroquine-resistant strains of *P. falciparum* and other malaria species. Other regimens for malaria chemoprophylaxis in regions with multidrug-resistant strains of *P. falciparum* are doxycycline and atovaquone–proguanil (Malarone).

    A Primaquine is the only antimalarial drug active against the hypnozoite stages of *P. vivax* and *P. ovale*. Because of this, some experts advocate the use of the drug after travel to an endemic area to markedly diminish the risk of relapse.

    B Metronidazole is not active against plasmodia.

    C, E Chemoprophylaxis with these drugs is not recommended because of frequent resistance.

    F Although most chloroquine-resistant strains of *P. falciparum* are sensitive to quinine, the drug is not used for prophylaxis because of its toxicity.

Learning objective: Describe the adverse effects of chloroquine.

21. **B** The patient was most likely treated with chloroquine, a quinoline derivative that is a first-line agent for *Plasmodium vivax* and *P. ovale* infections. All quinolines can prolong the QT interval on an electrocardiogram, increasing the risk of torsades de pointes. The arrhythmia is rare, but its occurrence may be increased in patients already at risk because of a concomitant disease, as in this case (see the patient's anorexia).

    A Quinine can cause torsades de pointes but is not used to treat *P. vivax* infection because chloroquine is more effective and less toxic.

    E, F These antimalarial drugs have a negligible risk of torsades de pointes.

    C, D These drugs are not effective against malaria.

Learning objective: Describe the adverse effect of metronidazole

22. **D** The patient's history and symptoms indicate that she was most likely suffering from oral candidiasis due to metronidazole, a first-line agent for amebiasis. The drug can cause a disruption of the normal biologic flora, favoring the appearance of opportunistic infections.

   A, B These antiamebic drugs have a very low risk of candidiasis.

   C, E, F These drugs are not effective against *Entamoeba* species.

ANTIPROTOZOAL DRUGS Answer key			
1. A	6. E	11. C	16. B
2. F	7. E	12. D	17. A
3. E	8. C	13. E	18. B
4. H	9. E	14. A	19. A
5. M	10. A	15. D	20. D
			21. B
			22. D

Answers and Explanations: VIII-8 Anthelmintic Drugs

Questions 1–5

1. **A**
2. **E**
3. **D**
4. **C**
5. **E**

Learning objective: Explain the anthelmintic mechanism of action of ivermectin.

6. **D** Strongyloidiasis is endemic throughout the tropics and subtropics, including rural areas of the southern United States. Ivermectin induces paralysis of worm musculature by activating a family of glutamate-gated Cl^- channels that are found only in invertebrates. This causes a slow and irreversible opening of the channels, leading to a long-lasting hyperpolarization of neurons or muscle cells. Ivermectin also activates (directly or indirectly) gamma-aminobutyric acid (GABA)-gated Cl^- channels, which leads to the same hyperpolarizing action. The ultimate effect is the paralysis of the worm. The drug, given for 1 or 2 days, is highly active against *Strongyloides stercoralis*. The drug does not cross the blood–brain barrier, so it cannot affect GABA neurotransmission in the human central nervous system.

   A–C, E See correct answer explanation.

Learning objective: Outline the appropriate pharmacotherapy for mixed nematode infections.

7. **E** Combined infections with two or even three different nematode species are not exceptional in people with inadequate personal hygiene living in a poor sanitation area, as in this case. Mebendazole is a drug of choice for roundworm and whipworm infection and is an alternative drug for threadworm infection. It is therefore the most appropriate drug in this case.

   A Metronidazole is effective against *Dracunculus medinensis* only.

   B Diethylcarbamazine is effective against filariasis only.

   C Ivermectin is very effective against *Strongyloides stercoralis* but is far less effective than mebendazole against *Ascaris lumbricoides* and *Trichuris trichiura*.

   D Praziquantel is used to kill trematodes and cestodes.

Learning objective: Identify the drug used in case of *Wuchereria bancrofti* infection.

8. **E** *Wuchereria bancrofti* infection affects 120 million people worldwide each year. More than 26 million cases of this infection are hydrocele. India bears the greatest burden of this disease, with more than 550 million people at risk. Infection often leads to microfilaremia without overt clinical manifestations. However, acute inflammatory filariasis can occur with fever and inflammation of lymph nodes, as in this case. Genitals and lower extremities are most commonly affected. Diethylcarbamazine is the first-line agent for filariasis infection. It kills both microfilariae and adult worms, but adults are killed more slowly, often requiring repeated courses of treatment.

   A–D These drugs are not active against *W. bancrofti*.

Learning objective: Identify the drug used to treat enterobiasis.

9. **E** The patient's signs and lab exam indicate that he was most likely suffering from enterobiasis, which is the most common helminthic infection in the United States, with an estimated annual incidence of 42 million. Mebendazole is a first-line agent against pinworm infection, and a single dose, repeated after 2 weeks, usually eradicates the infection. The drug has an oral bioavailability of less than10%, so it is nearly free of adverse effects.

   A–D, F These drugs are not active against *Enterobius vermicularis*.

Learning objective: Outline the appropriate therapy for schistosomiasis.

10. **A** The patient's history and lab exam (eggs with a lateral spine) suggest that *Schistosoma mansoni* was the most likely offending pathogen. This worm is the only schistosoma species present in the Western Hemisphere (Brazil, Venezuela, and some Caribbean islands). Humans are infected from cercariae present in fresh water. Acute schistosomiasis may occur 2 to 4 weeks after exposure and presents most of the signs and symptoms showed by the patient. Praziquantel is the first-line agent for treatment of most trematode infections, including schistosomiasis.

    B–F These helminths are incorrectly matched with the effective drug.

Learning objective: Explain the anthelmintic mechanism of action of praziquantel.

11. **D** *Diphyllobothrium latum* is a tapeworm found mainly in the northern temperate regions where freshwater fish are a major portion of the diet. Many freshwater fish species constitute the intermediate host of the parasite. Praziquantel is a drug of choice for diphyllobothriasis. It is thought to act by enhancing calcium influx, thus increasing worm muscular activity followed by contraction and spastic paralysis.

    A–C, E See correct answer explanation.

Learning objective: Explain the anthelmintic mechanism of action of mebendazole.

12. **F** *Trichuris trichiura* (whipworm) is a parasite with cosmopolitan distribution, although it is more common in warm, moist regions. The infection is usually asymptomatic, but heavy infection can cause abdominal pain, anorexia, and diarrhea and may retard growth. Mebendazole, albendazole, and thiabendazole are benzimidazole derivatives mainly active against nematodes. These drugs produce many biochemical changes in worm cells, but the main action seems to be inhibition of microtubule polymerization by binding to β-tubulin. The microtubular system of the host cells is unaffected. The inhibition of tubulin polymerization disrupts nematode motility and DNA replication, leading to immobilization and the death of the worm.

    A–E See correct answer explanation.

Learning objective: Identify the drug to be used in case of onchocerciasis.

13. **C** The patient's ocular signs and the skin biopsy indicate that she was suffering from a filarial infection, most likely due to *Onchocerca volvulus*. The infection causes a chronic skin disease and eye lesions that may lead to blindness (onchocerciasis is also called river blindness). Ivermectin is the drug of choice for onchocerciasis given as a single oral dose once or twice a year.

A, B Diethylcarbamazine and praziquantel are not active against onchocerciasis.

D, E Fluconazole and metronidazole are not anthelmintics.

Learning objective: Identify the drug used to treat paragonimiasis.

14. **E** The patient's history and lab exam indicate that she was most likely suffering from an infection by *Paragonimus westermani* (oriental lung fluke), a disease caused by ingestion of raw or poorly cooked crustaceans infected with encysted cercariae. The infection is endemic in Japan, Korea, China, and Taiwan, where people eat undercooked freshwater crabs or crayfish. The eggs of the helminth are large (80–100 millimicrons) and operculated. The infection affects the lung, as in this case. Praziquantel is effective for most trematode and cestode infections, and a 2-day course provides 90 to 100% cure rates for pulmonary paragonimiasis.

    A–D These anthelmintics are not active against trematode infections.

Learning objective: Identify the drug used to treat ascariasis.

15. **B** The patient's signs indicate that she was most likely suffering from an infection with *Ascaris lumbricoides*, one of the most common and cosmopolitan helminthic diseases. Benzimidazoles such as mebendazole and albendazole are first-line agents for this disease. Mebendazole, given for 3 consecutive days, achieves a cure rate of 90 to 100% for ascariasis.

    A, C–F See correct answer explanation.

Learning objective: Describe the adverse effects of ivermectin.

16. **A** The patient's history, signs, and symptoms suggest he was most likely suffering from a Mazzotti-like reaction, a syndrome due to killing of microfilariae by ivermectin. The drug does not kill adult worms but affects developing larvae and kills microfilariae in the worm uterus, markedly decreasing microfilarial counts in the skin and other tissues. The reaction is usually mild and lasts just a few days. Rarely, a more severe reaction can occur, as in this case. Antihistamines and nonsteroidal antiinflammatory drugs usually can control the syndrome. Glucocorticoids are indicated for the most severe cases.

    B, C Praziquantel and mebendazole are not active against onchocerciasis.

    D–F Ketoconazole, amphotericin B, and mefloquine are not anthelmintics.

Learning objective: Identify the drug used to treat cystic hydatid disease.

17. **E** The patient's exams indicate that he was most likely suffering from cystic hydatid disease due to *Echinococcus granulosus*. This type of infection occurs in sheep-raising areas of many parts of the world. Albendazole is the treatment of

choice for medical therapy of the disease. It provides only a modest cure rate when used alone, but it is a useful adjunct treatment in the preoperative period to reduce the risk of disseminated infection resulting from spillage of the cyst contents at the time of surgery or during aspiration.

C, D The anthelmintic drugs ivermectin and diethylcarbamazine are not active against echinococcosis.

A, B, F Metronidazole and chloroquine are not anthelmintics.

Learning objective: Identify the drug used to treat taeniasis.

18. **C** The history and signs of the patient, together with the lab results, indicate that he was suffering from taeniasis most likely due to *Taenia saginata* (unlike *Taenia solium, T. saginata* proglottids can emerge by means of their own motility through the anus and deposit the eggs in the perianal region). Praziquantel is currently a drug of choice for most cestode and trematode infections. A single dose results in nearly 100% cure rates for *T. solium, T. saginata,* and *Diphyllobothrium latum.*

A, B The anthelmintics ivermectin and artemisin are not active against cestodes.

D–F Metronidazole, amphotericin B, and fluconazole are not anthelmintics.

Learning objective: Outline the appropriate therapy for ancylostomiasis.

19. **E** The patient's signs and lab results indicate that he was suffering from a chronic helminthic infection (see the thin-shelled oval eggs) due to a worm able to cause iron deficiency anemia. Hook worms such as *Necator americanus* attach to the intestinal villi and suck blood. They periodically move from one place of the intestinal wall to another to suck blood from different villi. Because they locally inject anticoagulant compounds, the arteriole bleeds for a while, so occult blood is found in the stools. Mebendazole is the drug of choice for ancylostomiasis. A cure rate of more than 99% has been reported after a course of two tablets daily for 3 days.

A–D, F Infection with these helminths rarely causes anemia, and they are incorrectly matched with the effective drug.

Learning objective: Outline the therapeutic uses of pyrantel pamoate.

20. **A** When a drug therapy is not effective, an alternative treatment is appropriate. Pyrantel pamoate is a broad-spectrum anthelmintic that is highly effective for the treatment of enterobiasis and ascariasis. Pyrantel actions are neither vermicidal nor ovicidal. The drug inhibits cholinesterase and activates nicotinic acetylcholine receptors, thus acting as a depolarizing neuromuscular blocking agent in helminths. These actions cause extensive depolarization of the helminth muscle membrane, producing tension of the helminth's muscles that causes paralysis of the worms. Then normal peristalsis causes expulsion of the parasites from the gastrointestinal tract.

B, C The anthelmintics praziquantel and diethylcarbamazine are not active against *Enterobius vermicularis.*

D, E Metronidazole and fluconazole are not anthelmintics.

Learning objective: Describe the adverse effects of mebendazole.

21. **A** The patient's symptoms and laboratory values indicate that she was most likely suffering from an acute hepatocellular injury. The injury arose concurrently with signs and symptoms of hypersensitivity (rash and fever) within days of starting a second course of mebendazole. This pattern is typical of a drug-induced allergic reaction, immunoallergic hepatitis in this case. The disease usually resolves rapidly when the offending drug is withdrawn. The granulomas found on liver biopsy reflect the generalized hypersensitivity, and similar granulomas are likely to be found in other organs. Intestinal absorption of mebendazole is quite low (oral bioavailability is less than 10%), and dose-related adverse effects are rare. Although allergic reactions to mebendazole are also rare, they can occur, as in this case.

B, C Most drugs can cause allergic reactions, but the anthelmintic drugs praziquantel and diethylcarbamazine are not used to treat ascariasis.

D, E Metronidazole and fluconazole are not anthelmintics.

Learning objective: Describe the adverse effects of praziquantel.

22. **D** The patient's symptoms indicate that he was most likely suffering from adverse effects of praziquantel. This drug is the first-line agent for most trematode and cestode infections. Although serious adverse effects of the drug are rare, minor adverse effects are common and usually subside in 1 or 2 days.

A–C The anthelmintic drugs diethylcarbamazine, ivermectin, and pyrantel pamoate are not used against cestode infections.

E, F Metronidazole and miconazole are not anthelmintics.

ANTHELMINTIC DRUGS Answer key			
1. A	6. D	11. D	16. A
2. E	7. E	12. F	17. E
3. D	8. E	13. C	18. C
4. C	9. E	14. E	19. E
5. E	10. A	15. B	20. A
			21. A
			22. D

Answers and Explanations: VIII-9 Antineoplastic Drugs

Questions 1–4

1. **B**
2. **E**
3. **D**
4. **F**

Learning objective: Outline the anticancer use of trastuzumab.

5. **C** Trastuzumab is a monoclonal antibody against a surface protein called human epidermal growth factor receptor 2 (HER-2), which may be overexpressed in primary breast carcinoma. The drug binds with high affinity to this receptor, thus preventing the binding of HER to the same receptor. In this way, tumor growth is inhibited. Trastuzumab is used in HER-2 positive, metastasized breast cancer, alone or in combination with paclitaxel.

    A, B, D–F These drugs are not used in breast cancer chemotherapy.

Learning objective: Explain the concept of rescue therapy in anticancer drug treatment.

6. **E** Rescue therapy is a strategy aimed at alleviating some adverse effects of anticancer chemotherapy by the use of drugs that can "rescue" the normal cells exposed to the anticancer drug. Leucovorin (formyl tetrahydrofolate, also called folinic acid) is accumulated more readily by normal cells than by neoplastic cells. The administration of this drug results in rescue of the normal cells, as the drug bypasses the two steps in the purine synthesis that are blocked by methotrexate (i.e., folate to dihydrofolate and dihydrofolate to tetrahydrofolate).

    A Log kill is a rule that states that a given dose of an anticancer drug kills a constant proportion of the tumor cell population.

    B Recruitment refers to a strategy that involves initial use of cell cycle nonspecific (CCNS) anticancer drugs to achieve a significant cell kill. This kill "enrolls" previously resting cells in the G_0 phase of the cell cycle. At this stage, cell cycle specific (CCS) anticancer drugs are given. Because these drugs are active against dividing cells, maximal cell kill may be achieved.

    C Pulsing is a strategy that involves cycles of treatment with very high doses of an anticancer drug. Between cycles, normal cells can recover from the cytotoxic effects of the drug.

    D Combination therapy is the rule in anticancer treatment and is usually done with drugs having different mechanisms of action and (when possible) different toxic effects.

Learning objective: Explain why carmustine and other nitrosoureas are used to treat brain tumors.

7. **B** Carmustine belongs to the nitrosoureas group of drugs. These alkylating agents have a high lipophilicity that facilitates their entry into the brain. In fact, their concentration in the cerebrospinal fluid is 15 to 70% of the concurrent plasma values. Because of this, nitrosoureas are the main chemotherapeutic agents used in the treatment of brain tumors.

    A Nitrosoureas are alkylating agents that actually can kill both neoplastic and nonneoplastic cells.

    C Carmustine actually can cause encephalopathy when given in high doses.

    D The amine pump is specific for monoamines. Nitrosoureas are not monoamines.

    E The half-life of carmustine is actually short, about 15 to 30 minutes.

Learning objective: Explain the mechanism of anticancer action of doxorubicin.

8. **A** Doxorubicin is an anthracycline antibiotic, thus the A in the ABVD acronym; alternatively, the A may be considered to stand for Adriamycin, a brand name for doxorubicin. These anticancer drugs likely act with multiple mechanisms, including intercalation between adjacent base pairs of DNA, thus causing blockade of DNA replication; blockade of topoisomerase II, the enzyme that catalyzes DNA repair (it breaks and then reseals DNA strands); and generation of free radicals that can oxidize DNA bases. The end result of these multiple mechanisms is cell apoptosis.

    B This is the mechanism of action of taxanes.

    C This is the mechanism of action of vinca alkaloids.

    D This is the mechanism of action of alkylating drugs.

    E This is the mechanism of action of methotrexate.

Learning objective: Describe the adverse effects of doxorubicin.

9. **B** In the CHOP acronym, C stands for cyclophosphamide; H for hydroxydaunorubicin, which is another name for doxorubicin; O is for Oncovin, which is a brand name for vincristine; and P is for prednisone or prednisolone. The CHOP regimen has been considered the best treatment for the initial therapy of patients with diffuse non-Hodgkin lymphoma. Recently, it has been shown that the combination of CHOP with rituximab can improve response rates, disease-free survivals, and overall survivals compared with CHOP chemotherapy alone.

The signs and symptoms of the patient suggest the diagnosis of cardiac failure. Anthracyclines (doxorubicin, daunorubicin, idarubicin, etc.) are the anticancer drugs that have the highest risk of cardiac toxicity. They can cause a dose-dependent dilated cardiomyopathy associated with a potentially fatal cardiac failure. This toxicity appears to result from increased production of free radicals within the myocardium.

A, C–E These drugs have a low (cyclophosphamide) or negligible risk of cardiac toxicity. Other anticancer drugs that can cause cardiac toxicity are fluorouracil, paclitaxel, and trastuzumab.

Learning objective: Outline the chemotherapy for remission-induction of acute lymphoblastic leukemia.

10. **C** The patient's bone marrow biopsy confirmed the diagnosis of acute lymphoblastic leukemia. A combination of vincristine and prednisone (plus asparaginase) is a current therapy of choice to induce remission, as none of these agents is myelosuppressive to normal bone marrow elements. Over 90% of children enter complete remission with this treatment.

A This combination is currently used for lung and testicular cancers.

B This combination is currently used for prostate cancer.

D These drugs are used to treat breast cancer.

E This combination is currently used for head and neck cancers.

Learning objective: Explain the mechanism of cancer resistance to fluorouracil.

11. **A** Fluorouracil is a prodrug that is converted within cells to fluoro-deoxyuridine-monophosphate, which inhibits thymidylate synthase, thus causing a "thymineless death" of cells. A decreased ability of cancer cells to phosphorylate pyrimidines prevents the activation of the prodrug, thus causing drug resistance.

B–E All these mechanisms would decrease, not increase, the resistance to fluorouracil.

Learning objective: Outline the therapeutic uses of cisplatin.

12. **D** Testicular cancer is the most common malignancy in men between ages 15 and 35 years. The x-ray and computed tomography results indicate metastatic testicular cancer, and the patient should receive systemic chemotherapy. The combination of cisplatin, etoposide and bleomycin commonly controls the tumor long term and is widely used today.

A Carmustine is mainly used for brain tumors.

B, C, E Methotrexate, cytarabine, and mercaptopurine are mainly used for hematologic malignancies.

Learning objective: Describe the adverse effects of vincristine.

13. **A** The patient's paresthesias and loss of reflexes are signs of vincristine peripheral neuropathy, which often appears within the first few weeks of therapy. Areflexia is common in patients treated with high cumulative doses. Vinca alkaloids have certain toxicities in common (i.e., nausea and vomiting, diarrhea, alopecia), but other adverse effects differ. Vincristine causes a dose-limiting neurotoxicity but is a mild myelosuppressant, whereas vinblastine causes negligible neurotoxicity but gives rise to a severe, dose-limiting myelosuppression.

B–E The risk of peripheral neuropathy with these drugs is negligible.

Learning objective: Describe the local adverse effects of mechlorethamine given intravenously.

14. **D** The MOPP acronym is derived from: *M* for mustargen, also known as mechlorethamine; *O* for Oncovin, a brand name for vincristine; *P* for procarbazine; and *P* for prednisone. Mechlorethamine is an alkylating agent. All alkylating agents are strongly cytotoxic and can damage tissues at the site of injection. This is because they can form covalent bonds with many cell constituents, leading to cell death.

A–C Prednisone, vincristine, and procarbazine are devoid of vesicant properties.

Learning objective: Explain the mechanism of action of cytarabine.

15. **B** The standard treatment for acute myelogenous leukemia includes remission therapy with an anthracycline and cytarabine. Cytarabine is activated to a compound that is incorporated at the terminal position of a growing DNA chain, thus impairing elongation of DNA strands.

A This is the mechanism of action of etoposide

C This is the mechanism of action of pentostatin

D This is the mechanism of action of vinca alkaloids

E This is the mechanism of action of taxanes

Learning objective: Explain the mechanism of action of dactinomycin.

16. **D** Dactinomycin is a cytotoxic anthracycline antibiotic. The main mechanism of anticancer action of these drugs involves binding to double-helical DNA, thus preventing DNA transcription. The action is similar to that of alkylating drugs, but anthracyclines bind double-helical DNA by intercalation not by alkylation. Dactinomycin is used mainly in Wilms tumor, a kidney tumor that is the most common intraabdominal tumor of childhood and accounts for about 6% of all childhood malignancies.

A This is the mechanism of action of alkylating drugs.

B This is the mechanism of action of methotrexate.

C This is the mechanism of action of pyrimidine analogues.

E The formation, not the inhibition, of free radicals is one of the postulated mechanisms of action of some anticancer drugs, including doxorubicin and bleomycin.

F This is the mechanism of action of imatinib.

Learning objective: Explain the mechanism of action of cyclophosphamide.

17. **A** Cyclophosphamide is an alkylating agent. These drugs act by intramolecular cyclization to form either an ethyleneimonium or a carbonium ion which are strongly electrophilic (i.e., electron attracting). These intermediates can alkylate, that is they can transfer alkyl groups to various cellular constituents by formation of covalent bonds with nucleophile (i.e., electron donor) groups of these constituents. Alkylation of guanine of a single strand of the DNA molecule results in miscoding or in depurination by excision of guanine residues. Alkylation of guanines in both strands of the DNA molecule results in cross-linking, which appears to be of major importance to the cytotoxic action of alkylating agents.

      B This is the mechanisms of action of cytarabine.

      C This is the mechanisms of action of fluorouracil.

      D This is the mechanisms of action of topoisomerase inhibitors.

      E This is the mechanisms of action of vinca alkaloids.

Learning objective: Explain the mechanism of action of paclitaxel.

18. **C** Although adenocarcinoma of the lung is less sensitive than small cell lung cancer to chemotherapy, combination therapy can improve survival. A widely used first-line regimen includes a platinum compound (e.g., cisplatin), and a taxane (e.g., paclitaxel). Taxanes bind to tubulin and inhibits tubulin depolymerization, thus preventing microtubule disassembly.

      A, B, D–F These drugs are not used for lung cancer and they do not bind to tubulin.

Learning objective: Explain the mechanism of action of etoposide.

19. **C** Small cell lung carcinoma is one of the four main types of lung cancer and accounts for 15 to 20% of primary lung tumors. Because small cell lung carcinoma disseminates early in the disease, surgery is almost never indicated. Most chemotherapeutic regimens include high-dose cisplatin with etoposide. Etoposide inhibits topoisomerase II, one of the enzymes that reseals double-stranded DNA breaks. As a result, DNA breaks accumulate and lead to cell death. It is worth noting that quinolones are also able to inhibit topoisomerase II. However, quinolones inhibit only the bacterial cell enzyme and are therefore harmless to eukaryotic cells, whereas etoposide inhibits only eukaryotic cell enzymes and are therefore devoid of antibacterial activity.

      A This is the mechanism of action of methotrexate.

      B This is the mechanism of action of fluorouracil.

      D This is the mechanism of action of alkylating drugs.

      E This is the mechanism of action of taxanes.

Learning objective: Describe the adverse effects of bleomycin.

20. **E** The patient was at risk for several processes that could produce his symptoms, but the exam results ruled out bacterial infections and the progression of lymphoma. Therefore, pulmonary toxicity resulting from one or more of the drugs he received is the most likely hypothesis. Among the anticancer drugs, bleomycin most commonly causes pulmonary toxicity, mainly interstitial pneumonitis followed by pulmonary fibrosis. The mortality associated with bleomycin pulmonary toxicity is very high (about 50%).

      A Cyclophosphamide may cause pulmonary toxicity, but the risk is much lower than that of bleomycin.

      B–D The risk of pulmonary toxicity with these drugs is very low.

Learning objective: Describe the adverse effects of cisplatin.

21. **D** The patient's lab results suggest the diagnosis of renal failure. Cisplatin is the anticancer drug with the highest risk of nephrotoxicity, and hypomagnesemia is the most common electrolyte abnormality caused by cisplatin. However, the routine use of hydration and diuresis has largely reduced cisplatin-induced nephrotoxicity.

      A–C, E These drugs very rarely cause nephrotoxicity.

Learning objective: Explain the mechanism of action of mercaptopurine.

22. **F** Maintenance therapy of acute lymphoblastic leukemia is usually performed for 2½ to 3 years after remission, since early trials have shown that without maintenance, most children will relapse within 1 or 2 months. Impressive improvements in disease-free survival and cure rates are achieved with various maintenance regimens. Methotrexate and mercaptopurine are the drugs most often included in these regimens. Mercaptopurine is an antimetabolite anticancer drugs that is inactive in its parent form and must be metabolized by the enzyme hypoxanthine-guanine phosphoribosyl transferase into the monophosphate nucleotide 6-thioinosinic acid, which in turn inhibits several enzymes of de novo purine nucleotide biosynthesis. The monophosphate form is eventually transformed into the triphosphate form which can get incorporated into both DNA and RNA, blocking DNA and RNA synthesis.

      A–E See correct answer explanation.

Learning objective: Identify the drug to be used to treat colon cancer.

23. **E** Because of significant relapse rate in patients with extensive colon cancer, adjuvant therapy is usually performed in those patients who underwent potentially curative surgery. It has been shown that this therapy improves disease-free survival. The currently used adjuvant chemotherapy regimens contain

fluorouracil and leucovorin. Other drugs that can be used in combinations include oxaliplatin and capecitabine.

A–D These drugs are all cell cycle specific and are mainly used in tumors with a high growth fraction. Currently, they are not used to treat colon cancer, a tumor with low growth fraction.

Learning objective: Describe the effect of anticancer chemotherapy on blood cells.

24. **D** The decrease of peripheral blood cells after cancer chemotherapy depends upon the life span of that cell line. The life span of granulocytes, once released from the bone marrow, is 4 to 5 hours in the blood and another 4 or 5 days in the tissues. Platelets survive about 10 days. Therefore myelosuppression first results in granulocytopenia followed by thrombocytopenia

A Lymphocytes continually circulate throughout the body and have life spans of weeks, months or even years.

B See correct answer explanation.

C Monocytes, once in the tissues, become macrophages and can live for months or even years.

E Erythrocytes have a life span of about 120 days

Learning objective: Identify the pairs of drugs most frequently used to treat diffuse ovarian cancer.

25. **E** Ovarian cancer is the fifth most common cause of cancer and cancer death in women. Because the cancer is relatively asymptomatic, it usually has extended beyond the pelvis at the time of diagnosis. Chemotherapy is therefore indicated after surgery. Cisplatin or carboplatin plus paclitaxel are first-line regimens most commonly used in ovarian cancer.

A–D These drugs are not used to treat ovarian cancer.

Learning objective: Identify the drug to be used as a methotrexate antidote.

26. **E** Leucovorin can be given to counteract the adverse effects that methotrexate has on normal cells. Leucovorin (formyl tetrahydrofolate, also called folinic acid) is accumulated more readily by normal cells than by neoplastic cells. The administration of this drug results in rescue of the normal cells, because the drug bypasses the step in the purine synthesis that is blocked by methotrexate (i.e., dihydrofolate to tetrahydrofolate).

A–D See correct answer explanation.

Learning objective: Identify the drug to be used to treat acute myelogenous leukemia.

27. **D** The blood exam and the bone marrow biopsy are consistent with the diagnosis of acute myelogenous leukemia. This leukemia primarily affects adults (the incidence increases with age) and is characterized by the neoplastic proliferation of myeloblasts. The single most active agent for acute myeloid leukemia is cytarabine. For remission therapy, cytarabine is currently used together with an anthracycline.

A–C, E These drugs are not currently used for remission therapy of acute myelogenous leukemia.

Learning objective: Explain the meaning of the "log kill" rule in anticancer chemotherapy.

28. **B** The therapeutic strategy adopted in this case is based on the "log kill" rule. This rule states that a given dose of an anticancer drug will kill a constant proportion (not a constant number) of the tumor cell population as well as of sensitive normal cell populations. In other words, killing by anticancer drugs is a first order process, and the curve representing the number of killed cells with increasing dose of an anticancer drug is an exponential curve. This curve can be transformed into a straight line by plotting the logarithm of the number of killed cells against the dose. Remembering that the logarithm is the exponent required to produce a given number, it follows that 1 is the log of 10^1, 2 is the log of 10^2 (that is 100), 3 is the log of 10^3 (that is 1000) and so on. Therefore if a population of 10^3 tumor cells is reduced to 10^2 tumor cells it can be said that it is reduced by 1 log. This means that 900 cells are killed by the drug, resulting in a 90% decrease of cell number. Accordingly, a 2 log decrease means that 99% of the cells are killed, a 3 log decrease that 99.9% of the cells are killed, and so on. Usually a 2 log decrease is the strategy most often used, as a higher decrease would produce unacceptable toxicity to healthy dividing cells.

A, C–E See correct answer explanation.

Learning objective: Describe the adverse effects of cisplatin.

29. **E** Ototoxicity, characterized by a progressive hearing loss, commonly occurs with cisplatin and appears to be more pronounced in children. It most likely results from a direct toxic effect on the cochlea. The reversibility of this ototoxicity is questionable and seems substantial only with early cessation of cisplatin. Ototoxicity does not appear to be associated with other platinum analogues (carboplatin and oxaliplatin).

A–D The risk of ototoxicity with these drugs is negligible.

Learning objective: Identify the anticancer drug that acts in the G_2 phase of the tumor cell cycle.

30. **B** Bleomycin is the only cytotoxic antibiotic that is cell cycle specific (CCS). It has been shown that the drug causes accumulation of cells in the G_2 phase of the cell cycle.

A, D These drugs are cell cycle nonspecific (CCNS). The A in the ABVD acronym stands for Adriamycin, a brand name for doxorubicin.

C Vinblastine is CCS but acts in the M phase of the cell cycle.

Learning objective: Describe the adverse effects of cyclophosphamide.

31. **F** The patient presented with gross hematuria, which can be either painless or painful. Whereas the former can have many causes, painful hematuria is usually due to inflammatory disease of the urogenital tract (cystitis and prostatitis), renal infarction, or nephrolithiasis. Renal infarction and renal calculi are unusual in a very young child. Cyclophosphamide can cause bladder mucosa edema, ulcerations, and minor to severe hemorrhage. This toxicity is believed to be due to metabolites of cyclophosphamide, including chlorethylaziridine and acrolein, which are formed by hepatic microsomes and excreted in the urine. They can concentrate in the bladder and cause mucosal damage. The incidence of hemorrhagic cystitis from cyclophosphamide administered at conventional doses is unknown, but in patients receiving high-dose regimens, it is about 10%.

    A–C Adverse effects of these drugs do not include nephrotoxicity.

    D, E Cisplatin and, very rarely, doxorubicin can cause nephrotoxicity, but hemorrhagic cystitis has not been reported.

Learning objective: Outline the therapeutic uses of methotrexate in lymphoblastic leukemia.

32. **A** The blood test and the bone marrow biopsy are consistent with the diagnosis of acute lymphoblastic leukemia. Before central nervous system (CNS) preventive therapy was routine, the CNS was the most common site of leukemic relapse in children with acute lymphoblastic leukemia. Today, preventive therapy is performed with intracranial irradiation and intrathecal administration of anticancer drugs. Methotrexate with or without cytarabine and corticosteroids is the most common drug administered intrathecally to prevent relapse.

    B–F These drugs are not currently used to treat acute lymphoblastic leukemia and are not administered intrathecally.

Learning objective: Explain the mechanism of action of bleomycin.

33. **A** Bleomycin binds to DNA. The bleomycin–DNA complex reduces molecular oxygen to free oxygen radicals, which in turn causes DNA fragmentation.

    B This is the mechanism of action of vinca alkaloids.

    C This is the mechanism of action of fluorouracil.

    D This is the mechanism of action of alkylating drugs.

    E This is the mechanism of action of methotrexate.

Learning objective: Describe the adverse effects of anticancer combination chemotherapy.

34. **E** Nausea and vomiting are among the most common complications of chemotherapy administration. It has been shown that on the first day of chemotherapy, nausea is present in about 50% and vomiting in about 25% of patients. The most important factor influencing the frequency of nausea and vomiting is the emetogenic potential of the drug. Among the drugs administered to this patient, cyclophosphamide and doxorubicin are highly emetogenic, whereas the emetogenic potential of vincristine is low. Corticosteroids, by contrast, are effective antiemetics mainly in chemotherapy-induced nausea and vomiting, but the basis for this effect is unknown.

    A–D All of these listed adverse effects can occur (neuropathy with vincristine, hemorrhagic cystitis, and, rarely, pulmonary fibrosis with cyclophosphamide, congestive heart failure with doxorubicin), but they are much less frequent than nausea and vomiting and are not acute adverse effects.

Learning objective: Explain the molecular mechanism of action of methotrexate.

35. **A** Methotrexate is a folic acid antagonist that inhibits dihydrofolate reductase, the enzyme responsible for the reduction of dihydrofolate to tetrahydrofolate. The drug is biotransformed intracellularly to polyglutamated derivatives that are selectively retained within cancer cells and have a higher inhibitory effect on the enzyme. The inhibition of dihydrofolate reductase leads to decreased synthesis of tetrahydrofolate, which is a one-carbon unit carrier. These one-carbon units are used in the synthesis of purines, which in turn are essential for the synthesis of DNA and RNA.

    B This is the mechanism of action of cytarabine.

    C This is the mechanism of action of topotecan.

    D This is the mechanism of action of bleomycin.

    E This is the mechanism of action of vinca alkaloids.

Learning objective: Outline the pharmacotherapy of chronic myelogenous leukemia.

36. **A** The white blood cell count and the presence of the Philadelphia chromosome confirm the diagnosis of chronic myelogenous leukemia. The disease, which is associated with the Philadelphia chromosome in over 90% of cases, is characterized by increased granulocytes in peripheral blood and often increased platelets in early stages, as in this case. The goal of chemotherapy in newly diagnosed patients with very high leukocyte counts is to reduce leukocytosis and its associated symptoms. Hydroxyurea is still the most common agent used for initial leucocyte reduction. However, interferon-alfa and imatinib give better results in terms of remission and 5-year survival.

    B, C These drugs are hematopoietic growth factors.

    D–F These anticancer drugs are not used in chronic myelogenous leukemia.

Learning objective: Explain the mechanism of action of asparaginase.

37. **B** Asparaginase is an enzyme that hydrolyzes circulating asparagine. Because tumor cells in acute lymphoblastic leukemia have very low levels of asparagine synthetase, they require an exogenous source of asparagine for growth. Asparaginase depletes the existing supply of asparagine, inhibiting protein synthesis in the tumor cells. In contrast, normal cells can synthesize asparagine and are therefore less susceptible to the cytotoxic action of asparaginase. An increased asparagine synthetase activity of tumor cells is the cause of resistance to asparaginase.

    A, C–F All of these drugs can be used in acute lymphoblastic leukemia, but they have different mechanisms of action.

Learning objective: Identify the drug used concomitantly to increase the cytotoxic activity of fluorouracil.

38. **C** Fluorouracil is converted in cells to fluorodeoxyuridine monophosphate, which inhibits thymidylate synthase and causes a "thymineless death" of cells. Leucovorin is 5-formyltetrahydrofolate. By increasing the intracellular concentration of a reduced folate (i.e., leucovorin), the formation of a stable complex between the active fluorouracil metabolite, the reduced folate, and the enzyme thymidylate synthase is favored, thus increasing the cytotoxicity of fluorouracil.

    A Folic acid is not a reduced folate and does not increase the formation of the stable complex described above.

    B, D–F See correct answer explanation.

Learning objective: Describe the procedure to prevent cisplatin-induced nephrotoxicity.

39. **B** Cisplatin can cause nephrotoxicity, but this adverse effect has been largely abrogated by vigorous pretreatment with hydration and administration of diuretics. Loop diuretics are required in patients with compromised cardiac reserve, as in this case.

    A, C–E See correct answer explanation.

Learning objective: Explain the mechanism of multidrug resistance in cancer chemotherapy.

40. **E** Antineoplastic drug resistance can develop to a single drug or to a variety of drugs of different structures after the exposure to a single agent.

    Multidrug resistance is most likely due to

- Increased efflux of the drug from the cells, due to increased expression of a normal gene that encodes for a cell surface transporter glycoprotein (P-170) that uses the energy of adenosine triphosphate (ATP) to expel a variety of foreign molecules. This is the most common mechanism of multidrug resistance.

- Increased DNA repair, due to increased activity of topoisomerase enzymes

    A DNA repair is increased, not decreased, in cases of multidrug resistance.

    B–D These mechanisms can explain resistance to single drugs but cannot account for multidrug resistance.

Learning objective: Identify the drug used as an antidote against cyclophosphamide.

41. **C** Cyclophosphamide can cause hemorrhagic cystitis, which seems to be due mainly to acrolein, an active metabolite that is excreted in high concentration in the urine. Prevention consists of providing adequate intravenous hydration and administration of 2-mercaptoethane sulfonate (MESNA). This agent contains a free thiol group that can neutralize acrolein in the bladder. MESNA can prevent the bladder toxicity completely, so its use is the current standard of care.

    A, B, D, E None of these drugs can prevent cyclophosphamide-induced hemorrhagic cystitis.

Learning objective: Identify the appropriate combination chemotherapy for chronic lymphocytic leukemia.

42. **E** The lab results suggest that the patient was suffering from chronic lymphocytic leukemia, the most common form of leukemia in adults over age 50, which occurs twice as often in men as in women. The disease is high risk when lymphocytosis is accompanied by anemia and thrombocytopenia, as in this case. In the past, chlorambucil with or without prednisone had been the standard initial treatment of chronic lymphocytic leukemia, but today fludarabine gives better results. However, the combination of chlorambucil and prednisone can be useful in elderly patients with anemia and thrombocytopenia, as in this case.

    A–D These anticancer drug combinations are not used in case of chronic lymphocytic leukemia.

Learning objective: Identify the anticancer drug that acts by forming both inter- and intrastrand cross-links in DNA molecules.

43. **D** Cisplatin is the prototype of platinum analogues. These drugs have broad antineoplastic activity and are currently used for treatment of ovarian, head and neck, bladder, esophagus, lung, and colon cancers. Platinum analogues are activated inside cells, yielding positively charged and highly reactive molecules. These molecules can react with various sites on DNA, forming both inter- and intrastrand cross-links, which in turn block DNA replication.

    A–C, E See correct answer explanation.

Learning objective: Describe the adverse effects of bleomycin.

44. **E** Among the chemotherapeutic drugs, bleomycin has the highest risk of pulmonary toxicity. It can cause an interstitial pneumonitis followed by pulmonary fibrosis. The disease is very serious and is lethal in about 50% of cases. The main factor associated with the development of pulmonary toxicity is the cumulative dose of bleomycin. The higher the cumulative dose, the higher the risk.

    A Acute leukemias have been associated with cancer chemotherapy, but chronic myelogenous leukemia is not related to the previous use of anticancer drugs.

    B–D The drugs taken by the patient do not increase the risk of these diseases.

Learning objective: Identify the drug to be used for maintenance therapy in acute lymphoblastic leukemia.

45. **C** Maintenance therapy of acute lymphoblastic leukemia is usually performed for 2½ to 3 years after remission because early trials have shown that without maintenance, most children will relapse within 1 or 2 months. Impressive improvements in disease-free survival and cure rates are achieved with various maintenance regimens. Methotrexate and mercaptopurine are the drugs most often included in these regimens. Mercaptopurine is effective and well tolerated orally when administered daily.

    A, B, D, E All of these are cell cycle–nonspecific anticancer drugs, and they are not currently used in postinduction regimens for acute lymphoblastic leukemia.

Learning objective: Explain the mechanism of action of vinca alkaloids.

46. **A** Vincristine and vinblastine are vinca alkaloids. These drugs bind specifically to β-tubulin, the structural proteins that form microtubules, and block β-tubulin polymerization with α-tubulin, thus preventing microtubule assembly. In this way, they cause an arrest of the mitotic cycle in metaphase.

    B–E See correct answer explanation.

Learning objective: Describe the adverse effects of paclitaxel.

47. **C** Paclitaxel is the prototype of taxane derivatives. Peripheral neuropathy is a common adverse effect of taxanes, affecting more than 50% of patients under treatment. The effect is dose-dependent and cumulative.

    A, B The risk of these adverse effects is very low.

    D, E Paclitaxel causes a profound myelosuppression, which in turn increases the risk of opportunistic infections. These include candidiasis, cryptosporidiosis, cryptococcosis, and *Mycobacterium avium-intracellulare* infection, but urinary tract infections and tuberculosis have not been reported.

Learning objective: Outline the therapeutic uses of etoposide.

48. **F** The patient's symptoms and the bronchial biopsy are consistent with the diagnosis of a small-cell lung cancer. Although the risk of developing any type of lung cancer increases with cigarette smoking, the relative risk of small-cell lung cancer is among the highest. The cells of these cancers, also called "oat cell" carcinomas, contain a scanty amount of cytoplasm and rarely have nucleoli. These malignancies, which are of neuroendocrine origin, may cause a variety of paraneoplastic syndromes due to the synthesis and secretion of hormones such as adrenocorticotropic hormone (ACTH) and serotonin. Small-cell lung cancers carry a poor prognosis because they metastasize early and are already spread at the time of diagnosis. Etoposide, given together with a platinum compound, has been shown to significantly improve survival and is currently a drug of choice in this disease.

    A–C Isoniazid, ceftazidime, and streptomycin are antimicrobial agents and are therefore of no value in lung cancer.

    D, E Asparaginase and cytarabine are not used in small-cell lung cancer.

Learning objective: Outline the therapeutic uses of imatinib.

49. **F** Imatinib is the prototype of a new class of anticancer agents called tyrosine kinase inhibitors. These drugs specifically inhibit the tyrosine kinase activity of BCR-ABL (breakpoint cluster region–Abelson murine leukemia), the fusion product of the Philadelphia chromosome. BCR-ABL is a constitutively active protein kinase supporting cell proliferation; inhibition of the enzyme by imatinib blocks the kinase activity and downstream activation of cellular proliferation. Tyrosine kinase inhibitors cause apoptosis in cells that express the enzyme but do not affect normal cells. They are currently first-line agents in chronic myelogenous leukemia. They are not curative but can prolong survival and can achieve a complete hematologic remission.

    A–E These anticancer drugs are not used in chronic myelogenous leukemia.

Learning objective: Describe the adverse effects of asparaginase.

50. **E** Asparaginase is an enzyme that catalyzes the hydrolysis of plasma asparagine to aspartic acid and ammonia. Because it is a foreign protein, it has antigenic properties, and hypersensitivity reactions are common (up to 20%). They are usually mild, but fatal anaphylactic reactions have been reported.

    A–D The risk of these adverse effects after asparaginase administration is negligible.

ANTINEOPLASTIC DRUGS
Answer key

1. B	6. E	11. A	16. D	21. D
2. E	7. B	12. D	17. A	22. F
3. D	8. A	13. A	18. C	23. E
4. F	9. B	14. D	19. C	24. D
5. C	10. C	15. B	20. E	25. E
26. E	31. F	36. A	41. C	46. A
27. D	32. A	37. B	42. E	47. C
28. B	33. A	38. C	43. D	48. F
29. E	34. E	39. B	44. E	49. F
30. B	35. A	40. E	45. C	50. E